GYNECOLOGIC ONCOLOGY

GYNECOLOGIC ONCOLOGY

Larry McGowan, M.D.

Director, Division of Gynecologic Oncology
Professor, Obstetrics and Gynecology
Department of Obstetrics and Gynecology
The George Washington University Medical Center
Washington, D.C.

APPLETON-CENTURY-CROFTS / NEW YORK

78 79 80 81 82 / 10 9 8 7 6 5 4 3 2 1

Prentice-Hall International, Inc., London
Prentice-Hall of Australia, Pty. Ltd., Sydney
Prentice-Hall of India Private Limited, New Delhi
Prentice-Hall of Japan, Inc., Tokyo
Prentice-Hall of Southeast Asia (Pte.) Ltd., Singapore
Whitehall Books Ltd., Wellington, New Zealand

Library of Congress Cataloging in Publication Data
Main entry under title:

Gynecologic oncology.

    Includes index.
    1. Generative organs, Female—Cancer.   I.   McGowan,
Larry.
RC280.G5G883   616.9′94′65   78-2476
ISBN 0-8385-3529-1

Text design: Meryl Sussman Levavi

Cover design: Kristin Herzog

PRINTED IN THE UNITED STATES OF AMERICA

Contributors

Samuel C. Ballon, M.D.
Associate Director, Division of Gynecologic Oncology, Department of Obstetrics and Gynecology, UCLA Center for the Health Sciences, Los Angeles, California; City of Hope National Medical Center, Duarte, California

Hugh R.K. Barber, M.D.
Clinical Professor of Obstetrics and Gynecology, Cornell Medical College, Director, Department of Obstetrics and Gynecology, Lenox Hill Hospital, Attending Surgeon, Gynecologic Service, Memorial Hospital, Attending Obstetrician and Gynecologist, New York Hospital, New York City

William L. Benson, M.D., LTC, MC, USA
Chief, Gynecologic Pathology and Assistant Chief, Gynecologic Service Department of Obstetrics and Gynecology, Madigan Army Hospital, Tacoma, Washington

Michael L. Berman, M.D.
Director, Division of Gynecologic Oncology, Assistant Professor, Obstetrics and Gynecology, Department of Obstetrics and Gynecology, University of Pittsburgh, Pittsburgh, Pennsylvania

Luther W. Brady, M.D.
Hylda Cohn/American Cancer Society, Professor of Clinical Oncology, Professor and Chairman, Department of Radiation Therapy and Nuclear Medicine, The Hahnemann Medical College and Hospital of Philadelphia, Philadelphia, Pennsylvania

Ernest W. Franklin, III, M.D.
Director, Division of Gynecologic Oncology, Agnes Raoul Gleen Memorial Center of Crawford W. Long Memorial Hospital of Emory University, Atlanta, Georgia

Charles B. Hammond, M.D.
Director, Division of Gynecologic Endocrinology, Professor of Obstetrics and Gynecology, Director, Southeastern Regional Center for Trophoblastic Diseases, Department of Obstetrics and Gynecology, Duke Univesity Medical Center, Durham, North Carolina

Leo D. Lagasse, M.D.
Director, Division of Gynecologic Oncology, Professor, Department of Obstetrics and Gynecology, UCLA Center for the Health Sciences, Los Angeles, California; City of Hope National Medical Center, Duarte, California

David A. Lightfoot, M.A.
Technical Director, Treatment Planning Center, Associate Professor, Radiation Therapy and Nuclear Medicine, The Hahnemann Medical College and Hospital of Philadelphia, Philadelphia, Pennsylvania

John G. Maier, M.D., Ph.D.
Director, Division of Radiation Therapy, Professor of Radiology, Department of Radiology, The George Washington University Medical Center, Washington, D.C.

Richard A. Malmgren, M.D.
Director of Cytopathology, Professor of Pathology, The George Washington University Medical Center, Washington, D.C.

H. George Mandel, Ph.D.
Professor and Chairman, Department of Pharmacology, The George Washington University Medical Center, Washington, D.C.

John Marlow, M.D.
Assistant Professor, Department of Obstetrics and Gynecology, The George Washington University Medical Center, Columbia Hospital for Women, Washington, D.C.

Henry J. Norris, M.D.
Chairman, Department of Gynecologic Pathology, Armed Forces Institute of Pathology, Washington, D.C.

Robert C. Park, M.D., COL, MC, USA
Professor of Obstetrics and Gynecology, Uniformed Services, University of the Health Sciences, Chairman, Department of Obstetrics and Gynecology, Chief, Gynecologic Oncology Service, Walter Reed Army Medical Center, Washington, D.C.

Roy T. Parker, M.D.
F. Bayard Carter Professor and Chairman, Department of Obstetrics and Gynecology, Duke University Medical Center, Durham, North Carolina

Tim H. Parmley, M.D.
Associate Professor of Obstetrics and Gynecology, The John Hopkins Hospital School of Medicine, Baltimore, Maryland

Herbert J. Schmidt, M.D.
Director, Division of Gynecologic Oncology, Associate Professor, Department of Obstetrics and Gynecology, The University of Arizona Medical Center, Tucson, Arizona

Watson G. Watring, M.D.
Director, Division of Gynecologic Oncology, Associate Professor, Department of Obstetrics and Gynecology, Tufts New England Medical Center, Boston, Massachusetts

Contents

Preface

The diagnosis and treatment of cancers of the female reproductive organs have always been an integral part of the obstetrician's and gynecologist's education and medical practice. The many individuals who devoted their lifelong energies to the field of gynecologic oncology have left a rich legacy to the discipline of obstetrics and gynecology. Today, the gynecologic oncologist is recognized as the primary physician responsible for treatment planning, treatment, follow-up, rehabilitation, and terminal care of the woman with cancer of the female reproductive organs. This evolutionary process has been a logical response by the medical profession to centralize responsibility for the care of women with gynecologic cancers in those individuals who by training, experience, and current practice are most proficient. There is also a need to bring together sufficient clinical material to develop better diagnostic aids and therapies for several gynecologic cancers. Perhaps the most pressing demand for education and certification in gynecologic oncology is in the area of delivery of health care. No longer is it acceptable to make a patient fit into a fixed therapeutic modality or schedule; rather, the treatment—whether it be surgery, irradiation, or chemotherapy—must be individualized to the particular patient's needs.

The team approach in caring for the gynecologic cancer patient is desirable, and several disciplines of medicine are required to develop reasonable plans. The contributors to this edition are thus representative of several disciplines and, in an attempt to achieve balance, are drawn from a number of institutions with a wide geographic distribution. We have tried to present the current consensus in diagnosis and therapy of gynecologic cancer. Where opinion remains divided, we have given the rationale for each suggested form of management. At times the experience of the contributor has been extensive and consistent, which permits a particular form of treatment to be outlined. The objectives of this edition have been the creation of a gynecologic oncology text of sufficient scope to meet the needs of medical students, residents and fellows in gynecology, practicing obstetricians and gynecologists, physicians in closely allied fields, and gynecologic oncologists.

Chapter 1

Gynecologic Cancer: The National Problem

LARRY McGOWAN, M.D.

Cancer of the female genital tract has been subjected to more study over a longer period of time than any other major cancer in humans. Historical documentation of the compilation of knowledge regarding cervical cancer and its diagnosis and treatment is familiar.[1,2] There is no other major cancer in which more is known about the disease pattern and methods to markedly reduce morbidity and eliminate mortality than cervical cancer. The Papanicolaou cytosmear was one of the first broadly used cancer screening laboratory aids available to physicians to detect early cancer and remains today as one of the better screening aids.

Malignancies of the female genital organs are second in frequency only to breast cancer among women, and, if in situ carcinomas are included, they are the most frequently seen cancers.[3] Although it has been estimated that there are 387,000 women alive following a history of uterine cancer (excluding carcinoma in situ) in the United States,[4] a distressing figure is that in one year an estimated 248,927 person years are lost due to death from uterine cancer.[5] The American Cancer Society's estimation of cancer deaths and new cases in 1978 for the genital organs[6] is listed in Table 1–1. Cramer and Cutler, presenting data from the Third National Cancer Survey, noted that 6 of 10 newly diagnosed cancers of the female genital organs were invasive malignancies, and the remainder were in situ carcinomas. Of the invasive malignancies, 38 percent originated in the corpus, 30 percent in the cervix, and 25 per-

cent in the ovary; 94 percent of the in situ carcinomas originated in the cervix.[3] Carcinoma in situ of the cervix peaked at ages 25 through 34 and decreased rapidly thereafter. The age-specific incidence of invasive cervical cancer in whites increased more slowly than that for in situ carcinoma and plateaus at ages 45 through 49, though the rates at ages 65 through 80 are slightly greater. Cancers of the corpus are relatively infrequent until age 40, but increase rapidly, reaching a peak at 65 to 74 and declining thereafter. In all women younger than 45, cervical cancers, both in situ and invasive, are predominate. In black women, cancers of the cervix remain the most common cancers of the female reproductive organs throughout life. In white women, cancers of the corpus and ovary increase rapidly in the 45 to 50-year age group, and the incidence of cancers of the cervix, corpus, and ovary is similar in this period. After age 55, cancers of the corpus and ovary are more numerous than those of the cervix in white women.[3]

The average age of patients with epidermoid carcinoma (51.4 years) was significantly less than the average age of patients with adenocarcinoma of the cervix (56.2 years).[3] Sarcomas of the corpus also appeared at younger ages than adenocarcinoma of the corpus (56.5 versus 60.7 years). Cramer and Cutler observed that patients with germ cell malignancies of the ovary had a mean age of 37.5 years compared with the overall age of 57.7 years for women with ovarian cancer. Sar-

1

Table 1-1. ESTIMATED CANCER DEATHS AND NEW
CASES FOR ALL SITES—1978

SITE	ESTIMATED TOTAL DEATHS	ESTIMATED TOTAL NEW CASES
Genital organs	22,500	69,200
Cervix, invasive	7,400	20,000*
Corpus Uteri	3,300	28,000
Ovary	10,800	17,000
Other female genital	1,000	4,200

Incidence estimates are based on rates from NCI Third National Cancer
Survey 1969-71.
*Invasive cancer only.

comas of the vulva occurred at a younger age than that for all invasive malignancies of the vulva (32.9 versus 65.3 years). For cancers of the corpus, blacks showed a proportionately greater number of sarcomas and fewer adenocarcinomas than whites.

For ovarian cancer, blacks had a proportionately greater number of gonadal stromal and germ cell cancers, and fewer serous cystadenocarcinomas. Basal cell carcinomas and melanomas of the vulva were rare among blacks.[3]

Cramer and Cutler attached great importance to the observation that the crude rate in women 20 years of age and older for all invasive cancers of the genital organs had decreased from 118 cases per 100,000 in 1947, to 89 cases in 100,000 in 1969 and 1970. While the cervix accounted for one-half of the invasive malignancies in 1947, it now accounts for less than one-third of the cases.

The percentage of malignancies of the corpus has doubled, while ovarian cancers increased 40 percent.[3] The decrease in deaths due to uterine cancer is partly related to improved diagnostic methods for detecting cancer of the cervix, but the death rates were already on their way down when cervical cytology programs were being implemented, therefore, this decline cannot be totally explained by these programs.[4] A trend toward larger numbers of in situ carcinomas of the cervix is being observed in the United States.

The most common multiple primary cancers within the female reproductive tract were of the corpus and ovary. Cramer and Cutler report that the dominant malignancy in women is breast cancer, and, among women with multiple primaries, breast cancer was frequently found with cancers of the corpus and ovary.

REDUCTION OF MORBIDITY AND MORTALITY FROM GYNECOLOGIC CANCERS

There are only three avenues by which the toll of cancer illness and death can be controlled and reduced: prevention, earlier detection, and improvements in treatment. In women with a history of coitus, regular examinations that would include visualization of the cervix, a cervical cytosmear, prompt biopsy of an obvious lesion, and pelvic examination would have an even greater impact on the immediate reduction in cervical cancer morbidity and mortality. Visualization and more frequent biopsy of persistent lesions of the vulva and vagina would also reduce morbidity and

mortality from vulvar and vaginal cancer. Endometrial tissue aspiration in perimenopausal or postmenopausal women who are at risk for developing endometrial cancer (obese, hypertensive, diabetic, few to no children, or taking oral estrogens in high dosages over long periods of times) performed in the doctor's office will detect endometrial cancer at an earlier stage and reduce morbidity and mortality.

Although there should be very few deaths due to cervical cancer today, the fact remains that over 7000 occurred last year and with an overall five-year salvage that is only slightly better than 60 percent. Cervical cancer should serve as our model for delivery of cancer health care. Every physician's office should be a cancer detection center. Each obstetrician and gynecologist should be able to perform appropriate diagnostic procedures and basic surgical operations to establish the diagnosis of cervical cancer.

Screening for cervical cancer, whether it takes place in a physician's office or through a federal, state, or local program, must be intimately associated with the health delivery system (Fig. 1–1). An isolated or freestanding screening program can result in women with suspicious or positive cytosmears for cancer having a low percentage of follow-up and histologic study. These women then have a false sense of security that they are cancer free when, in fact, the opposite is true. Also, Schmitz and associates have documented that haphazard therapy for cervical cancer must not occur if women are to have the best chance to be cured of their disease.[7]

Three perceptions must be held before women will seek screening services for a gynecologic cancer: (1) The disease must be recognized as being serious, (2) a woman must believe herself to be susceptible to the disease, and (3) she must be convinced that early detection will lead to prevention of serious illness or that treatment will be effective. The absence of one or more of these beliefs in a group of women would indicate a need for cancer education.

In 1973, approximately three-fourths of all civilian, noninstitutionalized females 17 years and older had at least one Pap smear. Approximately 61 percent who had ever had a Pap smear had the examination during the preceding year. A higher proportion of females 25 to 44 years of age had a Pap smear than other ages (90 percent). Proportionately fewer females 65 years of age and over had ever had a Pap smear compared to other age groups, and these women were less likely to have had a recent examination.[8] This is an important observation, as the woman at age 65 today has an expected 17 more years of life and at age 55 about 25 more years of life.[9] The value of a complete physical examination, which must include a pelvic examination, cannot be too strongly stressed.

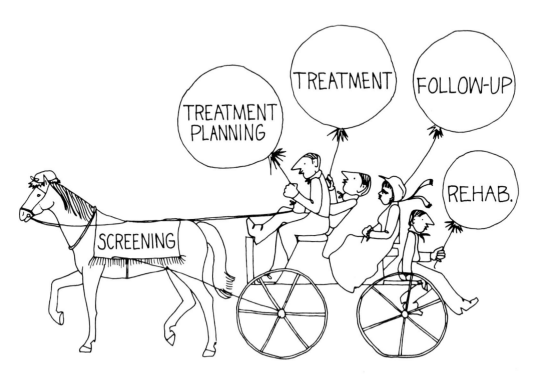

Figure 1–1. Screening for cervical cancer must be coupled with treatment planning, treatment, follow-up, and rehabilitation programs.

DELIVERY OF GYNECOLOGIC CANCER HEALTH CARE

The interaction between medicine and society, physicians and their patients are undergoing changes in several areas. Patients are becoming increasingly aware of their rights as consumers of health care and more commonly are exercising these rights. Costs of delivery of gynecologic cancer health care are under increasing public scrutiny, as well as the medical profession's concern as to who should deliver cancer care and where.

Informed Consent

Physicians must reveal the risks which, to a reasonable woman, would enable her to make her decision as to whether or not to undergo treatment. She has the right to have all the information that is necessary and relevant to give an informed consent. The physician must relate to his patient her medical problem in language that she can understand and be prepared to answer relevant questions. Areas to be covered in diagnosis are (1) what her condition is called, (2) how it affects her body, and (3) what her prognosis is with and without treatment.

Patients expect to be concisely informed on diagnostic and treatment procedures by knowing what the procedure is called, how it is performed, by whom, and where, what are the chances of it helping her and will it need to be repeated, and how long do these procedures take. If hospitalization is required, the patient should know how long will she be in the hospital, how painful the procedure is and will it limit her activity afterward, what are the possible side effects, complications, or risks and how often do these occur. Also, are there alternates to your suggested procedure and why is the one you have chosen better, is the treatment you are suggesting generally accepted or is it an experimental procedure, and if it is experimental, how often have you performed it. If surgery is to be used, will the anesthesiologist be available to visit your patient before operation and explain to her the type of anesthesia, risks, and how she will feel postoperatively.

With the use of drugs, particularly chemotherapy, patients need to know the name of the medication, how it is given, in what dosage and how often, and what does it do. Any side effects, restrictions, or limitations should be explained to the patient in terms she will understand. The risk involved in taking the medication and the frequency of these risks, as well as alternative medications and whether it is a generally accepted drug or an experimental one should be stated.[10]

The role and image of the physician in American society is changing. There is a suggestion that the physician is more of a technician than ever before, more likely to work as part of an institutionalized health care system, and subject, like other experts, to recurrent debunking of his once unquestioned authority. In our morally pluralistic, aggressively participatory society, physicians must first of all do no harm and respect the rights of patients in medical decision making beyond the strictly scientific level.

Costs

The costs of a catastrophic illness such as gynecologic cancer are significant. There are increasing professional and public concerns with the continued deaths from cervical cancer, which are almost universally preventable as are most endometrial cancer deaths. With approximately 7500 deaths due to cervical cancer last year in the United States[6] and a conservative estimate of $16,000 representing all expenses related to the disease and the death process,[11] a national figure of $120,000,000 each year is impressive.

All patients wish to know the costs of various diagnostic and treatment procedures in relation to the adequacy of their insurance coverage. Many people today would place national health insurance against catastrophic illness as an urgent demand. Over 96 percent of all women with gynecologic cancer are admitted to a hospital at some time during their illness to receive care.[4] Medicare and other "government" funds now finance about half of all hospital costs of all cancer patients.[12,13] Doctors must pay greater attention to governing themselves and particularly to overseeing the quality and costs of medical treatment.

Gynecologic Oncology

Every physician's office is a cancer detection center. Burkons and Willson, in a recent study in Michigan, found that 44 percent of women have no primary care physician and 86 percent see only their obstetrician-gynecologists for regular periodic examinations. Also, 41 percent of the women reported that their obstetrician-gynecologist either had treated them for non-gynecologic conditions or had decided that no treatment was necessary.[14] The U.S. Department of Health, Education and Welfare has defined obstetrics and gynecology as one of the disciplines of medicine included in primary care. The American Board of Obstetrics and Gynecology feels that the first year of graduate study should help prepare the physician to serve as the initial contact for entry into the health care system.

For at least the past two decades, there has been thoughtful inquiry within the field of obstetrics and gynecology, as to who should treat pelvic cancer,[15] where should gynecologic cancer be treated,[16] the need for advanced specialization,[17] and the responsibilities and training of the gynecologic oncologist.[18-21] Gynecologists have been involved for many years in formal education in gynecologic oncology, international collaboration in staging and end-result reporting, definition of uterine cancer precursors, devising combinations of surgical, irradiation, and chemotherapeutic regimes, and currently establishing standards for certification in gynecologic oncology.

The gynecologic oncologist today is the primary physician responsible for treatment planning, treatment, rehabilitation, follow-up and terminal care of the gynecologic cancer patient. No longer is it acceptable medical care to treat gynecologic cancer in an environment where there are not personnel and facilities to permit a team approach. On that team, to mention a few, are the obstetrician and gynecologist, cytopathologist, clergy, family or general practitioner, internist, medical oncologist, nurses, pharmacist, radiotherapist, social worker, surgical pathologist, and urologist. The public's demand for integrated medical care as well as the demand for identification of a coordinating physician has been met by the discipline of obstetrics and gynecology for cancers of the reproductive tract by the recognition and certification of the gynecologic oncologist. No woman with gynecologic cancer should be fitted into a treatment regime; rather, the treatment should be adapted to her particular needs and her disease. For example, she should not be referred to an institution or an individual who carries out only a surgical procedure or to another institution or individual who solely performs irradiation therapy for cervical cancer.

Although the gynecologic oncologist is the central figure to bring together treatment planning, treatment, follow-up, rehabilitation, or terminal care of the cancer patient, the obstetrician and gynecologist must be able to carry out basic diagnostic procedures and perform basic surgical operations for the diagnosis of gynecologic cancer. The obstetrician and gynecologist, along with the radiation therapist, family, or general practitioner, internist, or medical oncologist must share in the follow-up, rehabilitation, and terminal care of the gynecologic cancer patient.

The overall survival for most gynecologic cancers reflects a serious need for improvement. It is universally acknowledged that in situ carcinoma of the cervix is 100 percent curable. The overall survival for all cases of invasive cervical cancer is slightly better than 60 percent[4,22] and of all invasive cervical cancers 20 to 30 percent of them are in stages II to IV at the time of diagnosis. This latter figure has not changed in over 20 years. The survival rate for ovarian cancer has not changed in 30 years, with 70 percent of patients dying in 5 years.[22] Since there are approximately 17,000 new cases of ovarian cancer each year in the United States, it is obvious that more concentrated study of these women must be carried out. Epidemiologic studies, development of diagnostic aids, and improved therapies for this disease which now is the fourth leading cause of cancer deaths in American women are necessary. An overall five-year survival of 75 percent for endometrial cancer also reflects the need for more purposeful screening of women for endometrial cancer and an integrated team approach to therapy. The less frequent cancers, such as vulvar, vaginal, fallopian tube, as well as sarcomas of the female reproductive organs certainly could have an improvement in their generally poor prognosis by more organized medical care.

As the team approach for primary and continuing care of gynecologic cancer gives the patient a better chance for cure, it becomes readily apparent that increased training programs in gynecologic oncology must be developed so that there are sufficient health care delivery team leaders for all invasive gynecologic cancer patients in the United States.[23] Obstetrics and gynecology, with the support of the American Medical Association, has been a leader in the concept of regionalization of medical care. In 1971, both organizations supported centralized community and regionalized perinatal intensive care, and in 1976, they approved the concept of regionalization of obstetric care. Regionalization of gynecologic cancer care would seem to be the next logical step.

References

1. Martin A, Jung PH: Pathology and Treatment of Diseases of Women. New York, Rebman Co., 1912. English translation, written and edited by Henry Schmitz, M.D., 4th ed.
2. Speert H: Obstetric and Gynecologic Milestones. New York, MacMillan, 1958
3. Cramer DW, Cutler SJ: Incidence in histopathology of malignancies of the female genital organs in the United States. Am J Obstet Gynec 118:443, 1974
4. Levin DL, Devesa SS, Godwin JD, Silverman DT: Cancer Rates and Risks, 2nd ed. Bethesda, Md, U.S. Department of Health, Education and Welfare, Public Health Service, National Institutes of Health, 1974
5. Newell GR: Measuring improved survival of cancer patients. Ca 25:338, 1975
6. Cancer Facts and Figures. New York, American Cancer Society, 1978
7. Schmitz HE, Geiger CJ, Smith CJ, Blichert PA: Carcinoma of the cervix—failure of haphazard treatment. Obstet Gynec 4:75, 1954
8. Characteristics of females ever having a pap smear and interval since last pap smear, United States—1973. Monthly Vital Statistics Report from the National Center for Health Statistics. Rockville, Md, U.S. Department of Health, Education and Welfare, Public Health Service, Oct 7, 1975
9. Life Tables. Vital statistics of the United States, 1973, vol 2, sec 5. Rockville, Maryland, U.S. Department of Health, Education and Welfare, Public Health Service, National Center for Health Statistics, 1975
10. Soskis C: What to ask your doctor. Pennsylvania Health 36:8, 1975
11. Schneider J, Twiggs LB: The costs of carcinoma of the cervix. Obstet Gynec 40:851, 1972
12. Cutler SJ, Scotto J, Devesa SS, Connelly RR: Third national cancer survey—an overview of available information. J Natl Ca Instit 53:1565, 1974
13. Surgical operations in short-stay hospitals, United States, 1971. Rockville, Maryland, U.S. Department of Health, Education and Welfare, Public Health Service, National Center for Health Statistics, ser 13, no. 18, Nov, 1974
14. Burkons DN, Willson JR: Is the obstetrician-gynecologist a specialist or primary physician to women? Am J Obstet Gynec 121:808, 1975
15. Schmitz HE: Who should treat pelvic cancer? Am J Obstet Gynec 77:1161, 1959
16. Symmonds RE: Where gynecologic cancer should be treated. Obstet Gynec 35:144, 1970
17. Beecham CT: Advanced specialization. Obstet & Gynec 35:149, 1970
18. Rutledge FN: The gynecologic oncologist. Obstet & Gynec 40:749, 1972
19. Kolstad P: Gynecologic oncology: Present status and future aspects. Am J Obstet Gynec 115:597, 1973
20. Manka I: Where and by whom is ca cervicis uteri to be treated? Neoplasma 19:553, 1972
21. Gusberg SB: Education of a gynecologic oncologist. Obstet & Gynec 36:773, 1970
22. Recent trends in survival of cancer patients, 1960–1971. Bethesda, Md, U.S. Department of Health, Education and Welfare, Public Health Service, National Institutes of Health, National Cancer Institute, 1974
23. Brady LW: Advances in the management of gynecologic cancer—radiation therapy. Cancer 36:661, Suppl no 2, 1975

Chapter 2

Current Problems in Gynecologic Pathology

WILLIAM L. BENSON, M.D., LTC, MC, USA

HENRY J. NORRIS, M.D.

Communication of accurate, meaningful information between clinicians and pathologists is essential in providing optimal care for patients with gynecologic cancers. A deficiency in communication between clinician and pathologist may compromise the management of patients. Technical problems in the handling of tissues can reduce the accuracy and reliability of pathology reports, and problems in histologic interpretation and classification of tumors must be appreciated in order to make meaningful comparisons of data from different institutions. Each of these problem areas is examined below in anticipation that all members of the oncology team, and ultimately the patient, may benefit from an appreciation of the pathologist's viewpoint.

CLINICIAN–PATHOLOGIST COMMUNICATION

Pathology reports may contain so little information that planning of therapy is compromised. Examples of lapses in communication abound. For example, a diagnosis of "adenocarcinoma of the endometrium" is far from adequate. The pathologist should state the location of the tumor within the corpus, degree of differentiation, depth of myometrial penetration, and length of endometrial cavity, as prognosis and additional therapy often depend on these factors. It is as if the pathologist were unaware of the factors relating to the prognosis of endometrial carcinoma when he omits the essential information. Recognition of the prognostic factors is the key element of modern pathology and radical departure from prior decades when the pathologist was expected only to "pin a label" on the process. Now, a label is not enough and can be misleading. Our understanding of most histologic aspects of gynecologic cancer has progressed to the point that now the pathologist is required to identify not only the process but also its subtype, extent of growth, grade, and any unusual aspects or factors relating to prognosis, so far as the specimen is able to provide them.

The terms chosen to characterize a neoplasm should be current and their meaning unmistakable to the clinician reading the report. Certain diagnoses require explanation or amplification to avoid misunderstanding. If the diagnosis "adenocarcinoma in situ" is used, the pathologist must make clear what he means by that diagnosis, as it has had several meanings in the past. When reporting "microinvasive carcinoma" in a cervical cone, the pathologist must make clear to the clinician the specific characteristics of the lesion in question, since a uniform definition of this term has not been established. He should specifically state cell type, degree of differentiation, depth of stromal penetration, and method of measurement. Most important, he should indicate whether the margins of the cone contain invasive neoplasm. Since nearly half of cones may have invasion at the margins and in some of these cases the uterus will contain residual invasive neoplasm of unpredictable extent,[1] the clinician must have this information before planning further therapy. Proper diagnosis of epithelial ovarian tumors should include the degree of differentiation, cell type, and presence or absence of capsular invasion or external papillary processes.

Colposcopists are often frustrated by reports in which endocervical curettings are interpreted "insufficient for diagnosis" and those in which pathologists recommend a conization after colposcopically directed biopsy. Endocervical curettings are seldom truly insufficient, since the absence of malignant cells is significant. A report of "scanty fragments of benign endocervical mucosa" is meaningful. Colposcopists do not expect pathologists to exclude more significant lesions, as the colposcopic examination has already done that; colposcopists merely need to know what the pathologist *does* see. Pathologists should not recommend any procedure without stating the basis for their opinion.

Clinicians are often at fault in communicating adequate clinical information to the pathologist. The patient's age, menstrual history, duration of symptoms, any prior surgery or previous malignant condition, or any treatment that may have altered histologic findings must be given to assure that maximum benefit accrues from histologic study. A uterine leiomyoma might be misinterpreted as a sarcoma if the pathologist is unaware of hormonal therapy or pregnancy.[2] A condyloma acuminatum with frequent mitotic figures may be interpreted as dysplasia or even carcinoma if podophyllin therapy a few days previously is not mentioned. Knowledge of the surgical findings, including the precise location and gross extension of neoplasms, is often crucial to the pathologist; yet specimens are often labeled "pelvic mass." A neoplasm is sometimes given to the pathologist as an adnexal mass. It helps if the surgeon has an opinion as to which adnexal structure the mass was related. The same tumor interpreted as leiomyosarcoma in the broad ligament or pelvic soft tissues could be interpreted as cellular leiomyoma lacking metastatic potential if located within the uterus. A vaginal biopsy specimen showing adenosis might be interpreted "chronic cervicitis" if it is not stated that the specimen came from the vaginal wall. Sometimes the clinician does not record the important history of prior surgical procedures or malignant condition; a clinician who endangers his patient in that manner has earned the disrespect the pathologist might hold for him.

Good clinician-pathologist communication has several benefits, chief of which are more accurate diagnosis and better determination of the extent of disease, both of which lead to improved patient care. Communication is facilitated when clinicians examine slides from their patients. Both clinician and pathologist benefit through discussion and exchange of differing points of view, as they acquire further knowledge of the pathophysiology and clinical course of disease.

TECHNICAL PROBLEMS IN THE HANDLING OF TISSUES

Colposcopy has revolutionized the management of cervical neoplasia. The proficient colposcopist need not rely on the pathologist to identify the most severe process present; he visually selects the most abnormal area for target biopsy, greatly reducing the need for conization. The small biopsy specimens obtained, however, may lead to problems in histologic interpretation. It is essential that biopsy specimens be obtained with a sharp instrument to avoid tearing or crushing artifacts. The small, square-jawed biopsy instruments of the Kevorkian or Younge type are ideal, but to yield optimal specimens they must be kept sharp. The small specimens obtained must be properly oriented, since tangential cuts omitting surface epithelium will be obtained by routine imbedding. Occasionally, deeper cuts may reveal a satisfactory perpendicular section, but the pathologist may not think to do it, and an error may result. Biopsy specimens may be submitted floating freely in a jar of fixative, and from this they can be oriented by the interested pathologist with the aid of a dissecting microscope, but specimens submitted in this manner tend to curl and orientation may be difficult. Clinicians may aid in orienting the biopsy specimen by submitting it on filter paper with the plane of the epithelium perpendicular to the plane of the paper, as suggested by

Townsend et al.[3] Others place the specimen on cucumber[4] or cork[5] to orient it, but the principle—reflecting the need to orient the specimen—is the same.

Adequate processing of cone specimens is critical for proper interpretation. The entire cone should be processed. If a fixed cone is blocked radially, wedge-shaped fragments result in which the important epithelial edge is thin and may be lost in cutting the block. When a fixed, unopened cone is submitted to the pathologist, it may be blocked by the method of Foote and Stewart[6] or Sanerkin and Fraser[7] to avoid this problem. Alternatively, the unfixed cone may be opened and pinned flat, then covered with formalin, so that parallel blocks 2 mm wide may be cut later and none of the epithelium from the important transformation zone is lost. We frequently see cone specimens with much of the surface epithelium denuded. Avoiding vaginal scrubs, particularly vigorous ones, prior to conization may reduce the prevalence of this problem. Another procedure to be avoided is the "shave cone," as it yields multiple ragged fragments that are impossible to orient and judge the adequacy of its margins. Superficial biopsies and cones may leave tumor in cervical clefts below the level of excision. With the availability of colposcopy, the need for conization is greatly reduced, but when necessary it should result in an adequate cone.

When hysterectomy specimens are not promptly fixed, autolysis of the endometrium may preclude satisfactory examination. Uteri must be opened to allow adequate fixation of the endometrium. Pathologists usually prefer to examine unmutilated specimens, and ideally a pathologist is available in the operating room to examine and open the uterus, then place it in fixative. If a pathologist is not available and a delay is likely prior to fixation, the surgeon can open the uterus with least distortion by incising it along one lateral margin and then place it in fixative.

Histology includes the study of controlled artifacts, but excessive or unusual artifacts hinder the accurate interpretation of any specimen. Thin sections, adequately fixed, carefully cut by a sharp microtome knife and properly imbedded and stained, are essential in the identification of many gynecologic neoplasms. A good tissue technician is highly prized and should be carefully nurtured. The majority of problems in microscopic interpretation today are a result of artifacts occurring during processing. Good sections are especially important in distinguishing a leiomyoma

from a leiomyosarcoma, since thick sections and overstaining with hemotoxylin frequently makes accurate mitotic counts impossible.[8] Undifferentiated carcinoma of the ovary can be distinguished from dysgerminoma, lymphoma, and some poorly differentiated gonadal stromal tumors only with well-prepared sections.

The importance of adequate sampling cannot be overemphasized. For example, the diagnosis of malignant Brenner tumor requires the demonstration of a transition from benign to malignant Brenner epithelium,[9] easily missed if few blocks are taken. Ovarian tumors of germ cell origin must have adequate sampling, as admixtures of different malignant germ cell elements with varying degrees of malignancy are frequently found. The prognosis of dysgerminomas is reduced if the tumors contain areas of endodermal sinus tumor or choriocarcinoma.[10] The prognosis in patients with immature teratomas (and perhaps the need for ancillary chemotherapy) depends on the degree of immaturity of the elements,[11,12] and again, accurate determination depends on adequate sampling. For a cellular leiomyoma or a borderline ovarian tumor, one block of tissue is needed for every 1 or 2 cm of maximum tumor diameter, and for malignant germ cell tumors a block should be taken for every centimeter of maximum diameter.

In processing excisional and biopsy specimens from patients with vulvar lesions, the clinician must have confidence that the pathologist has examined the lesion thoroughly from two aspects: (1) whether the lateral and deep margins are free of tumor and (2) whether the neoplasm was adequately studied for invasion. In lesions less than 1 cm in diameter, the pathologist can be expected to take a cross section of the lesion and sections intersecting the transverse cut, producing three pieces of tissue containing four surface margins and good representation of the deep margins. Larger lesions should be processed by multiple transverse cuts similar to those taken in a pinned-out cone. The same procedure can be used for Paget's disease. Investigation for invasion of the dermis is important, as only those neoplasms with dermal invasion will develop metastases.

Most vaginal specimens are received as biopsies for diagnostic purposes, and in these cases the entire specimen should be submitted. In cases of vaginectomy for vaginal carcinoma, the clinician should mark the suspected area or identify it in the pathology laboratory, because vaginal carcinoma tends to spread along the mucosal folds, where only minor gross abnormalities may be visible. When this pattern of spread occurs in atrophic vaginal mucosa, recognition of the lesion becomes more difficult. The clinician can help de-

lineate the lesion by placing the patient on estrogens prior to surgery. The pathologist should submit sections from the lesion, from noncancerous but abnormal areas, and from the surgical margins.

CURRENT PROBLEMS IN HISTOLOGIC INTERPRETATION AND CLASSIFICATION

Ovary

Progress in the fields of embryology, cytogenetics, histochemistry, and morphology has resulted in new knowledge, necessitating frequent changes

in taxonomy. As new names appear, old names are discarded, and subdivisions within categories of tumors are found to have distinctive features that warrant separate designations. These changes take time to percolate through ranks of pa-

Table 2-1.   WHO HISTOLOGIC CLASSIFICATION

I. COMMON "EPITHELIAL" TUMORS	I. COMMON "EPITHELIAL" TUMORS (cont.)
A. Serous tumors	C. Endometrioid tumors
1. Benign	1. Benign
a) Cystadenoma and papillary cystadenoma	a) Adenoma and cystadenoma
b) Surface papilloma	b) Adenofibroma and cystadenofibroma
c) Adenofibroma and cystadenofibroma	2. Of borderline malignancy (tumors of low malignant potential)
2. Of borderline malignancy (tumors of low malignant potential)	a) Adenoma and cystadenoma
a) Cystadenoma and papillary cystadenoma	b) Adenofibroma and cystadenofibroma
b) Surface papilloma	3. Malignant
c) Adenofibroma and cystadenofibroma	a) Carcinoma
3. Malignant	1. Adenocarcinoma
a) Adenocarcinoma, papillary adenocarcinoma, and papillary cystadenocarcinoma	2. Adenoacanthoma
b) Surface papillary carcinoma	3. Malignant adenofibroma and cystadenofibroma
c) Malignant adenofibroma and cystadenofibroma	b) Endometrioid stromal sarcomas
B. Mucinous tumors	c) Mesodermal (müllerian) mixed tumors, homologous and heterologous
1. Benign	D. Clear cell (mesonephroid) tumors
a) Cystadenoma	1. Benign: adenofibroma
b) Adenofibroma and cystadenofibroma	2. Of borderline malignancy (tumors of low malignant potential)
2. Of borderline malignancy (tumors of low malignant potential)	3. Malignant
a) Cystadenoma	E. Brenner tumors
b) Adenofibroma and cystadenofibroma	1. Benign
3. Malignant	2. Of borderline malignancy (proliferating)
a) Adenocarcinoma and cystadenocarcinoma	3. Malignant
b) Malignant adenofibroma and cystadenofibroma	F. Mixed epithelial tumors
	1. Benign
	2. Of borderline malignancy
	3. Malignant
	G. Undifferentiated carcinoma
	H. Unclassified epithelial tumors

thologists and clinical oncologists as well, and attempts to define therapeutic progress suffer because of unstable and unstandardized terminology. Nowhere is this more apparent than with ovarian tumors. Earlier classifications were made with little knowledge of histogenesis and were often based on crude features such as whether tumors were cystic or solid—and the presence of endocrine effects. The World Health Organization (WHO) classification of ovarian tumors (Table 2–1) published in 1973,[13] provides a standard based on histogenetic origin that has already improved communication of cancer information. Pathologists who have not kept up with current concepts and modern terminology may be providing out-of-date diagnoses to modern clinicians.

Most chemotherapists, radiotherapists, and gynecologic oncologists have a fixed terminology in mind. More physicians will be using the WHO ovarian tumor classification from now on and will expect the pathologist to do the same.

Epithelial Tumors of Low Malignant Potential

The WHO classification adopted the International Federation of Gynecology and Obstetrics (FIGO) recommendation that borderline categories of epithelial tumors be recognized so that the low-grade tumors (Fig. 2–1) could be separated from the typically aggressive carcinomas of the ovary as well as from the benign neoplasms. In the past, reported five-year survival rates for pa-

OF OVARIAN TUMORS

II. SEX CORD STROMAL TUMORS
  A. Granulosa-stromal cell tumors
    1. Granulosa cell tumor
    2. Tumors in the thecoma-fibroma group
      a) Thecoma
      b) Fibroma
      c) Unclassified
  B. Androblastomas; Sertoli-Leydig cell tumors
    1. Well differentiated
      a) Tubular androblastoma; Sertoli cell tumor (tubular adenoma of Pick)
      b) Tubular androblastoma with lipid storage; Sertoli cell tumor with lipid storage (folliculome lipidique of Lecene)
      c) Sertoli-Leydig cell tumor (tubular adenoma with Leydig cells)
      d) Leydig cell tumor; hilus cell tumor
    2. Of intermediate differentiation
    3. Poorly differentiated (sarcomatoid)
    4. With heterologous elements
  C. Gynandroblastoma
  D. Unclassified
III. LIPID (LIPOID) CELL TUMORS
IV. GERM CELL TUMORS
  A. Dysgerminoma
  B. Endodermal sinus tumor
  C. Embryonal carcinoma
  D. Polyembryoma
  E. Choriocarcinoma
  F. Teratomas
    1. Immature
    2. Mature
      a) Solid

IV. GERM CELL TUMORS (cont.)
      b) Cystic
        1. Dermoid cyst (mature cystic teratoma)
        2. Dermoid cyst with malignant transformation
    3. Monodermal and highly specialized
      a) Struma ovarii
      b) Carcinoid
      c) Struma ovarii and carcinoid
      d) Others
  G. Mixed forms
V. GONADOBLASTOMA
  A. Pure
  B. Mixed with dysgerminoma or other form of germ cell tumor
VI. SOFT TISSUE TUMORS NOT SPECIFIC TO OVARY
VII. UNCLASSIFIED TUMORS
VIII. SECONDARY (METASTATIC) TUMORS
IX. TUMOR-LIKE CONDITIONS
  A. Pregnancy luteoma
  B. Hyperplasia of ovarian stroma and hyperthecosis
  C. Massive edema
  D. Solitary follicle cyst and corpus luteum cyst
  E. Multiple follicle cysts (polycystic ovaries)
  F. Multiple luteinized follicle cysts and/or corpora lutea
  G. Endometriosis
  H. Surface-epithelial inclusion cysts (germinal inclusion cysts)
  I. Simple cysts
  J. Inflammatory cysts
  K. Paraovarian cysts

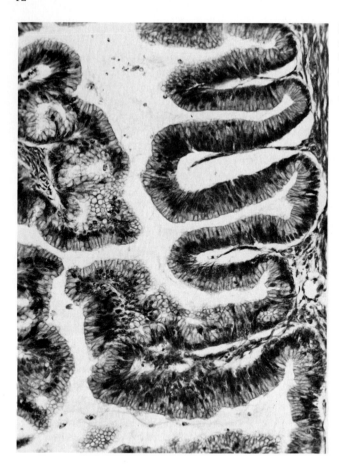

Figure 2–1. Mucinous tumor of low malignant potential (borderline tumor). Stratification and atypical cells are present, but there is no invasion of the supporting stroma. H&E, ×150; AFIP Neg. 75-13250.

tients with stage I mucinous carcinoma varied from 65 to 100 percent and from 20 to 75 percent when all stages have been included.[14] From 5 to 45 percent of mucinous tumors have been reported to be malignant.[14] These tremendous differences can be ascribed largely to the indiscriminate inclusion of borderline tumors with carcinomas in some studies and their exclusion in others. It has not been fully appreciated how large the borderline category really is. In the Armed Forces Institute of Pathology (AFIP) files, stage I serous borderline tumors are as common as stage I serous carcinomas. In stage I, borderline mucinous tumors are 2.5 times as common as carcinomas. In the material studied in the notable paper on ovarian carcinoma by Aure et al, there was one borderline tumor for every stage I carcinoma in both the mucinous and serous categories.[15] In stages II through IV the problem is less acute, for serous carcinomas are 16 times more common than borderline tumors and mucinous carcinomas are 5 times more common

than their borderline counterpart.[15] In an Armed Forces Institute of Pathology study,[14] the five-year survival in patients with stage I mucinous carcinomas was found to be 66 percent, as compared to 96 percent among those with borderline tumors of low malignant potential. Serous borderline tumors also have striking differences in behavior from serous carcinomas.[15] Since borderline serous and mucinous tumors are common and their behavior is so different from carcinoma, the borderline contingent must be recognized and isolated if one is to make sense out of ovarian cancer statistics. Not all clinicians and pathologists have become aware of the significance of the borderline category. Others make the mistake of assuming that peritoneal metastasis indicates that the neoplasm is behaving as if malignant, regardless of its microscopic appearance. Those holding this view ignore or are unaware of the striking differences in survival, stage for stage, of borderline and malignant tumors of the same cell type; this difference justifies their distinction, and the degree of spread does not enter into the question of whether a tumor is benign, borderline, or malignant.

Borderline tumors are most common in serous and mucinous categories, but all epithelial carcinomas have their borderline counterpart. The borderline counterparts of endometrioid carcinoma and clear cell carcinoma are usually variants of cystadenofibromas with stratification and atypicality of epithelial cells (Figs. 2–2 and 2–3). The borderline counterpart of the malignant Brenner tumor is a proliferative Brenner tumor (Fig. 2–4). To reduce the possibility of misinterpretation, we have recommended the noncommittal designation "tumor of low malignant potential" for borderline tumors—a name that avoids the terms "carcinoma" and "adenoma," as the behavior of these neoplasms is different from that of carcinomas and cystadenomas. A diagnosis by frozen section is often helpful at laparotomy. While formerly the pathologist had to concern himself with only the "benign" or "malignant" category, he must now also consider the borderline category. He may wish to state flatly whether it is benign,

borderline, or malignant. Some pathologists may prefer to state their diagnosis in these terms: (1) malignant, (2) probably malignant, possibly borderline, (3) probably benign, possibly borderline, (4) borderline, or (5) benign. Either way, the clinician is provided an impression for the aggressive potential of the disease and can plan his therapeutic strategy.

Germ Cell Tumors

Advances in the nomenclature and classification of ovarian germ cell tumors have paralleled those in the epithelial category, but here again, it takes time for the information to be disseminated and assimilated by clinicians and pathologists. In the past, reports on germ cell tumors often included mixtures of different germ cell tumors with varying behavior. Information on pure tumors, rather than mixtures, is now being collected. Asadourian and Taylor were among the first to recognize the importance of studying pure tumors. They noted that reported mortality rates for patients with dysgerminoma had varied from 27 to 75 percent,

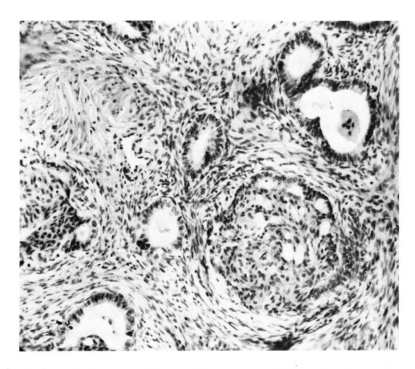

Figure 2–2. Endometrioid tumor of low malignant potential. The abundance of dense, fibrous stroma indicates that it is closely related to an endometrioid cystadenofibroma. This tumor should not be mistaken for endometrioid carcinoma. H&E, ×160; AFIP Neg. 76-1752.

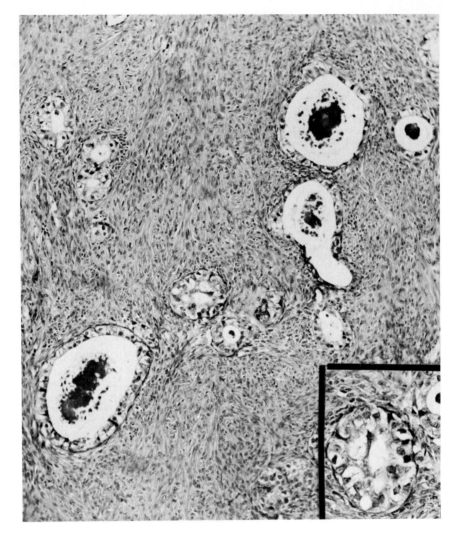

Figure 2–3. Low magnification of a clear cell or mesonephroid tumor of low malignant potential. H&E, ×70; AFIP Neg. 76-4056. **Insert:** Higher magnification showing atypicality of the epithelium. This tumor is closely related to a cystadenofibroma lined by clear cells. H&E, ×195; AFIP Neg. 76-4057.

and yet they found a five-year survival rate of 86 percent when tumors containing other germ cell elements were excluded.[10]

The classification of immature teratomas has been as confusing. According to current usage, these are tumors that contain immature elements (Fig. 2–5) and rarely occur in women past 40. Yet malignant teratomas have been reported to have a bimodal age distribution with a second peak in women over 70.[16] Scully noted that this could be explained by the inclusion of benign cystic teratomas containing adult types of malignancy or mixed mesodermal tumors (both occurring pre-

dominantly in older women) with the immature teratomas of younger women.[16] Mixed mesodermal tumors and benign cystic teratomas with malignant change have different biologic properties and must be separated from immature teratomas if useful information is to be obtained. Although some workers were unable to show a correlation between histologic features of immature teratomas and prognosis, they were reporting mixed germ cell tumors; investigators who evaluated pure teratomas found histologic grading useful in predicting the behavior.[11,12,17] In a study of 58 cases, five-year survival varied from 30 per-

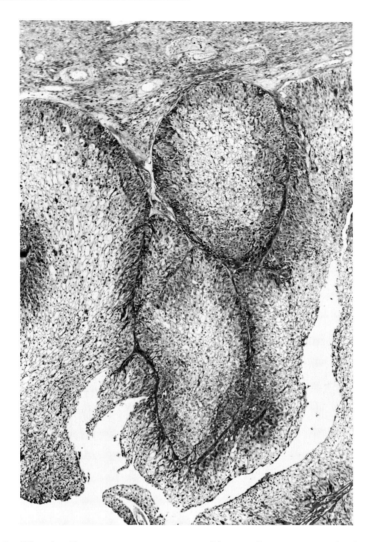

Figure 2–4. Proliferative Brenner tumor, a tumor of low malignant potential. Elsewhere, areas of benign Brenner epithelium merged with the proliferative epithelium illustrated here. H&E, ×145; AFIP Neg. 71-3925.

cent in grade 3 (most immature) to 81 percent in grade 1 (least immature) teratomas.[12] The correlation was obtained by excluding immature teratomas containing admixtures of other malignant germ cell elements.

The "mesonephroma" described by Schiller has been found subsequently to include two distinct types of tumor: one, the clear cell carcinoma (mesonephroid carcinoma) of epithelial origin, and the other, the endodermal sinus tumor of germ cell origin. These are also quite different in biologic behavior. The mesonephroid carcinoma occurs in older women and may have borderline

and malignant variants, as do the other epithelial tumors, with prognosis dependent on the degree of differentiation. In contrast, the endodermal sinus tumor occurs in girls and young women and until recently was almost universally fatal. The clinical and pathologic features of 71 pure endodermal sinus tumors have been recently described by Kurman and Norris.[18] The median age of patients with these neoplasms was 19 years, and neoplasms were stage I in 71 percent of patients, but 84 percent of those not given a modern chemotherapeutic regimen died nonetheless. The tumors grow rapidly, and the mean duration of

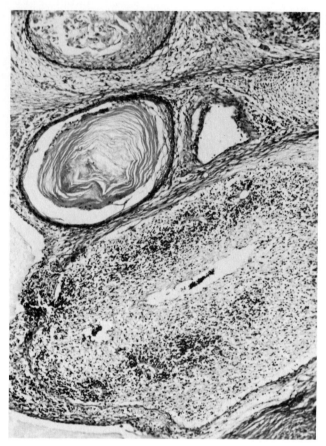

Figure 2–5. Immature teratoma, grade I. Immaturity conveys metastatic potential. H&E, ×76; AFIP Neg. 75-15087.

symptoms prior to diagnosis is only two weeks. Four histologic patterns as described by Teilum were identified, but mixtures of two or more patterns were common, and the predominant pattern had no relationship to survival. A characteristic feature was the presence of hyaline droplets, some of which contained α-fetoprotein by an immunohistochemical technique. As was the case in immature teratomas, no evidence of metastasis to the opposite ovary was seen in stage I tumors, so it is not surprising that unilateral salpingo-oophorectomy was as effective as hysterectomy with bilateral salpingo-oophorectomy. Smith and associates[19] have found startling improvement in survival with the use of immediate postoperative administration of a combination of vincristine, actinomycin D, and cyclophosphamide. Therefore, recognition of this tumor is important so that this therapy can be promptly instituted and unnecessarily radical surgery and irradiation can be avoided in these young patients. Furthermore, serial determinations of serum α-fetoprotein may aid in monitoring the effects of therapy and in the early detection of recurrences. Embryonal carcinoma analogous to carcinoma of the adult testis has been described recently in the ovary (Fig. 2–6).[20] Although similar to endodermal sinus tumor, patients with embryonal carcinoma tend to be younger (median age 15 years) and to have positive pregnancy tests and precocious puberty. Survival is better in these patients than in those with endodermal sinus tumor.

Gonadal Stromal Tumors

Gonadal stromal tumors include granulosa-theca tumors, Sertoli-Leydig tumors, lipid cell tumors, and stromal tumors of unspecified type. These neoplasms often show functional manifestations of endocrine activity, but a histologic classification is preferable to one based on function, because not all tumors of gonadal stroma have demonstrable functional activity and certain of these tumors may on occasion be associated with unexpected endocrine effect.[21] This group of tumors, more than any other, has been plagued by overclassification and imaginative subdivisions that have proved to have no significance or to be too complicated to gain acceptance. It is frequently possible to find patterns in one tumor that resemble those of another, suggesting that any subdivision of ovarian stromal tumors is to some extent artificial. Approximately 20 percent of gonadal stromal tumors cannot be classified into a specific category with any degree of certainty.[21]

The malignant potential of gonadal stromal tumors, particularly granulosa tumors, has been controversial, with widely varying mortality rates reported. This lack of agreement stems from several factors.

1. There has been little discipline over what constitutes the histologic features of granulosa-theca tumors. This is apparent from the imaginative and differing descriptions, which have resulted in a welter of terms and vague criteria for the various granulosa-theca histologic patterns. Poorly differentiated carcinoma accounts for most of the bilateral tumors and fatal cases reported in the past.

2. Since thecomas are nearly always benign, survival figures will vary according to the proportion of thecomas in the group.

3. Patient survival usually has been expressed as

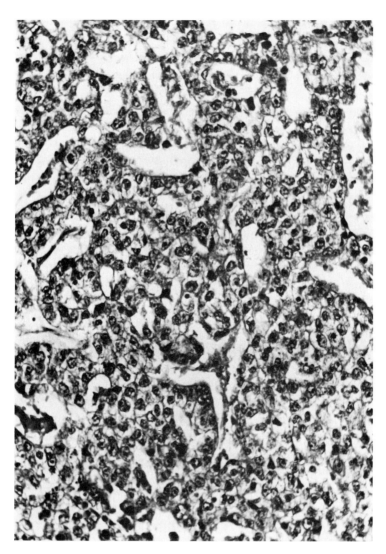

Figure 2–6. Embryonal carcinoma. Note the epithelial arrangement of this rare tumor, formerly confused with endodermal sinus tumor. H&E, ×200; AFIP Neg. 75-14212.

crude or "corrected," without mention of whether or not the patients died of the granulosa-theca tumors.

When rigid histologic criteria are used to exclude adenocarcinoma or other unclassified malignant tumors, it has become clear that granulosa tumors are seldom bilateral and carry relatively high survival rates (97 percent and 93 percent) at 5 and 10 years, respectively, in one study.[22] In the first 200 neoplasms with a granulosa pattern in the AFIP files, only 2 (1 percent) were bilateral. Nevertheless, they are prone to recur or metastasize over a protracted course; all granulosa tumors are malignant, but rather sluggishly so. The specific histologic pattern (e.g., trabecular or microfollicular) appears to have no bearing on prognosis—nor do such features as microscopic capsular invasion, degree of cellular atypism, or the presence of ascites.[22] The significance of apparent lymphatic invasion is unclear, and that mitotic activity may bear on prognosis has been both affirmed and denied.[22,23] Findings associated with an unfavorable prognosis include a short duration of symptoms, pain, weight loss, rupture or extension of tumor beyond the ovary at the time of surgery, age over 40, and tumor measuring over 15 cm in diameter. The relationship of different treatment modalities to survival is not known because of the variable criteria for diagnosis and varying proportions of thecomas in different series, but it is clear that unilateral salpingo-oophorectomy is as effective as more extensive surgery provided the opposite ovary is normal and there is no evidence of spread elsewhere. Because of the variability of the tumor and lack of uniformity in diagnosis, clinicians should not hesitate to request consultation when gonadal stromal tumors are diagnosed.

The associated endocrine activity also deserves comment. The estrogen produced by some of these tumors can be associated with precocious puberty in prepuberal girls and with the presence of endometrial hyperplasia or carcinoma in older women. Of 77 granulosa-theca tumors with endometrial findings available, 9 percent had an associated carcinoma and 22 percent had some form of endometrial hyperplasia associated with the ovarian tumor.[22] Granulosa tumors do not always produce estrogen, some unusually cystic tumors found mainly in young women have been associated with virilization.[24]

As with granulosa-theca tumors, it is important to distinguish Sertoli-Leydig tumors from adenocarcinomas, both primary and metastatic to the ovary. Carcinomas with their glandular elements amid a hyperplastic stroma, at times with stromal luteinization, may have a strong resemblance to Sertoli-Leydig tumors, as luteinized cells may closely resemble Leydig cells. The hyperplastic ovarian stroma accompanying some primary and metastatic carcinomas may also be functioning, producing either an estrogenic or androgenic effect. Fat and mucin stains may aid in differentiating carcinoma from Sertoli-Leydig tumors. Metastatic carcinomas, furthermore, are most often bilateral, whereas well-documented examples of bilateral Sertoli-Leydig tumors are so rare as to represent curiosities.[25]

The foregoing discussion of a few examples of ovarian tumors should alert the clinician and pathologist to the necessity for utilizing strict histologic criteria in the diagnosis of ovarian tumors. The use of the WHO classification, based on histologic features, furthers communication between pathologist and clinician and facilitates comparison of results among institutions.

Fallopian Tube

The major problem in the interpretation of fallopian tube lesions is failure to distinguish mucosal hyperplasias from carcinoma. Some pathologists do not realize that the tubal epithelium will become markedly hyperplastic and atypical in response to inflammation, and with the increase in incidence of tubal-ovarian inflammatory disease this problem is becoming more common. The inflammation can produce large masses of mucosal hyperplasia with superimposed atypism. The inflammation is often granulomatous or xanthogranulomatous but may be simply severe chronic inflammation. Invasion is the only sure criterion for carcinoma of the fallopian tube, and clinicians would be wise to request consultation if a diagnosis of carcinoma is rendered in the absence of invasion.

Uterus

Endometrium

The interpretation of hyperplastic and early neoplastic lesions of the endometrium is one of the major current problems in gynecologic pathology. As Gore has noted, "Not only are different names applied to the same lesion, but the same name is applied to different lesions, presumably of different malignant potential."[26] Also, there is little consistency in the diagnosis from one laboratory to another. Some have used the term "atypical hyperplasia" for all presumed precancerous lesions of the endometrium, while others have used "adenomatous hyperplasia" in a similar way. Others distinguish atypical hyperplasia from adenomatous hyperplasia, but use different criteria. Vellios, for example, distinguishes adenomatous hyperplasia as an architectural change with small glands budding from larger glands and atypical hyperplasia as denoting cellular atypism,[27] while the AFIP uses both architectural and cytologic atypias to distinguish different grades of hyperplasia. The term "adenocarcinoma in situ" has been applied variably also. Some have applied this term to carcinoma invading the stroma but not the myometrium, while others have used it to denote specific but varying atypias in the absence of stromal invasion. In the Vellios type of "adenocarcinoma in situ" there are pronounced nuclear changes but cytoplasmic alterations are not marked,[27] while in the Hertig type, nuclear atypicalities are not necessarily striking but there is abundant eosinophilic cytoplasm.[28] Thus, although an in situ phase is presumed to

occur, criteria for its recognition are not uniform, and the term "adenocarcinoma in situ" is perhaps best avoided in favor of a more descriptive term. If one uses "adenocarcinoma in situ" as a diagnosis, he must make the more subtle and subjective distinctions between atypical hyperplasia (Fig. 2–7) and adenocarcinoma in situ and between adenocarcinoma in situ and adenocarcinoma. We recommend that a diagnosis of carcinoma be reserved for those situations in which atypical glands replace or infiltrate the stroma. Atypical hyperplasia and "carcinoma in situ" do not require irradiation for eradication.

Endometrial stromal invasion may be difficult to identify with certainty because normal endometrial glands may be haphazardly distributed through the stroma. A determination that invasion is present is often subjective and sometimes must be presumed on the basis of virtual replacement of stroma by malignant-appearing glands. Contemplating a diagnosis of an atypical endometrial lesion or carcinoma, one must not be fooled by the back-to-back configuration of glands seen in menstrual-phase endometrium or from fragmentation of curettings. In menstrual endometrium, there is stromal dissolution from loss of fluid and ground substance with collapse of

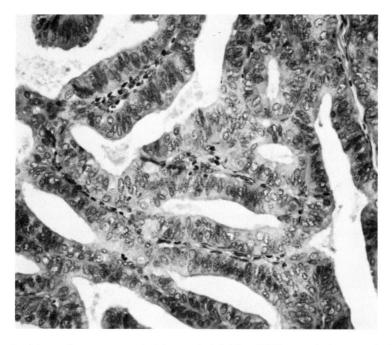

Figure 2–7. Is this carcinoma or atypical hyperplasia? The AFIP regards it as atypical hyperplasia, but there is no agreement or consistency over these lesions. H&E, ×250; AFIP Neg. 76-9376.

glands toward one another, thus the stroma appears dense and highly cellular and glands look crowded and irregular. More erroneous diagnoses of atypical hyperplasia and carcinoma occur with menstrual-phase endometrium than in any other condition. Another change that can be confusing is the eosinophilic, often stratified endometrial surface resulting from regeneration and prolonged cycles in the absence of progesterone.

Because of the variability in histologic criteria for diagnosis of hyperplasia and well-differentiated adenocarcinoma and because reports often are not adequately illustrated, it has been impossible to define accurately the malignant potential of what is being reported. Retrospective studies designed to evaluate this aspect may be criticized since only about 10 percent of women with adenocarcinoma have had prior endometrial specimens available for study and the earlier status of the endometrium in the other 90 percent is unknown. There are two major studies of the premalignant potential of hyperplasia. One, from the AFIP, concerned 90 women less than 36 years of age with hyperplasia or atypical hyperplasia, treated conservatively and followed for 1 to 30 years.[29] Of the 90, 14 (16 percent) subsequently developed what was regarded as adenocarcinoma, and 33 (37 percent) eventually had hysterectomy either for adenocarcinoma or for persistent bleeding; 80 percent had been followed for five years or more. The other major prospective study,[30] concerning women over 40 years of age, included 100 patients with atypical lesions referred to as adenomatous hyperplasia, and 12 percent of those followed for more than a year were found to have adenocarcinoma. The authors concluded that the cumulative risk of the development of carcinoma in patients with these atypical hyperplasias was about 30 percent in 10 years. In this study, however, six of the eight who developed carcinoma had had prior radiotherapy, and it may have played a role in the pathogenesis. Both studies can be criticized because the natural history of the disease could have been altered by the biopsy or curettage done for the diagnosis of the precursor lesion or modified by the therapy given.

Although the malignant potential of various histologic patterns is not known precisely, hyperplasia and atypical hyperplasia are widely believed to have some degree of malignant potential. This potential probably varies according to the degree of complexity of the pattern, being least in what has been termed "cystic hyperplasia" and greatest in lesions that are difficult to distinguish from invasive carcinoma. What has been called cystic hyperplasia in the past consists of two distinct entities, one a true hyperplasia with irregular, cystic glands lined by tall, sometimes stratified glandular cells without cytologic atypia, and the other, an atrophic change in which inactive, flattened cells line dilated cyst-like glands set in inactive stroma. The latter is not hyperplasia at all. The cystic aspect of both changes should be deemphasized by referring to the proliferative lesion simply as "hyperplasia" and to the atrophic lesion simply as "atrophic endometrium." Since all hyperplasias involve glands, it is superfluous to add the term "adenomatous." In the more complex hyperplasias, glandular cells may form intraluminal buds, bridges, and stratification; in the absence of cellular atypism, this lesion may also be designated simply "hyperplasia." When atypical cytologic features occur in a hyperplasia, mainly in the form of nuclear hyperchromatism and stratification of the cells, we believe the lesion should be designated "atypical hyperplasia" to denote a lesion of greater malignant potential (Fig. 2–7). This designation includes various patterns of preinvasive lesions, including what others have called "adenocarcinoma in situ." Finally, a proliferation showing unequivocal stromal invasion or replacement we designate adenocarcinoma.

It is of the utmost importance that a clinician become familiar with the terminology used by his pathologist. An individual pathologist's interpretation of degree of malignant potential will likely bear a closer relationship to that of another pathologist than a specific term will correlate to the same term in written reports. What terms are used in a single institution makes little difference as long as clinicians understand what those terms imply in terms of malignant potential.

Endometrial stromal tumors are benign or malignant, and the distinction is easy. Benign stromal tumors are expansile, circumscribed nodules that do not infiltrate vessels or myometrium. They do not metastasize. Endometrial stromal sarcomas, however, do infiltrate, and all have the capacity to metastasize to varying extent, depending on the degree of mitotic activity.[31] It is hoped that pathologists will use the modern terminology for stromal tumors rather than nonspecific and confusing terms like "stromatosis."

Myometrium

There is controversy over how to distinguish a leiomyosarcoma from cellular and atypical leiomyomas. A discrepancy in the five-year survival rates (0 to 68 percent)[32-34] in patients with leiomyosarcoma indicates a lack of uniform diagnostic criteria. Criteria for a diagnosis of leiomyosarcoma have included demonstration of invasion or metastasis, abnormal mitoses, smooth muscle giant cells, or simply a cellular area containing large and hyperchromatic nuclei of varying size, shape, and staining characteristics. To require invasion or metastases is too strict, since by this criterion 15 of 29 smooth muscle tumors that subsequently caused the patient's death would have been called leiomyomas, lacking evidence of invasion.[34] Several investigators have found the numbers of mitotic figures to be the most accurate and objective single criterion, and there is general agreement that neoplasms containing 10 or more mitotic figures per 10 high-power fields (HPF) are leiomyosarcomas.[35] In the AFIP series,[34] of 36 patients followed with tumors containing 10 or more mitotic figures per 10 HPF, 31 recurred or metastasized. Of 21 tumors with fewer than 10 mitotic figures per 10 HPF, none recurred or metastasized, regardless of the degree of atypism, but there were few in this group with mitotic counts in the range of 5 to 9 mitotic figures per 10 high-power fields. Others have found recurrence or metastasis with tumors containing 5 to 9 mitotic figures per 10 high-power fields.[33,36] Kempson and Bari have suggested utilizing cellular pleomorphism to distinguish sarcomas from leiomyomas in this borderline group.[36] Discrepancies in mitotic counts may occur for several reasons. Some neoplasms contain large numbers of leucocytes or pyknotic nuclei reflecting muscle cell degeneration, and these may be difficult to distinguish from mitotic figures if tissue is poorly preserved, sections are too thick, or slides are overstained. Furthermore, suspicious smooth muscle tumors must be adequately sampled (one block for every centimeter of maximum tumor diameter) and the most active areas counted.

Clinicians should know that some uterine smooth muscle tumors metastasize but still are not leiomyosarcomas. Intravenous leiomyomatosis and epithelioid leiomyomas have this capability,[37,38] and benign metastasizing leiomyomas do occur rarely. These do not progress as a leiomyosarcoma, however, and surgical excision of metastatic nodules will provide protracted relief if not cure. Adequate sampling, as mentioned earlier, is important.

Cervix

The advent of cytology and colposcopy as well as electron microscopy, cytogenetics, Feulgen microspectrophotometric DNA analysis, tritiated thymidine uptake studies and tissue culture have expanded our knowledge of squamous carcinoma of the cervix and its precursors. Carcinoma in situ and dysplasia were defined by an International Committee on Histological Definitions in Vienna in 1961, as follows:

> Carcinoma in situ. Only those cases should be classified as carcinoma in situ which, in the absence of invasion, show as surface lining an epithelium in which, throughout its whole thickness, no differentiation takes place. It is recognized that the cells of the uppermost layers may show some slight flattening. The very rare case of an otherwise characteristic carcinoma in situ that shows a greater degree of differentiation belongs to the exception for which no classification can provide.
>
> All other disturbances of differentiation of the squamous epithelial lining of surface and glands are to be classified as dysplasia. They may be characterized as of high or low degree, terms which are preferable to suspicious and nonsuspicious, as the proposed terms describe the histological appearances and do not express an opinion.[39]

The division of lesions into *carcinoma in situ* and *dysplasia* was thought to be justified because carcinoma in situ was thought to be irreversible, while dysplasias were thought to be capable of spontaneous regression. The definition of dysplasia allows side latitude in the histologic criteria for diagnosis, but there has been a trend toward limiting the diagnosis of dysplasia to those lesions with malignant atypical cytologic features, excluding benign atypias associated with inflammation and immature squamous metaplasia. The wide variability in the frequency with which dysplasia has been found to regress is due to variations in histologic criteria and problems in study design and statistical analysis. In studies attempting to circumvent these problems, it has been

shown that dysplasia rarely regresses spontaneously.[40-42] Thus the basis of distinguishing dysplasia from carcinoma in situ is a convenience rather
than a qualitative biological difference. Additional
evidence from electron microscopy, studies of
cervical epithelium by tissue culture, tritiated
thymidine uptake, and Feulgen microspectro-
photometry indicates that there is no qualitative difference between dysplasia and carcinoma
in situ,[43] and there is increasing acceptance of the
concept that carcinoma in situ and dysplasia are
not distinct diseases but represent different stages
of a continuum of change from normal to invasive carcinoma. The term "cervical intraepithelial neoplasia" used to encompass the dysplasia-
carcinoma in situ spectrum is more realistic and
avoids the implication that dysplasia and carcinoma in situ are different diseases. The use of
terms such as "mild," "moderate," and "severe
intraepithelial neoplasia" allows for grading of
quantitative severity and obviates the necessity of
telling the patient she has cancer when the lesion
is severe but not egregious carcinoma. An impor-

tant clinical implication of this concept is that the
histologic distinction between different degrees
of intraepithelial neoplasia is not important and
that all degrees may progress at unpredictable
rates in individual cases and, untreated, rarely regress. Therefore, both dysplasia and carcinoma
should be eradicated when discovered. The ease
of eradication depends more on the location and
extent of the lesion than upon the degree of histologic atypism.[43] Since the colposcopist is able to
localize and map the extent of the lesion, colposcopy has become increasingly important in the
modern management of dysplasia and carcinoma
in situ.

"Microinvasive carcinoma," a term introduced
in 1947,[44] originally designated a neoplasm invading to a depth of 5 mm or less. Since then, as
many as 18 different terms have been applied to
various early invasive carcinomas,[45] and a uniform, specific definition of the term "microinvasion" has not been established. The 1974 modification of the FIGO staging system[46] provides
that "microinvasive carcinoma" be assigned to

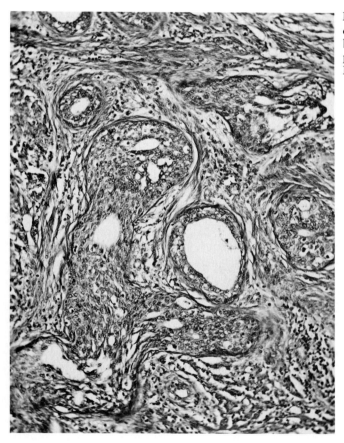

Figure 2–8. Adenosquamous carcinoma of the cervix. This tumor has
biphasic differentiation, and either
pattern may appear in metastases.
H&E, ×140; AFIP Neg. 76-5185.

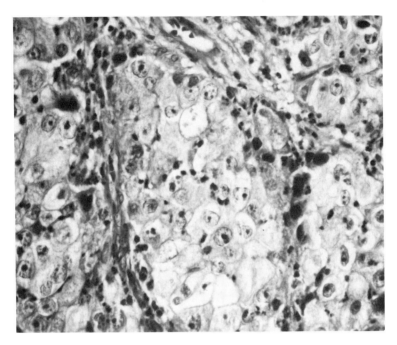

Figure 2–9. Glassy cell carcinoma of cervix. A rare form of carcinoma with a relatively unfavorable prognosis. H&E, ×310; AFIP Neg. 76-9384.

stage Ia, but no criteria for microinvasion were given. Because of the variation in definitions as well as techniques of measurement, it has been difficult to extract from the literature a sufficient number of cases similarly defined from which to base an estimate of the risk of metastasis to lymph nodes or death from tumor with "microinvasion." If neoplasms invading to a depth up to 5 mm, not excluding those with invasion of apparent lymphatic spaces or a confluent growth pattern, are selected from reports lacking various biasing factors, then only 98 cases are available from which to judge the frequency of nodal metastasis or death from tumor. Only one of the 98 showed nodal metastasis, a frequency of 1.0 percent, but 98 cases are too few to justify confidence that 1.0 percent is a good estimate.[47]

There are factors that might affect the risk of nodal metastasis. Some investigators have thought that invasion of lymphatic-like spaces or a confluent growth pattern is ominous and have excluded those cases from the category of microinvasion. Roche and Norris cast doubt on the significance of these features, noting the difficulty of proving that capillary-like spaces are, in fact, capillaries and that the separation of finger-like from confluent growth patterns is highly subjective.[48] There is a low frequency of metastases

whether or not capillary-like spaces are involved and whether the pattern is finger-like or confluent. Other factors, in addition to depth of invasion, that might affect the risk of metastases have not been adequately considered. These include volume of tumor, cell type, and degree of differentiation. Eventually an authoritative international body should establish specific histologic criteria for the diagnosis of microinvasive carcinoma, but until that is done it seems reasonable that all cases of early stromal invasion should be studied with respect to these factors in order to accumulate sufficient cases to establish reliably the risk of metastasis. Until a safe and specific definition of microinvasion is obtained, it is prudent to reserve judgment on whether hysterectomy or radical hysterectomy with lymph node dissection is more appropriate. Since clinicians may wish to treat microinvasive carcinoma differently from other invasive carcinomas, pathologists should use the diagnosis, but in addition must describe the histologic features so that the clinician will know exactly the features of the tumor.

There are rare special types of cervical carcinomas that the pathologist is just beginning to recognize. Formerly buried among diagnoses of squamous and adenocarcinomas are the newly recognized adenosquamous carcinoma, glassy cell carcinoma, basaloid carcinoma, argentaffin-positive apudomas, and verrucous carcinomas. The adenosquamous carcinoma (Fig. 2–8) has been particularly confusing because one biopsy specimen might be mostly squamous while a conization of the same specimen might be largely glandular, and a difference of opinion might arise when different specimens are viewed by different pathologists. It should be recognized that in adenosquamous carcinoma both the squamous and glandular epithelium appear malignant, in contrast to adenocarcinoma with squamous metaplasia, where the squamous epithelium is benign.

A special form of adenosquamous carcinoma is the poorly differentiated lesion termed "glassy cell carcinoma" (Fig. 2–9). In 1956, 41 examples were reported by Glücksmann and Cherry,[49] who described the characteristic features: (1) a moderate amount of cytoplasm of ground-glass appearance that stains faintly blue with hematoxylin, (2) a fairly distinct cell wall that stains with eosin or with PAS, and (3) large nuclei with prominent nucleoli. These features make it bear a superficial resemblance to decidua, and differentiation is important because 17 percent of adenocarcinomas of the cervix in pregnancy are adenosquamous in type.[49] The recognition of this pattern is also important because of the poor prognosis: None of the 32 patients followed and reported by Glücksmann and Cherry survived, whether treated by radiotherapy alone or radiotherapy followed by surgery, even though 19 of the 32 patients were in stage I or II. Recently, others have found a 30 percent survival rate in a series of 13 cases and noted that glassy cell carcinoma tends to metastasize frequently to pelvic lymph nodes and is prone to extrapelvic metastasis.[50]

The unusually well-differentiated adenocarcinoma or so-called "adenoma malignum" represents a major problem in histologic diagnosis. This tumor is composed of glands that show little or no atypia and are difficult to distinguish from normal endocervical glands except by their infiltrating pattern (Figs. 2–10 and 2–11). Diagnosis may be difficult or impossible from biopsy specimens or even cones, as the pattern cannot always be recognized. Moreover, most of the glands are uniform and cytologically normal, while rare ones show degrees of nuclear atypism. In spite of the good differentiation, the tumor has been found to infiltrate deeply, metastasize early, and have a low rate of cure.[51,52] Few cases, however, have been treated early by modern therapeutic techniques.[53]

Adenoid cystic carcinoma is a rare form of adenocarcinoma even in its most common sites, and it is especially rare in the cervix. It is composed of characteristic clusters of small uniform cells with darkly staining nuclei and little cytoplasm (Fig. 2–12). Of 12 examples in the AFIP files, 11 had invasion of capillary-like spaces, and all had deeply infiltrating margins, factors that may explain the relatively poor survival.[54] Most have basaloid features as well, a pattern similar to the "apudoma" of the cervix, a newly described carcinoma containing argyrophilic cells.[55,56]

The interpretation of papillary squamous lesions of the cervix also poses problems for the pathologist. In 1963, Pitkin and Kent, after reviewing 17 such lesions, wrote, "We believe it is not possible to distinguish histologically with any degree of accuracy between squamous papilloma, condyloma acuminatum, and well differentiated squamous carcinoma of the cervix."[57] This view is overly pessimistic, but it does reflect the difficulty of diagnosing and of reliably estimating the behavior of rare, unusually well-differentiated verrucous lesions of the vulva, vagina, and cervix. These lesions may have the gross and histologic features of benign papillary lesions, yet declare their malignant potential by recurrence or metastasis after multiple biopsy specimens have been interpreted as benign lesions. The term "verrucous carcinoma" was originally used by Ackerman in 1948,[58] to describe the same well-differentiated lesions arising in the oral cavity. In the vulva and vagina, the clinician tends to overestimate the malignant potential on gross inspection, and the pathologist tends to underestimate it on histologic examination.[59] Although these tumors invade locally and have a propensity for local recurrence, metastasis is unusual unless the lesion has been irradiated.[60,61] Recognition of this pattern is important so that adequate treatment can be given while the tumor is small and before extension or metastases occurs.

The misdiagnosis of malignant lesions as benign may occur in cases of verrucous carcinoma and well-differentiated adenocarcinoma, but benign lesions may as easily be misdiagnosed as malignant. The endocervical hyperplasia seen in pregnant women or in those taking oral contraceptives may develop after a progestin exposure of only a few weeks, or it may appear after several years.[62] It presents as a cervical polyp, and microscopically

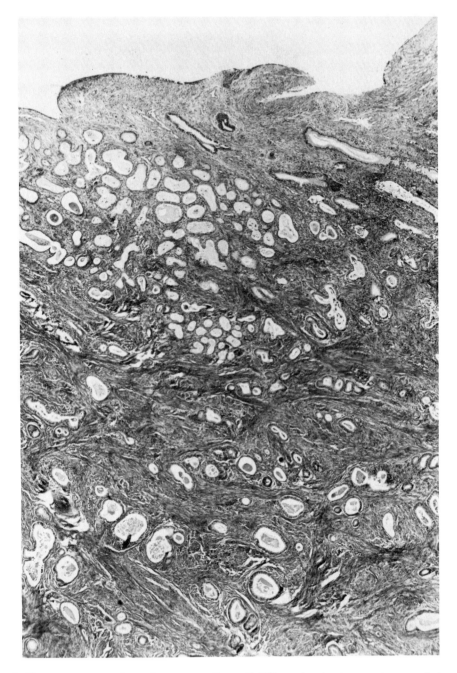

Figure 2–10. Low-power view of an unusually well-differentiated adenocarcinoma of the cervix, identifiable only by its invasive pattern. H&E, ×20; AFIP Neg. 75-13238.

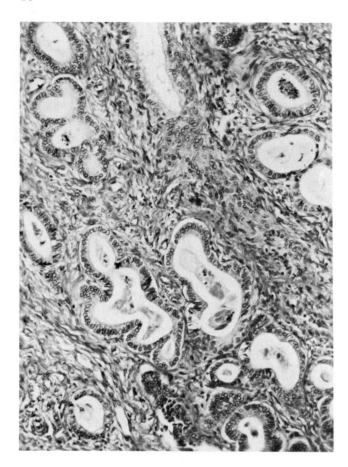

Figure 2–11. Higher magnification of Figure 2-10 showing well differentiated glands. H&E, ×160; AFIP Neg. 75-13239.

it is composed of tightly packed glandular or tubular elements lined by flattened or cuboidal cells. The cells are generally uniform, with finely dispersed chromatin, and mitotic figures are rare or absent, but they grow in dense clusters, causing concern as to possible malignancy. Experience has shown that the lesion regresses when the progestin influence ceases.

Clinicians should have patience with their pathologists as more lesions than they suppose are difficult to recognize reliably or consistently in gynecologic pathology. The diagnoses of intraepithelial and mucosal lesions of the vulva, vagina, cervix, and endometrium involve a degree of subjectivity that makes consistency difficult.

Vagina

There is great interest in the relationship of prenatal exposure to nonsteroidal estrogens and the subsequent development of vaginal adenosis and clear cell carcinoma of the vagina and cervix. The finding of clear cell carcinoma having an association with vaginal adenosis in 97 percent of instances[63] inevitably led to speculation that adenosis might be a precursor to the carcinoma in the same manner that dysplasia and carcinoma in situ of the cervix represent precursors to invasive squamous carcinoma. That adenosis might not play a precursor role is suggested by the disparity between the incidence of carcinoma (170 cases as of the last Registry report) and the incidence of adenosis (30 to 90 percent of those exposed).[64,65] Since some 250,000 to 1,000,000 persons are estimated to have been exposed to estrogens in utero, it is evident that only a small minority of those with adenosis have developed carcinoma (estimated to be less than 0.1 percent).[66] In contrast, about 33 percent of those with untreated carcinoma in situ of the cervix have developed invasive carcinoma in 10 years.[67] Furthermore, the cytologic features of dysplasia and carcinoma in situ are those of a malignant lesion, while ade-

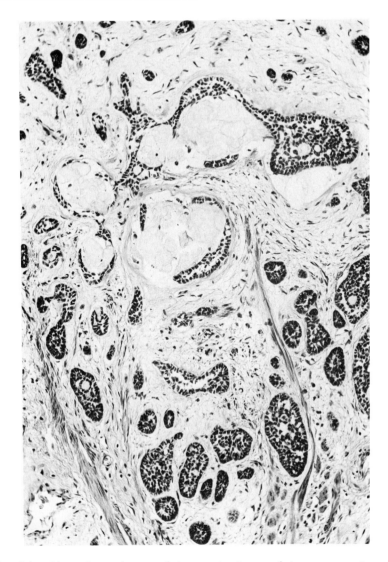

Figure 2–12. Adenoid cystic carcinoma of the cervix. Some of these tumors have basaloid features, and others resemble carcinoid and the newly described apudoma.[55,56] H&E, ×115; AFIP Neg. 70-7823.

nosis appears in every respect identical to normal endocervical or endometrial glandular cells without cytologic features of malignancy. Transitions between adenosis and carcinoma have not been documented. Until such time as there is evidence that adenosis carries significant malignant potential, pathologists should avoid implying that it does, thus influencing clinicians to utilize therapy more radical than necessary. Normal endocervical mucosa requires no treatment and it is unlikely that similar epithelium in the vagina will require treatment. On the other hand, the glandular epithelium of vaginal adenosis is subject to the same kinds of changes as seen in endocervical columnar epithelium, i.e., squamous metaplasia, dysplasia, and the microglandular hyperplasia associated with oral contraceptives. Adenosis greatly increases the surface area of epithelium subject to these changes and one must avoid regarding active, immature squamous metaplasia in adenosis as dysplasia (Fig. 2–13). There has been speculation that dysplasia occurring in adenosis might ultimately represent a more significant problem than clear cell carcinoma, but at present

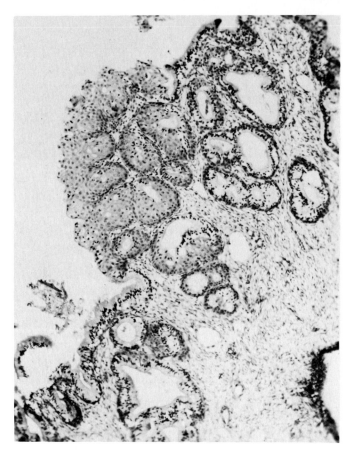

Figure 2–13. Squamous metaplasia occurring in vaginal adenosis. This metaplasia has been misinterpreted as dysplasia. H&E, ×80; AFIP Neg. 75-8407.

evidence to this effect is not available. As microglandular hyperplasia occurring in adenosis (Figs. 2–14 and 2–15) is increasingly encountered, it is important that this change not be misinterpreted as adenocarcinoma.[68]

Other vaginal lesions with potential for misdiagnosis and tragic consequences for the patient are benign vaginal polyps and benign rhabdomyomas. Both of these bear a resemblance to sarcoma botryoides and must be distinguished from it to avoid unnecessarily radical therapy. Vaginal polyps may occur in adults or in infants and present as polypoid, pedunculated, or grape-like masses, often with abnormal bleeding. Microscopically they are well circumscribed and covered by vaginal mucosa. The stroma is composed of loose fibrous connective tissue, often with large cytologically atypical cells.[69] When rhabdomyoblasts with cross striations are seen, the polyp is

designated as a benign rhabdomyoma (Fig. 2–16). In contrast to sarcoma botryoides, a cambium layer is absent, and infiltration of the overlying epithelium, common in sarcoma botryoides, is absent in vaginal polyps. Rapid growth is characteristic of sarcoma botryoides but not of vaginal polyps. Reports of vaginal "sarcoma" and "adult sarcoma botryoides" in adult and pregnant women have been in some instances misdiagnosed vaginal polyps and benign rhabdomyomas.

Vulva

Use of the term "leukoplakia" for certain lesions of the vulva has been discouraged by many, yet the term is still used and misused, confounding understanding between clinicians and pathologists. As a clinical diagnosis, a "white patch" on

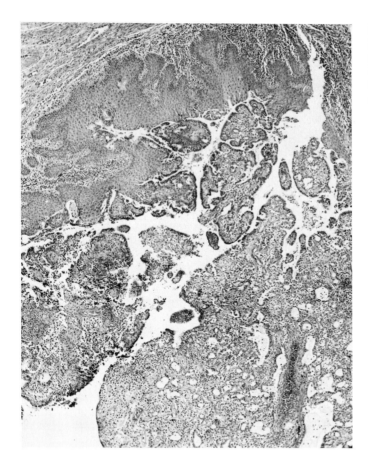

Figure 2–14. Microglandular hyperplasia occurring in vaginal adenosis. This lesion must be differentiated from adenocarcinoma arising in adenosis. H&E, ×42; AFIP Neg. 74-12097.

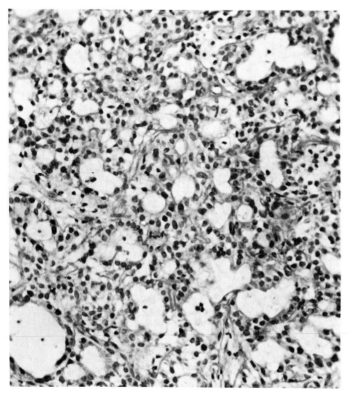

Figure 2–15. Higher view of the microglandular hyperplasia induced by oral contraceptives. H&E, ×180; AFIP Neg. 12096.

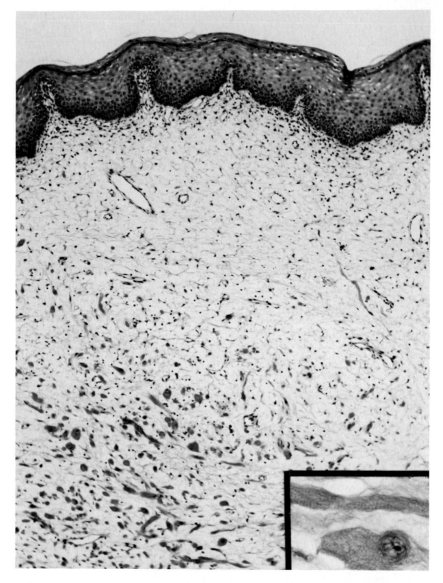

Figure 2–16. Vaginal polyp with striated muscle (vaginal rhabdomyoma). This lesion has been confused with sarcoma botryoides. Lower half of field shows striated muscle fibers, seen best in insert. H&E, ×50; AFIP Neg. 75-7634 (insert H&E, ×300; AFIP Neg. 75-3654).

the vulva may reflect a variety of histologic entities, listed in Table 2–2. The term "leukoplakia" should not be used in a pathology report. A specific diagnosis or the degree of atypism, when present, is what is important for the pathologist to note. Previous reports using variable terms and criteria for histologic lesions have resulted in confusion as to the malignant or premalignant potential of lichen sclerosis, one of the most common white lesions. Recent evidence based on follow-up studies of 107 cases of lichen sclerosis indicates that carcinoma does not occur very often.[70]

The important aspect of Paget's disease is whether or not there is an infiltrating carcinoma in the dermis and subcutaneous tissue underlying the Paget's disease. Involvement of the underlying sweat glands or hair follicles does not have the same significance as infiltration of the dermis.

Table 2–2. HISTOLOGIC BASIS FOR
"LEUKOPLAKIC" LESIONS OF THE VULVA

Inflammatory dermatoses (psoriasis, lichen planus,
  seborrheic dermatitis, neurodermatitis, etc.)
Lichen sclerosis et atrophicus
Squamous hyperplasia and hyperkeratosis*
Squamous dysplasia (atypical hyperplasia)
Paget's disease
Bowen's disease
Invasive squamous carcinoma

*Often found in combination with lichen sclerosis et
atrophicus.

Only with infiltration of the dermis is metastasis possible, and the prognosis is much worse. The expression "an underlying carcinoma is present" is not specific enough and may be misleading. To judge from recent reports,[71-74] about 85 percent of Paget's disease of the vulva is in situ (invasive carcinoma absent) and does not require lymphadenectomy.[72,73,75] Not all Paget's disease is of epidermal origin, some in AFIP files have been a result of an underlying urethral or Bartholin gland carcinoma.

The biologic behavior of microinvasive carcinoma of the vulva is less well defined than microinvasive carcinoma of the cervix. Two recent reports expressed opposite conclusions.[76,77] Of 25 patients reported by Wharton et al[76] with lesions less than 2 cm in diameter invading no more than 5 mm, none of 10 having lymphadenectomies had nodal metastasis, and none of the 25 had recurrences during the follow-up interval. In contrast, of 58 similarly defined neoplasms reported by Parker et al,[77] 3 of 40 having lymphadenectomies had nodal metastasis and 5 had recurrent invasive carcinoma. In two of the three cases with nodal metastasis, involvment of apparent vascular channels was seen in the vulvar specimen, and the third had an "anaplastic lesion." Another study found four patients with metastasis to lymph nodes from carcinomas invading less than 5 mm.[78]

Gestational Trophoblastic Disease

Gestational trophoblastic disease has been classified into three major varieties on histologic grounds: hydatidiform mole, invasive mole (chorioadenoma destruens), and choriocarcinoma.

The advent of curative chemotherapy without the necessity for hysterectomy has reduced the material available for histologic study. Frequently curettings are the only specimen available to the pathologist, and distinguishing the major varieties of disease can be difficult, particularly when curettings are scanty.[79] The presence of well-formed villi militates against choriocarcinoma,[79,80] but both invasive and noninvasive moles may contain proliferating trophoblast, and invasion, when present, may not be evident in the curettings. Small fragments of proliferating trophoblast in the absence of villi may be seen in a normal early gestation, so a subjective estimate that the quantity of trophoblast is sufficient to indicate choriocarcinoma must sometimes be made. All three varieties of trophoblastic disease may metastasize, so evidence of metastatic deposits cannot always be used to distinguish hydatidiform mole from choriocarcinoma. In addition, there is the problem of histologic classification used for estimating prognosis. Based on curettings, this estimate of behavior is not a reliable indicator of prognosis,[80,81] nor is it useful in managing patients undergoing therapy.[82] Many do not attempt to grade the malignant potential on the basis of histologic features because the morphologic diagnosis of trophoblastic disease variants has become less important, since assays for human chorionic gonadotropin (HCG) have allowed monitoring of therapy and because chemotherapy is used for metastatic disease regardless of the histologic picture. A classification into nonmetastatic (pelvic and extrapelvic) gestational trophoblastic disease provides practical subdivisions useful in planning treatment.[82] One should be aware of the poor prognostic features discussed by Hammond et al[83] (duration of disease greater than four months, initial HCG titer more than 100,000 IU/24 hours, and cerebral or hepatic metastasis), as survival in patients with these features can be improved by the initial use of triple-agent chemotherapy.

A new entity in the spectrum of trophoblastic disease has recently been described,[84] and it merits distinction because of its unique clinical and pathologic features. Termed "trophoblastic pseudotumor," it is characterized by cytotrophoblastic proliferation forming nodular masses in the myometrium (Fig. 2–17). Villi are rare, but—in contrast to choriocarcinoma—the trophoblastic proliferation is composed almost exclusively of cytotrophoblast, lacking the biphasic syncytial cells of choriocarcinoma. HCG

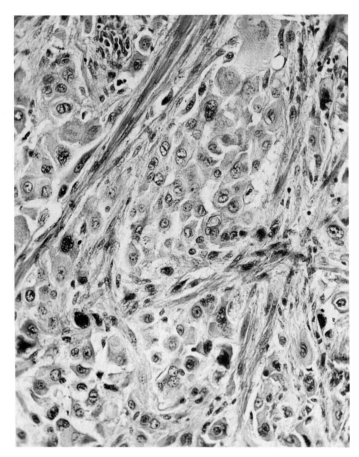

Figure 2-17. Trophoblastic pseudotumor.[84] This lesion has been misinterpreted as leiomyosarcoma and choriocarcinoma, but metastasis has not occurred. Cytotrophoblastic cells infiltrate stroma. H&E, ×210; AFIP Neg. 74-5113.

titers are low (usually less than 750 IU/1000 cc), and the hormone has been localized in scattered trophoblastic cells within the tumor. The trophoblastic infiltration resembles that of "syncytial myometritis" with individual cells and strands of trophoblast infiltrating between muscle fibers and invading the walls of blood vessels, but the process is exuberant, producing nodular tumor masses. Although infiltration may be extensive and uterine perforation with curettage is common, all patients who survived uterine perforation have survived during a follow-up interval of up to 12 years. If pathologists do not know of this entity, a false diagnosis of choriocarcinoma, leiomyosarcoma, or malignant mixed tumor is likely.

RESOLVING GYNECOLOGIC PATHOLOGY PROBLEMS

Improvements in clinician-pathologist communication and in the technical aspects of tissue processing can greatly improve accuracy of diagnosis, which in turn will improve the management of patients with gynecologic malignancies. Too often, pathologists are not given adequate clinical information, and pathologists do not always provide adequate descriptions or modern terminology in their reports. Utilization of modern terminology and classification of neoplasms by specific diagnostic criteria will greatly improve communication between individual physicians and facilitate comparisons of data among institutions, ultimately to the benefit of individual patients. In order to reduce errors in diagnosis, consultation between pathologists should be encouraged. Each clinician should form an opinion as to which pathologist he would like to refer his difficult or perplexing cases. Some pathology departments have standard forms to facilitate consultation, some send hundred of cases yearly to the AFIP. Registries of rare diseases have been formed at various centers for the sole purpose of obtaining a concentrated experience. Gynecologic oncologists would be wise to learn which pathologists in their community have had special training in gynecologic pathology and make use of the experience of those pathologists. The importance of the experienced gynecologic pathologist in accomplishing improvements in communication, tissue processing, consultation, and diagnosis is a strong argument for including such a pathologist on the gynecologic oncology team.

References

1. Leman MH, Benson WL, Kurman RJ, Park RA: Microinvasive carcinoma of the cervix. Obstet Gynecol 48:571, 1976
2. Fechner RE: The surgical pathology of the reproductive system and breast during oral contraceptive therapy. Pathol Annu 6:299, 1971
3. Townsend DE, Ostergard DR, Mishell DR, Hirose FM: Abnormal Papanicolaou smears. Evaluation by colposcopy, biopsies, and endocervical curettage. Am J Obstet Gynecol 108:429, 1970
4. Swan RW, Davis HJ: The biopsy-cucumber unit: a method to improve tissue orientation. Obstet Gynecol 36:803, 1970
5. Richart RM: The handling of small tissue samples for pathologic examination. Bull Sloane Hosp Wom 9:113, 1963
6. Foote FW, Stewart FW: Anatomical distribution of intraepidermal epidermoid carcinoma of the cervix. Cancer 1:431, 1948
7. Sanerkin NG, Fraser JMR: A technique for the orientation of blocks and sections from unbisected cervical cones. J Clin Pathol 28:202, 1975
8. Norris HJ: Editorial: Criteria for diagnosis of leiomyosarcoma. Hum Pathol 7:481–482, 1976
9. Miles PA, Norris HJ: Proliferative and malignant Brenner tumors of the ovary. Cancer 30:174, 1972
10. Asadourian LA, Taylor HB: Dysgerminoma. An analysis of 105 cases. Obstet Gynecol 33:370, 1969
11. Robboy SJ, Scully RE: Ovarian teratoma with glial implants on the peritoneum. Hum Pathol 1:643, 1970
12. Norris HJ, Zirkin HJ, Benson WL: Immature (malignant) teratoma of the ovary: A clinical and pathologic study of 58 cases. Cancer 37:2359, 1976
13. Serov SF, Scully RE: Histological Typing of Ovarian Tumours. Geneva, World Health Organization, 1973
14. Hart WR, Norris HJ: Borderline and malignant mucinous tumors of the ovary. Cancer 31:1031, 1972
15. Aure JC, Hoeg K, Kolstad P: Clinical and histologic studies of ovarian carcinoma: Long-term follow-up of 990 cases. Obstet Gynecol 37:1, 1971
16. Scully RE: Recent progress in ovarian cancer. Hum Pathol 1:73, 1970
17. Thurlbeck WM, Scully RE: Solid teratoma of the ovary: A clinicopathological analysis of 9 cases. Cancer 13:804, 1960
18. Kurman RJ, Norris HJ: Endodermal sinus tumor of the ovary: A clinical and pathologic analysis of 71 cases. Cancer 38:2040, 1976
19. Smith JP, Rutledge F: Advances in chemotherapy for gynecologic cancer. Cancer 36:669, 1975
20. Kurman RJ, Norris HJ: Embryonal carcinoma of the ovary: A clinicopathologic entity distinct from endodermal sinus tumor resembling embryonal carcinoma of the adult testis. Cancer 38:2420, 1976
21. Norris HJ, Taylor HB: The ovaries in en-

docrine disorders. In Bloodworth JMB (ed): Endocrine Pathology. Baltimore, Williams & Wilkins, 1968, p 478

22. Norris HJ, Taylor HB: Prognosis of granulosa-theca tumors of the ovary. Cancer 21:255, 1968

23. Fox H, Agrawal K, Langley FA: A clinicopathologic study of 92 cases of granulosa cell tumor of the ovary with special reference to the factors influencing prognosis. Cancer 35:231, 1975

24. Norris HJ, Taylor HB: Virilization associated with cystic granulosa tumors. Obstet Gynecol 34:629, 1969

25. Norris HJ, Chorlton I: Functioning tumors of the ovary. Clin Obstet Gynecol 17:189, 1974

26. Gore H: Hyperplasia of the endometrium. In Norris HJ, Hertig AT, Abell MR (eds): The Uterus. Baltimore, Williams & Wilkins, 1973, p 255

27. Vellios F: Endometrial hyperplasias and carcinoma in situ. Gynecol Oncol 2:152, 1974

28. Hertig AT, Sommers SC, Bengloff H: Genesis of endometrial carcinoma. III. Carcinoma in situ. Cancer 2:964, 1949

29. Chamlian DL, Taylor HB: Endometrial hyperplasia in young women. Obstet Gynecol 36:659, 1970

30. Gusberg SB, Kaplan AL: Precursors of corpus cancer. IV. Adenomatous hyperplasia as stage 0 carcinoma of the endometrium. Am J Obstet Gynecol 87:662, 1963

31. Norris HJ, Taylor HB: Mesenchymal tumors of the uterus. I. A clinical and pathological study of 53 endometrial stromal tumors. Cancer 19:755, 1966

32. Christopherson WM, Williamson EO, Gray LA: Leiomyosarcoma of the uterus. Cancer 29:1512, 1972

33. Saksela E, Lampinen V, Berndt-Johan P: Malignant mesenchymal tumors of the uterine corpus. Am J Obstet Gynecol 120:452, 1974

34. Taylor HB, Norris HJ: Mesenchymal tumors of the uterus. IV. Diagnosis and prognosis of leiomyosarcomas. Arch Pathol 82:40, 1966

35. Kempson RL: Sarcomas and related neoplasms. In Norris HJ, Hertig AT, Abell MR (eds): The Uterus. Baltimore, Williams & Wilkins, 1973, p 298

36. Kempson RL, Bari W: Uterine sarcomas: classification, diagnosis and prognosis. Hum Pathol 1:331, 1970

37. Norris HJ, Parmley T: Mesenchymal tumors of the uterus. V. Intravenous leiomyomatosis. A clinical and pathologic study of 14 cases. Cancer 36:2164, 1975

38. Kurman RJ, Norris HJ: Mesenchymal tumors of the uterus. VI. Epithelioid smooth muscle tumors including leiomyoblastoma and clear-cell leiomyoma. A clinical and pathologic analysis of 26 cases. Cancer 37:1853, 1976

39. Gore H, Hertig AT: Definitions. In Gray LA (ed): Dysplasia, Carcinoma In Situ and Microinvasive Carcinoma of the Cervix Uteri. Springfield, Charles C Thomas, 1964, p 84

40. Lerch V, Okagaki T, Austin JH, Kevorkian AY, Younge PA: Cytologic findings in progression of anaplasia (dysplasia) to carcinoma in situ: a progress report. Acta Cytol (Phila) 7:183, 1963

41. Richart RM, Barron BA: A follow-up of patients with cervical dysplasia. Am J Obstet Gynecol 105:386, 1969

42. Richart RM: Cervical neoplasia in pregnancy. A series of pregnant and postpartum patients followed without biopsy or therapy. Am J Obstet Gynecol 87:474, 1963

43. Richart RM: Natural history of cervical intraepithelial neoplasia. Clin Obstet Gynecol 10:748, 1967

44. Mestwerdt G: Probeexzision and kolposkopie in der frühdiagnose des portiokarzinomas. Zentralbl. Gynaekol 4:326, 1947

45. Nelson JH, Averette HE, Richart RM: Dysplasia and early cervical cancer. CA 25:134, 1975

46. Newton M: Staging classification of carcinoma of the cervix. ACOG Newsletter, March 1974, p 3

47. Benson WL, Norris HJ: A critical review of the frequency of lymph node metastasis and deaths from microinvasive carcinoma of the cervix. Obstet Gynecol 49:632, 1977

48. Roche WD, Norris HJ: Microinvasive carcinoma of the cervix. The significance of lymphatic invasion and confluent patterns of stromal growth. Cancer 36:180, 1975

49. Glücksmann A, Cherry CP: Incidence, his-

tology, and response to radiation of mixed carcinomas (adenoacanthomas) of the uterine cervix. Cancer 9:971, 1956

50. Littman P, Clement PB, Henriksen B, et al: Glassy cell carcinoma of the cervix. Cancer 37:2238, 1976

51. McKelvey JL, Goodlin RR: Adenoma malignum of the cervix. A cancer of deceptively innocent histological pattern. Cancer 16:549, 1963

52. Hertig AT, Gore H: Tumors of the Female Sex Organs. Supplement to Part 2. Tumors of the Vulva, Vagina, and Uterus. Atlas of Tumor Pathology. Washington, D.C., Armed Forces Institute of Pathology, 1968, p 312

53. Silverberg SG, Hurt WG: Minimal deviation adenocarcinoma ("adenoma malignum") of the cervix: A reappraisal. Am J Obstet Gynecol 121:971, 1975

54. Miles PA, Norris HJ: Adenoid cystic carcinoma of the cervix. An analysis of 12 cases. Obstet Gynecol 38:103, 1971

55. Tateishi R, Wada A, Hayakawa K, et al: Argyrophil cell carcinomas (apudomas) of the uterine cervix. Light and electron microscopic observations of 5 cases. Virchows Arch [Pathol Anat] 366:257, 1975

56. Albores-Saaveda J, Larraza O, Lopez SP, Rodriguez-Martinez H: Carcinoide primario del cuello uterino. Una Nueva entidad probablemente relacionade con las neoplasias del celular endocrino difuso. Sobretiro de Patologia 13:67, 1975

57. Pitkin RM, Kent YH: Papillary squamous lesions of the uterine cervix. Am J Obstet Gynecol 85:440, 1963

58. Ackerman LV: Verrucous carcinoma of the oral cavity. Surgery 23:670, 1948

59. Kraus FT, Perez-Mesa C: Verrucous carcinoma. Clinical and pathological study of 105 cases involving oral cavity, larynx and genitalia. Cancer 19:26, 1966

60. Lucas WE, Benirschke K, Lebherz TB: Verrucous carcinoma of the female genital tract. Am J Obstet Gynecol 119:435, 1974

61. Qizilbash AH: Papillary squamous tumors of the uterine cervix. A clinical and pathologic study of 21 cases. Am J Clin Pathol 61:508, 1974

62. Taylor HB, Irey NS, Norris HJ: Atypical endocervical hyperplasia in women taking oral contraceptives. JAMA 202:637, 1967

63. Herbst AL, Robboy SJ, Scully RE, Poskanzer DC: Clear-cell adenocarcinoma of the vagina and cervix in girls: analysis of 170 Registry cases. Am J Obstet Gynecol 119:713, 1974

64. Herbst AL, Kurman RJ, Scully RE: Vaginal and cervical abnormalities after exposure to diethylstilbesterol in utero. Obstet Gynecol 40:287, 1972

65. Stafl A, Mattingly RF, Foley DV, Featherston WC: Clinical diagnosis of vaginal adenosis. Obstet Gynecol 43:118, 1974

66. Yon JL, Lutz MH, Girtanner RE, Averette HE: Adenosis and adenocarcinoma of the vagina in young women: a review. Gynecol Oncol 2:508, 1974

67. Petersen O: Spontaneous course of cervical precancerous conditions. Am J Obstet Gynecol 72:1063, 1956

68. Kurman RJ, Norris HJ: Letter to the editor: Adenosis. Obstet Gynecol 46:373, 1975

69. Norris HJ, Taylor HB: Polyps of the vagina. A benign lesion resembling sarcoma botryoides. Cancer 19:227, 1966

70. Hart WR, Norris HJ, Helwig EB: Relation of lichen sclerosus et atrophicus of the vulva to development of carcinoma. Obstet Gynecol 45:369, 1975

71. Taylor PT, Stenwig JT, Klausen H: Paget's disease of the vulva. Gynecol Oncol 3:46, 1975

72. Tsukada Y, Lopez RG, Pickren JW, Piver MS, Barlow JJ: Paget's disease of the vulva. A clinicopathologic study of eight cases. Obstet Gynecol 45:73, 1975

73. Fetherston WC, Friedrich EG: The origin and significance of vulvar Paget's disease. Obstet Gynecol 39:735, 1972

74. Fenn ME, Morley GW, Abell MR: Paget's disease of vulva. Obstet Gynecol 38:660, 1971

75. Parmley TH, Woodruff JD, Julian CG: Invasive vulvar Paget's disease. Obstet Gynecol 46:341, 1975

76. Wharton JT, Gallager S, Rutledge FN: Microinvasive carcinoma of the vulva. Am J Obstet Gynecol 118:159, 1974

77. Parker RT, Duncan I, Rampone J, Creasman W: Operative management of early invasive epidermoid carcinoma of the

vulva. Am J Obstet Gynecol 123:349, 1975

78. Dipaola GR, Gomez-Rueda N, Arrighi L: Relevance of microinvasion in carcinoma of the vulva. Obstet Gynecol 45:647, 1975

79. Elston CW, Bagshaw KD: The diagnosis of trophoblastic tumours from uterine curettings. J Clin Pathol 25:111, 1972

80. Baggish MS: Gestational trophoblastic neoplasia. Clin Obstet Gynecol 17:259, 1974

81. Tow WSH, Yung RH: The value of histological grading in the prognostication of hydatidiform mole. J Obstet Gynaecol Br Commonw 74:292, 1967

82. Hilgers RD, Lewis JL: Gestational trophoblastic neoplasms. Gynecol Oncol 2:460, 1974

83. Hammond CB, Borchert LG, Tyrey L, Creasman WT, Parker RT: Treatment of metastatic trophoblastic disease: Good and poor prognosis. Am J Obstet Gynecol 115:451, 1973

84. Kurman RJ, Scully RE, Norris HJ: Trophoblastic pseudotumor of the uterus. An exaggerated form of placental site reaction (so-called syncytial endometritis) that simulates a malignant tumor. Cancer, 38:1214, 1976

Chapter 3

Cytopathology

RICHARD A. MALMGREN, M.D.

There is a generally held belief that early detection of cancer is one of the most important factors in achieving therapeutic success. At present, cytopathology represents the best single method for early detection of several gynecologic neoplasms. In addition, under certain circumstances, cytopathology can serve a diagnostic function. For cytopathology to reach its highest level of effectiveness, two conditions must exist. The first is a serious effort on the part of the clinician and the cytopathologist to develop and maintain meaningful communication. The cytopathologist needs to know as much about the clinical condition as possible if he is going to render the most accurate

evaluation of the specimen, and the clinician needs to be able to understand what pathologic entity he is dealing with in order to determine the appropriate therapy. This chapter will be devoted to a consideration of the application of cytopathology to the detection and diagnosis of gynecologic neoplasms with emphasis on the factors that are important in obtaining the optimum clinical effectiveness from the technique. Although the cytologic characteristics of the lesions will be included, this chapter is intended to improve clinician-cytopathologist communication rather than to be a text of cytopathology.

CYTOLOGY TECHNIQUES

Specimen Collection: General

Consideration of gynecologic cytopathology becomes an academic exercise unless the best methods are used for specimen collection and preservation. For that reason, these will be considered first.

The following basic principles are involved in collection of all gynecologic specimens for the best cytopathologic evaluation. (1) Obtain the diagnostically important cells. This is achieved by collecting the specimen from as close to the site of

origin of the cells as possible. That is, a direct scrape of the lesion is always better than collection of the cells that have spontaneously exfoliated and been transported in vivo in a fluid media to the collection site. In lieu of a direct scrape of the lesion, collection of the exfoliated cells from as close to the lesion as possible is the next best alternative. (2) Place the cells on a slide so that they maintain their morphologic integrity and remain on the slide. For most gynecologic specimens the mucus present in the specimen serves to hold the cells on the slide when fixed in the conventional ethyl or isopropyl alcohol fixative. Specimens collected in an irrigation fluid do not have the benefit of the mucus and require special laboratory procedures, such as albuminized slides, etched slides, filtration techniques, or carbowax in the fixative to keep the cells on the slide and to prevent drying. (3) Preserve the cells in such a way that their cytologic characteristics will be clearly visible when stained. *Prompt* exposure of the cells to fixative, either in a coplin jar or by one of the commercial spray fixatives is critical for optimal cell preservation. This is for the purpose of avoiding the damaging effect of drying, which seems to occur more rapidly with bloody, low-mucus specimens.

Specimen Identification and Clinical Information

At the time the specimen is collected, it is important that it be properly labeled with the patient's name. This is most easily done by the use of slides with one end etched where a lead pencil works very well for recording information that will not wash off in the fixative. The patient's name, her age, relevent menstrual history, clinical diagnosis, and any therapy she has received should be recorded on the request slip, along with what type of specimen it is. The major complaint one encounters in pathology and cytopathology laboratories is the incomplete request form. Since this represents the first communication between the physician and cytopathologist it is the occasion when a pattern for good information exchange should be established.

Fixative

An alcohol fixative, preferably 95 percent ethanol, is of particular importance to the cytologic technique because it is responsible for the clear cytoplasm and crisp nuclear detail which is so important for reliable results. The inclusion of carbowax in the fixative to prevent drying is an uncommon but optional addition. The use of an ether-alcohol mixture has been discontinued in most laboratories because of the explosive properties of ether and because the morphology did not seem to be altered by its omission. Once the cells have been fixed for at least one hour, they may be allowed to air dry for mailing purposes

and will retain their clear morphologic detail. In the laboratory, the smears should then be processed by the Papanicolaou technique.

Vagina, Cervix, Endocervix

There are several ways in which material is collected for cytologic evaluation, all of which seek to provide the maximum amount of information by providing the relevant cells in the highest number and best state of preservation. These include lateral vaginal wall scrape, vaginal pool smear, ectocervix scrape, and cervical os scrape and swab, and the endocervical swab and aspiration smear. The advantages and disadvantages of each must be considered when deciding which to use. After the clinician and cytopathologist have established which method or methods will be used, it is important that the clinician identify the type of collection method he has used for each smear he submits to the laboratory.

Lateral Vaginal Wall

The lateral vaginal wall scrape is taken for hormonal evaluation, to examine by cytology a grossly visible lesion, to localize the source of atypical cells found on a previous cytology specimen and thought to be of vaginal origin, or to demonstrate the presence of adenosis in a patient whose mother had taken diethylstilbesterol while pregnant. When the scrapings are taken for the last two reasons, in vivo contamination of the vaginal wall by cells shed from another area of the genital tract must be excluded by first wiping off the area to be examined with a cotton swab or gauze prior to collection of the specimen. If localization is important, quadrant scraping may be done and appropriately labeled. Lateral vaginal wall smears are *not useful for routine cancer detection.* The procedure involves scraping the vaginal wall with a wooden or plastic spatula and spreading the material on a glass slide. The spread may best be done with the spatula or the gloved fifth finger followed by immediate immersion of the slide in fixative.

Vaginal Pool

Vaginal pool material is collected for the detection of gynecologic malignancy, for hormonal evaluation, for assessment of radiation changes, or for information about inflammation involving the vagina and cervix. It has proved to be more useful for detection of endometrial carcinoma than the cervical scrape but much less reliable for the detection of cervical cancer. For this reason, when cervical cancer detection is the purpose for the cytologic examination, a cervical scrape specimen is recommended. If collection of vaginal pool fluid is done, either a pipet (glass or plastic) or a spatula is used to obtain the fluid from the posterior fornix. Material collected by spatula is placed on a slide in the same way as a vaginal wall scrape. When collected with a pipette the fluid is expelled from the pipette onto a slide and then smeared with a gloved finger followed by immediate fixation.

Cervical Scrape

The preferred method for detection of cervical cancer is a scrape from the ectocervix, at the squamocolumnar junction, and includes the immediately adjacent areas of the ecto and endocervix. This is best done with a spatula so constructed that it scrapes these areas all at one time and permits a 360 degree scrape of the entire region. The material collected on the spatula from the "transformation zone" is uniformly spread on the slide in order to avoid ridges and thick areas that cannot be fixed, stained, or screened properly and may be impossible to interpret (Fig. 3–1A).

Combined Methods

For routine cytology, Frost recommends a combination of the vaginal pool and cervical scrape material on one slide mixed and smeared together, the rationale being that a sample of the gynecologic system is obtained on a small area of the slide with the advantage that the vaginal pool sample will help prevent some of the drying effect

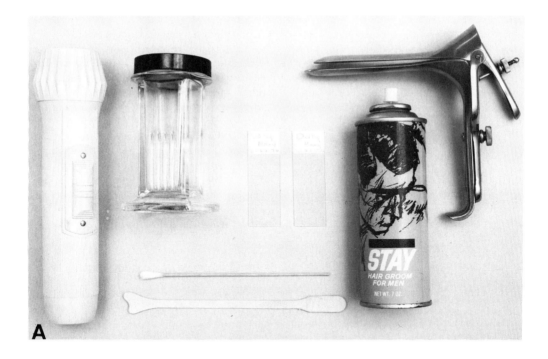

A

Figure 3–1A. Essentials needed for a Pap smear include an appropriate-sized speculum with an adequate source of light for direct visualization of the cervix. The Ayre spatula (bottom center) is for the ectocervical scrape, the cotton tip applicator for an endocervical swab. The cytologic specimens are placed on properly labeled microscope slides and then, preferably, placed in a coplin jar containing 95 percent ethyl alcohol or sprayed with a commercial fixative.

seen in the cervical scrape specimen alone.[1] Wied and Bahr suggest the vaginal, cervical (portio), and endocervical material be placed on one etched slide, but recommend keeping them separate so that certain hormonal information and localization of inflammation may be better determined.[2] To accomplish this without the material drying is not always easy. A third method,[3] which also used one slide, combines an aspiration taken from the os using a Papanicolaou pipet with a scrape of the squamocolumnar junction. Because of the improved detection of endocervical and endometrial cancer by this technique, it represents a combined method for detection of cancer of the cervix and endometrium. In each case, the use of one slide reduces the slide handling, the cover slipping, and screening by one-half while still maintaining accuracy. A careful study of this combination in which an additional comparison of endocervical swab and endocervical aspiration was made has substantiated the long-held view that the cervical scrape, which includes the squamocolumnar junction, is the most reliable technique for lesions of the cervix. The aspiration method seems superior to the swab technique although neither contributed significantly to cervical cancer diagnosis.[4] Removal of cervical mucus from the os with a cotton-tipped applicator before collection of endocervical material will reduce the number of unsatisfactory specimens.

Irrigation Smear

Because the time and personnel required for specimen collection has been thought by some to be a limiting factor in mass screening for the cytologic detection of gynecologic malignancy, a method that would permit the patient to collect the specimen herself and mail it to the laboratory was developed.[5] Although the results of the early studies with this method seemed promising,[6,7] later work indicated 40 to 50 percent of cervical cancer went undetected by this method.[8,9] Of the specimens collected by this method in one study, 19 percent were unsatisfactory, compared with 1 percent collected by cervical scrape,[10] and 13 percent of the women failed to return the kit.

The combination of unsatisfactory specimens and false-negative results with the irrigation method resulted in a detection rate of 73 percent as compared with 91 percent by the cervical scrape method. A number of laboratories have had similar results.[11,12] The method consists of instillation of a fluid containing a cell preservative

into the vagina through a pipet by means of an attached rubber bulb. The fluid is withdrawn and the whole kit sent to the laboratory where the fluid is centrifuged and the pellet of cells smeared on slides. Of course the most important disadvantage of this method is the fact that a complete gynecologic examination has been omitted and therefore at best, only a portion of the desired information will be obtained. If an automated device for cytology screening for cervical cancer became a reality, and if it were a flow system where the cells were presented to the equipment in a fluid suspension, such a collection method would certainly have merit, particularly if taken by the gynecologist at the time of examination. In summary, there are numerous disadvantages to patient-obtained smears that preclude their general use.

Endocervical Aspiration

Endocervical aspiration is a useful method for detection of endocervical and endometrial lesions. Although more time consuming, it is clearly better than vaginal pool specimens for the detection of endometrial carcinoma. With the increasing incidence of endometrial cancer, endocervical aspiration specimens should be considered on all women over the age of 45 who are having a gynecologic examination. The rationale is the same as the one that advocates cytologic examination for cervical cancer. The procedure involves gentle removal of cervical mucus from the os with a swab, followed by insertion of a plastic or glass pipet a few millimeters into the cervical canal. Material from this area is then aspirated with a rubber bulb attached to the pipet and then blown onto a glass slide, which is quickly placed in fixative.

Endometrium

Endometrial Aspiration

Disease of the endometrium can be evaluated by endometrial cytologic aspiration. The procedure may be indicated for routine detection purposes in women over the age of 45, as there is little discomfort or trauma. It is done on an out-patient basis with rapid and reliable results. The technique consists of the introduction of a cannula into the endometrial cavity via the precleaned cervical os (Fig. 3–1B). A 10-ml syringe is used to

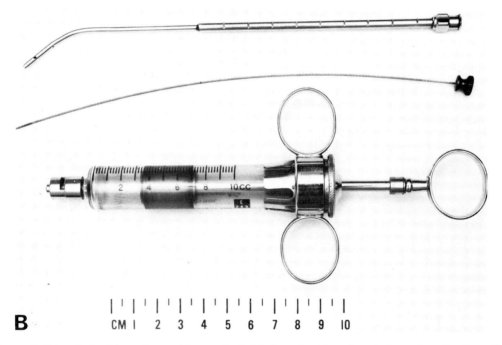

B

CM 1 2 3 4 5 6 7 8 9 10

Figure 3–1B. A flexible endometrial cannula (od 2.4 mm) with stylet. A three-ring glass-barrelled syringe with steel plunger and sana-lok tip attaches to the cannula to aspirate the cytologic specimen.

aspirate the endometrial cavity. The aspirated material is blown onto a glass slide and promptly fixed.[13,14]

Cytopathology Report

The cytopathology report should convey to the clinician as much information and as precise information as the cytopathologist is able to extract from the specimen. As experience has been acquired through the years it is expected that the cytologic interpretation will more and more anticipate the histopathologic findings. For this reason there is an effort being made to use histopathologic terms in the evaluation of cytologic specimens. It also makes a correlation between cytopathology and histopathology easier and should make for better understanding of what lesion is present when the histopathologic and cytopathologic terminology are the same. Since the histologic diagnosis is used as the bench mark and it represents only a sample of the lesion, it is to be expected that there will not always be absolute agreement between the two. However, when the cytology indicates a lesion of more serious sig-

nificance than the histopathology, careful follow-up of the patient is necessary.

The essential information in any report, regardless of the format, should include (1) an indication of the presence or absence of cancer, (2) the predicted histopathologic type, (3) a consideration of the possible cytopathologic explanation for any abnormal clinical information provided, (4) indication of the etiologic agent involved in any inflammatory response, and (5) the presence or absence of endocervical cells as a reflection of whether or not the specimen was satisfactorily collected from the squamocolumnar junction. Liberal use of notes to communicate information that the report would not otherwise bring to the attention of the clinician is to be encouraged.

Quality Control

All laboratory medicine has been involved in efforts to control the quality of the procedures they perform. This effort will certainly increase in the future with federal and state regulations added to those of the professional organizations. Cytopathology is no exception. It is more difficult to develop quality control techniques for cytology laboratories than it is for the more objective areas of laboratory medicine. However, present ways in which quality control is being instituted include the reexamination of 10 percent of the negative cases by the cytopathologist, retention of all slides from positive cases indefinitely and negative cases for five years, records of cytology-histology correlation, records of sources of stains and when prepared, used, and tested, as well as equipment maintenance records. The educational back-ground of the personnel working in the laboratory must meet certain requirements. Cervical cytology smears must be screened by qualified cytotechnologists working in accredited cytology laboratories under the direction of medically qualified personnel who have special training and expertise in the field of diagnostic cytology. All of this will provide the clinician with some assurance that the laboratory examining his specimen is qualified to do so.

CERVICAL CANCER

Cancer of the cervix is clinically a very important and relatively common disease, and it is especially important to the subject of cytopathology because it is the raison d'être for cytology in the beginning and is still the cancer most commonly detected and diagnosed by cytology. Cancer of the ectocervix is of the squamous cell variety. It most often occurs at the squamocolumnar junction and for this reason is best detected by specimen collection from that region. An Ayre spatula or similar device used under direct visualization of the cervical os is the method of choice for specimen collection.

Pathogenesis

The pathogenesis of cervical cancer has been a confusing subject because of the several "precancerous" changes that have been thought to give rise to this lesion and that may or may not be themselves interrelated. A consideration of the pathogenesis of cervical cancer is important because the so-called precancerous lesions are recognizable by cytopathology and a knowledge of their clinical significance effects the management of the lesions. One of the most comprehensive concepts that has been arrived at through the collection of a significant amount of data by Regan, Wentz, Patten and co-workers has been set forth in detail by Patten.[15] As a consequence of these observations certain terminology has developed which will be used in this text with the realization that the concepts are not universally accepted but the terms do describe cytologic entities.

The development of cervical cancer is thought to begin in two possible ways. Either with a premalignant lesion, dysplasia of the squamous epithelium, or reserve cell hyperplasia in the endocervical glands. The dysplasia of the squamous epithelium presents as a keratinizing dysplasia and is thought to give rise to well-differentiated keratinizing squamous cell carcinoma. The hyperplastic reserve cells in the endocervix are thought to develop either directly into small cell carcinoma in situ or into metaplastic squamous cells, the small cell carcinoma in situ leading to invasive small cell carcinoma while the metaplastic squamous cells develop into dysplastic cells, which go on to form large-cell carcinoma in situ and thus to nonkeratinizing squamous cell carcinoma.

Although reserve cell hyperplasia and squamous metaplasia are not usually considered preneoplastic lesions, because they are thought to preceed dysplasia and carcinoma in situ in the endocervix, they are included here.

Reserve Cell Hyperplasia

Reserve cells are the subcolumnar layer of cells lining the endocervix. They are not normally seen in cytopathology preparations unless the smear has been collected from the endocervical side of the os and the scrape has been vigorous enough to remove the columnar cells and the underlying reserve cells.

Reserve cell hyperplasia is thought to result from the effects of inflammation on endocervical cells with the consequence that the repair process causes hyperplasia of the reserve cells. Cytologic

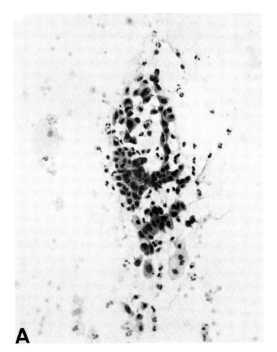

A

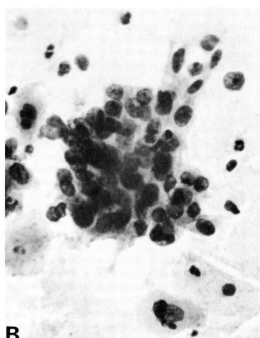

B

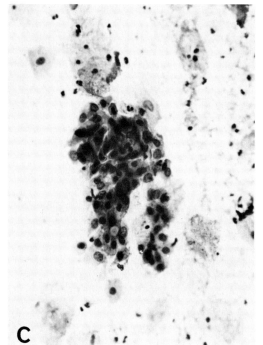

C

Figure 3–2. Reserve cells from endocervix. Note the slightly elliptical nuclei, scant amount of cytoplasm, and arrangement of the cells in a group. A. ×416 B. ×624 C. ×520.

preparations collected from the squamocolumnar junction would be the most likely to contain hyperplastic reserve cells. Cytologically, these cells retain, to a certain extent, the columnar-type cytoplasm and develop atypical nuclei still recognizable by the tendency to be oval. If seen singly they are difficult to distinguish from histiocytes, but when in groups and especially when associated with columnar cells, they are readily identified (Fig. 3–2ABC).[16-19]

Squamous Metaplasia

This is a very common lesion of the cervix considered to arise secondary to the effect of inflammation and subdivisible into a mature and immature variety.

Immature Squamous Metaplasia

The term "immature" was chosen because cells of this type are associated with persistence of the underlying reserve cells or with an overlying layer of columnar-like cells of the endocervix.

The reserve cell, as the precursor of the metaplastic cell, loses its endocervical, columnar cell cytoplasm and acquires a more squamous cytoplasm, which is more dense and more deeply cyanophylic. The cells tend to be single rather than in groups and have a round or oval outline often with one side flattened or with "spider-like processes." The nucleus is usually centrally located, not hyperchromatic and no nucleoli are evident (Fig. 3–3A–C). Obviously as a transition process, there are all gradations of cytologic features from the most immature metaplastic squamous cells to the most mature squamous cells. There is also a transition toward dysplasia. Nuclear enlargement, or an increase in the nuclear cytoplasmic ratio and increased hyperchromasia, is sometimes seen in the metaplastic cells and referred to as "atypical" metaplasia.

Mature Squamous Metaplasia

The point at which the immature metaplastic cell is considered mature is not sharp. Except for increased denseness of the cytoplasm and often two parts to the cytoplasm, an inner and outer zone recognized by different staining characteristics, the mature metaplastic cell is not distinguishable from normal squamous epithelium of the cervix (Fig. 3–3D).

Precancerous Lesions

Dysplasia

The cytologic feature that characterizes dysplasia is the presence of an "immature" or malignant nucleus in a cell with differentiated cytoplasm. The term dyskeratosis has been commonly used to describe this feature. The degree of "immatu-

Figure 3–3. Metaplasia. A. Immature metaplastic cells with relatively large nuclei and dense cytoplasm. A slight perinuclear clear area is present. ×800. B. Same as A with some vacuolization of the cytoplasm. ×800. C. Same as A and B with more cytoplasmic vacuolization. ×800. D. More mature metaplastic cells with cytoplasmic processes. ×416.

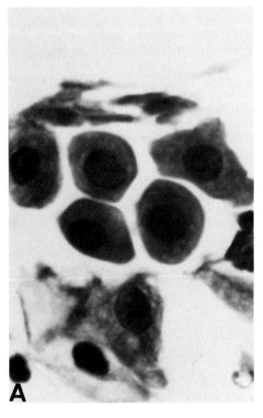
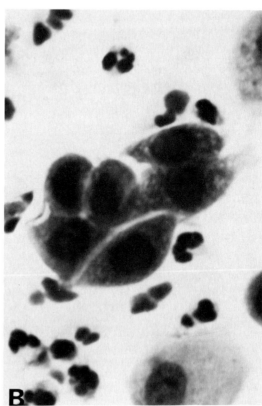

rity" can vary, as can the degree and type of differentiation of the cytoplasm. For this reason a classification has been devised which takes both of these variables into consideration. The cytoplasmic differentiation is described as keratinizing or nonkeratinizing, thus dysplastic lesions thought to arise in the ectocervix are keratinizing dysplasia while those arising in metaplastic epithelium are nonkeratinizing. The nuclear atypia is rated as mild, moderate, or severe, which may be expected to correlate in a general way with the progression of the lesion toward malignancy (Fig. 3-4ABCD). Another criteria for correlation of the severity of the dysplasia with the severity of the histologic lesion is the number of dysplastic cells per slide. The higher the number, the more severe the dysplasia.[20] Many feel that this subdivision into keratinizing and nonkeratinizing, mild, moderate, and severe is too fine, too subtle, and perhaps of no clinical significance. The fact that keratinizing and nonkeratinizing changes are commonly seen together certainly makes the clinical significance more difficult to evaluate.

Carcinoma in Situ

This lesion occurs near the cervical os extending out onto the ectocervix as well as up the cervical canal and it is, therefore, best detected by use of cervical scrapings. Long considered to be a premalignant lesion and often referred to as cervical cancer stage 0, carcinoma in situ is one of the most important lesions to be detected by cytology. Its importance lies in the fact that 100 percent survival can be expected from treatment of carcinoma in situ. Evidence that carcinoma in situ is in fact a precursor of invasive carcinoma comes from epidemiologic data and the frequent association of the two lesions on histologic section. Two types of studies have been done to demonstrate the association. In one case, patients with carcinoma in situ were carefully followed with cytology but without "treatment" and the number developing invasive lesions determined.[21,22] From these studies, it was evident that more than one quarter of the patients developed invasive lesions in a relatively short time. This was in spite of the

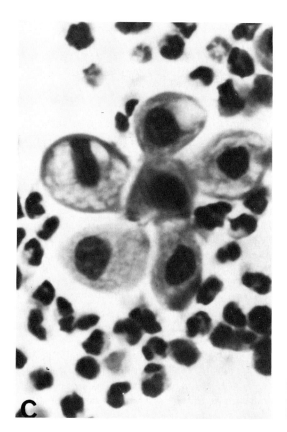

C

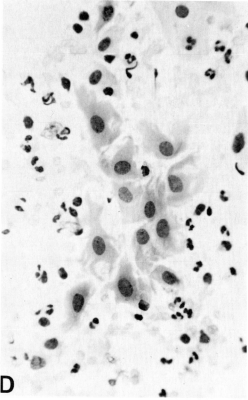

D

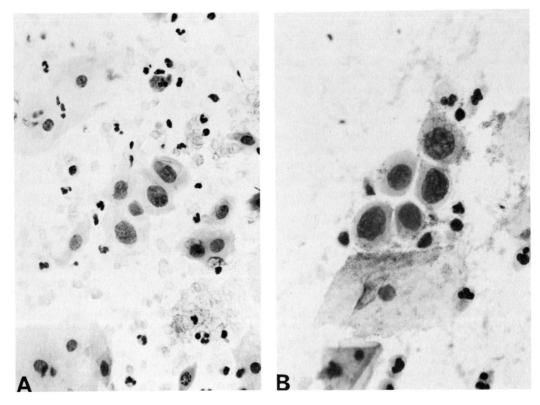

Figure 3–4. Dysplasia. A. Mild dysplasia. Intermediate cells with enlarged hyperchromatic nuclei with moderate chromatin clumping. ×520. B. Moderate dysplasia. Parabasal cells with enlarged hyperchromatic nuclei with chromatin clumping. ×624. C. Moderate dysplasia, same as B. ×800. D. Severe dysplasia. Marked nuclear enlargement with hyperchromatism. ×800.

fact that what might be considered minor local therapeutic measures, such as electrocautery and silver nitrate application, were done. The lesion disappeared in another quarter of the patients but persisted in about one-half. In another study similar results were obtained. The incidence of invasive lesions was much lower however and, because dysplasia as well as in situ carcinoma was studied, it was possible to conclude that they seemed to have a similar clinical course, the dysplastic lesions were somewhat less inclined to go on to invasion and disappeared slightly more frequently.[23] A second approach had been to observe the incidence of invasive lesions in a population that has been screened by cytology and the in situ lesions detected and removed. A comparison of this population with the incidence of invasive cancer in a similar population that was not screened by cytology revealed a significant decrease in the incidence of invasive cancer.[24] Similarly, a fall in the incidence of invasive cancer in

the same population following the institution of a cervical cancer screening program suggests an association between in situ carcinoma and invasive cancer.[23,25] The anatomic similarity of location of dysplasia, in situ carcinoma, and invasive cancer has been demonstrated.[26]

The peak prevalence of in situ carcinoma of the cervix has been reported to be in patients in their mid 30s;[27] it is of interest however that the incidence of the lesion seems to remain about the same even in the age group over 50. The cytologic characteristics of the lesion are different in the postmenopausal women.[28] In the premenopausal women the cytologic characteristic of in situ carcinoma is the "third type" cell of Graham, the "dysplastic" cell of Papanicolaou or the "impending prophase" cell of Regan. This is a round cell that is about the size of a parabasal cell with a markedly enlarged malignant nucleus for the size of the cells. The cells are most often found singly, although occasionally in small

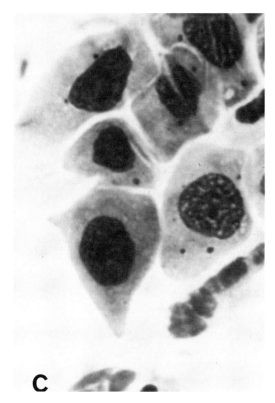

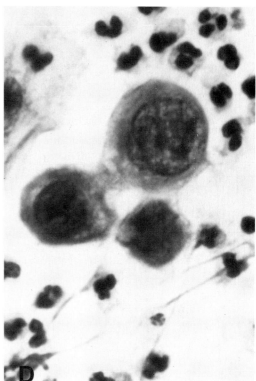

groups. The cytoplasm is cyanophylic and nucleoli are not seen. More in situ carcinoma cells are seen per slide than dysplastic cells (Fig. 3–5AB).

Two forms of in situ carcinoma are recognized. One is the large cell and the other the small-cell type. As the names imply the most prominent distinction between the two is their size. This is of some consequence because the large-cell type is thought to lead to a large cell nonkeratinizing squamous cell carcinoma while the small cell type is considered the precursor of the small cell carcinoma. These lesions have a rather different prognosis with the small cell variety being the more malignant.

In the postmenopausal woman the most common cell type associated with in situ carcinoma is a large keratinized cell with an angular outline, orangeophilic or eosinophilic cytoplasm, and a very hyperchromatic nucleus. The importance of this cytologic distinction between in situ carcinoma in the young and old woman is that the reliability of the method is high (80 to 90 percent) in the younger woman but less so in the older woman. The keratinized cells are likely to be interpreted as invasive cancer. It is uncertainty of

this sort that makes confirmation of the cytology by histology imperative.

Malignant Lesions

Squamous Cell Carcinoma

Carcinoma of the cervix unless otherwise specified refers to squamous cell carcinoma that develops in the same anatomic region as does metaplasia, dysplasia, and carcinoma in situ. Because it is usually visable if not symptomatic, there would seem to be less need for cytology in its detection and diagnosis. As it happens, the cytology is more often negative in cases of invasive cancer than for the preinvasive lesions, presumably as a result of the associated inflammation and cell necrosis. Because of its location, cervical scraping is the best method of specimen collection for carcinoma of the cervix, although vaginal pool specimens will also usually contain neoplastic cells in contrast to the more frequent absence of the significant cells in vaginal pool specimens of the premalignant lesions.

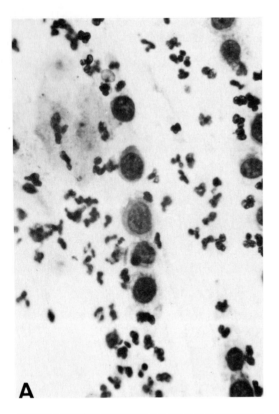

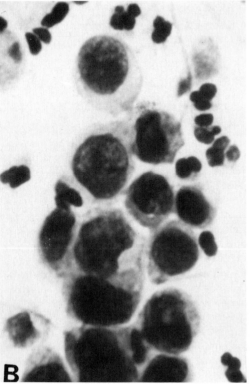

Low power microscopic examination of smears from cases of invasive carcinoma of the cervix are often characteristic because of the "tumor diathesis." This is a feature that is difficult to objectively describe, but in a general way refers to the presence of many degenerate red and white cells, tissue debris, and proteinaceous material. Even in the absence of cancer cells, a suspicion of the presence of a neoplasm should not only be thought of but should be verbalized on the basis of the diathesis. Some experience is required however in order to recognize the cytologic feature of tumor diathesis.

Microinvasive Squamous Cell Carcinoma

As the detection of carcinoma of the cervix has increased, more cases are being discovered at an early stage and microinvasive lesions have been reported to be present in between 5 percent and 63 percent of the in situ carcinomas,[29,30] and accounts for 6 percent to 10 percent of the squamous cell carcinomas.[31,32] As more lesions fall into the category of microinvasive and because the management of the case may be influenced by the diagnosis, it becomes important that the cytologic features of microinvasive squamous cell carcinoma be recognized. The cytologic characteristics of these lesions have been described.[33] They differ from in situ carcinoma in the following way. The cells are more numerous and are slightly smaller, and they occur less frequently as single cells and are more often seen in sheets of syncytia. There is significantly more irregular coursely granular chromatin as well as both micro- and macronucleoli, a feature that has been stressed in earlier studies as well.[34] A tumor diathesis is also seen in association with microinvasive lesions.

The ability to cytologically identify microinvasive carcinoma is reflected in a coded retrospective evaluation of in situ, microinvasive and invasive squamous cell carcinoma of the cervix, where 96 percent of the in situ lesions, 87 percent of the microinvasive, and 97 percent of the invasive carcinoma cases were correctly interpreted.[33]

Keratinizing Squamous Cell Carcinoma

There often seems to be less "tumor diathesis" on the smears from cases of this type of cancer than

Figure 3–5. In situ carcinoma. A. Scant cytoplasm and marked nuclear hyperchromasia. ×416. B. Same features as A. ×800.

with the others. It is also the tumor type with the greatest variability in numbers of cancer cells to be found on a smear. For this reason, it is the type most likely to be cytologically negative. The cells tend to be single although clumps do occur. The cytologic features, as the name suggests, are cytoplasmic differentiation in the form of keratin formation and a tendency toward cellular elongation with bizzare cell shapes. The nuclei present the usual characteristics of malignancy with chromatin clumping and irregular shape. Nucleoli are not a prominent feature (Fig. 3–6). Perhaps the most unusual aspect of these cells is the frequent occurrence of nuclear degeneration that is not of the usual pyknotic variety. Instead of the nuclear material becoming condensed in a small black mass it often assumes an irregular amorphous configuration, which is particularly evident when seen against the background of orangeophilic

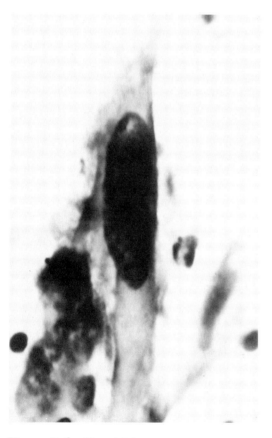

Figure 3–6. Keratinizing squamous cell carcinoma. An elongated cell with orangeophilic cytoplasm and an elongated hyperchromatic nucleus. ×800.

cytoplasm. "Snake cells," "fiber cells," and "tadpole cells," are names that have been applied to cells from this type lesion. Malignant epithelial pearls are occasionally seen.

Nonkeratinizing Squamous Cell Carcinoma

A tumor diathesis is frequently seen on slides from patients with this neoplasm, but does not seem to interfere with the presence of many identifiable tumor cells, which are seen both singly and in groups. However, they are more often in groups than are the keratinized squamous cell cancers. Bare or stripped malignant nuclei may also be a prominent feature. The cytologic feature that characterizes this lesion is the relatively large cell with cyanophilic cytoplasm, a malignant nucleus with clumped chromatin, and a prominent nucleolus (Fig. 3–7ABC).

Small Cell Carcinoma

As with the nonkeratinizing squamous cell carcinoma, a tumor diathesis is commonly present as are numerous tumor cells which tend to occur both singly and in groups. Again, as the name implies, these cells are identified by their small size. The cytoplasm is cyanophilic and scant. The nuclei tend to be slightly elongated rather than round and for this reason resemble reserve cells. The chromatin is granular and nucleoli are present (Fig. 3–8AB). This type of cancer is the most apt to escape diagnosis by the uninitiated.

Sources of Confusion

Tissue Repair

In smears from patients with severe cervicitis, following cautery or biopsy of the cervix or hysterectomy and after radiation therapy, "tissue repair" cells are often seen. These cells have on occasion been interpreted as cancer cells. Conversely, the presence of residual cancer cells may be overlooked both clinically and cytologically because of the presence of tissue repair.[35] The cells of tissue repair have been reported to occur in some patient populations with a frequency of 1.04 percent.[36] Although some believe the cells to be of epithelial origin, the resemblance to fibrolasts and their association with wound healing makes the latter a more likely explanation for the cell type of tissue repair cells. Cytologically, they have a

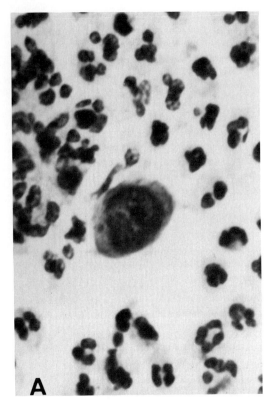

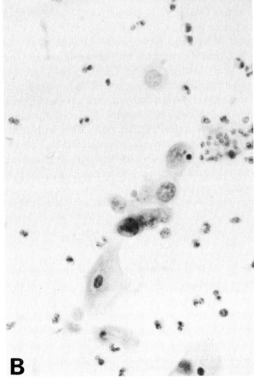

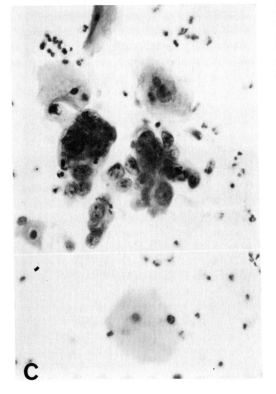

Figure 3–7. Large-cell nonkeratinizing carcinoma. A. Large cell with scant cytoplasm and a prominent nucleolus. ×800. B. A group of cells with pale cytoplasm and prominent chromocenters. ×416. C. Similar to B. ×520. (B and C supplied by Dr. Elizabeth Chu)

rather filmy cytoplasm, which is variable in staining characteristics and tends to have long, thin extensions. The overall shape of the cells is usually elongated with oval nuclei, which usually stain rather weakly, have a granular chromatin, and often large and/or multiple nucleoli (Fig. 3–9). The cells are sufficiently characteristic that a diagnosis of a healing lesion can be made when they are present.

Other cell types associated with benign ulcerative lesions of the cervix and/or vagina which may take on atypical features are the squamous cells, reserve cells,[37] and immature plasma cells.[38] Increased nuclear hyperchromasia of the reserve cells in the presence of an inflammatory background, which may be confused with a "tumor diathesis," may suggest a small cell carcinoma in situ. Similarly, squamous cells at the edge of an ulcer in the process of degenerating may have

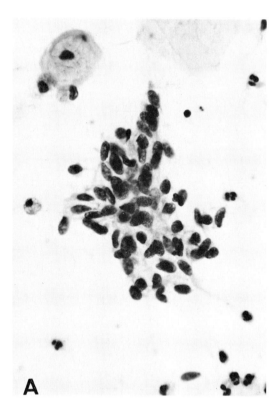

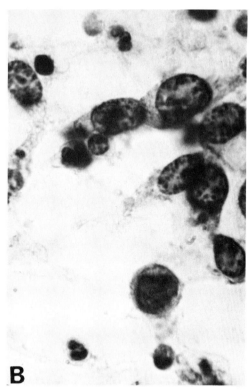

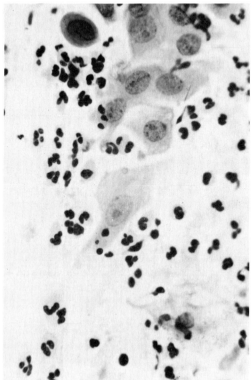

Figure 3–8. Small-cell nonkeratinizing carcinoma. A. Cluster of small cells with scant cytoplasm and rather elongated hyperchromatic nuclei. ×520. B. Cells similar to those in A. ×1125.

orangeophilic cytoplasm and a pyknotic nucleus, which may resemble dysplastic or carcinoma cells. Adequate clinical information, including evidence of cervical ulceration, use of a pessary, history of recent surgical procedures, following abortion or postpartum, irradiation therapy, or positive serology, is the most helpful way to alert the cytopathologist to the likelihood that atypical cells associated with benign ulcers and wound healing may be present.

Herpesvirus

Although of more historic than real importance at this time, the cellular alterations caused by her-

Figure 3–9. Repair cells. Resemble parabasal cells or fibroblasts. Pale, lacy cytoplasm with enlarged, often oval shaped, nuclei with prominent nucleoli and a finely granular cytoplasm. ×624.

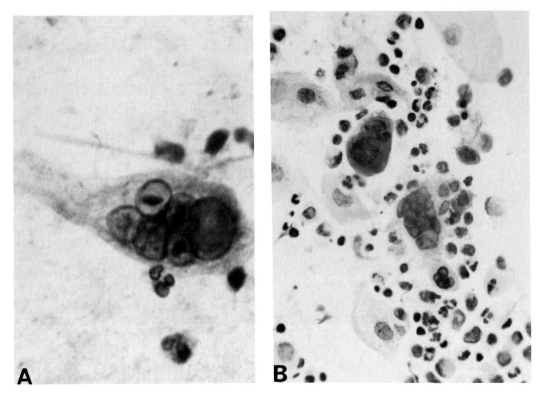

Figure 3–10. Herpes (virus) infected cells. A. Multinucleated giant cell with margination of the nuclear chromatin and intranuclear inclusions. ×800. B. Similar to A. The nuclei have the characteristic "ground glass" appearance. Nuclear inclusions are not seen. ×624.

pesvirus infection were, at one time, often mistaken for cancer cells. It was not until Stern and Longo[39] related these changes to herpes infection that their true significance was established. Because of the subsequent evidence[40,41] of an association between herpesvirus II and cervical cancer and because of the importance to the infant of this lesion in the maternal genital tract at the time of delivery, the cytologic diagnosis of herpes infection has become important over and above its former cytologic confusion with cancer. The cytologic features include multinucleation, frequently a "ground glass" appearance to the nucleus with margination of the chromatin, and occasionally an intranuclear inclusion body (Fig. 3-10AB).

Folic Acid Deficiency

Cellular changes on the vaginal-cervical smear which have been demonstrated to be the result of folic acid deficiency may, on occasion be interpreted as cancer.[42-44] These are most com- monly encountered during pregnancy, although not exclusively, and in many respects resemble changes associated with radiation. They include enlargement of parabasal cells, multinucleation, phagocytosis, and nuclear folds. These changes can be eliminated by folic acid therapy. Simple awareness of these changes, particularly in the pregnant patient, should eliminate the source of confusion.

Decidual Cells

Perhaps "reversal atypias" of pregnancy are the result of misinterpretation of decidual cells for dysplasia or malignancy. In any event, several authors have described cells believed to be decidual cells that suggested malignancy.[45-47] They resemble squamous cells having an acidophilic cytoplasm with variable shape from irregular to round. The nuclei are either pyknotic or enlarged but the chromatin is bland. Vacuolated cytoplasm is seen on occasion. As with folic acid deficiency, an awareness that the patient is pregnant should make the correct interpretation of these cells most likely.

Drug-Induced Cytologic Atypia

Following the observation that carcinogens and cancer therapeutic agents suppressed the immune response,[48] these agents have been used not only for cancer therapy but also for permitting successful organ transplantation and in the treatment of certain autoimmune diseases. Patients treated with a number of these agents, including cyclophosphamide, busulfan, and azathioprine, have been observed to develop dysplastic changes in a number of organs including the uterine cervix.[49-51] The cytologic changes seen on vaginal-cervical smears are those of dysplasia or carcinoma in situ. Without the clinical information of drug therapy, these lesions are cytologically and histologically indistinguishable from dysplasia and in situ carcinoma. It is estimated from radioautographic studies that the cervical epithelium is replaced every 5.7 days.[52] A drug-induced cytologic alteration might be expected within two weeks after the drug was given. This has been observed in the case of bladder epithelium.[53] Careful pulmonary, urinary, and gynecologic cytology follow-up of patients on such treatment is certainly indicated.

Pemphigus

It seems unlikely that the presenting evidence for pemphigus would be vaginal-cervical cytology, so the confusion of this disease with cervical cancer should not be a problem as long as adequate clinical information is transmitted to the cytopathologist. The cytologic features of pemphigus involving the cervix or vagina are similar to those of moderate to severe dysplasia.[54]

Radiation Therapy

CYTOLOGIC EFFECTS

Irradiation therapy for cancer of the cervix is often a very effective method of treatment. A way to separate the cases where it was effective from those where it was not would be most helpful. Since all the cells in the radiation field are exposed to the effects of irradiation, it was postulated that changes in the normal cells might be an indicator of how the tumor would respond. Graham[55] described the cytologic characteristics of radiation-induced cellular changes (Radiation

response [RR]) and correlated them with the prognosis.[56] The changes in the normal cells of an irradiated individual included cytoplasmic vacuolization, swelling of cytoplasm and nucleus, folding and wrinkling of the nucleus, and multinucleation (Fig. 3–11). These changes are most evident about two weeks after radium application and at the end of a course of external irradiation. The changes are the same regardless of the type of irradiation given but are more pronounced with radium and super-voltage radiation. A good RR and therefore a favorable prognosis depends upon 70 percent or more of the cells having these changes. Similar prognostic significance has been attached to changes in the buccal mucosal cells following irradiation,[57] where the potentially interfering effects of inflammation and tumor cells were not present and yet the effect of radiation on cancer of the cervix could be predicted. The duration of the RR changes seems to have prognostic significance with improved prognosis correlated with persistence of the cytologic changes.[58] These changes may persist for years. Not all studies of

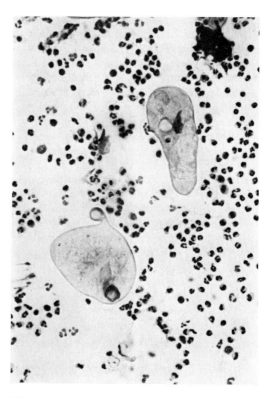

Figure 3–11. Radiation effect. Epithelial cells showing bizarre shape, overall enlargement and nuclear degeneration. ×312.

this phenomenon have reached the same conclusions,[59,60] and it is not a method that has gained popular use. However, it is important that the changes in normal irradiated cells be recognized for what they are and not be misinterpreted as cancer.

PRESENCE OF CANCER CELLS
FOLLOWING RADIATION

The cytologic effects of radiation on malignant cells have been studied to evaluate whether the cancer cells have been destroyed. The presence of intact neoplastic cells, degenerating neoplastic cells, and normal cells showing radiation effect must be distinguished. Neoplastic cells that have not been effected by the radiation have the same cytologic appearance as they have prior to radiation. When injured by radiation the changes are similar to those seen in normal cells. These include a swelling effect both of the nucleus and cytoplasm. The cells are larger, more pale, and take on bizarre shapes both of the whole cell and the nucleus. Although it is not possible to speak of the viability of neoplastic cells, it is possible to comment on their state of preservation, which may well be a reflection of their in vivo ability to grow. It is probably better to make repeated cytologic examinations over a period of time, for this will permit an assessment of the characteristics of any residual malignant cells and a more meaningful judgement can be made of the predicted biologic potential of the lesion. Studies of this sort have demonstrated that the persistence of cancer cells in cytologic preparations four weeks after the completion of radiation therapy indicates a poor prognosis.[61,62] This is particularly true for the stage I and II cases and when present 16 weeks postradiation. Radiation is a known carcinogen, the possible induction of a cancer by the therapy must be kept in mind and patients receiving x-ray therapy for a cancer of the cervix should be followed at six month intervals by cytology for evidence of dysplastic and neoplastic changes.

Dysplastic lesions are known to occur under these circumstances any time from 6 months to 21 days following x-ray therapy. The cytologic changes are the same as those for dysplasia seen without radiation therapy, but the biologic behavior of the lesion is not certain.[63]

Hormonal Influences

Vaginal cytology was first used for the determination of estrogen and progesterone levels. It is therefore not surprising that studies have been carried out to determine the relationship of these hormones to the presence of cervical cancer and to the effect of radiation therapy on cervical neoplasms. It appears that the presence of dysplasia, carcinoma in situ, or invasive cancer is, in general, associated with an elevated estrogen activity as measured by the karyopyknotic index.[64] It has been suggested that this would be a useful technique for detecting the incomplete irradication of a cancer or its recurrence.[65,66]

Cytology Automation

Work is in progress to develop equipment and techniques for machine analysis of samples of vaginal-cervical material for the presence of dysplasia, in situ, and invasive carcinoma. To accomplish this goal requires that some feature or features of the malignant cell be quantitatively or qualitatively different from the normal. Cellular characteristics that seem to differ and that are being investigated include DNA content and properties, nuclear cytoplasmic ratio, cell volume, and cell shape. The ratios between these features are also being studied.[67-74]

There are two general approaches. One consists of a flow or low-resolution system in which the cells from the vaginal-cervical area are suspended in a fluid media and passed through the sensing apparatus as single cells at a very rapid speed (several thousand per second). Sorting capability exists which permit cells with particular characteristics recognized by the sensing system to be separated from the rest. Once separated, they can be placed on a slide, stained, and examined by conventional cytologic methods. This aspect of the process is most useful at the research level and, although it would be hoped that the feature used for identification of the abnormal cells would be so specific that subsequent cytologic examination would not be necessary, it is conceivable that a persistent high level of false-positive results might necessitate the use of this sorting ability to prepare "enriched" specimens for cytopathologic evaluation. This would permit interpretation of the case by examination of one or a few microscope fields rather than several hundred.

The other approach is the static or high-resolution system in which cells on a slide are scanned by a high-resolution optical system and the image analyzed for its light-blocking or fluorescence features. A combination of the two methods has been considered in which the flow system would provide the rapid screening first stage followed by a high-resolution diagnostic system. The ultimate objective is application of cytology for cancer detection on a large population with a high level of accuracy at a low cost per case.

There is no proven clinically automated system at the present time, although high-resolution systems are being field tested in Japan. Work in this area is going on in Europe as well as Japan and the United States, and it may be anticipated that there is a reasonable prospect for the development of automated cytology techniques in the relatively near future. It is to be expected that this will result in an increase in the quality as well as quantity of cytology being done in the world.

Chromosome Analysis

Since all the cases of preinvasive lesions of the cervix do not seem to progress to cancer,[21,26] there has been an interest in finding features of the cells from such lesions which might correlate with the prognosis. The management of the case would then be determined by the presence or absence of these features. The chromosomal pattern of the preneoplastic lesions has been suggested as a method for making this determination.[75,76] The chromosome alteration associated with the development of neoplasia is a wide spread in the chromosome number. In dysplasia the pattern is distributed around the diploid, while in in situ carcinoma the chromosome number is more widely varied and often in the tetraploid and hypertetraploid range. In the case of invasive squamous cell carcinoma the number of chromosomes vary even more.[77,78] A shift in the chromosome number toward more chromosomes in a dysplasia or in situ lesion suggests a progression toward invasive cancer. The difficulties involved in chromosome analysis do not make this a generally available laboratory procedure. With the development of banding techniques where earlier changes and more definitive prognostic statements may be possible, this may become a more widely used method.

Trichomonas Vaginalis Neoplasia

There has long been observed an association between trichomonas vaginalis infection and cellular atypia. The argument in favor of this organism being more than casually associated with atypias has been circumstantial. That is, those factors known to be associated with an increased incidence of cervical cancer are also associated with increased trichomonas infections. In a study of 63,870 patients screened for cancer and for trichomonas, a statistically significant increase in trichomonas infection was observed in patients found to have dysplasia, in situ carcinoma, and invasive squamous cell carcinoma.[79] In general, the cellular atypicalities seen in association with trichomonas infection are not of a magnitude or quality to result in a false-positive cytologic interpretation.

CANCER DETECTION

Reliability of the Method

From the beginning, exfoliative cytology was used for the early detection of cervical cancer. Closely related to this was the awareness that carcinoma in situ was probably a premalignant disease and that it could be detected by cytologic examination. To be of value as a detection procedure it was necessary to know the reliability of the procedure, that is, how many cases of carcinoma in situ or invasive cancer would fail to be detected (false negative) and how many would be incorrectly interpreted as positive (false positive).

There have been innumerable reports of the results of screening programs on thousands of women. The false-positive results are probably accurate since these cases are thoroughly examined. It does not seem to exceed 5 percent. The false-negative rate on the other hand is difficult to know because cases considered cytologically negative are unlikely to be biopsied and if not symptomatic or reexamined for a year or more are considered to have developed the lesion after cytologic examination. In a most valuable study conducted by Young and reported by Friedell,[80] 14,859 women were examined and cytology taken as well as biopsy of all Schiller positive lesions. There were 143 cases of in situ carcinoma of which 16 had negative cytology (11.2 percent). Repeat examination of the slides failed to reveal abnormal cells. There were 53 invasive cancers and 6 of these had negative cytology (11.3

percent). One year later, 5292 patients were reexamined, and 7 cases of in situ cancer were discovered in patients who had negative cytology the year before. Thus the false-negative cytology for in situ cancer would seem to be between 11 percent and 22 percent for this study. Other studies have found between 1.4 percent[81] and 30 percent[82] false-negative cytology reports. Interestingly, the source of error in this case was not misinterpretation of the cells present but absence of atypical cells on the slide. The use of colposcopy is considered to be one way to help with this problem,[83] but it does not lend itself to a mass screening program. In a more recent report however, the difference between colposcopy and cytology was minimal.[84] The evidence indicates that carcinoma in situ remains as such for an average of seven years. The simplest solution to the false-negative problem would therefore seem to be an annual repeat smear beginning at age 20 and meticulous care in the technique of specimen collection.

Adenocarcinoma of the Cervix

Adenocarcinoma of the cervix arises from the glandular epithelium at the cervical os and within the cervical canal, being more commonly found within the canal. For this reason, although specimen collection by a scrape of the os will, in most cases, contain the endocervical cancer cells, an endocervical aspiration or swab specimen is to be preferred in suspected cases.

In Situ Adenocarcinoma

An uncommon lesion of the endocervical glands, in situ adenocarcinoma is recognized cytologically as endocervical cells with malignant nuclei which are seen both singly and in clusters. The nuclei may have prominent nucleoli and the cytoplasm may be vacuolated. Marked cell size variation is present. A differential between cells from this lesion and a low-grade endocervical adenocarcinoma may not be easy, although it is said the fact that the in situ cells retain their columnar character is the important clue.[17]

Adenocarcinoma

Cytologic features of adenocarcinoma of the cervix depend upon the degree of differentiation of the lesion. When very well differentiated the cytologic recognition of the lesion may be impossible. In the more common, less well differentiated lesions, the features include moderately large cells with ample cytoplasm, often vacuolated with an unusual almost purple color, and a malignant oval or round nucleus with clumped chromatin and often a prominent nucleolus (Fig. 3–12AB). It may be difficult to differentiate these cells from advanced endometrial carcinoma cells. Because of the different prognosis and different treatment for these two lesions, both the cytopathologist and clinician should be aware of the difficulties involved in this differential and depend upon the histopathology for the decision about therapy.

Adenosquamous Carcinoma

Rare metaplastic cells associated with an adenocarcinoma will develop atypical changes and may become neoplastic. Because the more common lesion involves a benign but atypical squamous component, when adenocarcinoma cells are seen in association with atypical squamous cells, very clear criteria of malignancy in the squamous-type cells must be evident before it should be given the cytologic interpretation of an adenosquamous carcinoma. The cytologic characteristics are the same as those already discussed for the independent lesions.

ENDOMETRIAL CANCER

The cytologic detection of endometrial cancer has not been as successful as detection of cancer of the cervix. This has been due primarily to the difficulty involved in developing a simple method for collection of the cytologic specimen from as close to the lesion as possible. The cancer cells are thought to be shed at irregular intervals so that a smear prepared from a cervical scrape has a good chance of not containing diagnostic cells. Vaginal pool smears are more valuable since the endometrial cancer cells can collect in the vaginal pool over a period of time and be available for examination. However, their state of preservation is poor under these circumstances. Cervical stenosis, a common postmenopausal condition, does not allow representative endometrial cells to descend to the cervical or vaginal areas. Ideally, collection of specimens for detection of endome-

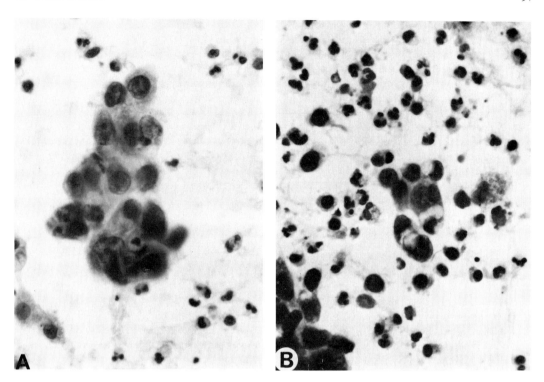

Figure 3-12. Adenocarcinoma endocervix. A. A group of neoplastic cells with some eccentricity to the nuclei, a granular cytoplasm, prominent nucleoli, and cellular and nuclear variability in size and shape. Phagocytosis of leucocytes is also evident. ×624. B. Similar to A but with more prominent cytoplasmic vacuolization. ×520.

trial carcinoma would best be accomplished by a technique that obtains the material directly from the endometrial cavity. A review of the literature revealed that of 2144 women with endometrial cancer, 68.5 percent were detected by the cytologic examination of samples containing desquamated cells (vaginal pool or cervical scrape), while 87.9 percent of 793 individuals with endometrial cancer were detected in material collected by methods which forcibly removed the cells.[85] The increase in the incidence of endometrial cancer makes it imperative that optimal methods be used for the detection of this neoplasm. A number of techniques have been described for collection of endometrial specimens by forceful removal of cells. These include endometrial aspiration,[86-91] intrauterine lavage,[92-94] endometrial brush,[95] aspiration curettage,[96-98] and jet wash.[99-104] Endometrial aspiration is done using a Kleegman cannula or similar device, inserted into the endometrial cavity, and by negative pressure with a syringe, endometrial cells are aspirated, smeared on slides, fixed, stained, and examined. The accuracy of this procedure has been reported to be 83 to 92 percent. Intrauterine lavage employs the same general procedure as the aspiration method except that saline is instilled and aspirated again, creating a lavage of the endometrium. The fluid is centrifuged and either cell blocked or smeared. The reported accuracy of this method is 87 to 90 percent. Endometrial brush techniques use a small brush, inserted through a cannula and a brushing of the endometrium is taken. The cells collected on the brush are smeared on a slide, fixed, and examined as a cytologic preparation. The accuracy of this method has been reported to be 60 to 90 percent. Aspiration curettage is done with a Novak device, which consists of a cannula with a small curette on the end. The curette is inserted into the endometrial cavity and the curettings are aspirated into the cannula. These are then either blown onto a slide or fixed and cell blocked. The accuracy of this method is 92 to 94 percent. The jet wash procedure employs a Gravlee jet apparatus, which consists of a cannula with a double lumen. Negative pressure is created within the endometrial cavity with a syringe attached to the cannula, which sucks fluid from a reservoir into the endometrial cavity. There it is aspirated by the open end of the cannula after having washed the endometrium. The fluid and cells that have been collected are either centrifuged and cell blocked or collected on a filter. Although some satisfactory results have been obtained using a millipore filter, there is universal agreement that the cell-block technique is satisfactory. The accuracy of this method is reportedly 93 to 100 percent. All of these methods have the drawback of being time consuming for the physician obtaining the sample and require special equipment either for collection or preparation of the specimen. They all have the advantage of being useful as an office procedure in contrast to the diagnostic dilatation and curettage, and therefore lend themselves to screening high-risk groups. In a recent review of the advantages and disadvantages of these methods for the cytologic detection of endometrial cancer, McGowan came to the conclusion that the simplicity, safety, low cost, and proven reliability of the aspiration smear technique made it the most useful of the methods when applied in a close gynecologist-cytopathologist working situation.[105]

Normal Endometrial Cells

Endometrial cells are frequently seen on vaginal pool and cervical scrape, or endocervical swab smears from the cyclic woman during and immediately following the menstrual period. They are not seen during the luteal phase of the cycle or in the postmenopausal woman. The normal endometrial cells seen on a cytology preparation consist of epithelial cells and stromal cells. They all have a scant amount of cytoplasm and are most easily recognized when in tight groups.

In the postmenopausal woman, age 50 and above, 20 percent of those who have normal endometrial cells on cytologic examination have been shown to have endometrial hyperplasia or neoplasia.[106] By the use of this nonspecific signal, that is, the presence of normal endometrial cells in a postmenopausal smear, one could expect to improve the detection rate of endometrial carcinoma even with the present specimen collection procedures.

Endometrial Hyperplasia and Adenocarcinoma In Situ

Cytologic changes in endometrial cells from hyperplastic lesions are not always easy to recognize.

They have been well analyzed and characterized by Ng et al.[107]

Cystic hyperplasia sheds cells that are slightly larger than normal endometrial cells and have an increased nuclear hyperchromasia with uniformly granular chromatin. Adenomatous hyperplastic cells are characterized by nuclear enlargement and a uniformly granular chromatin. Atypical hyperplasia has, in addition, micronucleoli. The chromatin becomes more coarse and unevenly distributed in adenocarcinoma in situ. These lesions are all very likely forerunners of adenocarcinoma of the endometrium. With advanced degree of atypia of the hyperplastic lesions, the distinction between them and adenocarcinoma in situ may be subtle.

Adenocarcinoma

Adenocarcinoma of the endometrium occurs in varying degrees of differentiation from well to poorly differentiated, and thus the ease with which it is recognized cytologically varies, the more poorly differentiated being easier to detect and identify than the well differentiated. In addition, the less well differentiated tumors seem to shed more cells, which also aids in their detection. Papillary carcinomas are more readily detected by cytology than nonpapillary varieties, and the more extensive the tumor the greater the likelihood it will be detected. Strangely enough, detection is facilitated by associated inflammation and necrosis of the tumor. The neoplastic cells are seen in groups as well as singly, although the cytologic evaluation should be based upon the single cells. As mentioned earlier, a variable amount of degeneration can be expected to have occurred before the cells are obtained for cytology, the amount depending in part upon the collection site and technique. In general, the cells are small, have a scant amount of cytoplasm and a round or slightly oval nucleus. With decreasing differentiation the cells become larger as do their nuclei. There are fewer cells with vacuoles in the less well differentiated cells and more of the cells have nucleoli and more have macronucleoli. There is also an increase in the amount of hyperchromasia in the less well differentiated group (Fig. 3–13AB).

Adenoacanthoma

The squamous component of an adenoacanthoma is usually not recognized cytologically and the le-

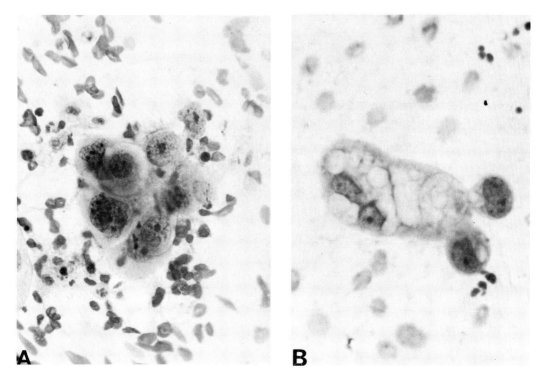

Figure 3–13. Adenocarcinoma of endometrium. A. Cluster of neoplastic cells exhibiting prominent nucleoli, chromatin clumping and a pale, slightly granular cytoplasm. ×624. B. A group of adenocarcinoma cells showing marked size variation and cytoplasmic vacuolization. ×1000. (Supplied by Dr. Elizabeth Chu)

sion is interpreted as an adenocarcinoma with about the same frequency as an adenocarcinoma that does not have a squamous component. A recently described cytologic feature of these tumors may make a definitive cytologic diagnosis possible.[108] This is the presence of "keratin bodies" on the smears. They are orange, psammoma-like bodies that may also stain blue or pink. They range from 10 to 70 microns in size and are usually associated with inflammatory cells, histiocytes, or endometrial cells.

Mixed Carcinoma

This is an increasingly important tumor as the incidence seems to be rising. Fortunately, it also would appear easier to detect than adenocarcinoma.[109] The cytologic characteristics are the same as those for an adeno- and squamous cell carcinoma. The less favorable prognosis associated with this lesion may herald an increased mortality from endometrial carcinoma associated with increased occurrence of this form of cancer.

Malignant Mixed Mullerian Tumor

This tumor presumably arises from the endometrial stroma and contains sarcomatous elements of mesenchymal origin and carcinomatous type cells of mullerian origin. The cytologic picture seems to be variable. Some cases present as myosarcoma cells while others have predominantly an adenocarcinomatous pattern, and on occasion a squamous carcinoma cell type coexists with the adenocarcinoma.[110]

Leiomyosarcoma

Cancer of the uterine musculature is a cytologically uncommon tumor. In order to be seen on a smear, there must be an ulceration of the neoplasm into the uterine cavity. When cells from a leiomyosarcoma are seen on a vaginocervical smear, they present as typical sarcoma cells or spindle shaped with malignant nuclei and either basophilic or slate gray cytoplasm on the Papanicolaou stain.

Choriocarcinoma

Trophoblastic cancer might be expected to shed rather readily into the vaginal fluid and be frequently detected by cytology. This in fact is not the case. During an intensive investigation of the chemotherapy of choriocarcinoma carried out at the National Cancer Institute, hundreds of smears were examined from patients with choriocarcinoma and two questionable malignant cytotrophoblastic cells were seen. The malignant cytologic features of these cells would make them easily identifiable as cancer and their cell type would be certainly high on the list of possible sources. It may be concluded that this is not a lesion that lends itself to cytologic detection or diagnostic efforts.

Sources of Confusion

Individuals using intrauterine contraceptive devices have been reported to have atypical endocervical cells and endometrial cells.[111] The changes include nuclear enlargement, chromatin clumping, some nuclear shape variation, and the presence of small multiple nucleoli. Presence of vacuolated cytoplasm creates the major problem however. Careful follow-up of these patients is indicated, for the relationship to neoplasia is not known.

FALLOPIAN TUBE CANCER

Carcinoma of the fallopian tube is a relatively rare tumor even though over 800 cases have been reported in the past 125 years.[112] There is no agreement on the value of cytology for the detection or diagnosis of these tumors, which no doubt means cytology is sometimes a diagnostic aid.[113,114] Cytology has been reported to be positive in 40 percent of the cases.[115] There are no cytologic features that permit the diagnosis of fallopian tube carcinoma. The presence of adenocarcinoma cells in a vaginal-cervical preparation following a negative curettage is considered highly suggestive of tubal cancer.[116] Although ovarian cancer cannot always be excluded, the subsequent steps in establishing a diagnosis would be the same. The presence of psammoma bodies, of course, would be a helpful clue that the malignant cells were of ovarian rather than tubal origin. It has been suggested that cytology will be positive only if the uterine end of the tube is patent and the distal end closed. Even when a neoplasm is in the fallopian tube, it is more commonly metastatic than primary.[117]

Primary carcinoma of the fallopian tube is an adenocarcinoma often papillary in nature and the cells shed from such a lesion may resemble those of an endometrial, endocervical, or ovarian carcinoma. That is, they may be relatively large with prominent cytoplasmic vacuolization or small and similar to endometrial carcinoma cells. As mentioned earlier, it is not always possible to make the differential diagnosis. This is an uncommon tumor and may be a diagnostic problem when malignant cells are observed on a vaginal smear in the absence of vaginal, cervical, or endometrial pathology. In a way, this situation puts the clinician's faith in the cytopathologist to the test, for an exploratory laparotomy may be the only recourse.

OVARIAN CANCER

Cancer of the ovary is said to be detected on the vaginal smear in 20 to 30 percent of the cases[17] and the papillary serous adenocarcinoma is the type most often observed. Those detected are the more far advanced cases, and therefore vaginal cytology is not useful as an early detection method. Although there is a cytologic resemblance between ovarian carcinoma cells and endometrial carcinoma, the former are larger, and psammoma bodies (calaspherites) are sometimes seen,[118,119] which aids in the diagnosis. Psammoma bodies are dark purple bodies when stained with the Papanicolaou stain. They are round in shape and have a laminated appearance (Fig. 3–14). They may be expected to be present in from 5 to 39 percent of the cases,[120,121] depending in part on the extent of involvement of mucosal surfaces.[120,122] On the other hand, psammoma bodies may be seen on

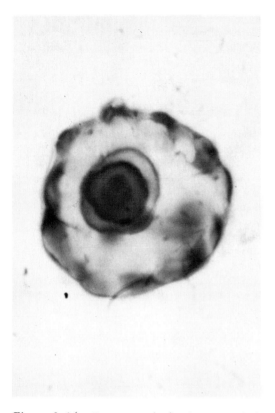

Figure 3–14. Psammoma body. A concentrically laminated basophilic staining structure. ×1000.

rare occasions in benign conditions,[123] so their presence is not pathognomonic of cancer and adenocarcinoma cells should be identified before a diagnosis of ovarian cancer is made. Fallopian tube carcinoma may also be a source of confusion. Mucinous adenocarcinoma may also be detected and the presence of mucus-containing malignant cells should suggest this possibility. Other types of ovarian cancer have been reportedly observed on vaginal cytology but are rare. The use of cul-de-sac aspiration for detection and follow-up of ovarian cancer has been carried out by a number of laboratories and will be discussed in detail in the chapter on ovarian cancer.

Hormonal Ovarian Tumors

Theca cell tumors, granulosa cell tumors, Sertoli-Leydig cell tumors, and arrhenoblastomas of the ovary may be suspected on the basis of their hormonal effect on the vaginal epithelium. Their presence in childhood or in the postmenopausal female is most readily appreciated. A high karyopyknotic index, an elevated estrogen effect, or a shift to the right in the maturation index is well correlated with the thecoma, granulosa cell tumor,[124] and Sertoli-Leydig cell tumor,[125] while the reverse is true for the arrhenoblastoma.[126]

VULVA

Neoplasms of the vulva are primarily squamous cell carcinomas, in situ carcinomas, and rare tumors of the adjacent glandular structures. They are not ordinarily detected or diagnosed by cytology because they are readily available to inspection and biopsy. However, the cytologic character of these lesions is the same as similar lesions in other sites, and it would therefore seem appropriate to examine cytologic preparations of vulvar lesions if biopsy was contraindicated.

Benign Tumors

Occasionally fluid will be aspirated from a benign Wolffian duct cyst for cytologic evaluation. The characteristic cells are similar to mesothelial cells with round, centrally located bland nuclei and ample clear cytoplasm. Smears taken from condyloma acuminatum present as parabasal cells sometimes with keratinization and mild nuclear atypia.

Adenoid Cystic Carcinoma

A technique which is widely used in many parts of the world for the diagnosis of cancer of nongynecologic sites is fine needle aspiration biopsy.[127] A situation in which a gynecologic tumor has been diagnosed by this method is the adenoid cystic carcinoma of Bartholin's gland.[128] Although this is an uncommon neoplasm, its metastatic potential and aggressive local behavior have been documented.[129,130] The use of fine needle aspiration cytology may be considered in the presence of a firm, enlarging, nontender, noninflamed mass in the region of Bartholin's glands. The cytologic characteristic of this lesion is uniform small cells grouped about homogeneous material that is metachromatic when stained with metachrome B.[126]

VAGINA

Smears prepared from direct scrapings of lesions observed at the time of pelvic examination are the ideal source of vaginal material for cytologic evaluation. If there is interest in localizing the source of abnormal cells, quadrant scrapings from the vagina may be collected, identified, and submitted for cytologic evaluation. Irrigation of the mucosa prior to scraping is recommended to eliminate contamination of the specimen by cells that had previously been shed from other locations in the vagina or cervix. For screening purposes, a vaginal pool specimen collected from the vaginal vault may be used.

Squamous Cell Carcinoma

Neoplasms of the vagina, like the vulva, are for the most part squamous cell carcinomas. Although less common than vulvar carcinomas, they are more likely to be detected or diagnosed by cytology. The cytologic characteristics of vaginal squamous cell carcinomas are the same as the cervix and because they are less common, a cytologic interpretation of cancer on a vaginal smear will invariably be assumed to be cervical cancer if a careful inspection of the vagina has not been made. Absence of confirmatory evidence of cervical cancer should lead the clinician to an examination of the vagina for an occult lesion. The vaginal neoplasms sometimes have cytologically larger cells with more bizarre nuclei and a more orangeophilic cytoplasm than their cervical counterpart. Carcinoma in situ and dysplasias of the vaginal mucosa are recognized cytologically by the same features as cervical lesions. Extension of epidermoid carcinoma of the cervix to the vagina is also encounted and may present with neoplastic cells being detected in the vaginal smear following therapy for cervical carcinoma. For this reason, cytologic follow-up of posttherapy cancer patients is recommended. Postradiation dysplasia arising in the vaginal epithelium is also detected in the vaginal smear. Cytology follow-up of patients treated surgically for in situ carcinoma of the cervix has occasionally revealed the presence of a "new" in situ lesion of the vagina.[131] In addition, invasive carcinoma in the vaginal cuff is occasionally seen.[132] A higher rate of cytologically detected recurrence has been reported in the case of radiation-treated cervical cancer than in the surgically treated group. This may reflect more a local recurrence in the cervix than a vaginal recurrence.[133] One must also consider the possibility of a radiation-induced neoplasm although presumably this would require a lengthy latent period.

Clear Cell Adenocarcinoma

A neoplasm that has recently become of special interest is the clear cell (mesonephric) adenocarcinoma of the vagina, because of the observed association between this cancer and the treatment of the patient's mother with diethylstilbestrol during pregnancy.[134–136] This lesion is being considered under the category of vaginal lesions, although 40 percent of the tumors appear to arise in the cervix, because the majority are vaginal lesions. The cytologic characteristics of this neoplasm correlate very well with the histologic features, consisting of large cells either single or in clusters with clear cytoplasm containing both large and small vacuoles. The nuclei are often hyperchromatic, some have large nucleoli, and often are irregularly shaped.[137,138] The relatively large cell size and large cytoplasmic vacuoles distinguish these tumors from other gynecologic neoplasms.

Of the 95 cases reported by Taft et al,[138] 11 were detected by cytology prior to clinical diagnosis, and 49 of 65 were cytologically positive after being detected clinically. The explanations offered for the relatively high false-negative figure were (1) an absence of cancer cells on the smear, (2) numerous interfering inflammatory cells, and (3) an unrecognized well-differentiated tumor in some cases.

The possible relationship of adenosis to clear cell carcinoma has been considered,[134,135,139] both because of its coexistence and because of the observation of adenosis in girls whose mothers received diethylstilbesterol while pregnant. To demonstrate the presence of occult adenosis in patients whose mother took diethylstilbesterol while pregnant and to follow these patients for evidence of clear cell carcinoma, cytologic evaluation of vaginal wall scrapings has been proposed.[140] It is unlikely that adenosis would be detected by cytology in the absence of a history of intrauterine exposure to diethylstilbesterol, because the presence of endocervical cells on routine vaginal aspiration smears is to be expected. To establish that they are of vaginal and not endocervical origin requires that scrapings be taken from the vaginal wall after removal of secretions overlying the mucosa.[140] The adenosis cells are seen in sheets and singly in these preparations and have a vacuolated or faintly eosinophilic cytoplasm often with cilia. They look like endocervical cells, occasionally with slightly atypical nuclei.

At the present time the relationship of adenosis to clear cell adenocarcinoma is not established. There is need for information about how frequently an adenocarcinoma develops in an area of adenosis and over how long a time span. The possible premalignancy of adenosis in girls whose mother received diethylstilbesterol while pregnant make cytologic follow-up of these individuals desirable. For this purpose a vaginal pool specimen, cervical scrape, and vaginal wall scrape smear should be taken probably every six to twelve months even though the therapy of the lesion remains in doubt.

Malignant Melanoma

The malignant melanoma is a tumor that may involve the vaginal mucosa. There were 35 cases of this lesion reported in the literature as of 1971.[141,142] Of these, 8 had been diagnosed cytologically, and all but 2 were amelanotic. Thus it is apparent that these tumors fail to shed cells that are identified cytologically. Certainly metastatic melanoma in other body fluids is readily recognized cytologically, so the most likely explanation for the poor cytologic detection of vaginal melanomas is that the cells do not shed or are rapidly destroyed in this site. The cytologic features, in the absence of the characteristic melanin pigment, are a malignant nucleus, usually spherical, which is large for the cell and contains a conspicuous, irregularly shaped nucleolus.

Sarcomas

Sarcoma botryoides occurs in the vagina of children usually as a submucosal tumor. When and if it grows through the mucosa, neoplastic cells may be detected on a vaginal smear. The cells are small and have malignant features occuring singly and in clusters. As a form of embryonal rhabdomyosarcoma, cross striation should be looked for in the cytoplasm of these cells.[17] Although cytology presents a reasonably acceptable form for specimen acquisition and diagnosis of this lesion in children, because sarcoma botryoides does not tend to become symptomatic until late, when it must break through the vaginal epithelium to be detected by cytology and is biopsied with less difficulty at that stage, the cytologic diagnosis of botryoid sarcoma is not usually the first-line diagnostic procedure.

METASTATIC CANCER

Many neoplasms may become established as metastatic lesions in the female genital organs and shed cells that are observed on a vaginal cervical smear. Cancer from other sites metastatic to the peritoneum may also appear in the endometrial cavity and vaginal cervical smear preparation, having arrived there via the fallopian tubes.[143] Such malignancies are recognized cytologically either by exclusion or by the lack of the usual tumor diathesis. "Exclusion" means neoplastic cells that are not identifiable as being of gynecologic origin.

This is often a difficult if not impossible differential to make. In addition, systemic neoplasms, such as Hodgkin's disease,[144,145] the leukemias, and lymphomas,[146] may have local deposits in the gynecologic organs. The tumors of other organs which have been reported to be found in vaginal cervical smears include breast,[147,148] stomach, anus, kidney,[143] urinary bladder and urethra,[149] malignant melanoma of the skin,[45] mesothelium, pancreas, gall bladder, and lung.[146] The possibility of extrauterine malignancy must be kept in mind when one has positive vaginal cervical cytology and negative cervical biopsy, colposcopy, and endometrial curettage. The expected frequency of extrauterine malignancy found on the vaginal cervical smear is 11/100,000.[146]

The frequency is probably higher, but vaginal cervical cytology is often not obtained on patients having a diagnosis of cancer of another organ since it is not considered contributory to the patients's care. In addition, the regularity with which cancer cells may reach the cervical os and vagina is no doubt variable. Consequently, finding cancer cells from an extrauterine site may be mostly a matter of chance.

References

1. Frost JK: Gynecologic and obstetric cytopathology. In Novak ER, Woodruff JD: Gynecologic and Obstetric Pathology. Philadelphia, Saunders, 1974, p 722
2. Wied GL, Bahr GF: Vaginal, cervical and endocervical cytologic smears on a single slide. Obstet & Gynec 14:362–367, 1959
3. Wilbanks GD, Ikomi E, Prado RB, Richart RM: An evaluation of a one-slide cervical cytology method for the detection of cervical intraepithelial neoplasia. Acta Cytol 12:157–158, 1968
4. Shingleton HM, Gore H, Straughn MJ, Austin JM, Littleton HJ: The contribution of endocervical smears to cervical cancer detection. Acta Cytol 19:261–264, 1975
5. Davis HJ: The irrigation smear. A cytologic method for mass population screening by mail. Am J Obstet Gynec 84:1017–1023, 1962
6. Davis HJ: The irrigation smear: Accuracy in detection of cervical smears. Acta Cytol 6:459–467, 1962
7. Koch F, Stakemann G: Irrigation smear: Accuracy in gynecologic cancer detection. Danis Med Bull 9:127–131, 1962
8. Richart RM, Vaillant HW: The irrigation smear. False-negative rates in a population with cervical neoplasia. JAMA 192:199–202, 1965
9. Muskett JM, Carter AK, Dodge OG: Detection of cervical cancer by irrigation smear and cervical scraping. Brit Med J 2:341–342, 1966
10. Coleman SA, Rube IF, Kashgarian M, Erickson CC: An appraisal of the irrigation cytology method for uterine cancer detection. Acta Cytol 14:502–506, 1970
11. Anderson WAD, Gunn SA: A critical evaluation of the vaginal irrigation kit as a screening method for the detection of cancer of the cervix. Acta Cytol 10:149–153, 1966
12. Regan JW, Lin F: An evaluation of the vaginal irrigation technique in the detection of uterine cancer. Acta Cytol 11:374–382, 1967
13. Jordan MJ, Bader G: New cannula for obtaining endometrial material for cytologic study. Obstet & Gynec 8:611–612, 1956
14. Oppenheim A, Hecht EL: The endometrial aspiration technique in a cancer detection and prevention center. Acta Cytol 10:296–298, 1966
15. Patten SF: Diagnostic Cytology of the Uterine Cervix. Baltimore, William & Wilkins Co., 1969
16. deBrux J, Dupré-Froment J: Exfoliative cytology of reserve cell hyperplasia, basal cell hyperplasia and dysplasia. Acta Cytol 5:142–144, 1961
17. Koss LG: Diagnostic Cytology and Its Histopathology Basis. Philadelphia, Lippincott, 1968, p 269
18. Song J: The Human Uterus: Morphogenesis and Embryological Basis for Cancer. Springfield, Thomas, 1964
19. Von Haam E, Old JW: Reserve cell hyperplasia, squamous metaplasia and epidermidization. In Gray LA (ed): Dysplasia, Carcinoma In-Situ and Microinvasive Carcinoma of the Cervix Uteri. Springfield, Thomas, 1964, pp 41–48
20. Regan JW, Hamonic MJ: Dysplasia of the uterine cervix. Ann NY Acad Sci 63:1236–1244, 1956
21. Peterson O: Precancerous changes of cervical epithelium in relation to manifest cervical carcinoma: clinical and histological aspects. Acta Radiol Suppl 127:1–168, 1955

22. Lange P: Clinical and histological studies on cervical carcinoma. Acta Path Microbiol Scand 50 Suppl 143:1–179, 1960

23. Christopherson WM: The control of cervix cancer. Acta Cytol 10:6–10, 1966

24. Ruch RM, Blake C, Abou A, Lado M, Ruch WA, Jr.: The changing incidence of cervical carcinoma. Am J Obstet & Gynec 89:727–731, 1964

25. Bryans FE, Boyes DA, Boyd JR, Fidler HK: The cytology program in British Columbia III. Management of preclinical carcinoma of the cervix. Canadian Med Ass J 90:62, 1964

26. Koss LG, Stewart FW, Foote FW, et al: Some histological aspects of behavior of epidermoid carcinoma in situ and related lesions of the uterine cervix. A long-term prospective study. Cancer 16:1160–1211, 1963

27. Day E: Evaluation of exfoliative cytology as a screening method for pelvic cancer. Clin Obstet Gynec 4:1183–1198, 1961

28. Gard PD, Fields MJ, Nobel EJ, Tweeddale DN: Comparative cytopathology of squamous carcinoma in situ of the cervix in the aged. Acta Cytol 13:27–35, 1969

29. Wheeler JD, Hertig AT: Pathologic anatomy of carcinoma of uterus. 1. Squamous carcinoma of the cervix. Am J Clin Path 25:345–375, 1955

30. Latour JP, Brown LB, Turnbull LA: Preclinical carcinoma of the cervix. Am J Obstet Gynec 74:354–360, 1957

31. Ng ABP, Regan JW: Microinvasive carcinoma of the uterine cervix. Am J Clin Path 52:511–529, 1969

32. Fidler HK, Boyes DA: Patterns of early invasion from intraepithelial carcinoma of the cervix. Cancer 12:673–680, 1959

33. Ng ABP, Regan JW, Lindner EA: The cellular manifestations of microinvasive squamous cell carcinoma of the uterine cervix. Acta Cytol 16:5–13, 1972

34. Alousi MA, Ballard LA, Reilly JV, Alousi SS: Microinvasive carcinoma and inflammatory lesions of the cervix uteri: histologic and cytologic differentiation. Acta Cytol 11:132–136, 1967

35. Montanari GD, Marconato A, Montanari GR, Gresmondi GL: Granulation tissue on the vault of the vagina after hysterectomy for cancer: diagnostic problems. Acta Cytol 12:25–29, 1968

36. Bibbo M, Keebler CM, Wied GL: The cytologic diagnosis of tissue repair in the female genital tract. Acta Cytol 15:133–137, 1971

37. Epstein NA: The significance of cellular atypia in the diagnosis of malignancy in ulcers of the female genital tract. Acta Cytol 16:483–489, 1972

38. Quizilbash AH: Chronic plasma cell cervicitis. A rare pitfall in gynecologic cytology. Acta Cytol 18:198–200, 1974

39. Stern E, Longo LD: Identification of herpes simplex virus in a case showing cytological features of viral vaginitis. Acta Cytol 7:295–299, 1963

40. Rawls WE, Tompkins WAF, Figueroa ME, Melnick JL: Herpes virus, type two: Association with carcinoma of the cervix. Science 161:1255–1256, 1968

41. Niab ZM, Nahmias AJ, Josey WE, Kramer JH: Genital herpetic infection association with cervical dysplasia and carcinoma. Cancer 23:940–945, 1969

42. Van Niekerk WA: Cervical cells in megaloblastic anemia of the puerperium. Lancet 1:1277–1279, 1962

43. Van Niekerk WA: Cervical cytological abnormalities caused by folic acid deficiency. Acta Cytol 10:67–73, 1966

44. Klaus H: Quantitative criteria of folate deficiency in cervicovaginal cytograms, with report of a new perimeter. Acta Cytol 15:50–53, 1971

45. Papanicolaou GN: Atlas of exfoliative cytology. Cambridge, Harvard University Press, 1954

46. Frost JK: Gynecologic and obstetric cytopathology. In Novak E, Woodruff D (eds): Gynecologic and Obstetric Pathology. Philadelphia, Saunders, 1974

47. Danos M, Holmquist ND: Cytologic evaluation of decidual cells: a report of two cases with false abnormal cytology. Acta Cytol 11:325–330, 1967

48. Malmgren RA, Bennison BE, McKinley TW: Reduced antibody titers in mice treated with carcinogenic and cancer chemotherapeutic agents. Proc Soc Exp Biol & Med 79:484–488, 1952

49. Gupta PK, Pinn VM, Taft PD: Cervical dysplasia associated with azathioprine (Imuran) therapy. Acta Cytol 13:373–376, 1969

50. Koss LG, Melamed MR, Mayer K: The ef-

fect of busulfan on human epithelia. Am J Clin Path 44:385–397, 1965

51. Schramm G: Development of severe cervical dysplasia under treatment with azathioprine (Imuran). Acta Cytol 14:507–509, 1970

52. Richart RM: A radioautographic analysis of cellular proliferation in dysplasia and carcinoma in situ of the uterine cervix. Am J Obstet & Gynec 86:925–930, 1963

53. Forni AM, Koss LG, Geller W: Cytological studies of the effect of cyclophosphamide on the epithelium of the urinary bladder in man. Cancer 17:1348–1355, 1964

54. Libcke JH: The cytology of cervical pemphigus. Acta Cytol 14:42–44, 1970

55. Graham RM: Effect of radiation on vaginal cells in cervical carcinoma. I. Description of cellular changes. II. Prognostic significance. Surg Gynec Obstet 84:153–165, 166–173, 1947

56. Graham RM, Graham JB: Cytological prognosis in cancer of the uterine cervix treated radiologically. Cancer 8:59–70, 1955

57. Jones HW, Goldberg B, Davis HJ, Burns BC: Cellular changes in vaginal and buccal smears after radiation: An index of the radiocurability of carcinoma of the cervix. Am J Obstet & Gynec 78:1083–1100, 1959

58. Ceelen GH: Persistent radiation changes in vaginal smears and their meaning for the prognosis of squamous cell carcinoma of the cervix. Acta Cytol 10:350–352, 1966

59. Rubio CA, Kottmeier HL, Olsson E, Zajicek J: Radiation response and sensitization response studies in 720 cases from Radiumhemmet, Stockholm. Acta Cytol 10:191–193, 1966

60. Sugimori H, Taki I: Radiosensitivity test for cervical cancer. Acta Cytol 16:331–335, 1972

61. Arrighi AA, Hopman CB, Koss LG, Von Haam E: Recurrent carcinoma and the presence of radiation cell changes. A symposium. Acta Cytol 3:415–419, 1959

62. Campos J: Persistent tumor cells in the vaginal smears and prognosis of cancer of the radiated cervix. Acta Cytol 14:519–522, 1970

63. Patten SF, Reagan JW, Obenauf M, Ballard LA: Postirradiation dysplasia of uterine cervix and vagina: an analytical study of the cells. Cancer 16:173–182, 1963

64. Rubio CA: Estrogenic effect in vaginal smears in cases of carcinoma in situ and microinvasive carcinoma of the uterine cervix. Acta Cytol 17:361–365, 1973

65. Rubio CA, Hvalec S, Pareja A: The value of cytohormonal studies (Karyopyknotic index) for detecting recurrence of carcinoma. Acta Cytol 11:176–178, 1962

66. Wachtel E: The prognostic significance of the karyopyknotic index after radical treatment for cancer of the female genital tract. Acta Cytol 11:35–36, 1967

67. Wagner D, Sprenger E, Blank MH: DNA content of dysplastic cells of the uterine cervix. Acta Cytol 16:517–522, 1972

68. Sprenger E, Moore GW, Naujoks H, Schluter G, Sandritter W: DNA content and chromatin pattern analysis on cervical carcinoma in situ. Acta Cytol 17:27–31, 1973

69. Atkin NB: Variant nuclear type in gynecologic tumors: observations of squash and smears. Acta Cytol 13:569–575, 1969

70. Valeri V, Cruz AR, Brandao HJS, Lison L: Relationship between cell nuclear volume and desoxyribonucleic acid of cells of normal epithelium, of carcinoma in situ and invasive carcinoma of the uterine cervix. Acta Cytol 11:488–496, 1967

71. Atkin NB: The desoxyribonucleic acid content of malignant cells in cervical smears. Acta Cytol 8:68–72, 1964

72. Mellors RC, Keane JF, Papanicolaou GN: Nucleic acid content of the squamous cancer cell. Science 116:265–269, 1952

73. Hrushovetz SB, Lauchlan SC: Comparative DNA content of cells in the intermediate and parabasal layers of cervical intraepithelial neoplasia studied by two-wavelength Fulgen cytophotometry. Acta Cytol 14:68–77, 1970

74. J Histochem Cytochem 24:1–414, 1976

75. Cellier KM, Kirkland JA, Stanley MA: Statistical analysis of cytogenetic data in cervical dysplasia. J Nat Cancer Inst 44: 1221–1230, 1970

76. Kirkland JA, Stanley MA: Chromosomes of cancer cells. Nature 223:623–633, 1971

77. Kirkland JA: Mitotic and chromosomal abnormalities in carcinoma in situ of the uterine cervix. Acta Cytol 10:80–96, 1966

78. Stanley MA, Kirkland JA: Chromosome and histologic patterns in preinvasive lesions of the cervix. Acta Cytol 19:142–147, 1975

79. Meisels A: Microbiology of the female reproductive tract as determined in the cytologic specimen III in the presence of cellular atypias. Acta Cytol 13:64–71, 1969

80. Friedell GH: Cancer of the cervix—a selective review and addendum. In Sommers, SC (ed): Genital and Mammary Pathology Decennial. New York, Appleton, 1975, pp 29–53

81. Richart RM: Evaluation of the true false negative rate in cytology. Am J Obstet & Gynec 89:723–726, 1964

82. Achenback RR, Johnstone RE, Hertig AT: The validity of vaginal smear diagnosis in carcinoma in situ of the cervix: A report of 60 cases. Am J Obstet & Gynec 61:385–392, 1951

83. Hill EC: Preclinical cervical carcinoma, colposcopy and the "negative" smear. Am J Obstet & Gynec 95:308–319, 1966

84. Ostergard DR, Gondos B: The incidence of false negative cervical cytology as determined by colposcopically directed biopsies. Acta Cytol 15:292–293, 1971

85. Regan JW: Cells observed in endometrial carcinoma. Presented at the International Conference on automation of uterine cancer cytology, Chicago, Illinois. Sponsored by the International Academy of Cytology, April 7–10, 1975

86. Hecht EL: The endometrial aspiration smear: research status and clinical value. Am J Obstet & Gynec 71:819–833, 1956

87. Boschann HW: Symposium on techniques for endometrial cytological examination. Acta Cytol 2:586, 1958

88. Jameson MH: A clinical appraisal and techniques for obtaining fresh cells for endometrial cytology. N Z Med J 60:316–332, 1961

89. Rascoe RR: Endometrial aspiration smear in diagnosis of malignancy of the uterine corpus. Am J Obstet & Gynec 87:921–925, 1963

90. Abramson D, Driscoll S: Endometrial aspiration biopsy. Obstet & Gynec 27:381–391, 1966

91. Papanicolaou GN, Marchetti AA: Use of endocervical and endometrial smears in diagnosis of cancer and other conditions of uterus. Am J Obstet & Gynec 46:421–422, 1943

92. Morton DG, Moore JG, Chang N: Lavage of the endometrial cavity as an aid in the diagnosis of carcinoma of the uterine corpus. J Intl College Surg 31:570–578, 1959

93. Torres JE, Holmquist ND, Danos ML: The endometrial irrigation smear in the detection of adenocarcinoma of the endometrium. Acta Cytol 13:163–168, 1969

94. Fox CH, Turner FG, Johnson WC, Thornton WN: Endometrial cytology: A new technique. Am J Obstet & Gynec 83:1582–1591, 1962

95. Ayre JE: Rotating endometrial brush: New techniques for the diagnosis of fundal carcinoma. Obstet & Gynec 5:137–141, 1955

96. Jordan MJ, Bader G, Nemazie AS: Comparative accuracy of preoperative cytologic and histologic diagnosis in endometrial lesions. Obstet & Gynec 7:646–653, 1956

97. McGuire TA: Efficacy of endometrial biopsy in the diagnosis of endometrial carcinoma. Obstet & Gynec 19:105–107, 1969

98. Palmer JP, Kneer WF, Eccleston HH: Endometrial biopsy: Comparison of aspiration curettage with conventional dilatation and curettage. Am J Obstet & Gynec 60:671–674, 1950

99. Dowling EA, Gravlee CC: Endometrial cancer diagnosis: A new technique using a jet washer. Ala J Med Sci 1:412–416, 1964

100. So-Bosita JL, Lebherz TB, Blair OM: Endometrial jet washer. Obstet & Gynec 36:287–293, 1970

101. Kanbour A, Klionsky B, Cooper R: Cyto-histologic diagnosis of uterine jet wash preparations. Acta Cytol 18:51–58, 1974

102. Bibbo M, Shanklin D, Wied G: Endometrial cytology on jet wash material. J Reprod Med 8:90–96, 1972

103. Abate SD, Edwards CL, Vellios F: A comparative study of endometrial jet-washing technique and endometrial biopsy. Am J Clin Path 58:118–122, 1972

104. Hilbard LT, Schwinn CE: Diagnosis by endometrial jet washings. Am J Obstet & Gynec 111:1039–1042, 1971

105. McGowan L: Cytologic methods for the

detection of endometrial cancer. Gynec Oncol 2:272–278, 1974

106. Ng ABP, Regan JW, Hawliczek S, Wentz WB: Significance of endometrial cells in the detection of endometrial carcinoma and its precursors. Acta Cytol 18:356–361, 1974

107. Ng ABP, Regan JW, Cechner RL: The precursors of endometrial cancer. A study of this cellular manifestation. Acta Cytol 17:439–448, 1973

108. Bushchmann C, Hergenrader M, Porter D: Keratin bodies: a clue in the cytological detection of endometrial adenoacanthoma. Report of two cases. Acta Cytol 18:297–299, 1974

109. Regan JW, Ng ABP: The cells of uterine adenocarcinoma, 2nd ed. Karger, Basal, 1973

110. Parker JE: Cytologic findings associated with primary uterine malignancies of mixed cell types (malignant mixed mullerian tumor). Acta Cytol 8:316–320, 1964

111. Fornari ML: Cellular changes in the glandular epithelium of patients using IUCD —a source of cytologic error. Acta Cytol 18:341–343, 1974

112. Boutselis JG, Thompson JN: Clinical aspects of primary carcinoma of the fallopian tube. Am J Obstet & Gynec 111:98–101, 1971

113. Brewer JI, Guderian AM: Diagnosis of uterine tube carcinomas by vaginal cytology. Obstet & Gynec 8:664–672, 1956

114. Larsson E, Schooley JL: Positive vaginal cytology in primary carcinoma of the fallopian tubes. Am J Obstet & Gynec 72:1364–1366, 1956

115. Sedlis A: Primary carcinoma of the fallopian tube. Obstet & Gynec Survey 16:209–226, 1961

116. Krugman PI, Fisher JE: Primary carcinoma of the fallopian tube. Am J Obstet & Gynec 80:722–726, 1960

117. Finn WJ, Javert CT: Primary and metastatic cancer of the fallopian tube. Cancer 2:803–814, 1949

118. Benson PA: Psammoma bodies found in cervico-vaginal smears. Acta Cytol 17:64–66, 1973

119. Beyer-Boon ME: Psammoma bodies in cervico-vaginal smears: An indicator of the presence of ovarian carcinoma. Acta Cytol 18:41–44, 1974

120. Rubin DK, Frost JK: The cytologic detection of ovarian cancer. Acta Cytol 7:191–195, 1963

121. Graham RM, Van Niekerk WA: Vaginal cytology in cancer of the ovary. Acta Cytol 6:496–499, 1962

122. Reagan JW, Ng ABP: The Cells of Uterine Adenocarcinoma. Baltimore, Williams & Wilkins, 1965, pp 109–111

123. Picoff RC, Meeker CI: Psammoma bodies in the cervico-vaginal smear in association with benign papillary structures of the ovary. Acta Cytol 14:45–47, 1970

124. Johnston WW, Goldston WR, Montgomery MS: Clinicopathologic studies in feminizing tumors of the ovary. II the role of genital cytology. Acta Cytol 15:334–338, 1971

125. deTorres EF: Feminization in tumors of Sertoli-Leydig cells. Acta Cytol 18:189, 1974

126. Rakoff A: Vaginal cytology of endocrinopathies. Acta Cytol 5:153–167, 1961

127. Franzen S, Zajick J: Aspiration biopsy in diagnosis of palpable lesions of the breast: critical review of 3,479 consecutive biopsies. Acta Radiol 7:241–273, 1968

128. Frable WJ, Goplerud DR: Adenoid cystic carcinoma of Bartholin's gland diagnosed by aspiration biopsy. Acta Cytol 19:152–153, 1975

129. Abell MR: Adenocystic (pseudoadenomatous) basal cell carcinoma of vestibular glands of vulva. Am J Obstet & Gynec 86:470–482, 1963

130. Eichner E: Adenoid cystic carcinoma of the Bartholin gland. Obstet & Gynec 21:608–613,1963

131. McIndoe WA, Green GH: Vaginal carcinoma in situ following hysterectomy. Acta Cytol 13:158–162, 1969

132. Frable WJ, Smith JH, Perkins BS, Foley C: Vaginal cuff cytology, some difficult diagnostic problems. Acta Cytol 17:135–140, 1973

133. Masubuchi K, Kubo H, Tenjin V, Ono M, Yamazaki M: Follow-up studies by cytology on cancer of the cervix uteri after treatment. Acta Cytol 13:323–326, 1969

134. Herbst AL, Scully RE: Adenocarcinoma of the vagina in adolescence: A report of seven cases including six clear-cell carcinomas (so-called mesonephromas). Cancer 25:745–757, 1970

135. Herbst AC, Ulfelder H, Poskanzer DC: Adenocarcinoma of the vagina. Association of maternal stilbesterol with tumor appearance in young women. New Eng J Med 284:878–881, 1971

136. Greenwald P, Barlow JJ, Nasca PC, Burnett WS: Vaginal cancer after maternal treatment with synthetic estrogens. New Eng J Med 285:390–392, 1971

137. Rosati LA, Jarzynski DJ: Clear cell (mesonephric) adenocarcinoma of the vagina. A case report. Acta Cytol 17:493–497, 1973

138. Taft PD, Robboy SJ, Herbst AL, Scully RE: Cytology of clear cell adenocarcinoma of genital tract in young females: Review of 95 cases from the Registry. Acta Cytol 18:279–290, 1974

139. Langmuir D: New environmental factor in congenital disease. New Eng J Med 284:912–913, 1971

140. Vooijs PG, Ng ABP, Wentz WB: The detection of vaginal adenosis and clear cell carcinoma. Acta Cytol 17:59–63, 1973

141. Ehrmann RL, Younger PA, Lerch VL: The exfoliative cytology and histogenesis of early primary malignant melanoma of the vagina. Acta Cytol 6:245–254, 1962

142. Lenthicum CM: Primary malignant melanoma of the vagina. A case report. Acta Cytol 15:179–181, 1971

143. Song YS: Significance of positive vaginal smears in extrauterine carcinomas. Am J Obstet & Gynec 73:341–348, 1957

144. Nasiell M: Hodgkin's disease limited to the uterine cervix. A case report including cytological findings in the cervical and vaginal smears. Acta Cytol 8:16–18, 1964

145. Uyeda CK, Stephens SR, Bridges WM: Cervical smear diagnosis of Hodgkins disease. Report of a case. Acta Cytol 13:652–655, 1969

146. Ng ABP, Teeple D, Linder EA, Regan JW: The cellular manifestations of extrauterine cancer. Acta Cytol 18:108–117, 1974

147. Liu W: Vaginal cytology in breast cancer patients. Surg Gynec & Obstet 105:421–426, 1957

148. Bhagavan BS, Weinberg T: Cytopathologic diagnosis of metastatic cancer by cervical and vaginal smears with report of a case. Acta Cytol 13:377–381, 1969

149. Isbel NP, Jewett JF, Allan MS, Hertig AT: A correlation between vaginal smears and tissue diagnosis in 1045 operated gynecologic cases. Am J Obstet & Gynec 54:576–583, 1947

Chapter 4

The Physics of Radiation Therapy for Gynecologic Malignancy

DAVID A. LIGHTFOOT, M.A.

The major concern of clinical radiation therapy physics is the relationship between the sources of radiation and the dose at the sites of interest within a patient. Once this relationship has been firmly established, it is possible to control the geometric arrangement of radiation sources, their strengths, and duration of application to obtain a clinically beneficial result.

DOSE SPECIFICATION

Dose in radiation therapy is the ratio of the energy deposited at the site of concern to the mass of material or tissue at the site of concern. The dose within any irradiated volume will tend to vary from point to point. Hence, the dose prescription is most certainly accurate at the site of prescription although other sites may happen to have the same dose. In order to duplicate or improve the results of accumulated clinical experience, it is important to know the site for dose specification and the factors that were employed to yield the stated value of dose. There are reports in the literature indicating that differences in dose as small as 5 percent may result, in some cases, in a noticeable increase in recurrences if the dose is too low, or complications if the dose is too high. Of course, many other details of treatment critically affect results. Perhaps chief among these factors is whether the dose is favorably distributed throughout all of the sites of concern. Additional factors such as dose rate, type of ra-

diation, and intermittant versus continuous irradiation will influence the total dose at the site of prescription necessary to achieve a desirable result.

The Rad

The most common unit in use for specification of dose at present is the rad. A rad is an absorbed dose of 0.01 J/kg. The energy deposited within a material ultimately appears as heat, and thus increases the average temperature. To appreciate the relationship between heat and absorbed dose it may be helpful to keep in mind that a thermally insulated volume of water irradiated in such a manner as to achieve a uniform dose of 418,400 rad at every point throughout the volume of water would experience a temperature rise of 1 C. Typical dose prescriptions in external beam radiation therapy are of the order of 200 rad delivered in a time period of a few minutes, repeated at daily intervals. Brachytherapy dose rates are usually much lower. In both cases, macroscopic temperature increase in the treated area is unquestionably negligible and cannot be named as the cause of the radiation effect. This is not to deny the current research interest in the biologic effects of hyperthermia and the possibility of some microscopic temperature increases having something to do with the biologic effects of particulate radiations with extremely high LET (linear energy transfer). Rather, it is to point out that the biologic effects of radiation therapy are initiated by ionization and excitation of the atoms and molecules within the irradiated volume. A dose of 200 rad results in the ionization of approximately 370 atoms per cubic micron in biologic soft tissue. Put another way, one out of every 261 million atoms within the soft tissue site of concern is ionized when the absorbed dose is 200 rad. Hence, the biologic effects of radiation are the result of physical effects, namely ionization, on a very small portion of the irradiated atoms.

The definition of dose applies only to a volume of sufficient size to give a meaningful ratio, yet sufficiently small to be considered an irradiated point. For example, the ratio formed for a volume centered about a site of ionization could eventually erroneously indicate an absorbed dose of extremely high values as the assumed volume for computation of dose is made progressively smaller. Conversely, the ratio formed for a volume centered about a site of no ionizations could eventually erroneously indicate a zero value as the volume employed in the ratio is made progressively miniscule. If the volume is made too large, it may smooth out meaningful variation in dose.

Since absorbed dose is a measure of energy deposited per gram, a statement that the treatment was 6000 rad in six weeks conveys no information about the total volume of tissue irradiated or the total energy imparted. Two tumors situated in a volume of uniform dose of 200 rad would both have the same percentage of cells affected even if one has a diameter of 2 cm and the other a diameter of 2 mm. Since the larger mass would have a larger number of viable cells it would require a larger dose for curative results. Since the percent survival of irradiated cells is logarithmically related to the dose, larger tumor masses require only slightly higher dose for curative results than small masses. This is quite fortunate since the tolerance of normal tissue decreases as the irradiated volume increases.

Mechanisms of Energy Absorption

Generally the word "radiation" is used in the sense that radiation is energy traveling outward from its source. This energy may be a pure form classified as electromagnetic radiation, or the energy may be attached to subatomic particles (electrons, protons, alpha particles, neutrons, mesons, pions, etc.) and classified as particulate radiation. The quantum theory of electromagnetic radiation states that the energy is not emitted continuously but discontinuously in discrete amounts or quantities, called quanta or photons. Each quantum or photon has a life history that begins at the instant it is released from the source of radiation and ends upon its interaction with one of the elementary particles or groups of elementary particles. A photon may be thought of as an energy particle.

The photons in a beam of electromagnetic radiation travel at the speed of light and have no rest mass. The subatomic particles in a beam of particulate radiation travel at a speed determined by their rest mass and kinetic energy. If either a single photon or single particle in a beam of radiation has sufficient energy to break the bond linking an electron to an atom the radiation is classified as ionizing radiation. Ionizing radiation may be alternately classified as indirectly ionizing radiation (comprised of photons or particles with zero net electric charge) or as directly ionizing radiation (comprised of particles with a net electric charge). The majority of atoms ionized during treatment are ionized by directly ionizing radiation regardless of the type of radiation emitted by the source. The explanation of how this is possible for x-rays and γ-rays follows.

Most of the photons directed toward a particular atom will go right past the atom with absolutely no effect. Since most x-ray beams and γ-ray beams contain an extremely large number of photons and since the human body contains an extremely large number of atoms, ultimately a substantial number of the photons will interact with some of the electrons. The amount of energy transferred by a single photon-electron collision is in the range of thousands to hundreds of thousands of electron volts of energy. This means that in a typical x-ray absorption interaction an electron travels away from the site of interaction with a very high velocity. Because of its electrical charge the high-speed electron is very much more likely to interact with electrons in other atoms than a photon would be. Ultimately, the high-speed electron will lose all of its energy through the ionization and excitation of atoms.

If one divides the total number of ion pairs formed by the high-speed electron into the total energy it lost, one obtains w, the average energy per ion pair. The value of w for the ionization of air is 33.73 eV/ip. Comparing this with the tens of thousands of eV of energy initially transferred to the high-speed electron leads to the conclusion that a photon-electron interaction that results in the ionization of a single atom ultimately results in the ionization of thousands to tens of thousands, perhaps even hundreds of thousands of additional atoms. And thus the explanation for the statement that "the majority of atoms ionized during treatment are ionized by directly ionizing radiation" is completed.

Linear Energy Transfer

Different types of radiation may have markedly different effects on biologic tissue for the same dose specification. The principle characteristic associated with the explanation of why the radiations differ in their effects is a characteristic of spacing between successive clusters of ionization created by the particular directly ionizing radiation associated with the radiation in question. This is usually measured by the ratio of energy lost by the directly ionizing particle per distance it travels. The resultant ratio is termed linear energy transfer or LET. Typical units are keV for energy and microns for distance. High LET indicates very close spacing of successive clusters of ionized atoms. The LET is a function of the energy as well as the type of directly ionizing particle. For example, a high-speed electron may travel past several atoms before it happens to come close enough to one of the electrons bound in an atom for there to be an interaction. Since the electrons bound in atoms are continuously in motion, they are much more likely to come close enough to an energetic electron for interaction to occur if the energetic electron is moving at a slower speed. As the energetic electron loses energy it begins to move slower. The likelihood of the electron ionizing an atom increases to the point where just before the high-speed electron loses all of its energy it deposits energy with a much higher LET or a much smaller spacing between clusters of ionizations than at the beginning of its travels. A very heavy particle such as an α-particle, which has approximately 7000 times the mass of an electron and

twice the charge, tends to move much more slowly than an electron of the same energy and is usually referred to as a very high LET particle.

Indirectly ionizing particles such as neutrons tend to interact with atoms by interacting with nuclei. As a result of this interaction between a neutron and an atomic nucleus, a charged nuclear fragment is often released. Since this charged nuclear fragment has a great deal more rest mass than an electron, it, like the α-particle, travels at a much slower speed and tends to be very densely ionizing. Hence the dose deposited by neutron irradiation has a high LET.

Since all directly ionizing particles slow down as they lose energy, there is no single value of LET that characterizes the entire microscopic distribution of dose. Furthermore, at any point of dose evaluation the absorbed dose results from ionization produced by many particles in various stages of the slowing down process and hence with a variety of LET values. Nevertheless, an average LET value can be stated and the dose qualitatively described as high LET dose or low LET dose. It is common in some cases to think separately about the high LET and low LET components of dose since any dose has a mixture of both.

The main difference in the effects of various types of radiation are to a considerable extent explainable by the relative amounts of the high and low LET components of dose for each type. For well-oxygenated tissues treated at dose rates of tens to hundreds of rads per minute, an absorbed dose of 10 rad from high LET radiation may be as damaging as 16 rad from low LET radiation. At very low dose rates the high LET radiation may be as damaging as 100 times the dose from low LET radiation, due to the very rapid drop in effectiveness of the low LET radiation. This is reasonable, since there tends to be less chance of recovery from the effects of high LET radiation than from low LET radiation.

High LET radiation is of interest because it also appears that the oxygen content of the cells has less of an influence on the response of the cell to the radiation if the radiation is high LET radiation. There are felt to be certain situations where tumor cells are protected to some degree from the effects of radiation by a low oxygen supply which is just sufficient to maintain their viability without being sufficient to give maximum sensitivity to the effects of radiation. Poorly oxygenated cells require approximately 2.3 times the dose of low LET radiation as well as oxygenated cells for equivalent damage. With high LET radiation, the oxygen enhancement ratio (OER) reduces from 2.3 to about 1.6.

Evaluation of LET is generally restricted to the planning stages in attempting to exploit a new modality of treatment with appropriate revision of dosage schemes. For purposes of recording treatment, it is sufficient to characterize the type and energy of the primary radiation and to state the resultant absorbed dose at a point without any comment about the LET. Qualitative comments about LET may be made in statements pertaining to the rationale for employing the new modality.

CONVERTING KNOWLEDGE OF SOURCE TO KNOWLEDGE OF ABSORBED DOSE

The sources of radiation employed in the treatment of gynecologic malignancies over the past 60 years have been usable primarily because of emitted photons. The photons may be classified as either γ rays, for those that originate from within the nucleus of an atom, or as x-rays, for those that originate from the portion of an atom external to the nucleus. Other than site of origin, there need be no other distinction between a γ photon and an x-ray photon. Photons do differ from one another, regardless of their origin, primarily in their energy content. The detailed aspects that must be understood to relate photon source strength, geometry, and duration of application to absorbed dose at a site of concern are divergence, attenuation, and the relationship between the exposure and absorbed dose.

Divergence

Divergence is a property that is the same for all photons regardless of their energy. Divergence refers to the gradual spreading apart of the photons as they travel outward from their source at the speed of light. As distance from the source increases the number of photons per unit area decreases. This is commonly embodied in the inverse square law referring to radiation which states that the intensity of the radiation is inversely proportional to the square of the distance from the source. If one is interested in the dose at two different sites and has knowledge of the distances from each site to a point on the source of radiation, it is a straightforward matter to compute the portion of the difference in dose due to difference in divergence. To reduce the effects of divergence, one places the source of radiation sufficiently far from both sites to achieve nearly equal divergence. For example, a site located at a distance of 0.5 cm from a point source of radiation would be exposed to 9 times as much radiation as a site located at a distance of 1.5 cm, in the absence of intervening material, due strictly to differences in divergence. If both distances are increased by 2 cm, the exposure rate to both sites is greatly reduced and the near site is then exposed to only about 56 percent more radiation than the far site. Few sources of radiation are truly point sources of radiation. The relationship of absorbed doses at two different sites of concern due to divergence considerations is determined by separately considering each portion of the source small enough to be considered a point. The net effect of divergence is then the appropriate average of the effect from each portion of the total source.

Attenuation

Attenuation is a term descriptive of the influence of the material between a source of radiation and the site of concern on the amount of radiation. Since attenuation refers to a reduction of intensity (the amount of energy per square centimeter per second incident at a point) other than by divergence, attenuation is often thought of as a reduction of energy. This is a valid conceptual framework provided the reduction in energy is thought of primarily as a reduction in the number of photons rather than a reduction of the energy of each photon.

Attenuation results from the absorption of the photons or the scattering of the photons away from their original direction of travel. The various types of processes involved are photoelectric absorption, Thomson scattering, Compton scattering, and pair production (Fig. 4–1). The probability of any given type of attenuation process is very strongly dependent upon the energy of a photon. Photons of low energy have a high probability of being completely absorbed. If they happen to be scattered, they tend to be scattered without significant change in energy. Photons with higher energies tend to be scattered rather

BEFORE INTERACTION   AFTER INTERACTION

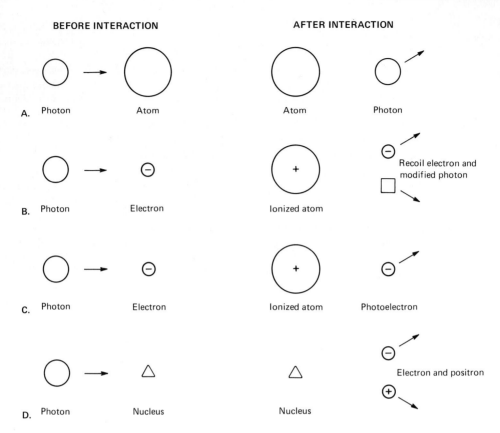

Figure 4–1. The basic processes most commonly occurring during the absorption of x and γ radiation. A. Thomson scattering of photon involves whole atoms and therefore essentially no change in characteristics of the photon. B. Compton scattering involves only a single electron resulting in modification of the photon and recoil of the electron. C. The photoelectric effect results in the complete disappearance of the photon with transfer of energy to the atom and electron. D. Pair production is the conversion of photon energy into the mass of an electron and a positron, occurring only if the photon energy is in excess of 1.02 MeV. In all but A, significant energy is transferred from a photon to a charged particle.

than absorbed. As they are scattered a substantial portion of their energy is transferred to the material resulting in the scattered photons having less energy than they had prior to scattering. Since scattering is actually an absorption and reemission of photon energy by orbital electrons, there is no conceptional difficulty in explaining how the photons can have a different energy after they are scattered.

The amount of attenuation of photons is a function of the energy of the photons, the type of material, and the thickness of material. Factors known as attenuation coefficients are used to predict the degree of attenuation. The negative of the product of the attenuation coefficient and the thickness of material (provided both are ex-

pressed in appropriate units) forms the natural logarithm of the fraction of the photons reaching a point with material present compared to the number that would reach the point without any material. This is commonly expressed by the formula

$$\frac{I}{I_0} = e^{-\mu t}$$

where I is the intensity with material present, I_0 is the intensity if no material is present, e is the base of the natural logarithms, μ is the absorption coefficient, and t is the thickness.

There are a variety of tabulated attenuation coefficients: mass attenuation coefficient, with and without coherent scattering effects included; mass energy-transfer coefficients; mass energy-absorption coefficients, to name a few. Each type of coefficient is intended for use in the solution of different types of problems of a physics nature. The "mass" part of the description enables the coefficient to apply to a material regardless of density.

As already mentioned, photons directed in such a manner that they would not normally strike the site of concern without material present may be scattered when material is present toward the site of concern. This fact may be accounted for by the attenuation coefficient selection or by the incorporation of a special factor known as a buildup factor. The net effect of attenuation and buildup is a function of the geometry of the situation. In treatment of patients with external sources of radiation the net effect of attenuation, buildup, material type, material thickness, geometry of irradiation, and energy of radiation may be accounted for by factors known as tissue-air ratios. If one can compute the amount of radiation that would be present at a site within a patient if only air were present between the site and source of radiation, then multiplication by the proper tissue-air ratio will yield the true value of the amount of radiation at the site with full accounting for the effects of the presence of the patient on the amount of radiation.

Relation Between Exposure and Absorbed Dose

The number of photons impinging upon a site of concern is usually not directly specified. It is customary to gauge the amount of photon radiation by a quantity termed exposure. Exposure is defined by the effect that the photons would have on air if air were present at the site of concern. The special unit of exposure is the roentgen. Practical difficulties make it impossible for national standardizing laboratories such as the U.S. National Bureau of Standards to provide exposure standards for photon energies above 3 MeV.

The relationship between exposure and number of photons is a complex function of the photon energy. However, the relationship between exposure and dose to air is a constant under conditions of charged particle equilibrium. Under conditions of charged particle equilibrium, also known as electron equilibrium, an exposure of one roentgen would result in an absorbed dose of

0.87 rad to air. Charged particle equilibrium is defined as a condition where the number and energy of energetic charged particles entering a site of interest is equal to the number and energy of energetic charged particles leaving the site of interest. This implies that any energy that is lost by the energetic charged particles is exactly compensated by transfers of energy from the photons to other "stationary" charged particles within the site of concern.

Interest in exposure is due to the development of equipment capable of measuring exposure very precisely in terms of the basic standards of mass, length, time, and charge. The conversion from exposure to absorbed dose in the simplest case is based on the assumption that the determining factor is the relative likelihood of interaction of photons with the material of concern compared to air. If the exposure at a site of concern in any material is known, and charged particle equilibrium is known to exist, the absorbed dose (rad) is computed by multiplying the exposure (R) by a factor known as the f factor. The f factor is defined by the equation

$$f = 0.87 \ u \Big|^{m}_{a}$$

where 0.87 is the rad/R factor for air, and $u\big|^{m}_{a}$ is the ratio of the mass energy absorption coefficients of the material, m, to air, a.

The use of f factors is a very necessary part of the methods of dose computation in the existing calibration systems. It must be appreciated, however, that there are many situations where this relationship is not so straightforward. Primarily, difficulty arises in locations close to the boundaries of the radiation field or at the interfaces of one material and another. For example, soft tissue inclusions in bone will generally have higher absorbed doses and lower exposure than they would if completely surrounded by soft tissue. This is due to an increased number of electrons being generated by increased photon interactions within bone compared to soft tissue.

Increased photon interaction means increased attenuation of photons, which accounts for the lower exposure of the soft tissue inclusions. Increased photon interactions means more electrons are set in motion in the bony matrix. These electrons are not totally stopped within the bony matrix, but rather, traverse the soft tissue inclusions resulting in the increased dose to the soft tissue. Some authors tabulate the f factor for soft tissue, and also the f factor for soft tissue inclu-

Table 4–1. VALUES OF f TO BE USED
IN THE CONVERSION,
DOSE (rad) = f EXPOSURE (R)*

PHOTON ENERGY (MeV)	MUSCLE	COMPACT BONE	SOFT-TISSUE INCLUSIONS IN BONE
0.05	0.926	3.58	2.27
0.1	0.949	1.46	1.36
0.2	0.963	0.979	1.03
0.5	0.957	0.925	
1.0	0.957	0.919	
2.0	0.955	0.921	

*From National Bureau of Standards: NBS Handbook 87, 1963.

sions in bone (Table 4–1). However, the f factor for soft tissue inclusions in bone does not fully describe the variation that exists between the exposure and the absorbed dose at various points within the soft tissue inclusions.

There are other examples pointing out that absorbed dose (a function of the concentration of energetic charged particles traversing the site) and exposure (a function of the photons directed at a point) are not always simply related by a single f factor appropriate to the irradiated material and the average photon energy. A familiar example is the skin sparing effect of high-energy radiation. Even though exposure is highest at the surface of a patient, the absorbed dose does not reach its maximum until electron equilibrium is achieved at a depth several millimeters below the skin surface (Table 4–2). The f factor relating exposure to absorbed dose based solely on the mass energy absorption coefficient does not apply until the depth of equilibrium is reached.

Another example of a complex relation between exposure and absorbed dose arises in the measured penumbra width for 35 MV x-ray beams. In external beam irradiation there is an area of rather uniformly irradiated material adjacent to areas that are shielded from the radiation. Between these two areas, there is a change in dose in a region known as the penumbra region. In most cases the width of the penumbra region is

felt to correspond very closely to a gradual change in exposure due to the size of the source and the degree of slope of the structures providing the shielding. One of the advantages of high-energy x-ray equipment is the potential to make source size very small, which should yield very small penumbral width. However, it has been found with measurements performed on a 35 MV linear accelerator, that the penumbra width is not as small as one would expect from geometrical considerations. The investigators responsible for the measurements of the dose distribution characteristics of the equipment report that the penumbra width is about as large as one would expect from a cobalt 60 unit. Furthermore, the penumbra width remains constant with depth. The conclusion of the investigators is that the penumbra is large because the energetic electrons set in motion in the irradiated area of the beam travel a distance approximately equal to the penumbra width before dissipating all of their energy.

The three examples of interfaces between soft tissue and bone, soft tissue and air, and irradiated and nonirradiated areas are intended to illustrate that a knowledge of exposure without additional information does not always yield a knowledge of absorbed dose. It is common practice in modern radiation therapy physics to focus attention on the absorbed dose at a site of concern rather than on the exposure at that site.

Table 4–2. TYPICAL DEPTHS OF PEAK
ABSORBED DOSE FOR VARIOUS
SUPERVOLTAGE BEAMS*

BEAM TYPE	DEPTH (cm)
Cobalt 60	0.5
4MV x-rays	1.2
6MV x-rays	1.5
8MV x-rays	2.0
10MV x-rays	2.5
22MV x-rays	4.0
45MV x-rays	5.0

*The exact depth is dependent on field size and type of absorbing material between source and skin.

RADIUM SOURCES

Historically, radium has played a very important role in the treatment of gynecologic malignancy. By placing the radium in encapsulated form as

close as possible to the cancerous mass, the cancerocidal effect is increased while the adjacent healthy tissue is spared by divergence effects.

Treatment failure is attributed to either the radio-resistance of the tumor cells or to inadequate arrangement of the sources to deliver an adequate dose to the deep seated portions of the tumor growth.

The radioresistant aspects of the typical malignant lesions of the uterine cervix require treatment doses as high as is possible to achieve without exceeding normal tissue tolerance. The analysis of treatment failure by Fletcher, et al. shows a high degree of correlation between recurrence or necrosis and cold or hot spots in the dose distribution. Hence, it is common practice nowadays to base treatment decision on computer-generated isodose curves for each radium placement.

A large variety of applicators have been developed to fix the relationship between the radium sources and the various anatomic structures in a favorable geometry. Many of these applicators, the so-called afterloading types, permit radioactive sources to be inserted after placement of the applicator to achieve an acceptable dose distribution.

Treatment results have also been improved by greater reliance on the use of external beams of radiation to deliver an adequate dose to those areas of likely tumor extension beyond the range of adequate radium dose.

The species of radium employed in medical radium sources is radium 226, which is part of the naturally occurring radioactive uranium 238 series. Within about a month after radium is sealed into a metallic capsule, decay equilibrium is established between the radium and at least 7 of the 11 radioactive daughter products. The eighth daughter product commonly referred to as radium D, also known as lead 210, has a half-life of 22 years. Hence, equilibrium with this daughter would be expected to occur over a much longer period of time. In 22 years, one-half of the equilibrium amount would be present. In 44 years, 75 percent of the equilibrium amount would be present. In 66 years, 87.5 percent of the equilibrium amount or radium D would be present, and so forth. The daughters of radium D have very short half-lives and would be expected to come to equilibrium level at about the same rate as radium D. The various materials included in the daughter products of radium 226 include isotopes of radon polonium, astatine, lead, bismuth, and thallium. The final daughter product of radium 226 decay is radium G (lead 206), which is a stable material. Since most of the important γ-ray photons arising from radium sources come from the decay of radium B (lead 214) to radium C (bismuth 214) and from the decay of radium C (bismuth 214) to radium C' (polonium 214), the exact level of radium D and its daughter products is of little concern to the dose from medical radium sources. The determining factor in the establishment of meaningful equilibrium activity in radium sources is the equilibrium activity of radon 222. Equilibrium with radon 222, the first daughter product of the decay of radium 226, occurs in a period of approximately one month due to the 3.83-day half-life of radon 222.

The chemical form of radium in modern sources is as an insoluble salt such as radium sulphate, to reduce the probability of biologic damage from accidentally ingested radium from a broken source. The specified radium content is based solely on the radium portion of the compound.

A variety of metallic shells have been employed, some of which do not hold up well. The best containment material is a platinum-iridium alloy.

Sources of unknown construction should be replaced.

Radium Exposure Rate Constant

Due to difficulties of measurement, the evaluation of the dose rate at various locations surrounding an encapsulated radioactive source is usually achieved by computation. Any measurements are usually restricted to simple checks at a few points. Calibration of the source is frequently accomplished by measuring the exposure rate in air at a large distance from the source in such a manner to exclude as much scattered radiation as possible. A key factor in the computation of dose rates and in source calibration is the exposure rate constant.

The exposure rate constant for any radioactive material is a number which, when divided by the square of the distance from a point source to a site of concern and multiplied by the activity of the source, will yield the true value of the exposure rate in air. Some exposure rate constants are based only on the γ emissions from the source, and ignore characteristic x-rays that are also contributing to the exposure. The preferred method of expressing exposure rate constants takes into account all photons emitted. Exceptions are noted. Typical units for exposure rate constants are R-cm^2/mCi-hour. The exposure rate constant for radium has some unique aspects. For radium sources the activity is indicated by specifying milligrams of pure radium 226. This is not a significant difference since the approximate activity of 1 mg of radium is 1 mCi. The exact value of millicuries per milligram for radium 226 is inversely proportional to the half-life of radium 226. In the relatively recent literature, recorded values of half-life for radium 226 range from 1590 years to 1620 years. The currently accepted value of half-life for radium 226 of 1600 years yields a value of 0.98873 millicuries per milligram. Another factor unique to the specification of the exposure rate constant for medical radium sources is the specification of the value for a source filtered by 0.5 mm of platinum rather than an unfiltered source. The value recommended by the International Commission on Radiation Units and Measurements (ICRU) is 8.25 R-cm²/mg-hour for a radium source filtered by 0.5 mm Pt. The exposure rate constant for an *unfiltered* 1 mg radium source is usually estimated by measuring the exposure rate from sources with different thicknesses of filtration and extrapolating to zero thickness. Using such a method, Shalek and Stoval derive a value of 9.09 R-cm²/mg-hour, which when combined with an effective filter thickness of .541 mm of platinum and a filter absorption coefficient of 0.170 per millimeter and a rad per roentgen conversion factor (f factor) of 0.957 yields good results in computing the dose rate in the vicinity of medical radium sources. Payne and Waggener, utilizing data compiled in nuclear data tables, compute an unfiltered exposure rate constant of 12.21 R-cm²/mg-hour. Their computation involves separate consideration of the effects of 72 tabulated x- and γ-ray energies. Since many of these energies are very low, they are rapidly absorbed by any filter. The computed value for a filtered radium source is thus essentially in agreement with the ICRU recommendation. The extremely complex spectrum of photons emitted by radium sources causes the carefully measured values of exposure rate constants to be more precise than the computed value. Accordingly, the value of the exposure rate constant for an unfiltered source and the effective wall thickness and absorption coefficient for the encapsulation metal are usually chosen to match reliable measurements.

Isodose Curves: Radium Sources

Typical construction for radium sources placed in vaginal or uterine cavities (intracavitary sources) consists of a platinum-iridium alloy capsule with external dimensions of 0.28 cm diameter by 2.17 cm total length. The radium is loaded into an internal space of 0.08 cm diameter by 1.5 cm active length. The total length is the dimension of importance when considering whether the information gleaned from radiographs of the source placement is sufficiently accurate to reconstruct the true geometric array of sources. The active length and the filtration of the source are most important dimensions in the determination of the true dose rate at any point of concern. Of course, the total amount of the radium and its uniformity of loading into the internal space are also factors affecting dose rate. The source just described has a filtration of 1.0 mm Pt. There are other available choices for active length, total length, and radium content.

The curves in Figure 4–2 depict surfaces of equal dose rate in the vicinity of a 10-mg radium capsule of the above construction. They are commonly referred to as isodose lines or curves. The entire figure would commonly be called an isodose chart. Since the drawing is two dimensional, it must be interpreted as only an indication of the three-dimensional shape of each isodose surface. In the case of a single straight radium source, the axis of the source is also the axis of symmetry about which the isodose curves may be spun in the mind's eye to comprehend the total surface geometry.

The isodose curves are computed rather than measured. This yields much better results than attempted direct measurement. The computer program is based on a Sievert intergral method employing an exposure rate constant of 8.25 R-cm²/mg-hour, an f factor of 0.957 rad/R, an attenuation coefficient of 1.50 cm⁻¹, an effective wall thickness of approximately 1.08 mm Pt, and a tissue attenuation correction of approximately 1 percent per centimeter. The program does not make full allowance for the details of the construction of the ends of the sources. The dose rates for which isodose lines are computed are specified by the computer operator. Maximum dose rates at the surface of the 10-mg sources are nearly 900 rad/hour. Dose rate at the surface of most applicators into which the radium capsules are loaded may be in excess of 300 rad/hour.

In reviewing the isodose chart of Figure 4–2, it should be noted that the distance between the 200 and 100 rad/hour surfaces is at most 0.25 cm. Halving the dose rate from 20 to 10 occurs in a distance of 0.75 cm, and from 10 to 5 in a distance of more than 1.0 cm. This leads to the general

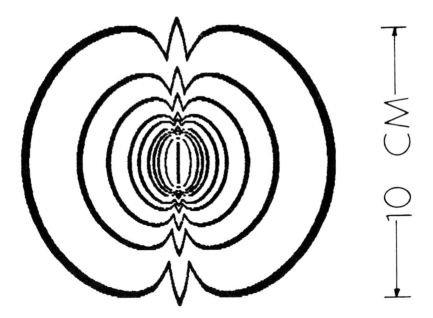

Figure 4–2. The isodose distribution curves for a 10 mg radium capsule. The vertical bar in the center represents the 1.5 cm active length of the source. The curved lines represent surfaces of equal dose rate. The highest dose rates are represented by the innermost curves. The values of dose rate shown are 200, 100, 70, 50, 30, 20, 10, 5, and 2 rad/hour. The thickness of each line represents the locus of points within ± 5 percent of the normal value. Gaps in the curves occur at points where the change in dose rate is greater than 10 percent in a distance smaller than 0.53 mm.

observation that the proper strategy to increase the thickness of tissue treated to an acceptably uniform dose the distance between the radium source and the tissue must be increased by an appropriately shaped spacer. In the case of treatment of cervix lesions the uniformity of dose to the lateral fornices of the vagina is improved by placing the radium in spacers, which are referred to either as ovoids in recognition of the shape required to match the source isodose surface, or as colpostates in recognition of their function to remain stationary in the colpos.

Another important aspect of the isodose curves of Figure 4–2 is the dip in the curves near the ends of the source. By proper orientation of the sources in the colpostats this region of low dosage can help to reduce the dose to bladder and rectum without reduction in the dose to the cervix or potentially involved lymph node groups. This orientation is generally assumed to be at right angles to the sources in the uterine tandem. However, several newer types of afterloading devices have colpostat sources oriented parallel to the uterine tandem with the argument that proper spacing and packing coupled with not positioning

sources too low in the uterine tandem produces resultant isodose summations that are completely acceptable. The distribution of dose from multiple sources is obtained by the summation of the isodose curves from each of the sources. It is common to refer to the diagram as either an isodose summation or dose distribution. Most such charts for brachytherapy are computed in terms of dose rate and are useful in deciding upon the time for removal of the radium sources. The comparison of alternate methods of treatment is achieved by comparison of the isodose summations.

Computer Techniques for Brachytherapy

The major change in brachytherapy in the past decade has been the increased reliance on computer techniques for establishing the dose rates at critical locations in the vicinity of brachytherapy sources. Prior to this development treatment was accomplished by adhering to a standard set of rules with computation of the dose to a few points, such as the junction of the ureter and uterine artery (point A), the obturator nodes (point B), bladder, and rectum. Due to the time requirements of hand computation few other points were ever evaluated. The rules defining the points of dose computation were frequently related to the geometry of the applicator and not anatomically reliable due to distortions of normal structural relationships by the disease present. Attempts to directly measure dose rate at the anterior rectal or posterior bladder wall were subject to error due to distortion of geometry by the placement of the probe.

With the advent of computer techniques it is now possible to obtain isodose summations in the plane containing any structures of interest, such as the external iliac, common iliac, and para-aortic lymph node groups. All that is required is a good set of AP and LAT radiographs with knowledge of magnification factors and structures such as cervix, bladder, and rectum visible, due to the presence of marking devices or contrast media. Points of greatest interest are simply marked directly on the film. Preparation for computer input performed by a competent operator yields results within a few hours. If the applicator is an afterloading type, the results of several potential loading arrangements are available in a matter of a few additional minutes (20 to 30) for each proposed change. The total time required is proportional to the total number of sources involved and the number of planes for which isodose summations are generated.

The limitations of computer techniques are the potential for the illusion of accuracy in the presence of serious errors. For this reason, most computer programs should be carefully evaluated for the results obtained with simple arrangements of one or two sources if they have not otherwise been documented. Items to check include investigation of the effects on results of the type applicator (many programs include no correction other than an "adjustment" of the source strength by the operator at time of data input), low dose rate truncation errors, and scaling of displays.

In some cases, such as Heyman packing of the endometrial space with multiple capsules, the computer technique will probably not accurately account for cross filtration effects of one source upon another. Hence, the tables derived by measurement for simulated packing are just as meaningful and easier to use.

There is little justification for computer techniques in the use of rigid vaginal applicators, since a set of isodose patterns for a few standard loadings need computation only once and may then be consulted forever after without gross error.

Implants of vaginal walls, etc., are normally planned to conform with Paterson-Parker rules. However, the results achieved are often not ideal. The computer generated isodose curves can be quite helpful in tough treatment decisions related to such implants. For guidance, a plan for an ideal distribution may be run. This is necessary to relate the Paterson-Parker roentgen with attendant hot and cold spots to the absorbed dose rate. Each Paterson-Parker roentgen per hour for an ideal implant is about 0.92 rad per hour for the same geometry. Appropriate tables must be consulted.

Radium Substitutes

Many radionuclides have been proposed as advantageous substitutes for radium. The principle advantages mentioned include the possibility to manufacture sources with smaller diameter, lesser shielding requirements, and lesser hazard in the event of breakage or loss. The disadvantage of the substitutes is the necessity to correct for their reduction in strength over a period of years and potential misunderstanding of whether their strength is specified in millicurie or milligram radium equivalent. Furthermore, the instruments of calibration may respond differently to the substitute, leading to additional error.

The substitute in most widespread use at present is cesium (Cs-137). The best method of employing it is to intercompare each source with a radium standard and assign a milligram radium equivalent. The sources are often used with the standard radium tables and computational methods. Greater accuracy requires the use of data developed specifically for Cs-137.

EXTERNAL PHOTON IRRADIATION

A major improvement in treatment results is obtained when intracavitary radiation therapy is combined with external irradiation of pelvic and/or abdominal structures. The intracavitary treatment is effective against accessible portions of the disease but is incapable of delivering adequate dose to likely areas of extension and spread of disease. External irradiation is capable of delivering fairly uniform dose over large volumes but is not as ideally suited as intracavitary source placement for delivering high dose in a localized volume. The optimum combination of both types of irradiation is a very significant factor in obtaining the best possible treatment results. Since the dose rates for the two types of irradiation are greatly different, simple addition of the total dose from each does not yield a meaningful index for comparing various combinations.

In the use of external photon radiation therapy for gynecologic malignancy, the types of problems that must be solved in the computation of machine settings to yield correct absorbed dose at the point of dose prescription include the influence of field shape, extended source skin distance, shielding bars, and multiple beam summation.

The resolution of these problems is mostly accomplished through the use of computer methods. Even so, it is helpful to understand the principles of hand computation so that the computer output may be verified at a few points. A variety of approaches have been developed. For brevity, the discussion in the section "Dosage Computations" will be limited to the tissue-air ratio (TAR).

Control of dose is ultimately achieved by setting a device that automatically terminates the exposure. In the case of cobalt 60 teletherapy units the device is a timer. If the dose rate in rad/minute is computed, the timer setting necessary to achieve the desired dose follows. The device to automatically terminate exposure for linear accelerators consists of an ionization chamber monitor with a digital readout. Each digit is commonly called a monitor unit, click, or RDL. If the dose rate in rad/RDL is computed, a monitor setting necessary to achieve the desired dose follows. In this case the number of RDL for a monitor-controlled machine is analogous to the number of minutes in a timer-controlled machine. However, the actual elapsed time for each RDL is usually a fraction of a second. In the following discussions related to computation of machine settings, it should be understood that the phrase "dose rate" usually has the special meaning for monitor-controlled machines of "rad/RDL" or its synonym, "rad/monitor unit." Whenever the true dose rate is of importance it will be specified as rad/minute.

Machine Calibration

Machine calibration is usually achieved by the use of an ionization chamber instrument. The size of the ionization chamber and magnitude and polarity of the collecting voltage are selected to suit the measurement conditions. Calibration factors to convert the instrument reading to exposure in roentgen are obtained through special calibration of the instrument at the National Bureau of Standards or at a Regional Calibration Laboratory. The factor is valid only for a specified beam quality and ambient air density. Corrections for variations in either are required. To convert the exposure to absorbed dose two alternate schemes are in use.

For cobalt 60 units with the chamber suspended in air the reading is converted to absorbed dose by employing the proper air density (temperature-pressure) correction, cobalt 60 calibration factor, an equilibrium attenuation factor, A_{eq} (0.985), and an f factor (0.957 rad/R for soft tissue). The resultant number is the absorbed dose at the center of a small sphere of tissue whose radius is equal to the depth of electronic equilibrium.

An alternate method replaces the A_{eq} and f factors with a C_λ factor to compute absorbed dose in water. An additional factor of approximately 0.99 is required to convert from absorbed dose in water to absorbed dose in tissue. The importance of C_λ is that values specific to the beam quality in question appear in standard tables and are always used in conjunction with the cobalt 60 calibration factor.

Either method results in about 0.94 rad at the center of the specified sphere for each R at the same point of irradiation by cobalt 60. For higher beam energies, equilibrium caps are placed over the ionization chamber to obtain a maximum reading and only the C_λ approach is valid.

Dosage Computations

Inverse square law computations are valid when considering the "dose rate" at the center of the equilibrium mass of tissue at different distances from the source. For extra precision, one may employ distances from a virtual source in the computations. However, this is not usually required. After computing this dose rate at the center of the equilibrium mass of tissue, the dose rate at the same position for a site of concern within a patient is determined by multiplication by the TAR. Tables of TAR for the beam quality in use (cobalt 60, 4MV, 6MV, etc.) are based on the beam size (normal to the central ray) and depth of overlying tissue (parallel to the central ray). The result is valid for sites of interest along the central ray.

If the TAR is considered to have independent components relating to attenuation of the primary radiation directed at the point and scattered radiation from other irradiated points, it is possible to deduce the absorbed dose for any beam shape. For points not on the central ray an additional factor describing the variation of primary beam intensity is also required. Several computer methods are based on the approach of separately considering primary and scattered radiation components to compute the dosage distribution.

For hand computations on the central ray the procedure would be as follows:

1. Approximate field shape by a rectangle.
2. Look up value of equivalent square for the rectangle.
3. Compute dose rate at the center of an equilibrium mass.
4. Look up TAR for beam quality, depth of overlying tissue, and equivalent square.
5. Multiply 3 by 4.

The computer approach is somewhat analogous, with the exception that approximations of shapes are eliminated and exact values of TAR rather than equivalent square values are employed.

Bibliography

Clarkson JR: A note on depth doses in fields of irregular shape. Brit J Radiol 14:265, 1941

Delclos L, Braun EJ, Herrera JR, Jr, Sampiere VA, Van Roosenbeck E: Whole abdominal irradiation by ^{60}Cobalt moving strip technique. Amer J Roentgen 96:75, 1966

Delclos L, Smith JP: Tumors of the Ovary. In Fletcher GH (ed): Textbook of Radiotherapy, 690. Philadelphia, Lea & Febiger, 1973

Durrance FY, Fletcher GH: Computer calculation of dose contribution to regional lymphatics from gynecological radium insertions, Radiol 91:140, 1968

Easson EL: Cancer of the Uterine Cervix. Philadelphia, Saunders, 1973

Fletcher GH: Textbook of Radiotherapy, 2nd ed. Philadelphia, Lea & Febiger, 1973

Fletcher GH, Wall JA, Bloedorn FG, Shalek RJ, Wooten P: Direct Measurement and isodose calculations in radium therapy of carcinoma of the cervix. Radiology 61:885, 1953

Hall EJ, Oliver R: The use of standard isodose distributions with high energy radiation beams —the accuracy of a compensator technique in correcting for body contours. Brit J Radiol 34:43, 1961

Hanks GE, Bayshaw MA: Megavoltage radiation therapy and lymphangiography in ovarian cancer. Radiology 93:649–654, 1968

Heyman J, Reuterwall O, Benner S: The Radiumhemmet experience with radiotherapy in cancer of the corpus of the uterus. Acta Radiol 22:14, 1941

Kottmeier HL: Surgical and radiation treatment of carcinoma of the uterine cervix. Gynaecol Clin Radiumhemmet 43, 1964

Krishnaswamy V: Dose distributions about ^{137}Cs sources in tissue. Radiology 105:181, 1972

Lewis GC, Jr, Raventos A, Hale J: Space-dose relationships for points A and B in the radium therapy of cancer of the uterine cervix. Amer J Roentgen 83:432, 1960

Linsley GS: Leakage Testing of Medical Radium Sources. Phys Med Biol 22:64, 1977

Meisberger LL, Keller R, Shalek RJ: The effective attenuation in water of the gamma rays of gold-198, iridium-192, cesium-137, radium-226, and cobalt-60. Radiology 90:953, 1968

National Bureau of Standards: Clinical Dosimetry. NBS Handbook 87, 1963

Payne WH, Waggener RG: A theoretical calculation of the exposure rate constant for radium-226. Med Phys 1:210, 1974

Radium Chemical Company, Inc.: Radium Radon Catalog. New York, Radium Chemical Co., 1973

Sampiere VA, Almond PR, Shalek RJ: Radiation measurement and dosimetric practices. In Fletcher GH (ed): Textbook of Radiotherapy. Philadelphia, Lea & Febiger, 1973

Shalek RJ, Stoval M: The M.D. Anderson method for the computation of isodose curves around interstitial and intracavitary radiation sources. I. Dose from linear sources. Am J Roentgenol, Rad Ther Nucl Med 102:662, 1968

Shalek RJ, Stoval M: Dosimetry in implant therapy. In Attix FH, Roesch WC, Tochlin E (eds): Radiation Dosimetry, vol III. New York, Academic Press, 743, 1969

Smoron GL: Strip-staggering: elimination of inhomogeneity in the moving-strip technique of whole abdominal irradiation. Radiology 104: 657–660, 1972

Stovall M, Lanzl LH, Moos WS: Brachytherapy isodose charts. Sealed radium sources. Atlas of Radiation Dose Distributions, vol IV. Vienna, International Atomic Energy Agency, 1972

Suit HE, Moore EB, Fletcher GH, Worsnop R: Modification of Fletcher ovoid system for afterloading, using standard-sized radium tubes (milligram and microgram). Radiology 81:126, 1963

Walstam R: The dose distribution in the pelvis in radium treatment of carcinoma of the cervix. Acta Radiol 42:237, 1954

Weast RC, Selby SM: Handbook of Chemistry and Physics, 47th ed. Cleveland, The Chemical Rubber Co, 1966

Wharton JT, Delclos L, Gallager S, Smith JF: Radiation hepatitis in ovarian carcinoma treated by whole abdominal irradiation. Amer J Roentgen 117:73, 1973

Wood RG: Computers in Radiotherapy—Physical Aspects. London, Butterworths, 1974

A Glossary of Terms Relating to Radiation Therapy

Absorbed dose. The energy deposited per unit mass, strictly definable for a localized area, with a size neither too large nor too small for changes in it to influence the ratio. Absorbed dose is never perfectly uniform throughout a clinically irradiated volume. Successful results in radiation therapy are dependent upon delivery of an adequate absorbed dose to all tumor-bearing structures. The tolerance, expressed in units of absorbed dose of unavoidably irradiated normal tissue, frequently is the basis for cessation of treatment of various regions of the body. There is good correlation between absorbed dose and the fraction of atoms at the site that are ionized. The most common unit of absorbed dose is the rad (1 rad = 100 erg/gm = 0.01 J/kg). The special name for the SI unit of absorbed dose, adopted in 1975, is the gray, symbol Gy, which has not as yet come into widespread use in medicine (1 Gy = 1 J/kg = 100 rad).

Absorption of radiation. This term refers to "collision-like" interactions between the individual particulate or quantum components of a beam of radiation and the subatomic parts of matter that occur at random during irradiation. Each interaction may result in partial or complete transfer of energy. Partial transfer of energy usually results in redirection (scattering) of the beam component. The total number of interactions determines the fraction of the radiation absorbed and depends upon the type of radiation and the thickness (total path length), density, and atomic number of the absorbing material. For some types of radiation, strategies to increase the absorption of radiation within cancerous tissue have been proposed, e.g., magnetic containment of electron beams or loading of target cells with material with high probability for interaction with neutron beams.

Accelerator (particle). A device that imparts kinetic energy to charged particles, such as electrons, protons, deuterons, and helium ions. These particles may be used in medical irradiation either directly or indirectly (via the production of x-rays or neutrons). See "Linear accelerator," "Van de Graaff Generator, Betatron," and "Cyclotron."

Afterloading techniques. The use of applicators for brachytherapy so designed that they may be quickly loaded with radioactive sources after placement within the patient. Such techniques have the advantage of eliminating radiation exposure of personnel involved in the operative placement of the applicator. Loading is usually performed in the patient's room a few hours after applicator placement. The most commonly used afterloading technique is that used in the treatment of carcinoma of the cervix.

Air dose. The absorbed dose that would be delivered to the center of an equilibrium mass of soft tissue were it situated at the point in question for the duration of treatment and otherwise surrounded by air only.

From CA: A cancer journal for clinicians. American Cancer Society 26:315, 1976

Arc therapy. External beam teletherapy in which the source of radiation is moved about the patient on an arc during treatment. Multiple arcs may be used. In some cases, the beam is stationary and the patient rotated in a vertical plane.

Attenuation of radiation. The reduction of intensity of radiation due to scattering and absorption of radiation. The effect on beam quality is dependent on the type of radiation and the conditions, e.g., a filter attenuates a photon beam usually with a resultant increase in the half-value layer; attenuation of a photon beam within a patient usually causes the half-value layer at depth to be lower than the half-value layer of the unattenuated beam due to the increased fraction of scattered radiation. Attenuation of electron beams always lowers the average beam energy.

Backscatter. Some of the radiation after entering the tissue will scatter back toward the surface. This portion of the radiation is called *backscatter*. Therefore, the peak absorbed dose may be equated to the air dose plus the backscatter dose.

Beam energy. *Beam energy* is usually stated only for particulate radiation beams (electrons, protons, neutrons, etc.). The average energy at the location where the entrance skin of the patient is placed is only one of many possible meanings of beam energy. Beam energy for x- or γ-ray sources is usually not stated directly but rather implied by stating the characteristics of the source and the half-value layer.

Beam quality. The spectral energy distribution of the radiation beam. *Beam quality* determines both the penetration of the beam through tissue and the relative absorption of the energy in different types of tissue. See "Beam energy," "X-ray voltage," and "Half-value layer."

Beam shaping. The use of special blocks, wedges, compensators, and other devices to create a treatment beam of the geometric proportions required for a treatment plan that is beyond the capabilities of the collimator.

Betatron. A megavoltage treatment machine capable of delivering high-energy x-rays and, in some instances, an electron beam. The electrons are accelerated in a circular orbit during a portion of the cycle of a low frequency alternating magnetic field.

Bolus. A material of density nearly equivalent to tissue placed within the treatment beam to compensate for unevenness of body contour or to enhance the absorbed dose to the skin.

Brachytherapy. The administration of radiation therapy by applying a radioactive material inside or in close approximation to the patient. This material may be contained in various types of apparatus, may be on the surface of plaques, or may be enclosed in tubes, needles, wire, seeds, or other small containers. Common materials for the administration of brachytherapy are radium, cobalt 60, cesium 137, iodine 125, and iridium 192. Brachytherapy is sometimes called plesiotherapy.

Brachytherapy—intracavitary application. The radioactive material, usually in the form of sealed sources, is placed into various types of applicators, which are then (or have been previously) inserted directly into a cavity in the patient through natural or surgically produced apertures. See "Internal sources of radiation" and "Afterloading techniques."

Brachytherapy—interstitial application. Direct insertion of sealed sources into tissue.

Buildup of absorbed dose. The initial increase in absorbed dose with depth. The depth of the peak absorbed dose may be several centimeters below the skin surface for high-energy radiation. This is due to the abrupt discontinuity in physical density between the irradiated tissue and air. The exact depth depends on the point at which there is a maximum concentration of charged subatomic particles that have been set in motion by absorption of radiation. The depth for cobalt 60 teletherapy is 0.5 cm.

Central axis depth dose. The relative dose along the central axis of a radiation beam usually expressed as a percentage of the peak absorbed dose.

Cesium 137 tubes. Used instead of radium for intracavitary insertions, especially in the treatment of carcinoma of the cervix. They are cylinders 2 cm in length and approximately 4 mm in diameter, usually calibrated as milligram equivalent of radium.

Cobalt 60 teletherapy. The administration of external beam radiation therapy by means of the 1.17 and 1.33 MeV γ rays of cobalt 60.

Collimator. The part of the radiation therapy machine that controls the size of the radiation beam usually through the use of movable blocks of heavy metal attached to a manual or motor-driven cranking mechanism. Some collimators have removable inserts usually called cones or diaphragms.

Conventional therapy. Treatment by x-ray beams other than supervoltage therapy.

Cyclotron. A circular accelerator used to produce

high-energy protons, deuterons, and other relatively heavy charged particles. Energies over 100 million eV may be achieved. Such particles may be used for basic physics research and to produce radionuclides for medical applications. They are sometimes used directly for experimental therapy or to produce neutron beams for therapy. The cyclotron utilizes high-frequency alternating voltage and a nonalternating magnetic field.

Depth dose. Dose at some specified depth or depths in tissue relative to the dose at a fixed reference point on the beam axis. Depth dose is usually expressed as a percentage.

Dose. See "Absorbed dose."

Dose distribution. See "Isodose distribution."

Dosimetry. Strictly, the measurement of dose; in practice, calculations, measurements, and other activities required for determining the radiation dose delivered.

Electrode. An x-ray tube component from which electrons emanate or to which they are attracted. The positive electrode is the anode, the negative one, the cathode.

Electron. The negatively charged part of an atom. When electrons strike a metal object at high energy, x-rays are produced.

Electron beam therapy. Treatment by electrons accelerated to high energies by a machine such as the betatron. Used mainly for lesions situated at or near the surface, electrons deliver maximum dose within the first few centimeters with the advantage, compared to x-rays, of rapidly diminished dose at greater depth. The depth of the high-dose region can be varied by varying the electron energy.

Electron volt. A unit of energy equal to 1.602×10^{-19} joule.

Entrance port. The area of the surface of a patient or phantom on which a radiation beam is incident.

Equilibrium mass. A spherical mass of tissue just sufficiently large to achieve a maximum absorbed dose at the center.

Exit dose. The dose at the point where the axis of the beam emerges from the patient.

Exposure. See "x-Ray and γ-Ray exposure."

External irradiation. A method of irradiation in which the source of radiation is outside the body. The radiation beam must always traverse the skin and some normal tissue except with a superficial lesion.

Field block. A quantity of attenuating material utilized to shape a treatment beam, especially to produce a beam of complex shape to shield

sensitive structures.

Field size. The measure of an area irradiated by a given beam. There are two most useful conventions. The first is the geometric field size; the geometric projection on a plane perpendicular to the central ray of the distal end of the collimator as seen from the center of the front surface of the source. The second is the physical field size, defined as the area included within the 50 percent maximum dose isodose curve at the depth of peak absorbed dose.

Filter. An insert, composed of various layers of different metals (aluminum, copper, tin), put in the x-ray beam to filter out the lower energy rays of the beam, and hence increase the half-value layer at the expense of reduced beam intensity.

Fractionation. A technique of administering radiation therapy in multiple doses over a number of days or weeks to achieve a maximum therapeutic ratio.

γ-Ray. A photon emitted from the nucleus of a radioactive atom, different from an x-ray photon only with respect to origin. A photon may be thought of as a moving electromagnetic disturbance that behaves sometimes as a wave and sometimes as a particle.

Gold 198. A radioactive isotope used in interstitial therapy encapsulated in metallic seeds or wire, or in intracavitary therapy in the form of a colloidal solution. The isotope has a half-life of 2.7 days and emits photons at 0.41 MeV, as well as electrons.

Half-life. The time required for the radioactivity to reduce to one-half of the value present at the start of the time period. After 10 half-lives the radioactivity will be reduced by a factor of 1024. Complete decay of a 1 mCi sample to a single undecayed nucleus depends on the decay constant and requires about 40 to 80 half-lives for medically useful materials. The effective half-life of an ingested source is determined by both the decay and excretion characteristics.

Half-value layer (thickness) (HVL). A measure of the quality of the radiation. Indicates the thickness of the specified material required to reduce the flux density of the radiation beam to one-half of its initial value. For example, the HVL of ^{60}Co is 11 mm of lead. Beams with identical geometry and HVL yield similar dose distributions.

High LET radiation. Energetic charged particles, or other radiation capable of liberating secondary charged particles, for which the spatial rate of energy loss (linear energy transfer of LET) is greater than about 10 keV/μ of particle path, i.e., a significantly higher rate than that for electrons. Examples are protons, pions, α-particles, and neutrons. Neutrons are uncharged but liberate protons and other charged particles in tissue.

Internal sources of radiation. See "Brachytherapy."

Removable implant. Radioactive material enclosed in needles, seeds, or tubes, which can be removed after the desired dose is given. Examples are radium 226 or cesium 137 needles and iridium 192 seeds or wire. The sources may be inserted directly into tissue or inside an applicator of some kind.

Distributed internal source. Intracavitary application of radiocolloids, such as Au-198, or P-32 (chromic phosphate), allows uniform distribution of radioactivity over serosal surfaces.

Inverse square law. The rule that accounts for the differences in dose rate or exposure rate at various distances from a point source of radiation due to the divergence of the radiation and not including any of the effects of absorption of radiation. Dose rate or exposure rate is inversely proportional to the square of the distance from a point source.

Isodose curve. A curve on which all points receive an equal radiation dose. A series of them will map out the relative intensities of a radiation field in a phantom or patient.

Isodose distribution. In a selected plane intersecting the treatment region, a representation of dose distribution by a set of curved lines, each line tracing the locations of points at which a specified dose is delivered. Its calculation is very time-consuming unless performed with the aid of a computer. The dose at each point is the sum of doses from all intersecting beams (in teletherapy) or from all implanted sources (in brachytherapy).

Isotopes. Atoms of identical chemical properties (same configuration of orbital electrons) but with a different atomic weight (different number of neutrons contained in the nucleus of the atom).

LD 50/30. A term that represents a single total-body irradiation lethal in 30 days to 50 percent of a group of animals. For man it is about 350 to 450 rads.

Linear accelerator. Essentially a pipe in which charged particles may be accelerated by applying a high-frequency potential difference during the particle transit along the pipe. In elec-

tron accelerators for radiotherapy, the pipe becomes a "waveguide," which may be a corrugated tube with continually increasing spacing between corrugations. Microwave frequency electromagnetic fields generated at one end travel down the waveguide in a wave of increasing velocity. A "bunch" of electrons injected at precisely the right time is accelerated by "riding the crest" of this wave. The electrons produce x-rays by striking a target at the far end of the tube.

Localization films. x-Ray films taken with various radiopaque markers in order to localize the position of the tumor relative to the external markings.

Megavoltage radiation. X or γ radiation with peak photon energies in excess of 1 MeV.

Multiple-port treatment. To deliver a high dose to the tumor volume at a depth without destroying the tissue near the surface, one may direct more than one radiation beam toward the tumor from different angles in order to increase the dose to the tumor relative to the skin.

NSD. The normal standard dose. The tolerance of normal tissue is influenced by dose rate, protraction and fractionation, as well as total dose. Computation of the NSD yields a value (measured in rets) that may correlate sufficiently well with late complications to permit more meaningful evaluation of alternate radiation therapy techniques.

Orthovoltage x-ray therapy. x-Ray therapy applied with a machine producing 140 to 600 kVp x-rays.

Peak absorbed dose. The highest value of absorbed dose on the central ray of a single radiation beam. The depth of peak absorbed dose ranges from several millimeters to several centimeters below the skin surface for megavoltage radiation beams. The exact depth depends on beam energy and field size.

Phosphorous 32. A radioactive isotope that emits β-rays and has a half-life of 14.3 days. It is administered internally, in solution, and tends to concentrate in the bone marrow, spleen, liver, and lymph nodes. Phosphorous 32 is used in colloidal form by injection into the serous cavities (pleural and peritoneal) in order to control the malignant accumulation of fluid.

Point A. An imaginary point described by Todd and Meredith as being 2 cm lateral to the cervical canal and 2 cm above the cervical os. The point is supposed to lie in the paracervical tissues.

Point B. A reference point that lies 3 cm lateral to point A and is used as a means of evaluating pelvic wall dosage.

Port film. A radiograph taken with the patient interposed between the treatment machine portal and an x-ray film. The purpose of this film is to demonstrate radiographically that the treatment field as externally set on the patient adequately encompasses the desired treatment volume and at the same time avoids adjacent critical structures.

Primary beam. The direct radiation beam emanating from the head of the irradiating unit. Scattered radiation is produced during the absorption of this beam.

Quality. The penetrating power of a photon beam, described in terms of half-value layer.

RAD. See "Absorbed dose."

Radioactivity. The property of certain nuclides of spontaneously emitting particles or γ radiation, or of emitting x radiation following orbital electron capture, or of undergoing spontaneous fission.

Radiation. The propagation of energy through space or matter. In radiology it can be divided into two main groups: charged particles (e.g., electrons, protons, α-particles) and electromagnetic (x-rays, γ-rays).

Radiation beam. A pathway of defined size and shape along which radiation is being propagated. The types of radiation involved include x-rays, γ-rays, electrons, and other particulate radiations.

Radium 226. A radioactive isotope commonly used for radiotherapy. It has historical importance in that it was the first isotope to be used medically and is used as a radiation standard. The half-life is about 1600 years and photons of many discrete energies are emitted up to a maximum of 2.2 MeV. Radium compounds are sealed in metal needles and tubes for interstitial and intracavitary insertions.

REM. (Roentgen-Equivalent-Man). Special unit of the radiation protection quantity "dose equivalent." Dose equivalent is obtained by multiplying absorbed dose by a "quality factor," which has higher values for higher LET radiations. When dose is expressed in rads, dose equivalent is in rems.

RET. See "NSD."

Roentgen (R). An x-ray or γ-ray exposure of 2.58 $\times 10^{-4}$ C/kg.

Rotation therapy. External beam teletherapy in which the source of radiation moves circumferentially around the patient while being centered in the volume of interest. Some devices allow the patient to rotate in the vertical plane within a stationary beam.

Scatter. When a material is in the path of a radiation beam, the material not only absorbs some of the radiation, it also scatters some in all directions, usually reducing the quality of the beam at the same time. Therefore, the radiation received at a point has two components: scattered and primary. It follows that the exposure rate at a point in air will be increased if a patient or phantom is placed behind it. This is caused by "backscattered" radiation.

Simulation film. x-Ray films taken with the same field size, source-to-skin distance, and orientation as a therapy beam in order to mimic the beam and for visualization of the treated volume on an x-ray film.

Simulator. A radiation generator operating in the diagnostic x-ray range with the mechanical capability to orient a radiation beam toward a patient with parameters imitating that proposed for therapy, and affording direct x-ray fluoroscopic visualization and roentgenographic images of the area. Machine is not capable of delivering radiation therapy.

Skin sparing. Because of the buildup of the absorbed dose in supervoltage radiation deep to the skin, the skin surface does not receive the maximum dose delivered. The skin reaction is therefore much less than would be expected from conventional radiation.

Source-skin distance (SSD). The distance from the source of radiation to the skin of the patient.

Split course. A course of radiotherapy delivered in two or more parts separated by planned rest periods.

Superficial therapy. Treatment with an x-ray machine of relatively low voltage, approximately 100 kV. Penetration is not large.

Supervoltage therapy. Treatment with x-rays or γ-rays with energies in excess of 600 KeV. Includes greater than 600 kVp x-rays, cesium 137, and cobalt 60.

Teletherapy. The delivery of radiation treatments to the patient from a source located far (usually more than 50 cm) from the region to be treated.

Tolerance dose. The maximum radiation dose that may be delivered to a given biologic tissue at a specified dose rate and throughout a specified volume without producing an unacceptable change in the tissue.

Treatment field. A plane section of a beam, perpendicular to the beam axis, as defined by the collimator of the treatment machine. Term often used synonymously with treatment port.

Tumor volume. That volume encompassing all known or presumed tumor.

Van de Graaf generator. An electrostatic machine that utilizes a moving belt to carry electrons to a high-voltage collector or terminal. The accumulation of electrons causes the high voltage, which may then be used to accelerate charged particles through electrostatic forces.

x-Ray and γ-ray exposure. A measure of the amount of x or γ radiation directed at a point. Knowledge of the exposure does not convey any information about the size of the radiation beam. Converting a knowledge of exposure to a knowledge of absorbed dose requires additional information about beam energy and the proximity to abrupt changes in material density and/or atomic number. Exposure is evaluated by measuring or computing the resultant ionization effect the same amount of radiation would have on air, expressed in units or electri-cal charge per unit mass. An exposure of 2.58×10^{-4} C/kg is an exposure of one roentgen, symbol R. Sometimes, the term exposure is used to mean exposure time.

x-Ray voltage. An indication of beam quality. The voltage stated may not actually be present in the machine unless the acceleration of the tube current is by electrostatic forces. Full specification of beam quality may be made by listing the x-ray voltage, the filtration, and the half-value layer. The peak voltage in KV is numerically the same as the peak x-ray photon energy in KeV. The average photon energy is much lower.

x-Rays or x-radiation. Electromagnetic radiation of energy greater than 100 eV, emitted when electrons (or other charged particles) experience a sudden loss of energy, either falling into a vacant orbital energy level of an atom (in which case "characteristic" x-rays are produced) or being sharply deflected in the field of an atomic nucleus (in which case "bremsstrahlung" x-rays are produced).

Chapter 5

Basic Aspects of Gynecologic Cancer Chemotherapy

H. GEORGE MANDEL, Ph.D.

GENERAL PRINCIPLES

The Present Status

Effective gynecologic cancer chemotherapy relies on the use of drugs that exploit characteristic differences between tumor cells and normal cells. Knowledge of such differences would be useful in designing agents that selectively kill the malignant cells without producing serious, irreversible harm to the vital tissues and organs of the patient. It is remarkable when one considers the immense talent, human effort, and financial resources that have been focused on such investigations, that no clear, qualitative biochemical distinction between tumor and nontumor cells has yet been uncovered to guide the oncologist in the selective eradication of cancer. Perhaps it is even more remarkable that in the absence of this knowledge, by relying on small quantitative differences between tumor cells and most types of normal cells, it has been possible to provide long-lasting remissions and occasional cures with antitumor drugs. This application of drugs in the treatment of cancer has,

more often than not, been quite empirical. It can only be hoped that with the greater knowledge that has been accumulating from these successes, a more rational underlying basis will be uncovered for the development of better drugs and, at least as important, for the more effective use of presently available chemotherapeutic agents.

Indeed, chemotherapy of human cancer has made major strides, especially in the last few years. It has been concluded that drugs can produce normal life expectancies in patients afflicted with one of 11 types of cancers (Table 5–1).[1] For example, for choriocarcinoma, where the level of urinary gonadotropins has provided a reliable index of tumor growth, up to 90 percent of patients with metastases are anticipated to achieve a normal life expectancy because of chemotherapy, and almost 100 percent are cured in the absence of metastases.[2] For the majority of tumors, however, there is no sensitive assay of the status of the malignancy. These tumors usually grow more slowly, and drug treatment has been palliative but not curative. It should be kept in mind, however, that because of the relative effectiveness of and greater experience with surgery and radiation, treatments that were available long before the advent of successful chemotherapy, chemotherapy

Supported by research grants CA 02978 from the National Cancer Institute, U.S. Public Health Service, and CI 110 from the American Cancer Society.

**Table 5–1.   TUMORS FOR WHICH
CHEMOTHERAPY PLAYS A CRITICAL
ROLE IN PRODUCING NORMAL
LIFE EXPECTANCY***

TUMOR	*% ESTIMATED TO HAVE ACHIEVED NORMAL LIFE EXPECTANCY*
Wilms' tumor	90
Choriocarcinoma	80
Retinoblastoma	75
Ewing's sarcoma	70
Burkitt's lymphoma	70
Acute lymphocytic leukemia	50
Hodgkin's disease	40
Mycosis fungoides	50
Rhabdomyosarcoma	50
Diffuse histiocytic lymphoma	25
Embryonal testicular cancer	10

*Adapted from Zubrod: In Pharmacological Basis of Cancer Chemotherapy, 1975, p. 11. Courtesy of Williams and Wilkins.

has been rarely evaluated early in the patient's disease. Even if drugs were used, the protocols would not be considered adequate by present-day standards. Only once it had become obvious that other treatment modalities had failed did the patient receive antitumor chemotherapy, and such a patient would be expected to be at a higher risk of drug failure as well. Recent reports on the treatment of breast cancer provide strong evidence that adjuvant chemotherapy immediately following mastectomy significantly prolongs the disease-free interval and probably survival.[3] This achievement confirms the belief in the efficacy of treatment of this disease with antitumor agents, especially if combined with other modalities of therapy.

Basis of Chemotherapy in Model Cell Systems

Animal models, which have permitted the elucidation of the selective inhibition of tumor growth, have been available for many years. Neoplasms have been developed for transplantation, mainly in the mouse and the rat. These implants grow as solid or ascites tumors and kill their hosts with remarkable reproducibility. Selective toxicity of antitumor drugs can thus be measured by observ-

ing the increase in survival time of the tumor-bearing rodents, or the reduction of the rate of progression of weight or size of the tumor while the host does not succumb to drug toxicity. These procedures have led to the discovery of numerous tumor-inhibitory drugs and have provided extremely valuable information regarding mechanism of drug action, pharmacokinetics, toxicity, and dose scheduling.[4] A remarkable correspondence in toxicity between the animal system and man has also been demonstrated (Fig. 5–1),[5] and toxicities observed in man have almost always been produced in laboratory animal systems.

Much basic understanding of the action of drugs has been derived from the kinetics of cell growth. For example, the L1210 mouse leukemia system has been studied most carefully because it is a relatively simple and reproducible line of malignant cells, which has served as a useful tool for selecting drugs later found to be effective against human cancer. It was observed that the survival time of mice receiving ascites tumor cells is inversely related to the number of tumor cells inoculated. A plot of this relationship (Fig. 5–2) demonstrates that for this model system cell death invariably occurs when the tumor cell population reaches a characteristic number, that cells grow at a logarithmic rate, and that the introduction of a single tumor cell eventually produces death from the neoplasm.[6] It should be noted that in this sys-

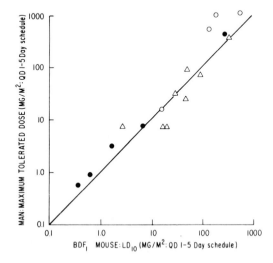

Figure 5–1.   Correspondence of toxicity of variety of antitumor drugs in man and the mouse, when calculated on a mg/m² basis. o, antimetabolites; Δ, alkylating agents; •, other drugs. (From Freireich et al: Ca Chemother Rep 50:219, 1966)

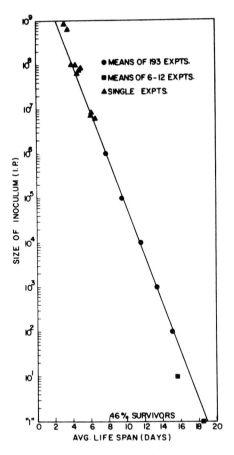

Figure 5-2. Survival time of mice inoculated with varying numbers of L1210 leukemic cells. Note ability of a single tumor cell to kill host. (From Skipper et al: Ca Chemother Rep 35:1, 1964)

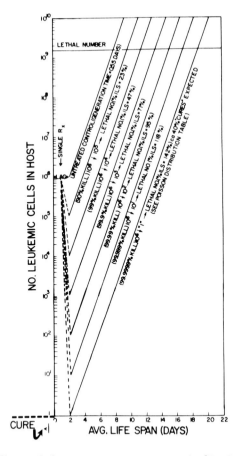

Figure 5-3. Prolongation in survival of L-1210 ascites tumor-bearing mice by drugs producing various percent cell kills. Note that animals die when certain tumor cell number is reached, unless tumor burden has been reduced below one, thereby resulting in cure. (Adapted from Skipper et al: Ca Chemother Rep 35:1, 1964)

tem there is little or no heterogeneity in the cells, that the cells are ascites cells with none of the vascular limitations of solid tumors, and there are few if any immunologic or other host interactions.

The addition of a tumor-inhibitory drug reduces the tumor population by a characteristic percentage (i.e., a "first-order" kill) regardless of the actual number or concentration of tumor cells present. Thus, a particular agent with a "one-log cell kill" reduces the cell concentration by 90 percent. The remaining 10 percent of cells, after a brief delay, then resume their former rate of proliferation, eventually leading to the death of the host, at the predicted time. Figure 5-3 demonstrates the enhancement in survival time with agents producing various percents of cell kill.[6] Once the kill exceeds the order of magnitude of

the cell population, so that, statistically, less than one cell remains, the drug becomes curative.

Unfortunately, for most clinical situations this cell kill potential of a drug is relatively limited, in comparison to the size of the cell population. Repeated administration of this drug may then permit an enhanced destruction of tumor cells, providing that host toxicity remains tolerable and resistant cell lines are not selected out by the drug. Figure 5-4[7] indicates how the repeated application of a chemotherapeutic agent killing only 90 percent of cells may be used to destroy a large tumor cell population, although concomitant toxicity probably would become prohibitive. On the other hand, if the tumor burden is relatively

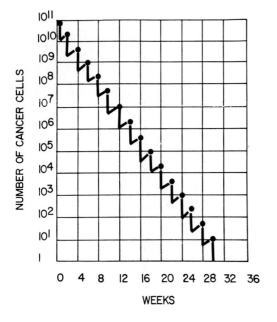

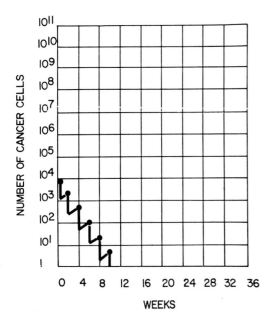

small, a few cycles of chemotherapy are more likely to be tolerated by the host and thus may produce a tumor-free animal. Unfortunately, at the present time the usual inability to detect tumors early in a clinical situation makes the model less realistic. For example, a 1-cubic-cm sample of tumor, a not uncommon size at the time of diagnosis, may represent 10^9 cells. Since death for cancer victims has been shown to occur at 10^{12} tumor cells, a relatively large proportion of the life of a clinically recognizable tumor has already taken place when it is finally detected. Therefore, the importance of early diagnosis of malignancy becomes even more essential. Alternatively, the tumor population may be reduced by surgery or radiation, so that adjuvant chemotherapy has a logical basis.

In the model ascites system, cell doubling time remains constant almost throughout the entire life of the tumor. In a solid tumor system, however, eventual interferences with tumor cell accessibility to nutrients gradually slows tumor doubling time and reduces the rate of proliferation of cells (Fig. 5–5).[8]

Dividing cells may be viewed as undergoing a sequence of functional phases that make up the mitotic cycle. Time spent in mitosis takes up only a limited proportion of this cell cycle, which is the only phase of the cycle that can be identified microscopically. Following the completion of mitosis, cells enter the G_1 phase which permits ribonucleic acid (RNA) and protein synthesis in preparation for the S phase, or deoxyribonucleic acid (DNA) synthesis phase. This phase is followed by the G_2 phase where there is additional RNA and protein synthesis, leading again to mitotic division and a repetition of the cycle (Fig. 5–6).[9] Alternatively, a cell may reach maturity, or may enter a G_0 phase where cells capable of cell division are temporarily resting while not traversing the cell cycle. These cells in G_0 may eventually return to the active mitotic cycle or they may die without further division.

Most antitumor drugs inhibit only proliferating cells, malignant or normal. Thus, a major difference between tumor and normal cells may relate to the relative percentage of the cell population in mitotic cycle (i.e., the growth fraction), and the selective effect of drugs may well be explained by the increased sensitivity of tumor cells with their characteristic high growth fraction, compared to normal cells. For the model ascites system, the growth fraction stays at approximately 100 percent, whereas for the solid tumor it diminishes

Figure 5–4. Top: Repeated treatment (●) should reduce tumor burden by a constant percentage each time, while permitting some regrowth between treatments. Eventually all tumor cells will be killed, but toxicity to normal tissue would probably intervene. Bottom: With lower initial tumor cell burden, likelihood is greater that tumor cells may be completely destroyed before toxicity becomes limiting. (Adapted from Connors: In Harris: What We Know About Cancer, 1970. Courtesy of Allen and Unwin)

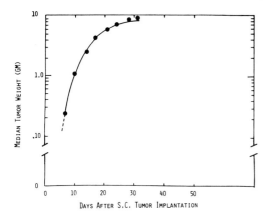

Figure 5-5. In contrast to ascites tumor cells growing in suspension at a constant but logarithmic rate, solid tumor doubling time decreases progressively with proliferation. (Adapted from Griswold: Ca Chemother Rept, Pt 2 3:315, 1972)

with increasing enlargement. Toxicity, on the other hand, results from the effects of the drugs on normal cells in mitotic cycle. Knowledge as to the localization of action of antitumor drugs within the mitotic cycle, therefore, can help explain the mechanism of their effectiveness and may suggest means of enhancing their carcinostatic properties.

Drugs which interfere with DNA formation

thus kill the cell in the S phase of its cycle. Antimetabolite drugs, such as methotrexate, fluorouracil, the thiopurines, as well as the drug, hydroxyurea, block tumor growth during this phase of the cell cycle. Drugs which block RNA synthesis will inhibit during the S phase, as well as the G_1 and G_2 portions of the cycle. Thus, drugs like methotrexate, the thiopurines, and fluorouracil, which in addition to limiting DNA synthesis, also block RNA formation, are "self-limiting" inhibitors of cell growth because they reduce the ability of the cell to enter S phase. The vinca alkaloids and colchicine act on spindle formation and inhibit mitosis specifically. All of the above drugs are termed cell-cycle specific, since they require a cell in cycle.

Cells in the nonproliferative or G_0 phase are impervious to the action of these drugs, and thus, tumors with a low growth fraction are resistant to antimetabolites. Other antitumor drugs, especially alkylating agents and certain antibiotics, may be active during the G_0 phase, as well as during the cell's progression through the cycle. These cell cycle nonspecific drugs therefore may be useful against tumors with a large fraction of resting cells. Their application may reduce the tumor burden sufficiently so as to encourage the remaining G_0 cell population to return into mitotic cycle, at which time the cells may then become vulnerable to other drugs.

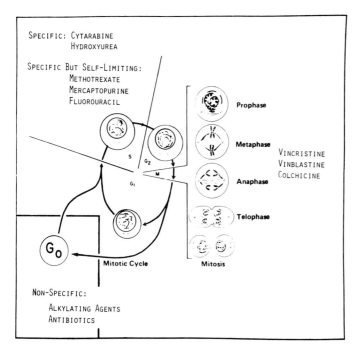

Figure 5-6. Attempt to localize action of antitumor drugs at specific phases of mitotic cycle. Certain drugs are effective during the resting or G_0 phase. (Adapted from Karnofsky, Clarkson: Annu Rev Pharmacol 3:357, 1963)

Problems Limiting Success of Cancer Chemotherapy

A review of some of the problems the physician faces in applying chemotherapy may explain why it has taken so long to develop cures for cancer patients. A better appreciation of the adversities hampering successful therapy may assist in devising a more effective chemotherapeutic program for a particular patient.

Antitumor Effectiveness Versus Inherent Toxicity

There is a lack of a recognized qualitative biochemical difference between malignant and normal tissue, which can become the rational basis for producing destruction of the tumor selectively. The existence of major biochemical dissimilarities between microorganisms and mammalian tissue, for example, now explains the effectiveness of most antimicrobial chemotherapy. Penicillin inhibits bacterial cell wall formation, a process that has no analogy in man. Tetracycline and streptomycin interfere with microbial protein synthesis, a process that differs from that in most mammalian tissue. Antifungal antibiotics interact with the membranes of susceptible microbes selectively, and the sulfonamides competitively inhibit a biochemical reaction required by sensitive bacteria which does not exist in man. It should be kept in mind, of course, that these biochemical differences were not recognized until several decades after the drugs had been introduced into clinical practice.

The problem of selectivity of action is obviously greater when differentiating between a microbial and a mammalian cell on the one hand, and two eukaryotic cells on the other hand. Although cancer cells may be characterized by a failure of normal mechanisms of growth regulation, no such abnormality is presently recognized which appears exploitable by the use of a drug. In specific instances where a tumor has derived from an organ characterized by a distinct biochemical feature, such as the thyroid gland's ability to accumulate iodine, the sensitivity of the adrenal cortex to mitotane, or the selective destruction of the pancreatic island cells by streptozotocin, chemotherapy can be devised which attacks that tumor preferentially and with limited general systemic toxicity. The use of the sex hormones similarly is valuable because of their relative action on specific target tissue. Usually, however, there will be

toxicity in biochemically similar normal tissues that may increase in severity as the malignancy becomes less differentiated and less sensitive to chemotherapy. One biochemical difference, exploited for its possible antitumor selectivity, is based on a requirement for the amino acid asparagine by some tumor cells in contrast to normal cells. This discrepancy has been responsible for the clinical introduction of asparaginase; however, this enzyme, which interferes with the availability of asparagine to the tumor requiring this component for its nutrition, has shown success limited only to acute lymphocytic leukemia.

In practice, many individual differences between a particular tumor cell and a normal cell have been uncovered, but there has been no single biochemical feature that pertains only to one or the other category exclusively. More careful examination, usually aided by the availability of effective anticancer agents, has suggested numerous potential sites where small quantitative differences between tumor and normal tissue could be exploited. The specific features of cells that have suggested such potential opportunities, and that will be described more extensively under those drugs where applicable, include selective uptake of drugs into tumors, enhanced anabolism in tumors of "pro-drugs" requiring activation, diminished catabolism of drugs by tumors, diminished repair of tumor cell damage, and reduced availability of a protecting metabolite in tumor tissue.[10]

The limited selectivity of action of anticancer drugs is typified in Figure 5–7, where antitumor effectiveness is expressed as an enhancement of survival time of tumor-bearing mice. As the dose of such a drug is increased, there is an increase in life span compared to control animals bearing the tumor. Further increases in the drug dose, however, will eventually reduce survival time again due to lethal drug toxicity.[11]

Recently, it has been recognized that recovery from the damage to the tumor cells produced by a tumor-inhibitory drug may be more protracted than that of normal host cells. The judicious application of a second dose of drug during the interval following return of normal tissue functions but prior to recovery from drug treatment of tumor cells has been successful in further promoting increased antitumor selectivity. It would appear at the present time that this approach of selective recovery from cell damage after chemotherapy may be of enormous potential benefit in enhancing the antitumor activity of presently

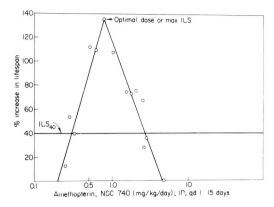

Figure 5–7. Effect of increases in dosage of methotrexate (amethopterin) on survival time of L-1210 tumor-bearing mice. Low drug doses increase survival time by inhibiting tumor growth, higher doses reduce survival time due to host toxicity. ILS_{40} refers to dose producing a 40 percent increase in life span. (From Goldin, Carter: In Holland, Frei (eds): Cancer Medicine, 1973, p 611. Courtesy of Lea and Febiger)

available drugs. Evidence of the occurrence of this phenomenon will be presented during the subsequent discussion on anticancer agents.

For a long time it was believed that human tumor cells grow more rapidly than normal cells. This view was based in part on the models for chemotherapy of animals bearing malignancies transplanted under standardized laboratory conditions. Although many rodent tumor lines do proliferate rapidly, certain normal cell populations do likewise, frequently growing even more rapidly than tumors. Partly because these model systems have served as screens, the identified antitumor drugs are most active against rapidly growing cells and usually are found to inhibit the biosynthesis of nucleic acids. The application of these drugs in clinical chemotherapy undoubtedly explains their relative success against tumors with short doubling times, such as in acute leukemia, in contrast to the slower growing solid tumors, such as those of the breast or lung (Table 5–2).[12] For identical reasons, however, bone marrow, intestinal epithelium, hair roots, and a few other normal cell populations with rapid turnover are also sensitive to the inhibitory actions of the drugs. Consequently, the typical toxicity of most anticancer drugs is directed against the hematopoietic and gastrointestinal systems, and may include alopecia (Table 5–3).[13] Nevertheless, it should be appreciated that these drugs, under precisely de-

fined protocols, have also produced successful selective chemotherapy in many instances where tumor growth was not rapid. It appears that this area of research must be further explored to fully exploit the drugs' potential.

There are some extremely significant distinctions between populations of tumor and normal cells with respect to their relative growth fractions, and exploitation of these differences appears extremely promising. As described before, drugs that act as cellular growth inhibitors because they block biosynthesis may therefore inhibit preferentially those cell populations having a higher growth fraction. Although bone marrow cells, like tumors, have a relatively high growth fraction, usually the stem cell population of bone marrow has enough resting cells that its growth fraction is less than that of the tumor. Precise dose scheduling is required to optimize conditions so that inhibitory drug levels will prevail during that cell cycle phase when tumor populations are maximally sensitive to the drug, in contrast to normal cells. The large pool of normal stem cells out of cycle will then repopulate the host and provide preferential protection. Scheduling of drug dosages is usually arrived at empirically, but there is rationale for exploitation for selective toxicity. At the present time this approach is being explored extensively because of its likelihood of greater therapeutic benefit in man.

Table 5–2. DOUBLING TIMES OF HUMAN TUMORS AND REGIME REQUIRED FOR EFFECTIVE CHEMOTHERAPY*

TUMOR	DOUBLING TIME (DAYS)	REGIMEN GIVING LONG SURVIVAL
Burkitt's lymphoma	1.0	Single drug
Choriocarcinoma	1.5	Single drug
Acute lymphocytic leukemia	3–4	Drug combination
Hodgkin's disease		Drug combination
Colon	80	—
Lung	90	—
Breast	100	—

*From Zubrod: Proc Nat Acad Sci 69:1042, 1972. Tumors with long doubling times are much less responsive to chemotherapy.

Table 5–3.   CHARACTERISTIC TOXICITY OF ANTITUMOR DRUGS
TO BONE MARROW AND GI TRACT*

DRUG	BONE MARROW	GI TRACT	HAIR ROOT	LIVER	OTHERS
Alkylating agents					
Nitrogen mustard	++++	+			
Melphalan	++++	+			
Cyclophosphamide	++	+	+++		Bladder
Busulfan	+++				Endocrinological Addison-like syndrome Pulmonary fibrosis
Chlorambucil	+++	+			
Dibromomannitol	+++				
Mitomycin C	++++	++			
Antimetabolites					
Methotrexate	++++	++++	+	+++	Osteoporosis
6-Mercaptopurine	+++	+	0	++	
6-Thioguanine	++		+		
5-Fluorouracil	++++	++++		0	Neurological
Cytosine arabinoside	+++	+	0	+	
Mitotic inhibitors					
Vincristine	+	+	++++		Myoneural junction Dorsal root ganglion
Vinblastine	++	+++	+		
Antibiotics					
L-Asparaginase		+		+++	Pancreatitis Diabetes mellitus Anaphylaxis, CNS Clotting defects
Actinomycin D	+++	+++	+++		Skin
Daunorubicin	++++				Cardiac failure
Doxorubicin	+++		++		Cardiac failure
Mithramycin	++++	+		++	Clotting defects
Streptozotocin				+	Renal tubular acidosis Diabetes mellitus
Miscellaneous synthetics					
BCNU	++++	+			
Procarbazine	+++	++	+		CNS
Dacarbazine	+++	+			
Hydroxyurea	+++	+			

*Adapted from Zubrod: In Sartorelli, Johns (eds): Antineoplastic and Immunosuppressive Agents I, 1974, p. 4. Courtesy of Springer.

Imperfect Models for Human Tumors

Another difficulty that complicates the search for better therapeutic agents is the lack of pertinent animal model systems that mimic human tumor(s). Although several such laboratory models have been used extensively, one wonders how many agents that would have been effective in man have failed in the animal screens and are now beyond consideration. Fortunately, there is a strong similarity in the effectiveness of drugs against transplanted and spontaneous tumors. The relative slowness of the disease in man, the usual absence of biochemical markers that permit a rapid quantification of the status of a tumor, the individualities of tumors, and even the heterogeneity of a particular tumor population require that readily reproducible and serviceable animal model systems be available for evaluating chemotherapeutic agents. It has been fortunate that many additional drugs have become established by serendipity.

Incomplete Knowledge About Pharmacokinetics

It is becoming increasingly clear that the scheduling of a drug can have enormous impact on its antitumor selectivity. Because of the relatively low therapeutic index of the drugs, it is essential that the tumor be exposed to relatively high concentrations of the active drug moiety for at least a minimum time period and that normal tissue may tolerate these conditions. Putting this principle into practice is further complicated for those anticancer agents that must first be metabolized to active derivatives, such as the purine and pyrimidine antimetabolites.[14] Although the overall pattern of pharmacokinetics including metabolism may be recognized for the administration of a single dose of an individual drug, multiple-dose scheduling may produce major alterations in the physiologic disposition of anticancer drugs and needs to be better understood to materially improve the clinical application of the drugs.

Poor Host Defenses

The normal body's immunologic defense against an invading tumor cell population is unreliable and still inadequately understood, operates only if the tumor mass is relatively small, and becomes even less effective with age. In contrast to the analogous situation with most microbial infections, which the body's defense mechanisms usually can control effectively with only a bacteriostatic drug, in most clinical situations an antitumor agent must virtually kill all tumor cells to prevent a lethal recurrence of the tumor. Drug therapy therefore, should be more intensive, but actually must be practiced sparingly because of the lack of antitumor selectivity. Attempts are currently in progress to enhance immunologic host defenses by the use of adjuvant therapy with immunostimulants such as Bacillus Calmette-Guerin (BCG).

In addition, most of the antitumor drugs have immunosuppressant properties, which further reduce the body's natural capacity to protect itself against tumor infiltration. As tumor growth progresses, the body's diminishing immunosurveillance ability compounds the difficulties of therapy, often leading to death by secondary microbial infections that no longer respond to any treatment. Treatment schedules, therefore, must be developed to minimize immunosuppression while permitting adequate therapeutic effectiveness.

Protected Tumor Sanctuaries

Frequently antitumor drugs fail to reach all sites of tumor cells, and sanctuaries may exist that permit the establishment and unimpeded proliferation of a tumor once it has been successfully annihilated from the remainder of the system. This problem may develop because of the metastatic spread of tumors to distant sites, and is accentuated by the lack of knowledge regarding drug susceptibility of such secondary neoplasms. The central nervous system (CNS), which is impervious to many drugs, often represents such a protected site, and major efforts are required to contact such sequestered cells. Attempts to solve this problem have included intrathecal drug administration, or the use of more lipid-soluble drugs capable of rapid penetration of the blood-brain barrier. The success in the peripheral chemotherapy of the leukemias is due in part to the ease of providing high concentrations of drug at the sites of tumor cells. In contrast, those leukemic cells that have penetrated the CNS can no longer be reached by most of the drugs, and the disease progresses.

Some solid tumors may have a diminished blood supply, which curtails the delivery of antitumor drugs to the core of a solid tumor that, even though necrotic, may still contain active tumor cells. Those cells would respond to treatment if they could be exposed to the drugs.

Resistance

A tumor usually consists of a heterogenous population of cells. The selection pressure of an effective antitumor drug leads to the destruction of those tumor cells susceptible to that drug, but permits the overgrowth of populations inherently resistant to it. Successive generations of tumor cells then emerge that no longer respond to the drug. Thus, with time, drugs lose their effectiveness and need to be replaced by other and unrelated compounds.

Overwhelming Tumor Cell Populations

If it were possible to initiate chemotherapy at a time when the tumor burden is relatively small, many of these problems of chemotherapy could be prevented or at least diminished in severity. Such a situation, however, requires early recognition of the disease, which is rarely possible. At the time of patient presentation, usually the tumor is well advanced. The lack of a simple and early diagnostic test for most tumors, therefore, delays the onset of treatment and geometrically magnifies the requirements for effective chemotherapy.

Carcinogenesis

It should be added that many of the present day antitumor drugs also have carcinogenic potential. The validity of this threat has become recognized only recently because of the limited prolongation of life previously provided by anticancer drug treatment. With increasing success of chemotherapy, however, patients are surviving longer, and secondary tumors have been observed. Future research will have to be devoted to this emerging problem.

DRUGS USED AGAINST GYNECOLOGIC CANCERS

The following sections describe the major agents used in the chemotherapy of gynecologic cancers. In order to better understand some drugs in current use, agents not commonly used but that are very similar and have provided relevant basic clinical experience are mentioned. Drugs that are in the various phases of clinical investigation for gynecologic cancers as well as those currently regularly utilized are presented. Many of these compounds are not exclusively effective for particular organs only, and their successful application to gynecologic tumors can be anticipated. As a general overview, a recent tabulation on anticancer agents, published by The Medical Letter, is included (Table 5–4).

The purpose of the presentation has been to provide a description of the agents in women, with a principal focus on their mechanism of action as influenced by their physiologic disposition.* Particular emphasis has been devoted to the basis of the drug's antitumor selectivity whenever possible. Fundamental biochemical information has been stressed heavily since this information is so essential for understanding the action of the drugs, and is the basis for the rational use of the drugs in clinical practice. It is not the intent to provide a detailed description of the clinical applications or optimal dosing schedules associated with the agents. Since cancer chemotherapy has

become a highly specialized and sophisticated discipline, an experienced oncologist should be consulted. Improper chemotherapy during the early phases of a patient's disease will limit the individual's opportunity for successful treatment later.

Alkylating Agents

Alkylating agents refer to various groups of drugs which covalently attach electrophilic (positively charged) "alkyl" groups to nucleophilic (negatively charged) centers of cellular constitutents. This interaction with the various molecules, especially macromolecules, then leads to alteration in biological function, expressed as toxicity or cell death, depending on the change produced in the target molecule. As a rule, the metabolically active tissues are most susceptible to the alkylating agents, and consequently in addition to tumors, cytotoxicity is also expressed against the bone marrow, lymphoid tissue, and gastrointestinal epithelium. Nondividing cells may also be susceptible to the alkylating agents once these cells are stimulated to divide. Thus, although these agents are most destructive to cells in the late G_1 or S phases of the cell cycle, they are also cell cycle nonspecific. Because of this comparative nonselectivity, intermittent treatment using relatively high single or rapidly repeated doses of these drugs, with sufficient interval spacing to allow for host recovery, may be preferred to chronic therapy.

These drugs arose from secret observations during World War I of the leukopenia produced by the war gas, sulfur mustard, $S(CH_2CH_2Cl)_2$.

*Data provided on plasma half-life of anticancer drugs should be considered as a general guide only, since considerable discrepancies have been reported in humans. This diversity is largely due to variations in assay techniques used, different approaches to measuring parent drug versus inactive metabolites, dissimilar classifications in separating the drug distribution phase (α) from the disappearance phase (β), as well as variable experimental conditions.

Table 5-4.   CANCER CHEMOTHERAPEUTIC DRUGS*:

COMMERCIALLY AVAILABLE DRUGS

| DRUG | MAJOR TOXICITY† | | SOME PRECAUTIONS |
	Acute	Delayed	
Alkylating Agents			
Busulfan (Myleran—Burroughs Wellcome)	Nausea and vomiting; diarrhea	Bone marrow depression; pulmonary fibrosis; hyperpigmentation of skin; alopecia; gynecomastia; impotence; sterility	
Chlorambucil (Leukeran—Burroughs Wellcome)		Bone marrow depression	
Cyclophosphamide (Cytoxan-Mead Johnson)	Nausea and vomiting	Bone marrow depression; alopecia; hemorrhagic cystitis; possible secondary malignancy; sterility (may be temporary); pulmonary fibrosis; hyperpigmentation	Maintain adequate fluid intake to avoid cystitis
Dacarbazine (DTIC; DIC; DTIC-Dome)	Severe nausea and vomiting	Bone marrow depression; flu-like syndrome; alopecia; renal impairment; liver damage	
Mechlorethamine (nitrogen mustard; HN2; Mustargen-Merck)	Severe nausea and vomiting; local reaction and phlebitis	Bone marrow depression; alopecia	Unstable (use immediately after reconstitution); strong local irritant, administer through a running IV infusion; protect eyes and skin of person administering the drug
Melphalan (1-phenylalanine mustard; Alkeran-Burroughs Wellcome)	Mild nausea	Bone marrow depression (especially platelets)	Check platelets before each dose
Thiotepa (triethylenethiophosphoramide; Thiotepa-Lederle)	Nausea and vomiting; local pain	Bone marrow depression; anorexia	
Antimetabolites			
Cytarabine HCl (cytosine arabinoside; Cytosar-Upjohn)	Nausea and vomiting; diarrhea	Bone marrow depression; megaloblastosis; oral ulceration; hepatic damage	Use with special caution in hepatic disease

(continued)

*From: The Medical Letter 18:109–116, 1976. Courtesy of The Medical Letter, Inc., 56 Harrison Street, New Rochelle, New York, 10801.
†Information is preliminary; additional or more severe adverse effects may be reported.

Table 5–4. (cont.)

DRUG	MAJOR TOXICITY		SOME PRECAUTIONS
	Acute	*Delayed*	
Fluorouracil (5 FU; Fluorouracil-Roche)	Nausea and vomiting; diarrhea; may precipitate angina	Oral and gastrointestinal ulceration; stomatitis; bone marrow depression; neurological defects, usually cerebellar; pigmentation; alopecia; dermatitis	Decrease dose in patients with impaired hepatic or renal function, or after adrenalectomy; do not exceed daily dose of 800 mg; contraindicated in poor nutritional state
Lomustine (CCNU; cyclohexyl chloroethyl nitrosourea; CeeNU-Bristol)	Nausea and vomiting	Delayed (4 to 6 weeks) leukopenia and thrombocytopenia (may be prolonged); stomatitis; alopecia	
Mercaptopurine (6MP; Purinethol-Burroughs Wellcome)	Occasional nausea and vomiting, usually well tolerated	Bone marrow depression; hepatic damage	Since allopurinol potentiates mercaptopurine, if it is given to prevent hyperuricemia dosage of mercaptopurine should be reduced to no more than one-third of usual dose
Methotrexate (MTX; Methotrexate-Lederle)	Nausea; diarrhea	Oral and gastrointestinal ulceration; bone marrow depression; hepatic toxicity including cirrhosis; renal toxicity; pulmonary infiltration; osteoporosis	Normal renal function must be present and urine output must be maintained
Thioguanine (6TG; Thioguanine-Burroughs Wellcome)	Occasional nausea and vomiting, usually well tolerated	Bone marrow depression; possible hepatic damage	Use lower doses in patients with impaired renal or hepatic function
Natural Products Plant Alkaloids and Antibiotics			
Bleomycin (Blenoxane-Bristol)	Nausea and vomiting; fever	Pneumonitis and pulmonary fibrosis; cutaneous reactions; stomatitis; alopecia; anorexia (may be prolonged)	Anaphylactic reactions may occur in patients with lymphoma—two 2-unit test doses are recommended; use with extreme caution in renal or pulmonary disease; do not exceed total dosage of 400 units
Dactinomycin (actinomycin D; Cosmegen-Merck)	Nausea and vomiting; diarrhea; local reaction and phlebitis	Stomatitis; oral ulceration; alopecia; folliculitis; bone marrow depression	Administer through a running IV infusion; use with special caution in hepatic disease
Doxorubicin (Adriamycin-Adria)	Nausea and vomiting; red urine (not hematuria); severe local tissue damage at infiltration site; diarrhea	Bone marrow depression; cardiotoxicity (may be irreversible); alopecia; stomatitis; hepatic damage; cutaneous toxicity	Administer through a running IV infusion; special caution in patients with heart disease; reduce dose if hepatic function is impaired; do not exceed total dosage of 550 mg/ sq meter

Table 5–4. (cont.)

| DRUG | MAJOR TOXICITY | | SOME PRECAUTIONS |
	Acute	Delayed	
Mithramycin (Mithracin-Pfizer)	Nausea and vomiting; diarrhea	Hemorrhagic diathesis, probably related to abnormalities of clotting factors; bone marrow depression (thrombocytopenia); hepatic damage; hypocalcemia and hypokalemia; stomatitis	Very toxic drug; strict adherence to monitoring of LDH, BUN, prothrombin time and platelet count before each dose; contraindicated in hepatic and kidney dysfunction and in patients with coagulation disorders
Mitomycin C (Mutamycin-Bristol)	Nausea and vomiting; local reaction if extravasation; fever	Bone marrow depression (cumulative); stomatitis; renal toxicity; alopecia	Administer through a running IV infusion (acts as alkylating agent)
Vinblastine sulfate (Velban-Lilly)	Nausea and vomiting; local reaction and phlebitis	Bone marrow depression; alopecia; stomatitis; loss of deep tendon reflexes	Administer through a running IV infusion or inject with great care to prevent extravasation
Vincristine sulfate (Oncovin-Lilly)	Local reaction is extravasation	Peripheral neuropathy; neuritic pain; alopecia; bone marrow depression (leukopenia); constipation leading to paralytic ileus	Administer through a running IV infusion or inject with great care to prevent extravasation; omit or decrease dose if reflexes diminish or paresthesias appear; patients with underlying neurologic problems may be more susceptible to neurotoxicity; hyperuricemia can be treated with allopurinol; prophylactic cathartics may be helpful
Other Synthetic Agents Hydroxyurea (Hydrea-Squibb)	Mild nausea and vomiting	Bone marrow depression; hyperkeratosis and hyperpigmentation; stomatitis	Decrease dose in patients with renal dysfunction
Mitotane (o,p'-DDD; Lysodren-Calbio)	Nausea and vomiting; diarrhea	CNS toxicity, mental depression; visual disturbances; dermatitis; adrenal insufficiency	Low dose should be used initially with gradual build-up to maximum tolerated dose (usually 8-10 gm per day); discontinue following shock or severe trauma; decrease dose in patients with hepatic disease

(continued)

Table 5–4. (cont.)

| DRUG | MAJOR TOXICITY | | SOME PRECAUTIONS |
	Acute	Delayed	
Procarbazine HCl (Matulane-Roche)	Nausea and vomiting; CNS depression	Bone marrow depression; stomatitis; dermatitis	Decrease dose in patients with hepatic or renal dysfunction; synergism with CNS depressants (phenothiazines, barbiturates) may occur as well as an Antabuse-like reaction with ethanol; acts as MAO inhibitor—sympathomimetic drugs and foods with high tyramine content should be avoided
Hormones Calusterone (Methosarb-Upjohn)	Nausea and vomiting	Fluid retention; masculinization; hypercalcemia	
Diethylstilbestrol (DES)	Nausea and vomiting; cramps	Fluid retention; hypercalcemia; feminization; uterine bleeding; if given during pregnancy, may cause vaginal carcinoma in offspring; increased frequency of vascular accidents	Use low doses in patients with prostate cancer; do not use in premenopausal breast cancer patients; serum calcium can rise rapidly in breast cancer patients shortly after therapy is started, especially with bone disease
Dromostanolone propionate (Drolban-Lilly)		Fluid retention; masculinization; hypercalcemia	Contraindicated in patients with prostate cancer; immobilized patients are especially likely to develop hypercalcemia; use with care in patients with cardiac, hepatic, or renal disease
Ethinyl estradiol (Estinyl-Schering; and others)		Fluid retention; hypercalcemia; feminization; uterine bleeding; increased incidence of vascular accidents	
Fluoxymesterone (Halotestin-Upjohn)		Fluid retention; masculinization; cholestatic jaundice; hypercalcemia	Contraindicated in patients with prostate cancer; immobilized patients are especially likely to develop hypercalcemia; use with care in patients with cardiac, hepatic or renal disease
Hydroxyprogesterone caproate (Delalutin-Squibb)	Local abscess, pain	Hypercalcemia; cholestatic jaundice	Contraindicated in patients with impaired hepatic function, breast cancer

Table 5–4. (cont.)

DRUG	MAJOR TOXICITY		SOME PRECAUTIONS
	Acute	*Delayed*	
Medroxyprogesterone acetate (Provera-Upjohn; and others)	Orally, nausea (rare); IM, local pain, abscess at site of injection	Fluid retention; hypercalcemia	Use with care in hepatic dysfunction
Megestrol acetate (Megace-Mead Johnson)		None reported	
Prednisone or prednisolone		Hyperadrenocorticism	
Testolactone (Teslac-Squibb)		Hypercalcemia	Immobilized patients are especially likely to develop hypercalcemia
Testosterone propionate (Oreton-Schering; and others)		Fluid retention; masculinization; hypercalcemia	Contraindicated in cancer of prostate and hepatic disease; immobilized patients are especially likely to develop hypercalcemia

INVESTIGATIONAL DRUGS

Asparaginase (Elspar; Crasnitin)	Nausea, fever, and possible anaphylaxis; abdominal pain; diabetes leading to coma	Hepatic damage; pancreatitis; CNS depression; coagulation defects	Epinephrine should be available; rise in BUN and ammonia is due to action of the enzyme and is not evidence of toxicity
5-Azacytidine	Nausea and vomiting; diarrhea; fever	Leukopenia (may be prolonged); thrombocytopenia; hepatic damage unrelated to dosage	Change infusion solution every 3 to 4 hours to avoid loss of potency
Carmustine (BCNU; bischlorethyl nitrosourea)	Nausea and vomiting; local phlebitis	Delayed leukopenia and thrombocytopenia (may be prolonged)	Slow infusion rate to prevent local pain
Cis-platinum diammine dichloride	Nausea and vomiting	Bone marrow depression; renal damage; ototoxicity	Maintain adequate fluid intake; use lower dose in patients with impaired renal function; do not repeat until recovery of baseline renal function
Daunorubicin (Daunomycin; Cerubidin)	Nausea and vomiting; fever; red urine (not hematuria)	Bone marrow depression; cardiotoxicity; alopecia	Administer through a running IV infusion; avoid giving to patients with heart disease
Dibromomannitol (Mitobromitol; Myelobromol)	Gastrointestinal disturbances	Bone marrow depression; alopecia; skin pigmentation	
Ftorafur	Nausea and vomiting; diarrhea	Oral and gastrointestinal ulceration; cerebellar ataxia; pigmentation	Decrease dose in patients with diminished hepatic or renal function, or after adrenalectomy

(continued)

Table 5–4. (cont.)

| DRUG | MAJOR TOXICITY | | SOME PRECAUTIONS |
	Acute	Delayed	
Hexamethylmelamine	Nausea and vomiting	Bone marrow depression; CNS depression; peripheral neuritis	
Nafoxidine	Nausea	Phototoxicity; ichthyosis; alopecia; may induce hypercalcemia in patients with bone metastases	
Razoxane (ICRF-159)	Mild nausea	Bone marrow depression; alopecia	
Semustine (methyl-CCNU)	Nausea and vomiting	Delayed leukopenia and thrombocytopenia (may be prolonged)	
Streptozocin (Streptozotocin)	Nausea and vomiting; local pain	Renal damage	Slow infusion rate to prevent local pain; contraindicated in patients with renal disease; albuminuria used to monitor toxicity; do not repeat dose until renal function recovers
Tamoxifen citrate	Nausea		
VM-26 (epipodophyllotoxin demethyl-thenylidene-glucoside)	Nausea and vomiting	Bone marrow depression; alopecia	
VP-16213 (epipodophyllotoxin ethylidine glucoside)	Nausea and vomiting	Bone marrow depression; alopecia	

Indeed, this agent was found to have some antitumor activity almost 50 years ago. Structural modifications to reduce toxicity provided nitrogen mustard (I), a drug that was found to produce valuable remissions in the treatment of malignant lymphoma. Numerous related β-chloroethylamine derivatives were then synthesized, many of which are currently still in use as carcinostatic agents. This group of drugs thus represents the beginning of the more rational chemotherapy of cancer. At the present time most of these drugs are used extensively in gynecologic cancers, very often in combination with other antitumor drugs.

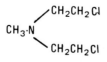

I   Mechlorethamine

Nucleophilic targets for the alkylating agents in the cell are numerous, and these drugs interact with RNA, DNA, proteins, many varieties of organic anions, amines, sulfhydryls, and even water. For example, the reaction of an alkylating agent with hydroxyl ion, or with the N-7 position of guanine (one of the most nucleophilic centers in the cell) is shown in Figure 5–8.[15]

The groups of alkylating agents vary in chemical structure, and particularly in the rates at which they react with their targets. Although the nucleophilic chemical groups with which the drugs interact are qualitatively similar regardless of the type of drug used, the more reactive drugs will never reach certain tissues intact because they will already have reacted with more available nucleophilic centers. In other words, for better infiltration into certain sites, less reactive agents may be superior. In spite of the availability of drugs that were designed to react preferentially with

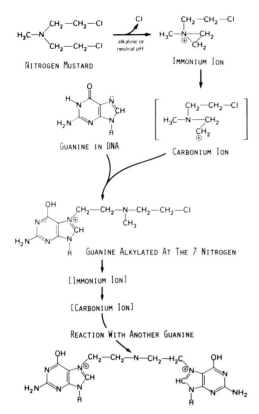

Figure 5–8. Structural rearrangement of nitrogen mustard to reactive cyclic immonium ion which, among several reactions, interacts with N-7 position of guanine and eventually cross-links two molecules of guanine in different DNA chains. (Adapted from Pratt: Fundamentals of Chemotherapy, 1973, p 272. Courtesy of Oxford)

specific biochemical targets, there is no selective concentration of the drugs in any characteristic site, including the tumor. However, it has been possible to apply these drugs directly by regional perfusion of selected tumor sites. Unfortunately, technical analytical difficulties have discouraged the more intensive exploration of the actions and fate of these agents that are being used so extensively in tumor patients.

The efficiency of cell kill with the alkylating agents depends on the concentration of the drug and the time of exposure. It is still controversial whether the mechanism of carcinostasis or cytotoxicity is alkylation of DNA, since so many other constituents are also alkylated and the drugs inhibit such a large number of biochemical reactions. The extent of alkylation, expressed per mg dry weight of DNA, RNA, protein, and various smaller molecules, generally is of the same order

of magnitude. Because of the limited number of high molecular weight DNA molecules, however, an interaction with that macromolecule would be expected to be more closely associated with inhibitory effects, since few if any DNA molecules can escape alkylation altogether even at low concentrations of alkylating agents. In addition, because of the specificity associated with DNA molecules, any incapacitation could have grave consequences. The larger number of lower molecular weight molecules, such as RNA, protein, and all of the biochemical intermediates, on the other hand, suggest that sufficient function would still be available to the cell, by the randomness of alkylation, even if the number of such molecules were slightly reduced.

Although the evidence is far from convincing, it is generally believed that alkylation of purines and pyrimidines of DNA is the most severely damaging action on the cell. Most of the alkyl groups are recovered on the N-7 position of guanine, although other positions alkylated include N-3 of adenine, N-3 of cytosine, and O-6 of guanine. Alkylation of N-7 of guanine of DNA may lead to chain scission, depurination, and miscoding. Because of the bifunctional nature of alkylating agents, it is also known that the second β-chloroethyl group may interact so as to complex another guanine molecule, thus forming intrachain or interchain cross-links. This process would be expected to prevent the separation of DNA chains, leading to failure in the normal replication process (Fig. 5–9).[16] This latter action, which should have profound consequences to an actively dividing cell, may explain the greater biologic activity of difunctional compared to monofunctional alkylating agents.

It has been extremely difficult to associate cellular susceptibility to the drugs, with cross-linking of DNA, or with binding of alkylating agents to any macromolecule. DNA from cells sensitive or resistant to an alkylating agent will usually bind similar quantities of that drug.[17] It has also been difficult to establish differences in the subsequent rate of recovery from this binding effect in strains of tumors of widely varying sensitivities to the drug. The antitumor effectiveness of various monofunctional alkylating agents, which cannot cross-link DNA chains, remains unexplained. It is possible that more specific analytical techniques will have to be employed to discriminate among the many sites of drug binding to macromolecules. For example, recently it has been proposed[18] that the retention of alkylating agents on the O-6 position of DNA guanine has been corre-

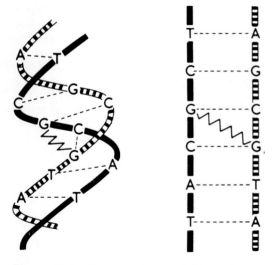

Figure 5–9. Interstrand cross-linking of guanine components of 2 DNA chains by nitrogen
mustard, resulting in failure of strand separation
for cell division. A, C, T, and G refer to DNA
bases adenine, cytosine, thymine, and guanine,
respectively. Hydrogen bonding of normal base
pairs, − − − −; covalent cross-links, ʌʌʌʌ. (From
Brookes: In Plattner (ed): Chemotherapy of
Cancer, 1964, Courtesy of Excerpta Medica)

lated with carcinogenicity. Perhaps the specific
binding of drugs at that or another site has implications with respect to carcinostasis.

The role of repair of alkylated DNA undoubtedly complicates the assessment of damage to this
macromolecule. Correction of a small number of
cross-links may protect against low levels of alkylation, depending on the functional state of the
repair system. When the repair process can no
longer cope with the alterations in structure of
DNA, however, permanent damage to DNA
function may result. Cells resistant to alkylating
agents may have increased capacity for this repair
function. More commonly, however, resistant
cells may have decreased permeability to the
drugs, or may contain higher numbers of nucleophilic targets (such as sulfhydryl compounds)
which compete with the more vital macromolecules for the alkylating agents and thereby protect
these cellular constitutents. In general, there is
cross resistance between the members of each
category of alkylating agents.

In addition to the direct cytotoxic effects of the
alkylating agents on proliferating tissue, such as
the bone marrow, gastrointestinal tract, and hair
follicles, some of the drugs will produce central

nervous system stimulant effects and some will
produce a delayed vesicant action. The compounds are also teratogenic, mutagenic, and
carcinogenic, and all have immunosuppressive
properties.

The alkylating agents used in cancer chemotherapy fall into several chemical categories:
(1) the nitrogen mustards, compounds characterized by a bis-β-chloroethyl amine group, (2)
the closely related ethylenimines, (3) the alkyl
sulfonates, (4) the nitrosoureas, which lack one or
both of the β-chloroethyl arms, and (5) methylating agents, such as the dimethyltriazenes or procarbazine. Older alkylating agents, such as epoxides, are no longer employed clinically.

Nitrogen Mustards

MECHLORETHAMINE

This alkylating agent, also called nitrogen mustard, mustargen, or HN2, was the first such drug
used clinically, because of its potential in producing leukopenia. HN2, a most reactive and vesicant drug, must be used with great care, and is
normally given during intravenous infusion by injecting it directly into the tubing. The drug has an
extremely short half-life in plasma (about four
minutes), and disappears rapidly from blood and
tissues. Because of this very high reactivity and
the difficulty of drug delivery to various tissue
sites, alkylating agents with diminished reactivity
have been preferred. The parent compound is still
employed in the treatment of Hodgkin's disease,
other lymphomas, bronchogenic carcinoma, and
carcinomas of the breast and ovaries, frequently
in combination with other agents. It may also be
used directly by intracavitary instillation against
malignant effusions.

The drug's major toxicity is on the bone marrow. Lymphocytopenia occurs during the first day
and precedes granulocytopenia and thrombocytopenia. Erythrocytopenia may be noticed only
after two to three weeks. Hematologic recovery
may require a month or more. Emesis is extremely common and is usually controlled by coadministration of prochlorperazine and a short-acting
barbiturate.

MELPHALAN (PHENYLALANINE
MUSTARD, ALKERAN) (II)

This compound is the phenylalanine derivative
of HN2 which was synthesized in the hope of
producing a selective action against malignant

NH_2
$CH_2CHCOOH$

CH_2CH_2Cl
N
CH_2CH_2Cl

II Melphalan

O $CH_2CH_2\cdot Cl$
$P-N-CH_2CH_2\cdot Cl$
N
H

III Cyclophosphamide

melanoma because of the structural relationship to melanin. Even though such selectivity is not marked, the drug is useful against various tumors because of its slower reactivity compared to HN2, its greater infiltration into tissues, and its oral effectiveness. The drug is well absorbed and remains active in blood for about six hours. Qualitatively, toxicity mainly against the bone marrow is similar to that of HN2, with a greater likelihood of thrombocytopenia, but much less emesis. Response rates for melphalan from 20 to 60 percent have been reported in the treatment of ovarian cancers of epithelial origin. Because the agent can be given by mouth, has low toxicity, and produces as favorable a response as any other single or combination drug regime, it is the most frequently used primary drug for ovarian cancers of epithelial origin. Melphalan is also used in combination with other drugs such as hexamethylmelamine for women with ovarian adenocarcinomas who have stages 3 or 4 with significant residual disease or for women who have recurrent ovarian adenocarcinoma. Melphalan plus immunotherapy (Corynebacterium parvum) is being investigated as a treatment for women with stage 3 and small residual disease whose ovarian cancers are of the epithelial type. In combination with megestrol acetate and 5FU, melphalan is being studied for treatment of recurrent endometrial cancer.

CYCLOPHOSPHAMIDE (CYTOXAN) (III)

This drug was designed to take advantage of the higher levels of phosphatase and phosphamidase in tumors compared to other tissue. The drug was known to depend on activation by cleavage of the phosphamide linkage, and the difference in enzyme activities then was to be exploited to produce selective antitumor activity. The drug does possess considerable carcinostatic selectivity, but not for the reason described.

Actions and uses. Cyclophosphamide has become one of the most popular alkylating agents of the nitrogen mustard type. Since it is less reactive than HN2 and can be given either orally or parenterally, its benefit to risk ratio can be better controlled. In women with ovarian adenocarcinomas of stages 3 and 4 and with significant residual disease or with recurrent disease, cyclophosphamide is combined with doxorubicin (Adriamycin) in current treatment studies. Cyclophosphamide in combination with dactinomycin and vincristine is being employed against the uncommon germ cell ovarian cancers, embryonal and malignant teratomas with and without neural elements. A maintenance regimen with cyclophosphamide is utilized following dactinomycin and vincristine given concomitantly with radiotherapy for mixed mesodermal ovarian cancers. A combination of cyclophosphamide, dactinomycin, and 5-fluorouracil for the treatment of women with malignant ovarian stromal cancers, such as granulosa cell cancer, granulosa-theca cell cancers, and arrhenoblastomas is currently being evaluated. As a second-line treatment regimen for uterine sarcomas, cyclophosphamide is combined with vincristine and dactinomycin. Cyclophosphamide in combination with other agents has long been used in the treatment of very advanced epidermoid cancer of the cervix, vulva, and vagina, and recurrent endometrial cancer. The compound also has been considered clinically useful because of its strong immunosuppressive properties.

Pharmacokinetics. Cyclophosphamide is well absorbed after oral administration. In plasma it has a half-life of approximately six hours, and maximal plasma concentrations are reached about one hour after oral administration. Cyclophosphamide is activated by the cytochrome P_{450} system of liver microsomes to 4-hydroxycyclophosphamide, which is in equilibrium with its tautomer, aldophosphamide (Fig. 5-10). This compound can be converted nonenzymatically to the cytotoxic

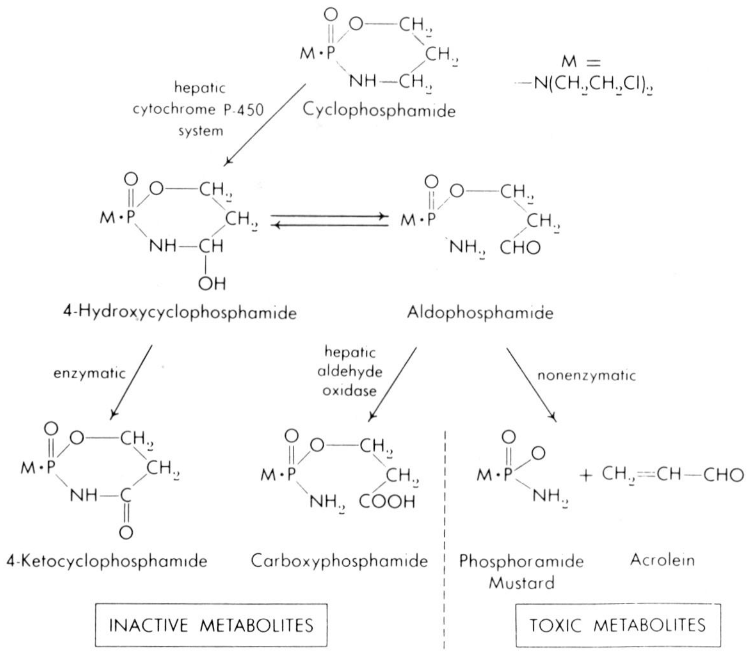

M =
—N(CH$_2$CH$_2$Cl)$_2$

hepatic
cytochrome P-450
system

Cyclophosphamide

4-Hydroxycyclophosphamide   Aldophosphamide

enzymatic   hepatic
aldehyde
oxidase   nonenzymatic

+ CH$_2$=CH—CHO

4-Ketocyclophosphamide   Carboxyphosphamide   Phosphoramide   Acrolein
Mustard

INACTIVE METABOLITES   TOXIC METABOLITES

Figure 5–10. Microsomal metabolism of cyclophosphamide to 4-hydroxycyclophosphamide, which is in equilibrium with aldophosphamide. 4-Ketophosphamide and carboxyphosphamide are nontoxic end products formed enzymatically, whereas highly toxic phosphoramide mustard and acrolein are produced spontaneously in tumors where detoxifying enzymes are absent. (Adapted from Connors et al: Biochem Pharmacol 23:115, 1974)

phosphoramide mustard, or it can be inactivated enzymatically to form ketocyclophosphamide and carboxyphosphamide. Phosphoramide mustard, the metabolite now held responsible for the cytotoxicity of cyclophosphamide, is believed to be formed in tumor tissues sensitive to the parent drug, which apparently lack the degradative enzymes. For other organs, such as in liver, there is little cytotoxicity because rapid enzymatic catabolism prevents the formation of phosphoramide mustard. It is now held unlikely that the acrolein simultaneously released from aldophosphamide has selective carcinostatic potency. Phosphoramide mustard is extremely cytotoxic in vitro,[19] although in vivo its antitumor effect is less than that of the parent compound. This apparent discrepancy may be related to the sustained preferential localized release of the phosphoramide mustard after the administration of cyclophosphamide, in contrast to the many complicating factors related to its disposition following direct administration. It is very important to appreciate, however, that cyclophosphamide itself is inactive as a drug unless it is activated by the liver, and that this drug, unlike HN2, therefore is unsuitable

for intracavitary administration for malignant effusions.

Toxicity. In addition to the anticipated toxicity of bone marrow depression and gastrointestinal (GI) toxicity, therapy with cyclophosphamide, like other alkylating agents, has been associated with sterility, amenorrhea, drug-induced ovarian fibrosis, and probably malignant tumors. Compared to other alkylating agents, thrombocytopenia may occur less commonly, but alopecia is more often observed with this drug than with other alkylating derivatives. A corresponding effect in animals has led to the use of this drug in the shearing of sheep. Teratogenic effects have also been seen in humans. Cardiac toxicity has been reported from high doses of the drug. Occasional hepatotoxicity, hyperpigmentation, and mucosal ulcerations have been observed. Bladder hemorrhage and hyperplasia with cystitis have resulted from the high concentration of active metabolites in the urinary tract. This toxicity may be counteracted by hydration, bladder irrigation with acetylcysteine, and frequent voiding. Impairment of water excretion, which should be carefully

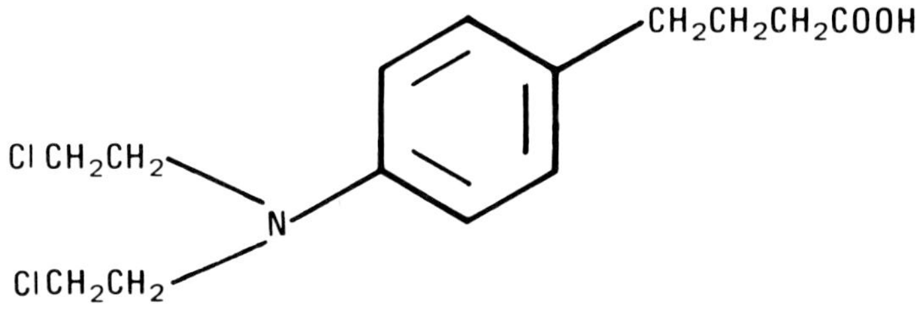
CH2CH2CH2COOH
Cl CH2CH2
N
ClCH2CH2

IV Chlorambucil

monitored by the physician, may result from a direct action of an active drug metabolite on the kidney tubule.

CHLORAMBUCIL (LEUKERAN) (IV)
This alkylating agent is only slowly reactive and thus is relatively low in toxicity, particularly for the GI tract. Its myelosuppressive activity is only moderate, but qualitatively its cytotoxic effects are typical of other alkylating agents. Hepatotoxicity and exfoliative dermatitis occur rarely. Chlorambucil is used to treat adenocarcinoma of the ovary. In combination with dactinomycin and methotrexate, chlorambucil is utilized against ovarian germ cell cancers containing choriocarcinoma. Chlorambucil has also been tried in advanced endometrial cancer. The drug can be administered orally and can be used for maintenance therapy when bone marrow is already depressed.

Ethylenimine Derivatives

THIOTRIETHYLENE PHOSPHORAMIDE (THIO-TEPA) (V) AND TRIETHYLENEMELAMINE (TEM) (VI)
These drugs are examples of ethylenimines that closely resemble the ethylenimmonium ion, a cyclic intermediate in the initial reaction of a nitrogen mustard (Fig. 5–8). TEM is used in the treatment of ovarian adenocarcinomas and as in other malignancies has been largely replaced because of its erratic oral absorption, occasional toxicity, and

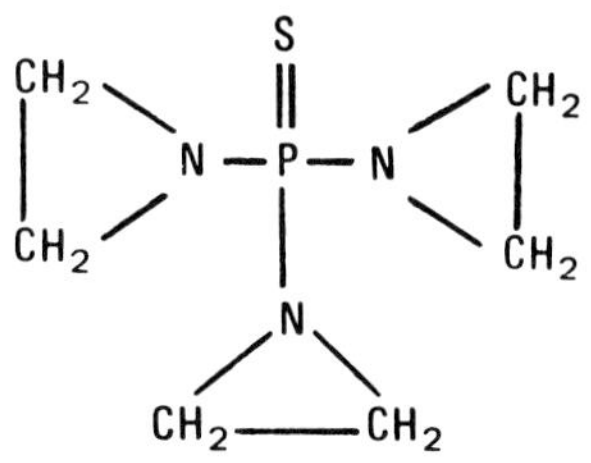
S
CH2
CH2
N — P — N
CH2
CH2
N
CH2
CH2

V Thiotriethylene phosphoramide

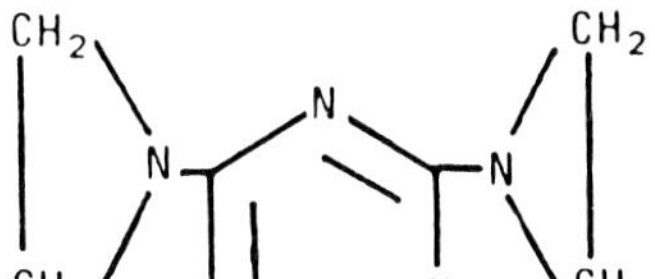
CH2
CH2
N
N
N
N
N
CH2
CH2
N
CH2
CH2

VI Triethylenemelamine

clinical unpredictability. The pharmacologic response to thio-TEPA is slow, and hematopoietic toxicity, mainly to white cells and platelets, may be delayed one to four weeks. It is now used parenterally.

Alkyl Sulfonates

BUSULFAN (MYLERAN) (VII)
This drug, which is the only clinically used compound in this category, differs in chemical structure from the nitrogen mustards HN2, melphalan, chlorambucil, or cyclophosphamide, in that it does not possess the characteristic β-chlorethyl groups. Nevertheless, like those drugs, the compound alkylates nucleophilic targets, and a butyl group becomes attached to the N-7 position of guanine. Evidence for cross-linking at two gua-

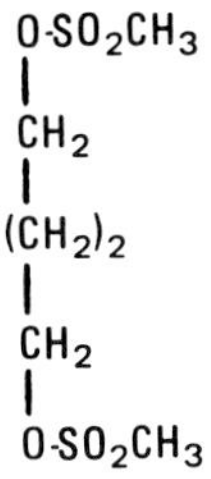
O-SO2CH3
CH2
(CH2)2
CH2
O-SO2CH3

VII Busulfan

nines by a four-carbon chain has also been provided.

The pharmacologic actions of busulfan differ somewhat from those of the nitrogen mustards. In contrast to the effects of HN2, busulfan acts selectively to produce granulocytopenia and some thrombocytopenia, but it has little if any action on lymphoid cells. There is little gastrointestinal toxicity. Ovarian function may be selectively depressed, resulting in amenorrhea. A characteristic skin hyperpigmentation and pulmonary fibrosis have been reported after busulfan treatment. Busulfan is rapidly absorbed orally, disappears rapidly from the systemic circulation, and is extensively metabolized.

Nitrosoureas

There are, at the moment, at least four carcinostatic nitrosourea agents that are being used clinically: carmustine or bischloroethyl-nitrosourea

$$Cl\text{-}CH_2CH_2\text{-}N\text{-}\overset{\overset{\displaystyle O}{\|}}{C}\text{-}NH\text{-}CH_2CH_2\text{-}Cl$$
$$\underset{NO}{|}$$

VIII   BCNU

$$\text{cyclohexyl}\text{-}NH\text{-}\overset{\overset{\displaystyle O}{\|}}{C}\text{-}N\text{-}CH_2CH_2\text{-}Cl$$
$$\underset{NO}{|}$$

IX   CCNU

$$CH_3\text{-}\text{cyclohexyl}\text{-}NH\text{-}\overset{\overset{\displaystyle O}{\|}}{C}\text{-}N\text{-}CH_2\ CH_2Cl$$
$$\underset{NO}{|}$$

X   Methyl-CCNU

XI   Streptozotocin

(BCNU) (VIII); lomustine or cyclohexylchloroethyl nitrosourea, (CCNU) (IX); semustine (methyl-CCNU) (X); and streptozotocin (XI). The drugs behave most like alkylating agents, and indeed, BCNU, analogous to HN2, has two β-chloroethyl groups. However, its antitumor spectrum differs considerably from that of the classical bifunctional alkylating agents and includes solid tumors that do not respond well to the nitrogen mustards.

Actions and uses. BCNU, CCNU, and methyl-CCNU have been used in the treatment of advanced ovarian adenocarcinoma (BCNU) and widespread epidermoid cancer of the cervix, vagina, and vulva (methyl CCNU and CCNU). The relative effectiveness of these drugs has recently been compared.[20]

Pharmacokinetics. An outstanding feature of BCNU, CCNU, and methyl-CCNU is their relative lipid solubility. Thus, they can cross the blood-brain barrier and inhibit brain tumors. Their greater penetration into other solid tumors may also explain partially their different antitumor spectrum compared to the nitrogen mustards. CCNU and its methyl analog are readily absorbed orally, whereas BCNU is usually administered intravenously. The compounds are so rapidly metabolized that they cannot be detected in plasma or urine.

Mechanism of action. It is remarkable that BCNU should resemble in its pharmacologic actions CCNU and methyl-CCNU, which have only one β-chloroethyl arm, especially since the latter two drugs may have clinical superiority in certain instances to BCNU. In the nitrogen mustard series, for example, major reductions in pharmacologic activity have been noted in comparing mono- to bifunctional alkylating agents, and only the latter are useful as carcinostatic drugs. Since streptozotocin (a naturally occurring fermentation product) has no β-chloroethyl group, but instead bears a methyl group, it is apparent that the drug's effectiveness must rest on a principle different from that of the nitrogen mustards. The exact mechanism by which these drugs act is still unknown (Fig. 5–11).[21] Although they alkylate DNA, with the exception of BCNU they cannot cross-link. Nevertheless, alkylating activity appears to correlate with antitumor effectiveness. In addition, an isocyanate metabolite of the drugs interacts with protein. Thus carbamoylation of protein and inhibition of DNA repair have been

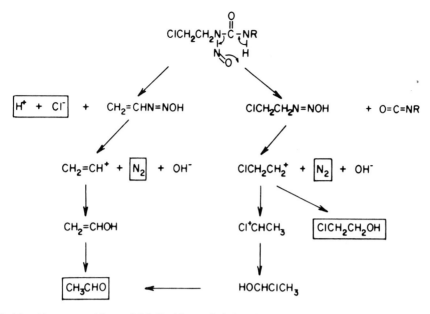

Figure 5–11. Decomposition of N-(β-chloroethyl)-N-nitrosoureas to various reactive species, including vinyl carbonium ions acting as alkylators, and as isocyanate (RNCO) carbamoylating intermediary. (From Montgomery: Ca Treat Rept 60:651, 1976)

proposed to contribute to the drug's cytotoxic actions, but the significance of these observations with respect to drug action is very much disputed. It is interesting that following therapy with these agents DNA synthesis of bone marrow and gastrointestinal tract may be able to recover more rapidly than that of tumor, suggesting a likely reason underlying the antitumor selectivity of these drugs.

The rather selective cytotoxic effect of streptozotocin on pancreatic islet cells is remarkable. This action is not shared by the nonglucose-containing nitrosoureas. Apparently the glucose moiety acts as a carrier to permit the nitrosoureas to enter islet cells and to produce a rapid reduction in pyridine nucleotide concentration.

Toxicity. Toxicity of BCNU, CCNU, and methyl-CCNU are very similar. Leukopenia and thrombocytopenia, which may be profound, are characteristically delayed in onset until three to five weeks after drug administration and may not reach their peak effect until somewhat later. Myelosuppression is usually dose limiting and cumulative. Hepatotoxicity has also been reported after BCNU. In sharp contrast, streptozotocin has very little bone marrow toxicity but produces renal damage. A newer derivative, chlorozotocin, also has a bone marrow–sparing effect, but is not diabetogenic. It is being explored for its antitumor potential, possibly in combination with other myelosuppressive antitumor drugs.[22]

Methylating Agents

DACARBAZINE (XII)

This drug, also known as dimethyltriazenoimidazole carboxamide, DTIC, or DIC, is a recent addition to the commercially available alkylating agents. It was at first believed that the imidazolecarboxamide moiety of dacarbazine is responsible for some antimetabolite action of the drug. However, since it can be replaced by other aromatic groups without loss of antitumor effectiveness, the drug must owe its pharmacologic effectiveness to the dimethyltriazene portion of the molecule.

XII Dacarbazine

Actions and uses. DIC is primarily used in the treatment of malignant melanoma and soft tissue sarcomas. Dacarbazine plus doxorubicin is being investigated in women with residual or recurrent biopsy-proven nonresectable uterine sarcomas.

Pharmacokinetics. In man, DIC appears to be incompletely absorbed after oral administration. Given intravenously DIC has a biphasic disappearance from plasma, with $t_{1/2}\,\alpha$ and β values of 20 minutes and 5 hours, respectively. The drug is secreted by the renal tubules, and almost half of the dose may be excreted unchanged in the urine within 6 hours. An inactive normal intermediary metabolite, 4-amino-5-imidazolecarboxamide, is also recovered in urine after DIC administration.

Mechanism of action. The drug behaves biochemically and pharmacologically like the nitrogen mustards, but it lacks β-chloroethyl groups. Instead, it is postulated[23] (Fig. 5–12) that the drug

DIC

Liver Microsomes
+ NADP + O_2

MIC

Nonenzymatic

AIC

$CH_3^+ + N_2$

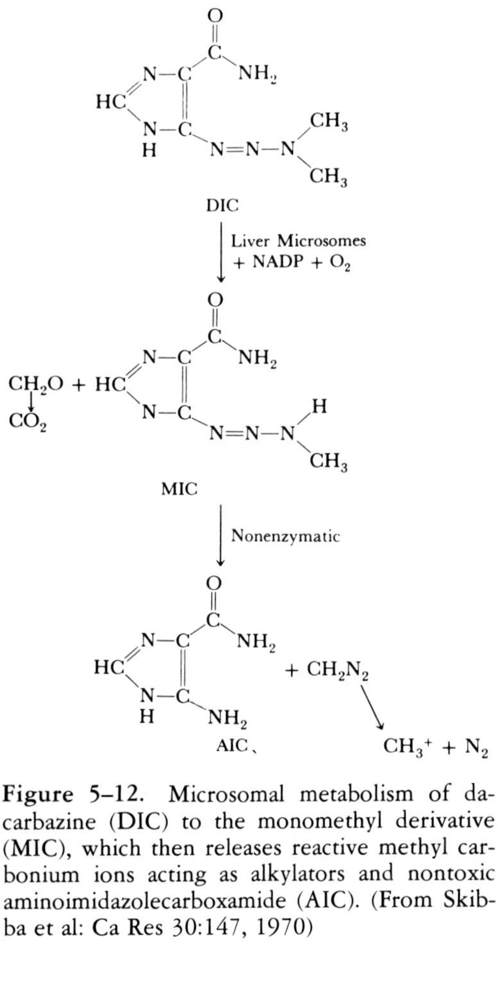

Figure 5–12. Microsomal metabolism of dacarbazine (DIC) to the monomethyl derivative (MIC), which then releases reactive methyl carbonium ions acting as alkylators and nontoxic aminoimidazolecarboxamide (AIC). (From Skibba et al: Ca Res 30:147, 1970)

is activated first by liver microsomal enzymes whereby one methyl group is oxidized to formaldehyde. The remaining unstable molecule then releases a carbonium ion that interacts with cellular nucleophilic targets, as do the other alkylating agents.

Toxicity. The major toxicity of dacarbazine includes leukopenia, thrombocytopenia, sometimes gastrointestinal and hepatotoxicity, and a flu-like syndrome.

PROCARBAZINE
(NATULAN, MATULANE, MIH, XIII)

Procarbazine was originally prepared as one of several methylhydrazine derivatives being examined for monamine oxidase (MAO) inhibitory properties when its antitumor activity was discovered. Although its MAO inhibition was weak, the drug had useful carcinostatic properties.

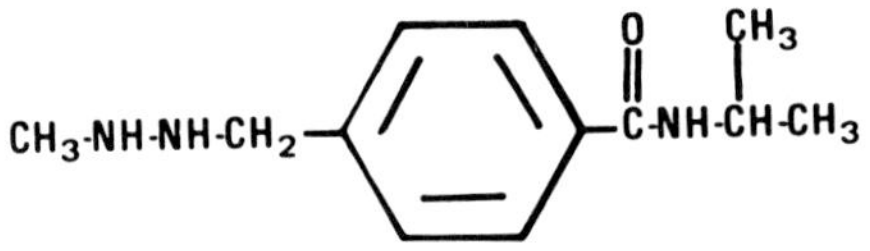

XIII   Procarbazine

Actions and uses. Procarbazine is employed in the combination therapy of Hodgkin's disease. It is now being tested for its wider antitumor spectrum in women. It is interesting that ethyl substituted hydrazines are inactive.

Pharmacokinetics. Oral absorption of procarbazine appears to be rapid and complete since the drug is equally effective if given orally or parenterally. Passage across the blood-brain barrier occurs readily. Metabolism is extensive since only about 5 percent of the original drug is recovered unchanged in the urine, and the $t_{1/2}$ of the drug has been estimated as about 10 minutes. Between 30 and 70 percent of the total drug is excreted into the urine. The major metabolite recovered is N-isopropylterephthalamic acid. Although the exact nature of the steps involved in the metabolism of procarbazine is still unclear, several reactions are recognized. The hydrazine moiety of the parent drug is oxidized to the azo compound, which apparently retains pharmacologic activity. This reaction is mediated largely by erythrocytes and liver microsomes, but also proceeds nonenzymatically in the presence of water, and is accompanied by the production of H_2O_2. Isomerization to the hydrazone is then followed by cleavage to the aldehyde and acid products as shown in Figure 5–13,[24] together with the production of methylhydrazine or a similar unstable derivative. Breakdown products of this intermediary include methane, CO_2, formaldehyde, methylamine (?), and methyl carbonium ion, or N-hydroxymethyl derivatives. The latter compounds then methylate guanine and other nucleic acid bases like other alkylating or methylating agents.

Mechanism of action. Although numerous biochemical effects of procarbazine have been recognized, the mechanism by which the drug produces its antitumor effects is still uncertain. The compound remains inactive in vitro for a long time before inhibiting nucleic acid synthesis, implying metabolic activation. In vivo the drug inhibits RNA and DNA synthesis, with blockade of protein synthesis a secondary event. Polysome function appears to be altered, and complexes of this fraction with the parent drug have been isolated. The role of H_2O_2, if any, in the effects of procarbazine to produce degradation of DNA and inhibiting RNA and DNA polymerase is doubtful. It has been suggested that the drug acts directly on cell division rather than on nucleic acid

or protein synthesis. Tumors resistant to alkylating agents may still respond to procarbazine.

Toxicity. Leukopenia and thrombocytopenia occur as dose-limiting responses. Nausea and vomiting are common, especially during the initiation of a course of therapy. Central nervous system effects, such as ataxia, confusion, and somnolence, occur at somewhat higher doses, and may be due to depression of pyridoxal phosphate levels. Other CNS drugs, such as alcohol, barbiturates, and phenothiazines, may aggravate the sedative effects. Sympathomimetic amines and other drugs, including specific foods, which interfere with other MAO inhibitors, may provoke a hypertensive crisis. The drug is also immunosuppressive, carcinogenic, and teratogenic.

Antimetabolites

Antimetabolites, or substrate analogs, are compounds that closely resemble in chemical structure and physical properties a constituent of normal tissue. The analog may replace the natural metabolite in one or more of its normal reactions, eventually leading to a metabolic block. Actually, only a portion of the antimetabolite molecule

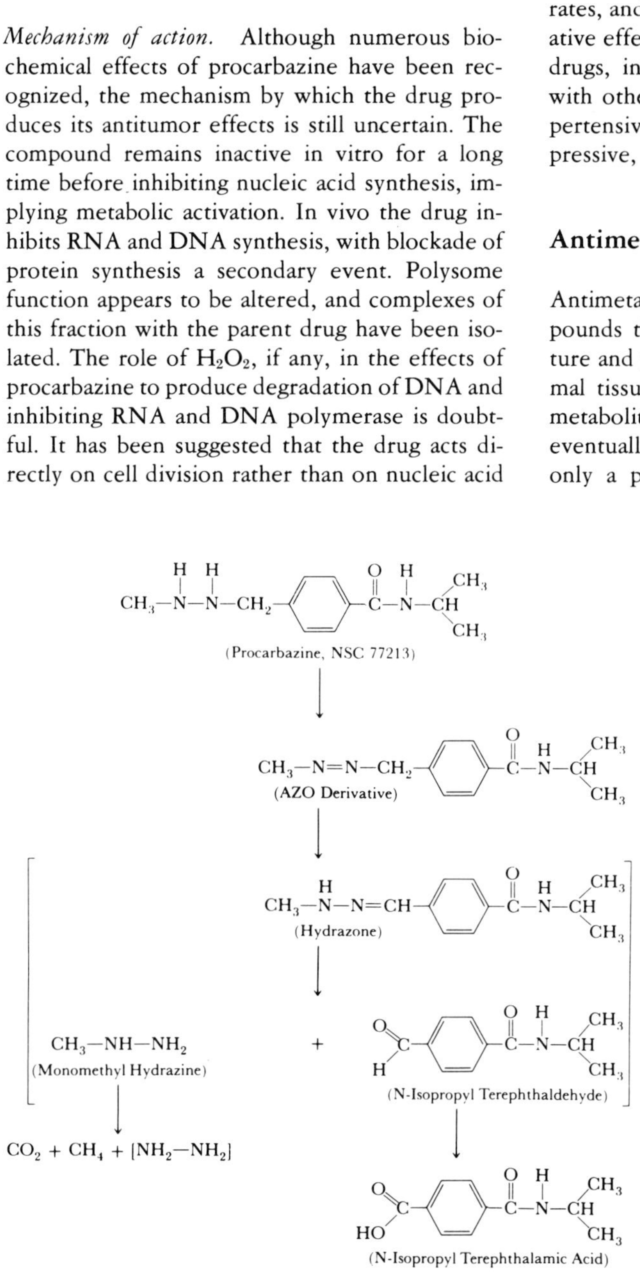

Figure 5–13. Metabolism of procarbazine, including autoxidation to azo derivative with formation of H_2O_2, and methylhydrazine. Final products include active methyl carbonium ions and hydrazine. (From Oliverio: In Holland, Frei: Cancer Medicine, 1973, p 812. Courtesy of Lea and Febiger)

need be analogous for competition with the corresponding normal substrate at a particular enzyme binding site. Because the analogs usually use the same biochemical pathway as their normal counterparts, they are frequently metabolized to derivatives of much greater pharmacologic potency than the parent analog. This process is termed "lethal synthesis."

A number of antitumor agents have been developed on a rational basis because of the early successes of such drugs in tumor screens, in association with our increasing knowledge of cellular biochemistry. When it was observed that folate exacerbated leukemia, the folate antagonists were introduced in clinical trials and were found to have useful antitumor properties. Research in the nucleic acid field provided many purine and pyrimidine analogs, which have carcinostatic effects in animals exploitable for man. Investigations on antimetabolite drugs have, in addition, enlarged our knowledge of nucleic acid function in the normal and malignant cell, and led to the introduction of other valuable therapeutic agents in fields unrelated to cancer: allopurinol in gout, azathioprine as an immunosuppressant, iododeoxyuridine as an anti-viral compound, methotrexate in psoriasis, etc.

METHOTREXATE

Methotrexate (Amethopterin, MTX) (XIV) is a more recent member of one of the older groups of anticancer agents, the folic acid (XV) antagonists. At the present time amethopterin has almost completely replaced aminopterin in the clinical use of these agents. It should be noted that methotrexate was the first cancer chemotherapeutic agent used successfully to cure choriocarcinoma in women.[2]

Actions and uses. In addition to choriocarcinoma and related trophoblastic diseases in women,

methotrexate is being used in combination with dactinomycin and chlorambucil for ovarian germ cell cancer containing choriocarcinoma. Methotrexate in combination with other agents is utilized for the treatment of widespread ovarian adenocarcinomas as well as advanced epidermoid cancer of the cervix, vagina, and vulva.

Pharmacokinetics. Although at high doses of methotrexate absorption is inefficient, at low doses the drug is readily absorbed orally. An active uptake system exists which permits methotrexate to enter cells against a concentration gradient, and the drug competes with folate and reduced tetrahydrofolates for this transport system. This process appears to be of considerable importance in the action of methotrexate, and may be a determinant for the selective action of the drug. About 90 percent of the drug is rapidly excreted in the urine as methotrexate. There is very little, if any, systemic metabolism but intestinal bacteria degrade a small percentage of the total drug given. Plasma disappearance is triphasic in man, with half-lives of 0.8, 3.5, and 27 hours, respectively. Various drugs given concomitantly, such as salicylates, phenylbutazone, and sulfonamides, displace methotrexate from plasma protein binding sites. There is extensive enterohepatic circulation, apparently followed by reabsorption, since only little of the intravenously administered drug is recovered in the feces. Tissue levels may remain appreciable over several weeks and months, especially in kidney and liver, because of drug binding to dihydrofolate reductase. The drug penetrates the blood-brain barrier poorly, and intrathecal administration may be required to attack leukemic cell sanctuaries in the CNS. However, this procedure is not without danger. In the kidney the drug is filtered and actively secreted. Salicylate and p-aminohippurate compete with methotrexate for this secretion.

XIV   Methotrexate   A: $-CH_3$; B: $-NH_2$

XV   Folic acid   A: $-H$; B: $-OH$

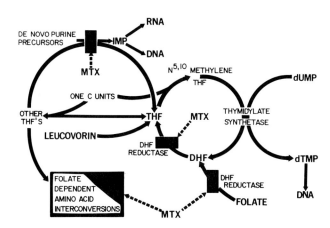

Figure 5–14. Major sites of action of methotrexate (MTX) indicated as shaded blocks connected to MTX by broken arrows. Interaction with dihydrofolate (DHF) reductase reduces concentration of tetrahydrofolate (THF) and other THF cofactors, thereby limiting (right) the conversion of deoxyuridylate (dUMP) to thymidylate (dTMP) and DNA synthesis, formation of inosinate (IMP) and of RNA and DNA purines (top left), and certain amino acids (bottom left). Leucovorin, a THF derivative, acts as rescue agent by overcoming THF deficiency.

Mechanism of action. Methotrexate interferes in the reduction of dihydrofolate to tetrahydrofolate, a biochemical intermediate which forms various other cofactors involved in the transfer of one-carbon moieties in biosynthesis. One of these cofactors, $N^{5,10}$ methylene tetrahydrofolate, stoichiometrically converts deoxyuridylate to thymidylate, and thus a deficiency of this cofactor leads to diminution in the synthesis of thymidylate and thus DNA. The formation of DNA and RNA purines from formate is also depressed, as is the biosynthesis of methionine and serine, which require various other tetrahydrofolates (Fig. 5–14).

Methotrexate has an extremely strong affinity for the enzyme dihydrofolate reductase and competes with the normal substrate dihydrofolate for binding sites on the enzyme. Eventually one molecule of the drug will bind to and inactivate one enzyme molecule. The complexing of methotrexate to the enzyme can be so avid that it is termed "pseudoirreversible" but actually the complex will dissociate slightly at physiologic pH. The resulting deficiencies of $N^{5,10}$ methylene tetrahydrofolate and other methylated tetrahydrofolates then prevent the formation of thymidylate and purines respectively. Of the sites of drug action, the effect on DNA synthesis may be more important to the cell, especially in the human, and is caused by the lethal effect of DNA deficient unbalanced growth. However, the inhibitory effect on purine synthesis can also be of critical significance in specific tumor systems, even though the resulting inhibition of RNA synthesis concomitantly slows the entry of cells into the S phase, thereby "self-limiting" the inhibition of DNA synthesis.

It has been difficult in the past to demonstrate a direct correlation between the formation of the methotrexate-dihydrofolate reductase complex and inhibition of DNA synthesis, probably because the enzyme occurs in great excess of that needed for thymidylate synthesis. It is now recognized that unbound methotrexate, in addition to that bound to the enzyme, is necessary to inhibit DNA synthesis, probably because only in the presence of free drug can methotrexate bind maximally to the enzyme and continue to inhibit it quantitatively. Free drug has been found to persist longer in mouse tumor tissues than in small intestine, which parallels the favorable therapeutic index (Fig. 5–15),[25] and probably explains the preponderance of antitumor effect over toxicity. An impressive relationship has now been established between the levels and persistence of the unbound methotrexate, and the resulting drug damage to the tissues.[26]

Resistance to methotrexate in animal systems has been associated with increased levels or turnover of dihydrofolate reductase in tumor cells, and/or decreased transport of the drug into the cell. Alteration in the conformation of the dihydrofolate reductase has also been postulated to account for a decreased affinity of the drug for the enzyme, leading to the diminished effectiveness of the analog. Much less information is available to explain tumor refractoriness to methotrexate in women.

Rationale for dose scheduling. The destructive effect of methotrexate will be greatest for those cells whose dihydrofolate reductase pools are low or depleted, which synthesize the new enzyme relatively slowly, or which have a high requirement for the cofactors because of a short generation time. Methotrexate is most efficacious if ad-

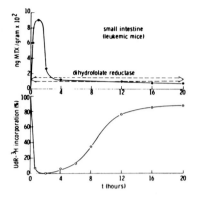

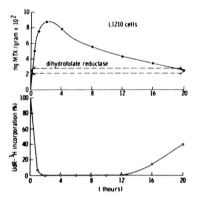

Figure 5–15. Relationship between intracellular levels of methotrexate (MTX) (•) and inhibition of deoxyuridine incorporation (o) into mouse DNA. (**Top**) small intestine, (**bottom**) L1210 cells. Note that recovery takes place only when the level of free MTX (i.e., not bound to dihydrofolate reductase) returns to low values, even though quantity of drug bound to enzyme does not change appreciably. Also note earlier recovery in intestine than tumor, in agreement with selective antitumor activity of MTX. (From Sirotnak and Donsbach: Ca Res 33:1290, 1973)

ministered against tumor cells with a high growth fraction, delivered just long enough so that all cells will be exposed to a lethal drug concentration as they traverse the S phase. Bone marrow and GI cells, on the other hand, with a lower growth fraction than tumors, will have their G_0 cells protected from the drug, and hence the drug action becomes more selective against the tumor. It has been observed, for example, that high tissue levels of methotrexate can be tolerated by women for 48 hours; longer exposure, however, will permit stem cells of the bone marrow and GI cells

to become recruited into mitotic cycle, at which point they also become vulnerable to the drug, and major toxicity ensues. Thus toxicity is more closely related to duration of drug action than to dose of drug, although both factors play important roles.

In order to make available sufficient methotrexate in tumor cells to exceed that bound to dihydrofolate reductase, larger doses of drug must be given which will then have greater effectiveness against the tumor. Consequently, instead of smaller doses of methotrexate repeated frequently, the newer regimens of administration specify high doses of the drug, repeated intermittently to permit recovery of normal tissue.

Toxicity. Toxicity to methotrexate involves mainly the GI tract, the bone marrow, and oral mucosa. Damage to the intestinal tract includes ulceration and, if severe, can lead to hemorrhagic desquamating enteritis. Bone marrow depression is characterized by granulocytopenia, thrombocytopenia, and reticulocytopenia, with some lymphopenia. The appearance of oral or gastrointestinal mucosal toxicity is usually a forerunner of more serious damage which should halt further use of the drug. Skin rash and alopecia have been observed, and the drug is extremely embryotoxic. With high doses of methotrexate liver damage may be produced or accentuated. Renal injury may also result from large drug dosage, perhaps because of deposition of methotrexate in the kidney tubules. Liquids and alkalinization may avoid insolubility of the drug in the kidney. Since this drug is excreted almost entirely by renal excretion, systemic toxicity may develop, especially after large doses or because of drug accumulation in individuals with kidney disease. The dose of methotrexate should be reduced under those conditions.

When large doses of methotrexate are given, toxicity may be reduced by the coadministration of leucovorin (N^5-formyl-tetrahydrofolate) which appears to protect selectively mainly against the myelo-, oral-, and gastrointestinal toxicity. This "rescue" agent may then allow the preferential recovery of normal tissue and thus permits the use of higher doses of methotrexate as required for tumor growth inhibition. Although the exact mechanism for the preferential tissue protection is not clear, leucovorin by supplying a usable biochemical alternative negates the block in synthesis of tetrahydrofolates. It also competes with the antifolate drug for intracellular transport, and may accelerate the efflux of intracellular methotrexate.

THIOPURINES—MERCAPTOPURINE AND THIOGUANINE

The sulfur-containing purines, 6-mercaptopurine, purinethol (6MP) (XVI) and 6-thioguanine (6TG) (XVIII) will be discussed together because of their strong similarity. Characteristically like other purine or pyrimidine analogs, 6MP and 6TG follow closely the metabolic pathways available for the normal metabolites, hypoxanthine (XVII), and guanine (XIX), respectively. However, there are also some significant differences between the two purine analogs with respect to antitumor effectiveness, many of which still remain unexplored. These drugs are described in some detail because they may be prototypes of the class of purine antimetabolites.

XVI   6-Mercaptopurine   A: –SH

XVII   Hypoxanthine   A: –OH

XVIII   6-Thioguanine   A: –SH

XIX   Guanine   A: –OH

Actions and uses. *6MP* has been extremely useful in the maintenance therapy of acute lymphoblastic leukemia, especially in children. It has been tried in the treatment of advanced endometrial cancer. *6TG* has been used mainly in the induction of remission in acute granulocytic leukemia. Both drugs are powerful immunosuppressive agents, and the commonly used immunodepressant drug, azathioprine, is a derivative of 6MP, which it slowly releases in vivo.

Pharmacokinetics. At a moderate dose, *6MP* is absorbed after oral administration, and has a plasma $t_{1/2}$ of about one hour. It crosses the blood-brain barrier with difficulty and is ineffective in CNS leukemia. Most of the drug is metabolized, and some is converted to several anabolite derivatives. Without these activation steps the drug would be totally ineffective. The first and probably most significant reaction is the formation of the ribose-phosphate adduct, 6-mercaptopurine ribonucleoside monophosphate, or thioinosinate (TIMP) (Fig. 5–16). This product is an analog of inosinate, the natural intermediate in purine biosynthesis corresponding to the ribose phosphate derivative of hypoxanthine. The same enzyme, hypoxanthine-guanine-phosphoribosyltransferase (HGPRT) mediates both reactions. 6MP also forms several S-methyl metabolites, but no di- or triphosphate derivatives from TIMP have been isolated in vivo. Some 6MP is converted to derivatives of 6TG, which has been recovered from nucleic acids following treatment with 6MP. Apparently no 6MP is incorporated into nucleic acids as such.

6MP is also degraded by the liver via the enzyme xanthine oxidase, forming thiourate. Urinary excretory products, in addition to thiourate, include the parent drug, sulfate, and various other products. Inhibition of xanthine oxidase by the antihyperuricemic drug, allopurinol, therefore leads to toxic concentrations of 6MP and its anabolites in tissues. In the presence of allopurinol, which is frequently used during cancer chemotherapy to prevent the extensive formation and deposition of urates, the administered dose of 6MP therefore must be greatly reduced to avoid toxicity.

6TG also is administered orally. Following intravenous administration most of the drug is cleared within 24 hours with a $t_{1/2}$ of about one hour, whereas following oral administration excretion is slower. The drug is anabolized by HGPRT to its ribonucleoside monophosphate, thioguanosine phosphate (TGMP) which, as distinct from the parent drug, has pharmacologic activity. Unlike TIMP, however, TGMP forms di- and triphosphates, and is condensed into polynucleotides. Thus TG has been isolated from RNA and DNA following treatment with this drug.

Figure 5–16. Interrelationship between anabolism of mercaptopurine (6MP) to thioinosinate (TIMP) via hypoxanthine-guanine-phosphoribosyl transferase (HGPRT) and interference in nucleic acid formation at various sites: (1) ribosylamine-5-phosphate and inosinate (IMP) synthesis (center), (2) guanylate (GMP) and adenylate (AMP) synthesis and thus RNA and DNA formation (right), and (3) formation of 6TG-containing nucleic acids via intermediaries thioguanosine mono-, di-, and triphosphates (TGMP, TGDP, and TGTP, respectively). For thioguanine (6TG) there are many similar inhibitory effects. Degradation to thiourate is blocked by allopurinol, a xanthine oxidase inhibitor, when that enzyme catalyzes breakdown. Inhibitory drugs or metabolites connected by broken arrows to shaded blocks indicate sites of inhibition.

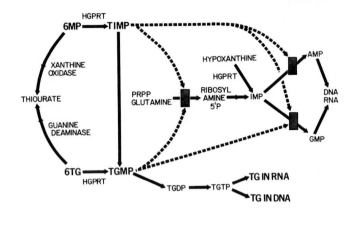

In the urine, much of the TG is recovered as S-methylated products, together with some sulfate and a small quantity of thiourate. Unlike the degradation of 6MP, however, TG is catabolized by guanine deaminase. Thus, allopurinol does not directly alter the metabolism of TG when coadministered, and no toxicity has been reported due to that drug combination.

Mechanism of Action. Undoubtedly anabolism of the drugs is essential for their pharmacologic activity[27] (Fig. 5–17) and it is likely that the drugs' overall actions represent a composite of the many biochemically detrimental effects produced by the persistence of drug anabolites in specific tissues. Both drugs are considered to act as self-limiting S phase inhibitors of the cell cycle, since in addition to DNA synthesis other biosynthetic reactions such as RNA synthesis are also inhibited.

The recovery of 6TG integrally associated with RNA and DNA in susceptible tumors following the administration of 6MP has led to the conclusion that 6MP owes at least a part of its antitumor actions to incorporation into polynucleotides as 6TG. Other actions of this analog, which probably are less responsible for antitumor action, include a reduction in the synthesis of RNA and DNA by TIMP or its S-methylated derivative. This drug action is due to pseudo-feedback inhibition of the formation of ribosylamine-5-phosphate, a reaction analogous to the normal biosynthetic regulatory mechanism asserted by the natural purine ribonucleoside phosphates and thus controlling the formation of additional purines for nucleic acid synthesis. In addition, 6MP acting through TIMP also partially blocks in the interconversion of purine nucleotides from inosinate to both (1)

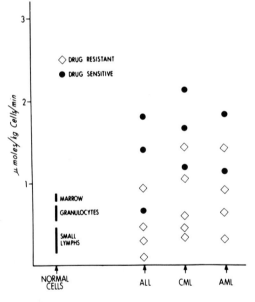

Figure 5–17. Correlation between phosphorylation of 6MP of normal human and various leukemic cell types and response to drug therapy. Leukemic cells unable to anabolize 6MP usually are resistant (◇) to treatment by this drug, whereas cells inhibited by 6MP (●) formed phosphorylated drug derivatives. (Adapted from Kessel, Hall: Ca Res 29:2116, 1969)

adenylosuccinate and adenylate and (2) xanthylate and guanylate.

There has been extensive evidence of a close and perhaps causal relationship between incorporation of 6TG into DNA and tumor growth inhibition,[28] although there still exist some major discrepancies so that the mechanism of antitumor action is still unclear. For the same degree of tumor growth inhibition, however, the direct incorporation into nucleic acids of 6TG, and the incorporation of 6TG formed from 6MP have provided similar levels of 6TG in polynucleotides (Fig. 5–18).[29] It is likely that the incorporated analog in the DNA then leads to failure of replication of the cells. Other effects of 6TG acting through TGMP, which may contribute to its pharmacologic action, include again the pseudo-feedback inhibition of the synthesis of ribosylamine-5-phosphate and thus of RNA and DNA, and inhibition of the conversion from inosinate to xanthylate and guanylate.

Acquired resistance to the thiopurines in animal models has involved deletion of enzymes required for activation, such as HGPRT, which forms the highly active anabolites TIMP or TGMP from 6MP or 6TG, respectively. Other mechanisms of resistance probably of greater significance in the human include the decreased permeability to the drugs, and the enhanced deactivation of the drugs and/or their ribonucleoside monophosphate anabolites in comparison with susceptible cell lines. A few instances have been described where there was no cross-resistance between 6MP and TG.

Toxicity. Clinically the two drugs are very similar, except that TG may be somewhat more deleterious than 6MP in man. TG is toxic mainly to bone marrow where it is extensively incorporated into nucleic acids. Both agents slowly produce leukopenia and thrombocytopenia. GI disturbances, including jaudice and liver damage, are more common after 6MP than 6TG and occur more readily in the adult than in children.

FLUOROURACIL

5-Fluorouracil, FU (XX), was designed as a potential anticancer agent to exploit the observation that tumor cells utilized the normal pyrimidine base, uracil (XXI), for biosynthesis more effectively than did nontumor cells. Hence, such an antimetabolite was believed to have antitumor selectivity. In addition, it was anticipated that substitution of the stable carbon-fluorine bond for the carbon-hydrogen at position C-5 of uracil would prevent methylation at that site, thereby blocking thymidylate synthesis and preventing DNA formation.[30]

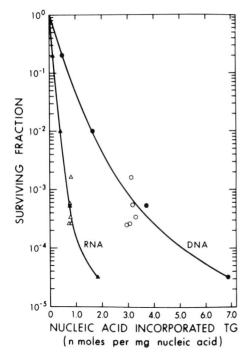

Figure 5–18. Relationship between thioguanine (6TG) content of nucleic acids and surviving fraction of thiopurine treated L5178Y cell cultures. Note that incorporation of 6TG into RNA or DNA is quantitatively related to cell death, and that for similar cell kill, direct incorporation of 6TG, and incorporation of 6TG after conversion from mercaptopurine (6MP) to 6TG compounds, are identical. 6MP administration Δ,ο; 6TG administration ▲,●. Circles refer to incorporation into DNA, triangles into RNA. (From Tidd, Paterson: Ca Res 34:738, 1974)

XX   5-Fluorouracil   A: –F

XXI   Uracil   A: –H

Actions and uses. The compound has demonstrated useful anticancer activity when given systemically. It has been used in combination with other agents for the treatment of metastatic ovarian adenocarcinoma and endometrial cancer. Also when combined with various other drugs, FU has been utilized against advanced epidermoid cancer of the cervix, vulva, and vagina. Fluorouracil in combination with dactinomycin and cyclophosphamide is being used in the treatment of women with malignant ovarian stromal tumors, granulosa cell cancers, granulosa-theca cell cancers, and arrhenoblastomas, which are not completely resectable. The drug has also been used successfully as a topical agent against skin neoplasms, such as carcinomas in situ of the vulva and vagina as well as some dysplastic lesions of the vulva.

Pharmacokinetics. Oral absorption of the drug is erratic and therefore the intravenous route is preferred. When administered by this route, FU is rapidly cleared from the plasma, with a $t_{1/2}$ of about 15 minutes, and plasma concentrations remain measurable for about 3 hours at the usual therapeutic doses. The drug enters the CNS to a significant degree, and therapeutic levels remain in the cerebral spinal fluid (CSF) for many hours. The drug and its metabolites persist much longer in malignant peritoneal and pleural effusions than in plasma, a factor that may explain the drug's usefulness in intracavitary instillation.

The drug mimics the biochemical pathways available for uracil and forms several products that are responsible for its pharmacologic properties. As shown in Figure 5–19, FU is anabolized to a variety of ribose and deoxyribose derivatives. Fluorouridine phosphate (FUMP) is further phosphorylated to the di- and triphosphate derivatives, and FU is incorporated into RNA. An analogous series of reactions are applicable for uridine phosphate (uridylate, UMP) and FU thus replaces uracil in RNA. Undoubtedly of even more importance is the formation of fluorodeoxyuridine phosphate, FdUMP. This derivative is retained for long periods of time in tumors and other organs sensitive to the actions of FU.[31] Unlike most antitumor drugs, there is more anabolism of FU to active compounds in tumors than in normal tissues. At the same time, the capacity of tumor to degrade FU to inactive metabolites is less than that of normal tissue.

The catabolism of FU follows the metabolic breakdown of uracil, and several inactive fluorine-containing fragments have been identified in the urine. The degradation of FU takes place mainly in the liver, but other organs also contribute. Because of this rapid metabolism, FU has been infused directly into the portal vein or hepatic artery for the treatment of hepatic metastases, without excessive systemic toxicity.

Mechanism of Action. FU acts only as a "prodrug," which by a process of lethal synthesis is converted to the active agent. Without this activation, FU would have little if any pharmacologic properties. A remarkable correlation was found between the anabolism of FU in tumors and the degree of susceptibility of these tumors to the inhibitory actions of FU (Fig. 5–20).[32] Biochemical studies have revealed the much greater potency of the drug anabolites of FU, such as FdUMP, than the parent drug in inhibiting DNA synthesis. Probably the formation of FdUMP is most closely linked to the antitumor action of FU.

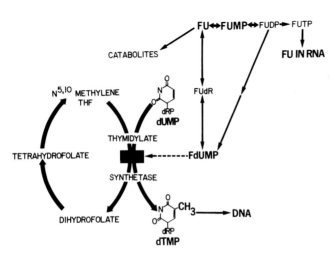

Figure 5–19. Interrelationship between anabolism of fluorouracil (FU) and actions of the drug. (1) Inhibition of thymidylate synthetase and DNA synthesis by fluorodeoxyuridylate, FdUMP (center), and (2) incorporation of FU into RNA (right). FUdR, fluorodeoxyuridine; FUMP, fluorouridylate; FUDP + FUTP, fluorouridine di- and triphosphates, respectively, and dRP, deoxyribose phosphate. Broken arrow from FdUMP connects to shaded block at enzyme site methylating deoxyuridylate (dUMP) to thymidylate (dTMP).

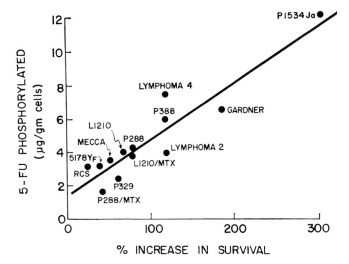

Figure 5–20. Correlation between extent of anabolism of FU to inhibitory compounds by phosphorylation in a series of animal tumors, and response of those tumors to the drug. Survival of animals bearing those tumors increases as tumor burden is reduced by effective chemotherapy with FU. (From Kessel et al: Science, 154:911, 1966. Copyright © by the American Association for the Advancement of Science.)

FdUMP is a potent inhibitor of the enzyme, thymidylate synthetase, and it binds with great affinity to this enzyme. A stable complex of FdUMP, the enzyme and the cofactor, $N^{5,10}$ methylene tetrahydrofolate has been isolated. The enzyme normally is responsible for the methylation of deoxyuridylate to thymidylate, and thus plays a major role in DNA synthesis. Inhibition of DNA synthesis by this anabolite of FU leads to imbalanced growth and results in cell death.

The formation of fluorine-containing RNA leads to numerous changes in biochemical functions that undoubtedly play a role in the drug's toxicity, if not its antitumor effect as well.[33] Probably because of the constellation of biochemical effects produced by FU, localization of the action of FU at a precise step in the cell cycle has not been possible, and the drug acts as a self-limiting inhibitor of S phase.

The selectivity of FU as an antitumor drug has recently been demonstrated in experiments that reveal the slower recovery of DNA synthesis of tumors than bone marrow and intestinal mucosa following FU treatment of mice (Fig. 5–21).[34] This recovery was associated with the loss of intracellular FdUMP from these tissues. With this information it has been possible to design dose schedules maximizing the therapeutic index of FU.

Tumor cells with acquired resistance to FU have been demonstrated to have deficient capacities to convert FU to the phosphorylated de-

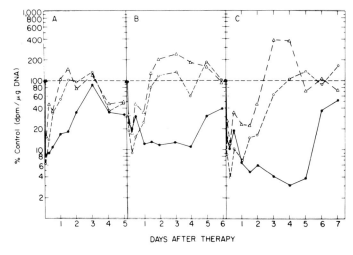

Figure 5–21. Differential effect of fluorouracil (FU) on formation of DNA from deoxyuridine in various mouse tissues: P1534 ascites cells (●), gastrointestinal mucosa (Δ), and bone marrow (○). Doses of FU were (A) 15, (B) 50, and (C) 100 mg/kg. Note the differential recovery of DNA formation in intestine and bone marrow compared to tumor which becomes more apparent as dose of drug is increased, explaining antitumor selectivity. (From Myers et al: Ca Res 36:1653, 1976)

rivatives, compared to sensitive tissues of the same tumor. An alteration in response to FdUMP by thymidylate synthetase has also been reported.

Toxicity. The major toxic effects of FU are myelosuppression, especially leukopenia, which may be delayed. Thrombocytopenia and anemia may also result in addition to gastrointestinal ulceration, diarrhea, and particularly anorexia and nausea, stomatitis, hair loss, cerebellar dysfunction, and hyperpigmentation. Toxicity to the oral mucosa and diarrhea are usually predictors of more serious bone marrow depression, and therapy should be withheld. This drug has to be administered with great care during the initiation of therapy because of variation in patient tolerance to it. Chemotherapeutic efficacy, which appears to lead to an increase in survival, is usually associated with some incipient toxicity. Drug catabolism may be impaired in patients with extensive liver metastases, resulting in increased anabolism of FU to toxic compounds.

ARABINOSYLCYTOSINE

Ara-C (1-β-D-arabinofuranosylcytosine, cytosine arabinoside, cytarabine, cytosar) (XXII) is an analog of cytidine (XXIII) in which the 2′ hydroxyl is in the inverse steric configuration so that arabinose replaces the normal ribose constituent. It is of greater significance that the drug is also an analog of deoxycytidine (XXIV).

Actions and uses. Ara-C is most useful in the treatment of the adult acute leukemias, particu-

XXII   Ara-C   A: –OH ; B: –H
XXIII   Cytidine   A: –H ; B: –OH
XXIV   Deoxycytidine   A: –H ; B: –H

larly the granulocytic variety. It has been beneficial in Hodgkin's disease and lymphomas. Arabinosylcytosine has been used in women with recurrent ovarian cancer and ascites.

Pharmacokinetics. Ara-C is poorly absorbed after oral administration because of extensive breakdown. After intravenous administration satisfactory plasma levels can be obtained but again the drug is extensively catabolized. The parent drug crosses into the cerebrospinal fluid in significant amounts, and the level of the drug in the CSF reaches about 50 percent that of plasma. The $t_{1/2}$ for the α and β phases are 10 minutes and 2 hours, respectively. Ara-C is rapidly deaminated to uracil arabinoside (ara-U) which is biologically inactive. Cytidine deaminase, which mediates this reaction, is present mainly in liver but also in gastrointestinal tract and kidney, while very little is present in plasma. Ara-U is the major drug catabolite in the blood, and about 90 percent of the total drug is excreted as ara-U in the urine.

Of greater significance to the action of ara-C is the anabolism to the phosphorylated derivative, ara-CMP, and its di- and triphosphates, ara-CDP and ara-CTP respectively (Fig. 5–22). Small amounts of the arabinoside derivative are also incorporated into DNA and RNA.

Mechanism of action. Ara-C mainly acts as an antimetabolite of deoxycytidine in that its mono- and triphosphate derivatives are antagonists of deoxycytidine mono- and triphosphate, respectively. Arabinoside triphosphate competes with normal deoxycytidine triphosphate for DNA polymerase and inhibits this enzyme. The resulting cessation of DNA synthesis, which is probably the parent drug's major biochemical effect, then explains the S phase specificity of ara-C. Chromatid breakage, which results from this action, may be most closely associated with the lethal effects of the drug. The pharmacologic consequences of the incorporation of the analog into DNA and RNA are still unclear. Another but much less important site of action of ara-C, acting through its diphosphate derivatives, is inhibition of the reduction of cytidine to deoxycytidine compounds.

Again, as with other pyrimidine or purine analogs, an interesting correlation has been demonstrated between the ability of various rodent tumors to anabolize ara-C to phosphorylated derivatives, and the sensitivity of these tumors to inhibition by ara-C. Tumors were found to reach

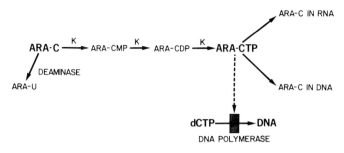

Figure 5–22. Interrelationship between anabolism of arabinosylcytosine (ara-C) via several kinases (K) to the mono-, di-, and triphosphates ara-CMP, ara-CDP, and ara-CTP, respectively, and interference with DNA polymerization. There is also direct incorporation of ara-C into RNA and DNA. Ara-C is readily deactivated by a deaminase to arabinosyluracil (ara-U). The broken arrow connects to the shaded block of DNA polymerase, which usually converts deoxycytidylate (dCTP) into DNA.

and retain higher levels of ara-CTP than intestine and other normal tissue, whereas concentrations of ara-CMP or ara-C are more similar in most tissues examined.[35] It is likely that the drug's antitumor effect, at least in the rodent, is related to the selective formation and retention of ara-CTP in the tumor, leading to a prolonged inhibition of DNA synthesis (Fig. 5–23).

Activation by deoxycytidine kinase and deamination by cytidine deaminase as well as the ratio of these enzyme activities have been proposed as indicators of tissue susceptibility to ara-C, but none of these parameters serve as a reliable predictor of human tumor sensitivity to ara-C.

Acquired resistance to this drug has been closely associated with diminished deoxycytidine kinase levels. In addition, resistance may also be brought about by changes in the affinity of ara-CTP to DNA polymerase, and by alteration in the pool size of dCTP.

Currently experiments are underway to delay the catabolism of ara-C by the concomitant administration of the deaminase inhibitor, tetrahydrouridine, in an effort to prolong carcinostatic plasma levels. It is still unknown, however, whether this combination alters the antitumor selectivity of ara-C.

Rationale for dose scheduling. Because of the short $t_{1/2}$ of the drug and its relative specificity in inhibiting DNA synthesis, it has been possible to elaborate drug dosages in a mouse model system that permitted cytotoxic drug concentrations of sufficient duration to expose all clonogenic tumor cells as they traversed S phase and synthesized DNA (Table 5–5).[36] During this period, less than 100 percent of the host's clonogenic hematopoietic and intestinal crypt cells were exposed because of the lower growth fraction in those tissues. In addition, the repeated and frequent administration of ara-C during every fourth day was shown to be curative, since this schedule permitted sufficient recovery of the normal tissue to limit host toxicity. On the other hand, single but

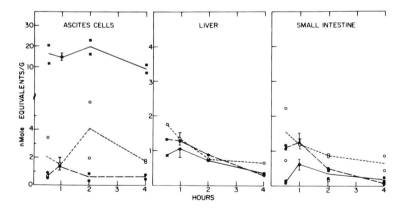

Figure 5–23. Relative tissue levels of ara-C (○), ara-CMP (●) and ara-CTP (■) following administration of ara-C to leukemic mice. Antitumor selectivity of ara-C may be related to higher levels of ara-CTP in ascites cells than in liver or small intestine. (From Chou et al: Ca Res 35:225, 1975)

Table 5–5. CRITICAL NATURE OF INTERVAL BETWEEN PERIOD OF EFFECTIVE BLOOD
LEVEL OF ARA-C AND THE RESPONSE OF MICE BEARING L-1210 LEUKEMIA*

mg/kg/ DOSE	NO. OF DOSES	INTERVAL BETWEEN DOSES	INTERVAL BETWEEN DOSES DURING WHICH THE BLOOD LEVEL WAS <0.3 µg/ml (hr)	% "CURES" IN ANIMALS BEARING DIFFERENT NUMBERS OF LEUKEMIC CELLS 10^6	10^5	10^4	COMMENTS
15	8	10 min	0	0	0	0	Periods of effective blood
15	8	30 min	0	0	0	0	concentration were too
15	8	1 hr	0	0	0	0	short (i.e., 4–10 hr)
15	8	3 hr	0.2	0	10	60	Optimal interval between
15	8	4 hr	1	—	10	70	15 mg/kg doses = <9
15	8	5 hr	2	—	20	60	hr; optimal interval
15	8	6 hr	3	0	10	40	between periods of
15	8	7 hr	4	—	30	40	effective blood
15	8	8 hr	5	—	20	30	concentration = <6 hr
15	8	9 hr	6	—	0	0	Interval between periods
15	8	10 hr	7	—	0	0	of effective blood
15	8	11 hr	8	0	0	0	concentration was too
15	8	12 hr	21	0	0	0	long

*From Skipper et al: Ca Chemother Rep 54:431, 1970.

much larger doses on the same days have produced only little therapeutic effect (Table 5–6).[37] Qualitatively similar results have been demonstrated in the human, in whom prolonged exposure to cytotoxic levels of the drug administered by continuous infusion with an interval for recovery has been more effective than single or infrequently administered doses.

Toxicity. The toxicity of ara-C is expressed mainly against the bone marrow and gastrointestinal tract. Hepatic dysfunction, phlebitis, and fever have also been reported. The drug is also a potent immunosuppressive agent.

Antibiotics and Other Drugs

Largely by chance, numerous naturally occurring compounds isolated from plants or microbial fermentation media have been found to possess antitumor properties in animal model systems and the human. There are also a few synthetic products that have demonstrated activity in tumor screens and have been introduced into clinical treatment. Of interest against solid tumors are mainly the antibiotics actinomycin, doxorubicin, bleomycin, mitomycin, and mithramycin; other compounds include hydroxyurea and the vinca alkaloids, vincristine and vinblastine.

Table 5–6. SUCCESS VS FAILURE:
IMPORTANCE OF SELECTION OF
PROPER DOSE SCHEDULE DURING
REPEATED TREATMENT WITH
ARA-C OF TUMOR-BEARING ANIMALS

DOSE (mg/kg)	TIME OF INJECTIONS	TOTAL DOSE	NUMBER OF ANIMALS CURED	LEUKEMIC CELLS AT END OF TREATMENT
240	Days 2,6,10,14	960	0/10	10^9
15	8× daily on days 2, 6, 10, 14	480	10/10	None

*From Skipper et al: Ca Chemother Rep 51:125, 1967.

DACTINOMYCIN

Dactinomycin, actinomycin D, or Cosmegan (XXV), was one of the first useful antibiotics with tumor-inhibitory properties derived from streptomyces cultures.

XXV   Dactinomycin   Sar, Sarcosine; Meval, N-methylvaline

Actions and uses. Dactinomycin has been used successfully in choriocarcinoma resistant to methotrexate. The drug is being used in combination with vincristine and cyclophosphamide in the treatment of women with ovarian cancer of embryonal types and malignant teratomas with and without neural elements. Also dactinomycin in combination with methotrexate and chlorambucil is being utilized for ovarian germ cell cancers containing choriocarcinoma. In the treatment of women with mixed mesodermal ovarian cancers a combination of dactinomycin and vincristine given concomitantly with radiotherapy followed by a maintenance regimen with cyclophosphamide is being studied. Women with malignant tumors of the ovarian stroma such as granulosa cell cancers, granulosa-theca cell carcinomas, and arrhenoblastomas that are not completely resectable are being evaluated with a treatment combination of dactinomycin, 5-fluorouracil, and cyclophosphamide. Unresponsive uterine sarcomas may be treated with dactinomycin, vincristine, and cyclophosphamide.

Pharmacokinetics. The drug is poorly absorbed orally and is normally administered parenterally, frequently through the tubing during intravenous infusion to avoid subcutaneous toxicity. The compound disappears rapidly from the blood but none enters the CNS. Much of the drug is excreted by bile, and very little is recovered in urine. No metabolic alterations have been reported. The drug is distributed in liver, kidney, spleen, and salivary gland, but not all of the drug in tissues is actually bound to DNA.

Mechanism of action. The compound binds strongly to double-stranded DNA in the cell nucleus, and actually inserts itself (intercalates) between base sequences (Fig. 5–24).[38] It usually positions itself adjacent to guanine, i.e., a dG-dC base pair, and then inhibits RNA polymerase. The inhibition of DNA-dependent RNA synthesis is directly caused by drug complexing with template DNA. The formation of ribosomal RNA appears to be preferentially blocked, but all RNA synthesis is inhibited. With large doses of the drug, there may also be inhibition of DNA and protein synthesis. Cytotoxicity is usually related to uptake and especially retention of the drug, in a particular tissue, and tumors resistant to actinomycin normally demonstrate reduced permeability of the antibiotic.

Toxicity. Toxicity is directed against the gastrointestinal tract and the hematopoietic system. Thrombocytopenia may precede other hemato-

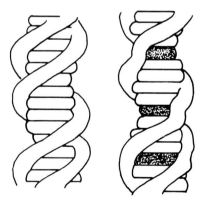

Figure 5–24. Model of (left) normal DNA with two deoxyribose phosphates chains wound around base pairs, and (right) DNA with a drug sandwiched between pairs of bases, thereby changing the configuration of DNA (intercalation). (From Fishbein et al: Chemical Mutagens: Environmental Effects on Biological Systems, 1970, p 30. Courtesy of Academic Press)

logic toxicity, but bone marrow suppression may be complete and rapid. Other toxicity includes oral ulceration, alopecia, skin reactions, as well as liver and kidney abnormalities. There may be enhanced toxicity and sensitization when radiation therapy is used concurrently.

DOXORUBICIN

Doxorubicin or Adriamycin (XXVI) is an anthracycline antibiotic discovered in certain streptomyces fermentation broths. The drug is very similar structurally and pharmacologically to the antileukemic drug, daunorubicin, which it has replaced clinically because of its greater effectiveness against solid tumors.

XXVI Doxorubicin

Actions and uses. Doxorubicin alone or with dacarbazine is used in the treatment of women with residual or recurrent biopsy-proven nonresectable uterine sarcomas. In combination with cyclophosphamide, doxorubicin is being evaluated in the treatment of women with ovarian adenocarcinomas stages 3 and 4 with significant residual disease or with recurrent ovarian adenocarcinoma. Either alone or in combination with various agents, doxorubicin is utilized for advanced epidermoid cancer of the cervix, vagina, and vulva and endometrial adenocarcinoma. It has been administered with irradiation therapy for cervical cancer. Doxorubicin is usually given directly into the tubing of an intravenous infusion because of its tissue necrotic properties. An assessment of its gynecologic antitumor spectrum has been prepared.[39]

Pharmacokinetics. Studies on the disposition of doxorubicin have been complicated by the difficulties in analytic methodology which have permitted variable interpretations. The drug is not absorbed orally since it is too readily degraded. The disappearance of doxorubicin from plasma has an initial $t_{1/2}$ of less than one hour, and most of the drug is rapidly cleared from the blood. Thereafter, there is a much slower $t_{1/2}$, about 28 hours. Because of this drug retention and slow elimination, the effectiveness of the drug is not very schedule dependent, and drug-free intervals of three weeks are often recommended. Biliary excretion following hepatic metabolism represents the major route of elimination, and only about 6 percent of adriamycin and its numerous metabolites are excreted in the urine.

A major metabolite formed through the mediation by a ubiquitous aldo-keto reductase is the reduction product, doxorubicinol, which has pharmacologic activity. Various inactive aglycones are also formed which are excreted in conjugated form in bile and urine. The enzyme that catalyzes this degradation is a microsomal glycosidase which, at least in animals, appears to be inducible by drugs like phenobarbital. The resulting increase in doxorubicin breakdown leads to reduced antitumor effectiveness. Correspondingly, impairment of liver function has been associated with toxicity because of diminished detoxication and delayed excretion of active drugs.[40] Therefore, the dose of doxorubicin must be sharply reduced in patients with hepatic disease. Renal disease is not associated with increased drug toxicity. Doxorubicin is taken up by many organs, including spleen, kidney, lung, and small intestine, but little penetrates into the CNS. Liver and heart also contain some of the drug.

Mechanism of action. The drug binds extensively to DNA in the cell nucleus and intercalates between adjacent base pairs. This drug insertion causes an uncoiling of the DNA helix, the inhibition of both DNA and RNA polymerases and thus, inhibition of DNA and RNA synthesis. Maximal antitumor action is observed during S phase, but the antibiotic is also effective at all other phases of the cell cycle as well as for G_0 cells. The precise mechanism of action of doxorubicin is not known, since many of the drug's inhibitory effects are not associated with inhibition of nucleic acid synthesis. Major chromosomal alterations, probably independent of the inhibition of DNA synthesis, have been observed. Resistance to doxorubicin probably rests on inability of penetration of the drug into the cell.

Toxicity. The major adverse effects are myelo-suppression which occurs acutely, and cardio-myopathy which is related to total dose and may be delayed six months or longer. Leukopenia may be dose limiting, and thrombocytopenia, anemia, gastrointestinal disturbances, stomatitis, and par-ticularly alopecia may occur. The myocardial ef-fect results in fragmentation and reduction in myofibrils, myocardial mitochondrial swelling and congestive heart failure. Symptoms include tachy-cardia, arrhythmias, and electrocardiographic changes. Cardiac symptoms are frequently ob-served at a total drug dosage of 550 mg/sq meter and appear more frequently in elderly individuals with preexisting heart disease. The mechanisms of this cardiac toxicity, which may be fatal, is not known, but is probably not directly related to binding of the drug to myocardial DNA. Cardiac glycosides apparently have little effect on cardiac toxicity produced by doxorubicin. Skin injury and hyperpigmentation of nails has been reported.

BLEOMYCIN

Bleomycin (XXVII) is a mixture of glycopeptide antibiotics isolated from cultures of certain strep-tomyces strains. The drug consists of an unknown number of products, one of which, bleomycin A2, has been isolated in purified form. However, this ingredient does not produce the full therapeutic effect of the mixture.

Actions and uses. The mixture has been effec-tively used against squamous cell carcinoma of the head, neck, and genitourinary tract. Bleomycin has been used with various combinations of drugs for the treatment of advanced epidermoid cancer of the cervix, vagina, and vulva, plus metastatic sarcomas of the uterus and ovarian adenocarci-nomas. Also topical bleomycin for carcinoma in situ of the vulva is under study.

Pharmacokinetics. Bleomycin is normally given parenterally. It is not surprising, considering the complexity of the molecular structure of just one component of this mixture, that there is still only fragmentary information available on its disposi-tion. The antibiotic is rapidly cleared from plas-ma, and localizes in tumors, lung, and skin. It produces its major inhibitory or toxic effects in those tissues, apparently because of low levels of a peptidase that usually catabolizes the drug. Topical bleomycin in a 5 percent cream is being evaluat-ed as a treatment of Paget's disease of the vulva.

Mechanism of action. The antibiotic binds to DNA, causing scission of DNA, and inhibits DNA repair, resulting in fragmentation of DNA and chromosomal abnormalities. DNA synthesis is markedly inhibited whereas the effects on RNA are less pronounced. The drug inhibits during the S phase and also blocks progression from the G_2

XXVII Bleomycin

to the mitotic phase of the cell cycle. The drug may sensitize to subsequent irradiation, perhaps by preventing repair of sublethal irradiation damage.

Toxicity.   The major and occasionally fatal toxicity of the drug, which at the present time limits its usefulness, is pulmonary fibrosis. This effect may be encountered even after relatively low doses of the drug but occurs more frequently at higher doses. The pulmonary toxicity appears to be more pronounced in the elderly, particularly after a total dose of 400 mg. Additional toxicity includes hypotension and fever, especially for the lymphoma patient who therefore should be carefully tested before the full dose of drug is administered. Alopecia, stomatitis, and cardiac arrest have been reported, and cutaneous toxicity of the fingers and hands is frequently observed. Subsequent therapy with some other antitumor drugs may enhance the toxicity of previously administered bleomycin.

The value of bleomycin in chemotherapy has not yet been fully explored, but its unusual lack of toxicity to bone marrow compared to most antitumor drugs suggests that it should be used in combination with other antitumor drugs.

MITOMYCIN C
Mitomycin C (XXVIII) is an antibiotic isolated from a strain of streptomyces. Its actions as an alkylating agent explain why the drug can also be grouped with those anticancer agents.

Actions and uses.   Mitomycin is effective in the treatment of various solid tumors including those of the breast, stomach, pancreas, lung and osteogenic sarcoma. In combination with vincristine and bleomycin, mitomycin C is being evaluated against very advanced epidermoid cervical cancer.

XXVIII   Mitomycin

Pharmacokinetics.   The drug is variably absorbed after oral administration and disappears rapidly from plasma. It is quickly inactivated.

Mechanism of action.   Mitomycin is a "prodrug" that needs to be activated before it exhibits its antitumor properties. In vivo the quinone ring is reduced and the tertiary methoxy group is eliminated. A three-membered ring is unmasked which alkylates like an ethylenimine ring. The reaction is analogous to that of bifunctional nitrogen mustards, and both the quinoid oxygen and the ethylenimine group interact with nucleophilic targets such as DNA. This effect leads to crosslinking of DNA, inhibition of DNA synthesis, and breakdown of RNA.

Toxicity.   Leukopenia and thrombocytopenia are usually the limiting toxic effects of mitomycin. The myelosuppression is delayed and cumulative. Gastrointestinal effects are also common and neuromuscular toxicity has been reported. Local tissue necrosis results from extravasation of the drug during intravenous therapy.

MITHRAMYIN
Mithramyin or Mithracin (XXIX) is an antibiotic isolated from cultures of *streptomyces atroolivaceous* and is closely related chemically to two other tumor-inhibitory fermentation products, olivomycin A and chromomycin A_3. Mithramycin is more effective when administered intravenously than orally, suggesting poor absorption.

Actions and uses.   Mithramycin is frequently valuable against trophoblastic neoplasms. The drug does have an additional action of lowering plasma calcium levels in hypercalcemic patients at nontoxic concentrations. Thus, the drug is also used in cases of hypercalcemia associated with metastatic carcinoma involving bone.

Mechanism of action.   The drug, in the presence of Mg^{2+}, forms a complex with DNA by a process not unlike the intercalation of dactinomyin with polynucleotides. This interaction results in the inhibition mainly of RNA synthesis, which is believed to be the mechanism of tumor inhibition.

Toxicity.   In addition to major toxicity to bone marrow, kidney, and liver, mithramyin interferes with the clotting process and produces generalized hemorrhage. The drug should be discontinued if these toxicities are persistent.

XXIX Mithramycin

HYDROXYUREA

Hydroxyurea or Hydrea (XXX), a carcinostatic compound with a very simple chemical structure, was first synthesized as long as a century ago and has been known for 50 years to produce hematopoeitic depression.

XXX Hydroxyurea

Actions and uses. The compound's effectiveness in the treatment of leukemias has led to its evaluation of other human malignancies, such as in women with advanced epidermoid cancer of the cervix, vagina, or vulva. It has also been combined with irradiation therapy for cervical cancer.

Pharmacokinetics. Hydroxyurea is well absorbed after oral administration and produces a peak in blood level at about 2.5 hours. About half of the drug is recovered unchanged in the urine within 3.5 hours and another 30 percent is excreted dur-

ing the next 8 hours. The remainder probably is excreted as degradation products. Acetoxyhydroxamic acid may be a drug metabolite in plasma.

Mechanism of action. The most likely effect of hydroxyurea is the inhibition of ribonucleoside diphosphate reductase, the enzyme that probably is rate limiting for DNA synthesis. The drug therefore blocks the reduction of ribonucleoside diphosphates to the corresponding deoxyribonucleoside diphosphates, leading to inhibition of DNA formation. This inhibition is partially competitive with ferrous iron, suggesting that the drug interferes with or complexes the nonheme iron portion of a protein subunit of the enzyme system. Consequently, hydroxyurea inhibits specifically during the S phase of growth. The effect is marked, rapid, and reversible once the drug is removed. There may still be additional mechanisms by which the drug inhibits tumor growth.

Toxicity. Hydroxyurea produces leukopenia, megaloblastic anemia, and occasionally thrombocytopenia. Recovery from these toxicities occurs promptly after cessation of therapy because of the ready reversibility of the drug effects. Gastrointestinal disturbances, alopecia, and neurologic toxicities have been reported. The drug is teratogenic and immunosuppressive in animals.

VINCA ALKALOIDS

Several alkaloids have been isolated from the periwinkle plant, *Vinca rosea,* two of which have useful antitumor properties. Although the chemical structures of vincristine or Oncovin (XXXI) and vinblastine or Velban, (XXXII) are extremely similar (the sole difference between these complex molecules rests on a methyl vs a formyl group) their pharmacologic properties and antitumor spectra exhibit certain important differences.

Actions and uses. Vincristine in combination with dactinomycin and cyclophosphamide is being used in the treatment of germ cell ovarian cancers, embryonal, and malignant teratomas with and without neural elements. In the treatment of women with mixed mesodermal ovarian cancers, vincristine with dactinomycin is given concomitantly with radiotherapy and followed by a maintenance regime with cyclophosphamide. Vincristine with dactinomycin and cyclophosphamide is utilized for the treatment of unresponsive uterine

XXXI   Vincristine   A: –CHO
XXXII Vinblastine   A: –CH₃

sarcomas and endometrial carcinomas. Vincristine, mitomycin C, and bleomycin are being evaluated in advanced squamous cell carcinoma of the cervix. Women with advanced epidermoid carcinoma of the cervix and choriocarcinoma have received some benefit. Vinblastine is used more frequently in the therapy of choriocarcinoma and advanced ovarian germ cell cancers. It is interesting that there is little cross-reistance between the two drugs. The different antitumor spectra may be related to differences in the penetrability of the drugs.

Pharmacokinetics. Vinblastine and vincristine must be given intravenously since oral absorption has been erratic. Both drugs have a sclerosing action and their administration has to be handled with great care. Clearance for both drugs from the blood is rapid, and excretion is primarily in bile. Patients with biliary obstruction should therefore receive a reduced dosage of these drugs. Little information on the pharmacokinetics of the drugs is available, but the drugs appear to be extensively metabolized. Vincristine is rapidly cleared from the blood, and has $t_{1/2}\alpha$ and β of five minutes and three hours, respectively.

Mechanism of action. The mechanism by which these two drugs produce their effects has not been clarified in great detail. Both drugs act mainly during mitosis, and block cells at metaphase. In this regard the compounds resemble colchicine and its derivative, demecolcin, drugs formerly used in cancer chemotherapy. The vinca alkaloids form a complex with the spindle protein, tubulin, leading to dissolution of the microtubules, chromosomal alterations, and arrest of cell division. In addition, effects on nucleic acid and protein biosynthesis have been reported.

Toxicity. Significant differences in toxicity between the two compounds have also been established (Table 5–7).[41] Vincristine has relatively little toxicity to the bone marrow and the gastrointestinal tract, and therefore is frequently applied in combination with myelosuppressive antitumor drugs. The limiting toxicity of vincristine is usually neurologic, and may take several weeks to be expressed even after a single dose. Peripheral neuropathy includes paresthesias of the extremities, loss of deep tendon reflexes, foot drop, neurogenic constipation, and other muscular weaknesses. The neuromuscular effects may be

Table 5–7. DIFFERENT INCIDENCES
OF HUMAN TOXICITY OF
TWO VINCA ALKALOIDS*

% INCIDENCE	VINBLASTINE	VINCRISTINE
>50		Paresthesias
30–50	Leukopenia	Loss of deep tendon reflex
10–30	Nausea; vomiting; anorexia	Constipation; hoarseness
5–10	Neurotoxicity; hair loss	Weakness; hair loss; slapping gait
<5	Stomatitis; diarrhea; constipation; lethargy and depression; phlebitis; ileus	Abdominal pain; muscle cramps; depression; phlebitis; cranial nerve palsy

*From Creasey: In Sartorelli, Johns (eds): Antineoplastic and Immunosuppressive Agents II, 1975, p. 686. Courtesy of Springer.

more severe in the elderly. Leukopenia is rare, but alopecia can be seen frequently.

Limiting vinblastine toxicity is usually on the bone marrow, but some muscle weakness and neurotoxicity may be observed. Constipation and alopecia also may occur.

The Hormones

Although it was first recognized about 50 years ago that estrogenic hormones could produce mammary tumors in mice, it was the early work of Huggins and Clark in 1940[42] that demonstrated that estrogens, like orchiectomy, could also reduce the size of prostatic enlargement in the dog. These observations have rapidly led to the use of sex hormones in the treatment of sex organ–related malignancies. It is now recognized that estrogens, androgens, progestins, and glucocorticoids all have a distinct role in the chemotherapy of cancer. In spite of the extensive use of these drugs, and the immense attention they have received in the laboratory, it is remarkable how many of the basic questions on the mechanism by which these compounds produce carcinostatic effects remain unanswered.[43] Consequently their employment in a particular patient still relies

largely on an empirical basis. Hormone therapy is usually terminated when no beneficial effects are observed, or, as occasionally happens, if the consequences are actually detrimental. Table 5–8[44] represents a recent summary account of the various modalities of treatment in the therapy of breast cancer.

Probably the most significant development in the field of hormonal anticancer agents has been the elucidation by Jensen and Jacobson[45] of the observed complexing of these steroids with specific target proteins in organs that normally respond to hormones. It is now becoming evident that breast hormone–dependent tumors contain substantial quantities of these specific target proteins, although the presence of these receptors does not guarantee sensitivity to hormonal treatment.[46] The further elaboration of this concept has permitted a more rational selection of patients for hormonal therapy of tumors, and may provide an essential step in explaining the mechanisms of the drugs' effectiveness.

For various reasons usually related to reliability and ease of oral administration, ratio of beneficial to adverse effects, and cost, hormones have been replaced by synthetic derivatives with more desirable characteristics. Unfortunately, there is relatively little information available to discriminate among the various derivatives available in a particular category. Differences in potency and plasma half-life are usually taken into account by the dose schedules for each drug, and information on comparable side effects at equieffective doses is scant and usually controversial.

ESTROGENS

The use of estrogens in the treatment of metastatic prostatic carcinoma in the male is based on the successful therapy of orchiectomy and the more

Table 5–8. COMPARISON OF
THERAPEUTIC MODALITIES
IN HUMAN BREAST CANCER*

MODALITY	RESPONSE (%)
Oophorectomy	40–50
Hormonal ablative surgery	30–40
Androgens	20
Estrogens	35
Single-agent chemotherapy	30
Combination chemotherapy	56–75

*From Carter and Slavik: Annu Rev Pharmacol 14: 157, 1974

rapid progression of the disease following androgen therapy. Similarly, estrogens have often been effective in postmenopausal women with advanced breast cancer, whereas such treatment in premenopausal women is generally contraindicated since it may actually accelerate the neoplastic process. It appears, therefore, that tumors of organs dependent on or controlled by hormones for growth and function may retain these requirements until the neoplasms become more undifferentiated. Alterations of the hormonal environment of tumors therefore may be beneficial in controlling their proliferation.

Actions and uses.   The major indications for estrogens is in the treatment of advanced breast cancer and in prostate carcinoma. When the compounds are effective they will produce regression of the tumor, an increase in life expectancy, relief of pain, and a general improvement of well-being. Therapy is palliative rather than curative, and eventually the tumor will become refractory to further estrogen treatment.

Mechanism of action.   The fundamental mechanisms by which estrogens produce their antitumor effects is still unclear. Pharmacologic doses of estrogens may inhibit pituitary control, or they may produce a direct cellular action. In the past few years, major progress has been made in the elucidation of the interaction of these compounds with

the appropriate target tissue. It had been observed earlier that more estrogen could be bound by a breast neoplasm in a patient who had a favorable response from ablative surgery than one who did not respond. Estrogen-responsive tissue of uterus, vagina, mammary gland, hypothalamus, and anterior pituitary are now known to contain a characteristic cytoplasmic protein, called estrophilin, which binds estrogen. This binding is selective, in that progesterone, testosterone, and corticosteroids do not compete with the estrogen. The steroid-protein complex that is formed then moves to the nucleus, and accumulates in the chromatin (Fig. 5–25).[47] An unmasking of restricted regions of DNA of chromatin may result from the steroid-chromatin interaction, which then produces the various responses associated with estrogen action, via the intermediary synthesis of messenger RNA and proteins. The longer the duration of contact between the hormone and chromatin the greater the intensity of estrogenic action anticipated.

It has been concluded that mammary tumors that have little or no estrophilin usually do not respond to endocrine ablation and/or estrogens, whereas a majority of, but not all, patients with tumors with high estrophilin levels will respond to such treatment (Fig. 5–26). An appreciation of this concept should permit a more accurate prediction as to which patients should be candidates for estrogen therapy, and those who should re-

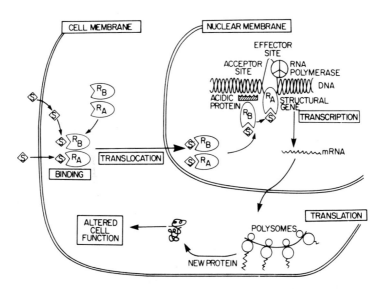

Figure 5–25.   Schematic representation of the subunit structure of model steroid hormone receptors. After binding of steroid S to receptor subunits R_A and R_B in cytoplasm, complex then translocates to nucleus and interacts with DNA, resulting in variety of molecular alterations. (From Chan, O'Malley: N Eng J Med 294:1322, 1976)

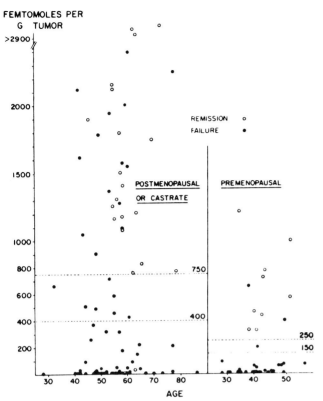

Figure 5–26. Correlation of tumor estrophilic level with response to endocrine therapy for breast postmenopausal (left) and premenopausal (right) cancer patients. Note that tumors responsive to hormone therapy usually have high level of hormone binding to receptor. (From Jensen: Ca Res 35:3362, 1975)

ceive alternative therapy. A reliable indication as to those patients who will respond poorly to estrogens will save them valuable time before more effective treatment can be instituted, and would avoid needless toxicity. This problem has been reviewed recently.[48]

Therapeutic agents. The major estrogens used in therapy today are synthetic since the isolated natural steroids such as estradiol (**XXXIII**) cannot be given orally. Diethylstilbestrol or DES (**XXXIV**), a nonsteroid, is used most extensively because it can be given by mouth, is extremely effective, and quite inexpensive. In animal model systems, this derivative binds more avidly to uterine protein than do the natural estrogens. Diethylstilbestrol diphosphate and polyestradiol phosphate have been designed in the expectation that following their intravenous administration in prostatic tumor patients, there will be a selective intracellular release in the tumor of diethylstilbestrol or estradiol, respectively, because of preferential hydrolysis by what are believed to be relatively high levels of prostatic phosphatase. Chlorotrianisine (Tace) (**XXXV**), is an orally effective triphenylethylene derivative. However, this drug apparently first needs to be activated

XXXIII Estradiol

XXXIV Diethylstilbestrol

XXXV Chlorotrianisine

metabolically and is extensively stored in adipose tissue, so that its actions are slower, more protracted, and more difficult to control. Ethinyl estradiol (Estinyl) (XXXVI) is more potent than diethylstilbestrol and may be given orally, whereas estradiol dipropionate and benzoate are parenteral preparations.

Toxicity. Typical toxicities of estrogens are nausea and vomiting, which are complaints in the majority of elderly female patients, but usually disappear after one to two weeks; vaginal bleeding; urinary incontinence; sodium and water retention with edema, possibly leading to congestive heart failure; hypercalcemia; thromboembolic disease; hypertension; and an increase in gall bladder disease.

ANDROGENS

The therapeutic effects of castration in women with breast cancer suggested the application of androgens in the treatment of this disease. Indeed, these compounds have contributed in slowing the disease, even though the exact mechanism of this effect still remains obscure.

Actions and uses. In addition to producing objective remissions in breast cancer in women, there is

XXXVI Ethinyl estradiol

usually a decrease in bone pain of the osseous metastases following treatment with androgens.

Mechanism of action. It seems likely that by suppressing pituitary function, the androgens limit gonadotropin secretion, although inhibition of tumor growth may be achieved without significant changes in gonadotropin levels. Some of the actions of the compounds may be related to interference with prolactin secretion. It is also possible that the carcinostatic action is related to the rather nonspecific anabolic response of these compounds, since these substances are known to favor protein synthesis or inhibit its breakdown, probably by acting directly on the cell.

Androgens, like other steroid hormones, are known to interact with special receptor proteins in the cytoplasm of sensitive tissue, such as prostate, seminal vesicles, pituitary, and hypothalamus. Following the administration of testosterone, dihydrotestosterone is recovered as a complex with a specific binding protein, whereas dihydrocortisone, progestins, or estradiol do not interact with the protein receptor. Again, the steroid receptor complex moves into the nucleus and interacts with chromatin to produce its endocrinologic effects.

Therapeutic agents. It has been possible by suitable molecular modification to separate, in part, the virilizing properties of androgens from the compounds' anticancer and anabolic effects, since in the treatment of malignancies excessive masculinization is undesirable. By addition of a methyl group in position 2 of testosterone (XXXVII) or the addition of a fluoro group in position 9, for example, the selectivity of action against advanced breast cancer has been increased. Because these newer compounds have less virilizing characteristics, they have largely replaced testosterone in the treatment of breast cancer in women. The major drugs are listed in Table 5–9.

Toxicity. Unwanted drug effects, which are usually not too serious, may include virilism, hepatic dysfunction, biliary stasis, jaundice, sodium retention, and hypercalcemia. Virilization may involve hirsutism, increased musculature, voice deepening, alopecia, as well as clitoral hypertrophy, acne, and increased libido. Hypercalcemia is a more dangerous side effect that may occur in some 10 percent of patients, and plasma calcium levels should therefore be monitored carefully. These drugs are contraindicated in patients with car-

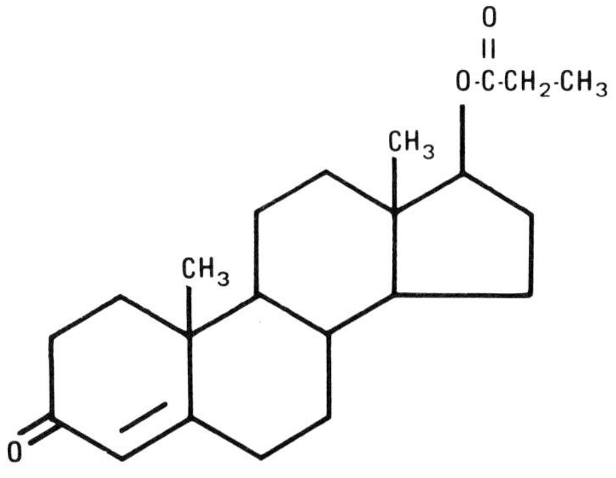

XXXVII   Testosterone propionate

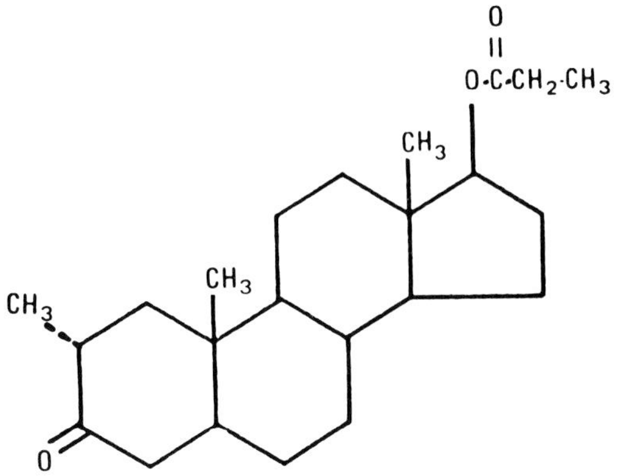

XXXVIII   Dromostanolone propionate

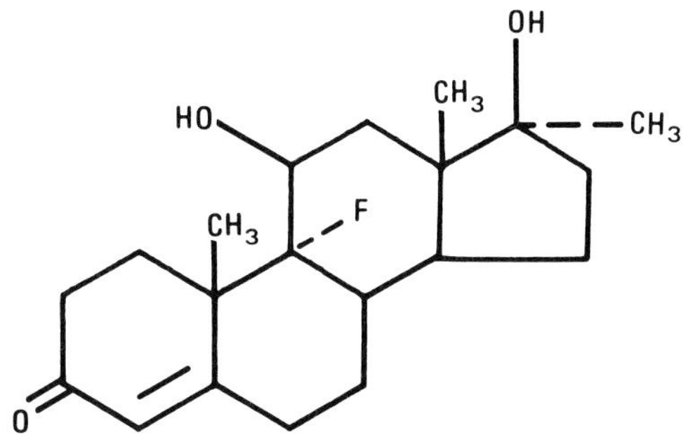

XXXIX   Fluoxymesterone

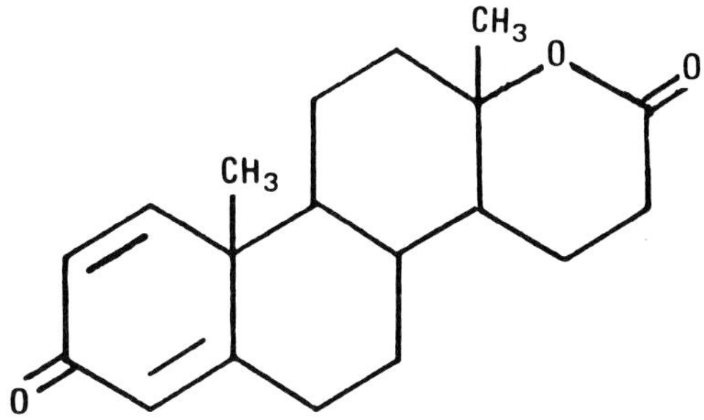

XL   Testolactone

Table 5–9.   ANDROGENS USED IN CANCER THERAPY

NAME	ROUTE	COMMENT
Testosterone propionate (Oreton propionate, XXXVII)	Intramuscular	Virilization
Dromostanolone propionate (Drolban, XXXVIII)	Intramuscular	Less virilization than testosterone, same anti-tumor action
Fluoxymesterone (Halotestin, XXXIX)	Oral	Not as virilizing as other androgens, may be used for maintenance once remission has occurred; cholestasis and jaundice
Testolactone (Teslac, XL)	Intramuscular and oral	Little or no virilizing effect, good antitumor efficacy

diorenal disease, persistent hypercalcemia, and during pregnancy.

PROGESTINS

Because of the physiologic balance in function between estrogens and progestins, progestational agents have been used in the therapy of endometrial carcinoma, a disease state perhaps related to prolonged overstimulation by estrogens without the normal cycling effect of progesterone. Progesterone, which normally promotes the maturation and secretory activity of the endometrium, was demonstrated to produce beneficial effects in certain of these tumors. The development of newer derivatives that promote differentiation and maintenance of the normal endometrial tissue has provided several drugs with antineoplastic activity, which appear to be more reliable than progesterone and also are easier to administer.

Actions and uses. In endometrial cancer, the progestins often produce a favorable response, producing regression of the lesions, especially pulmonary metastases. With higher doses other metastases may also respond. Megestrol acetate in combination with melphalan and 5FU or with doxorubicin, cyclophosphamide, and 5 FU are being studied in women with recurrent endometrial cancer.

Mechanism of action. The mechanism by which these drugs act is unclear. The action may be a direct one, since progesterone produces an inhibitory effect on endometrial cells in culture, though at high concentrations. The possibility also exists that the drug may act through the pituitary to interfere with sex hormone secretion. However, not all of the progestins are effective in inhibiting gonadotropic activity. Progesterone and its synthetic substitutes interact with specific cytoplasmic receptors present in appropriate target tissues, such as uterus, vagina, and pituitary. Estradiol, hydrocortisone, and testosterone do not compete with progesterone for binding to its receptor, but estrogens increase progesterone binding. The binding complex moves into the nucleus leading to increases in chromatin template activity and the synthesis of RNA and protein. This drug-receptor interaction is quite analogous to that described for the other hormones.

Therapeutic agents. The major progestins used against malignancies, in addition to progesterone (XLI) are methoxyprogesterone acetate (XLII)

(either as an oral preparation, Provera, or an intramuscular preparation, Depo-Provera), hydroxyprogesterone caproate (an intramuscular preparation, Delalutin) (XLIII), and the oral preparation, megestrol acetate (Megase; XLIV). Hydroxyprogesterone acetate is active for about two weeks after intramuscular administration, while methoxyprogesterone may be effective somewhat longer, especially as the depot preparation.

Toxicity. Usually there is little toxicity associated with the progestins. Androgenic and corticoid properties are minimal, but fluid retention and hypercalcemia have been reported occasionally.

CORTICOSTEROIDS

The effectiveness of cortisone in controlling the growth of various rodent tumors prompted the application of glucocorticoids in human cancer treatment, whereas mineralocorticoid activity was not required.

Actions and uses. These drugs have been most useful in the induction and maintenance of remission in the lymphatic leukemias, and in the therapy of various lymphomas. The steroids may also be of value in the treatment of hypercalcemia produced by osteolysis resulting from metastatic spread and other forms of hypercalcemia. The edema resulting from brain metastases also usually is well controlled with the glucocorticoids, which are able to penetrate into the CNS, although additional therapy is usually indicated.

Mechanism of action. Lymphoid cells are particularly sensitive to these agents, and hydrocortisone receptors have been identified on such cells. Leukemic lymphocytes contain more receptors than normal lymphocytes, and it is provocative that leukemic cell populations with acquired resistance to the lympholytic effects of glucocorticoids bind less of the hormone to cytoplasmic receptors. A strong lympholytic effect is particularly true in the rodent, but is less likely in man. Its exact mechanism remains unclear, but may involve the induced synthesis of an inhibitory protein which then blocks glucose transport, phosphorylation, and nucleic acid synthesis. In breast cancer the drugs may act on the pituitary to inhibit ACTH secretion and therefore suppress adrenal production of androgens and estrogens, although this mechanism is insufficient to explain

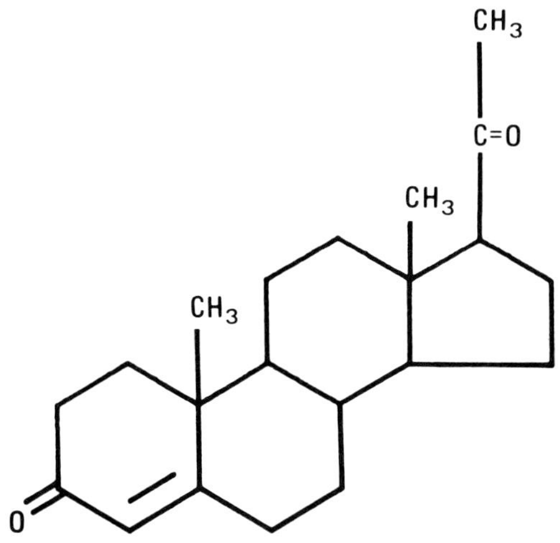

XLI Progesterone

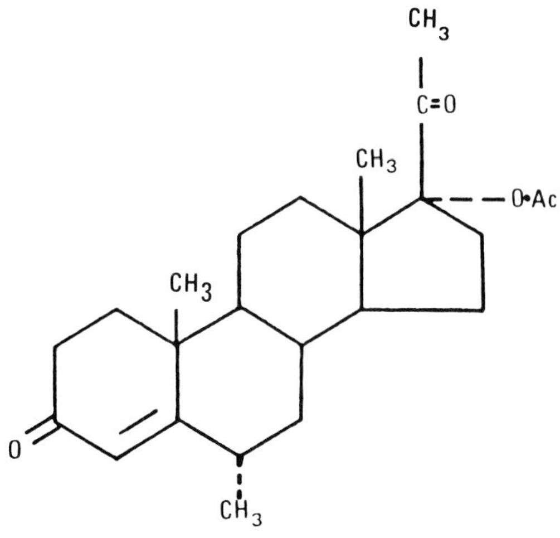

XLII Methoxyprogesterone acetate

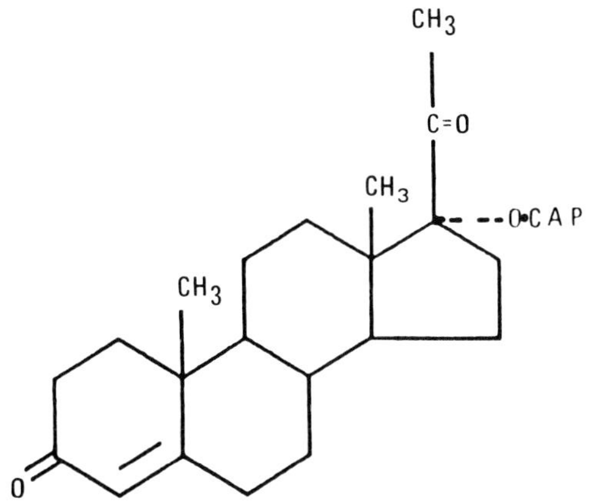

XLIII Hydroxyprogesterone caproate

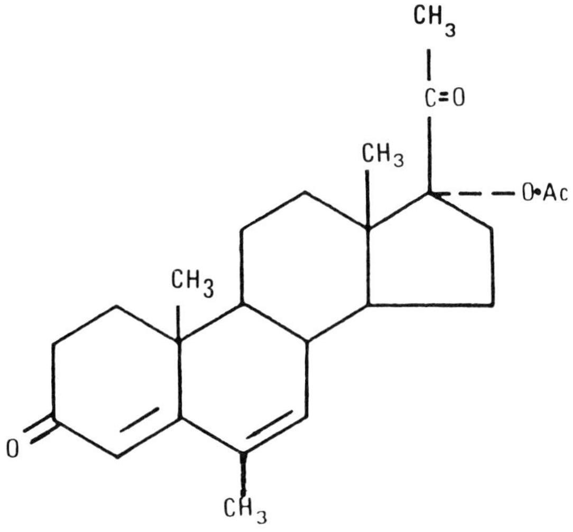

XLIV Megestrol acetate

their actions. The pituitary release of prolactin may also be inhibited by the corticosteroids. The euphoric and appetite stimulant actions of the compounds probably play a significant role in their effectiveness. Their value in the symptomatic palliation of bone marrow depression produced by disease, chemotherapy, or radiation, and their anti-inflammatory actions may produce an improved sense of well-being.

Therapeutic agents. Cortisone and hydrocortisone have useful glucocorticoid activity, but these are accompanied by mineralocorticoid function that leads to sodium and water retention, hypertension, and hypokalemia. Some of the newer derivatives lack these undesirable effects. The major drugs of this group are listed in Table 5-10.

The drugs are normally well absorbed after oral administration, although several may also be administered intravenously when rapid action is desired, such as in the treatment of hypercalcemia. Blood levels decline slowly; hydrocortisone has a plasma $t_{1/2}$ of about two hours, and is extensively bound to an α-globulin protein, transcortin. Many of the hydrocortisone derivatives have a more

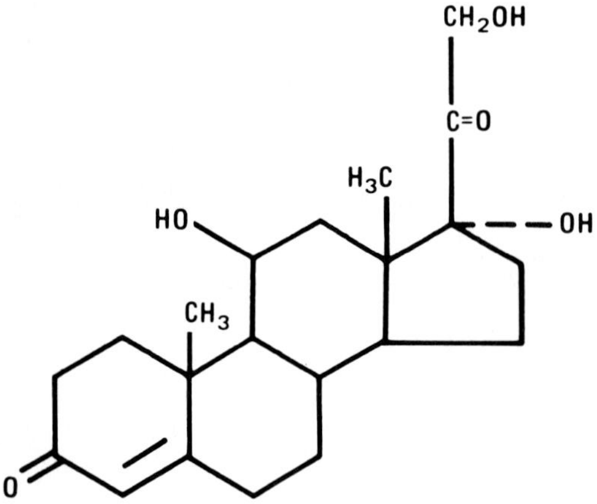

XLV   Cortisol

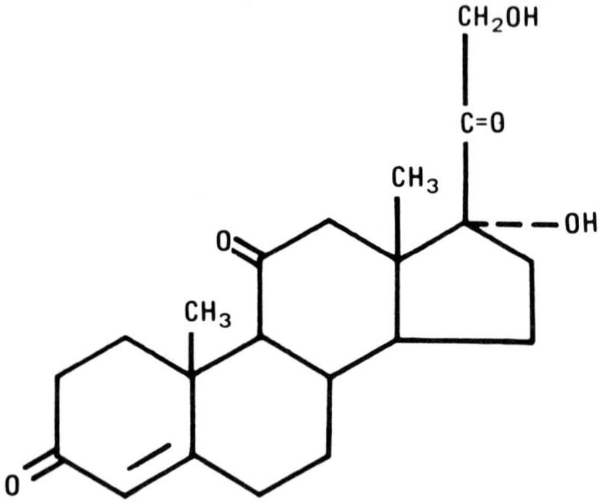

XLVI   Cortisone

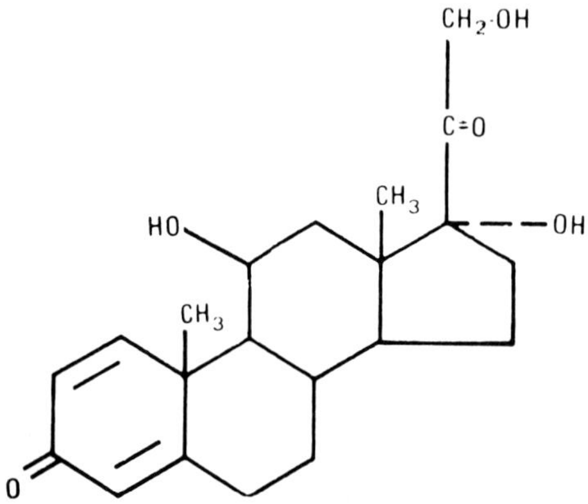

XLVII   Prednisolone

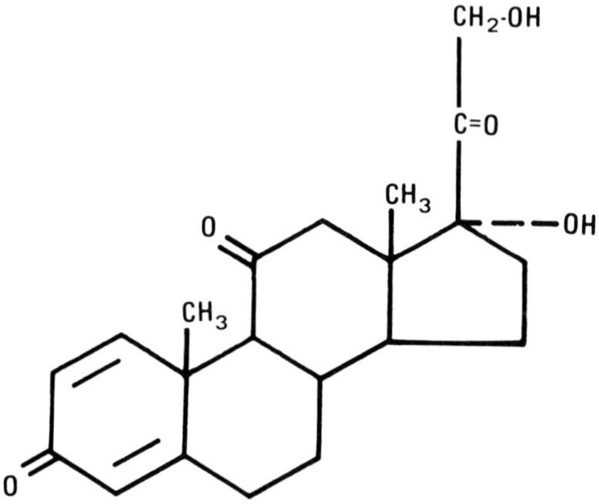

XLVIII   Prednisone

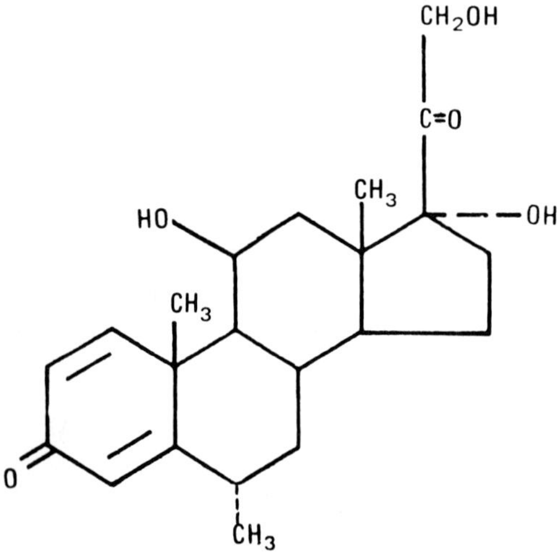

XLIX   Methylprednisolone

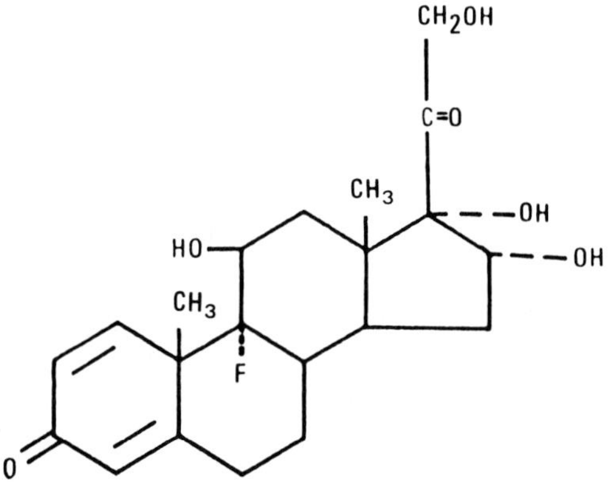

L   Triamcinolone

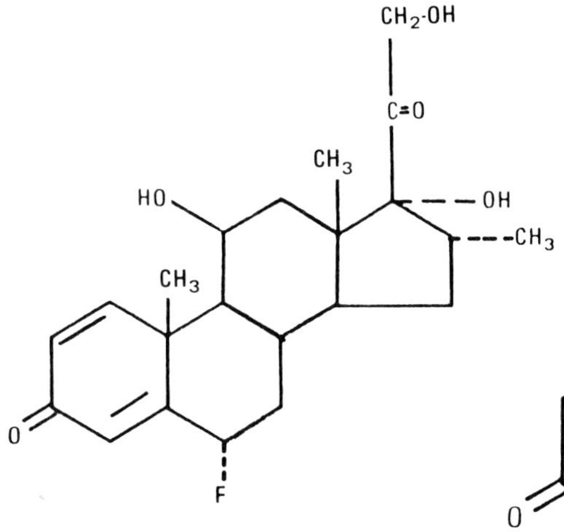

LI   Paramethasone

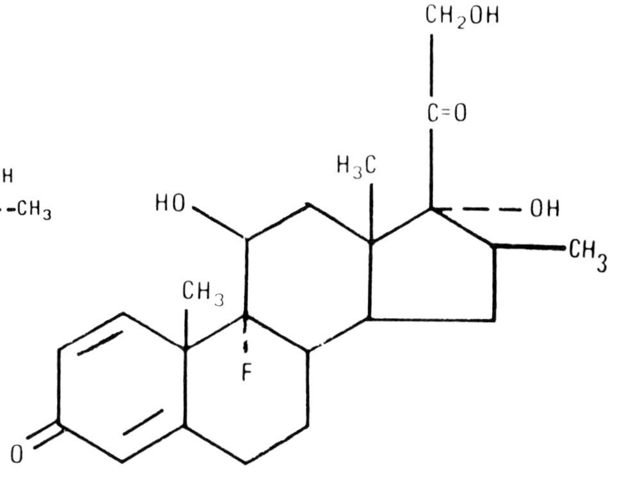

LII   Betamethasone

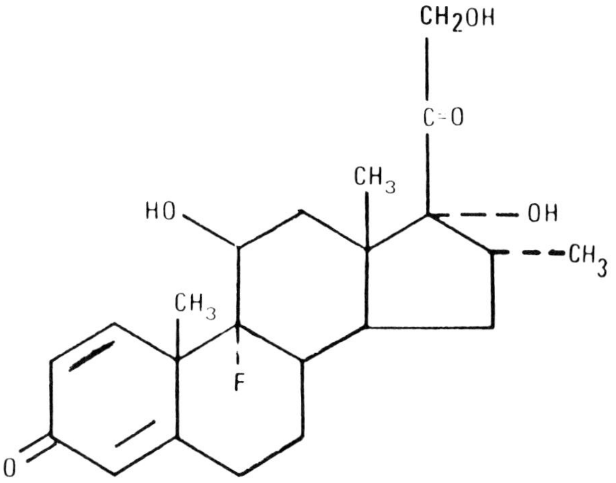

LIII   Dexamethasone

prolonged $t_{1/2}$, e.g., 3.5 hours for prednisolone. Most of the hydrocortisone and its derivatives are catabolized or conjugated by liver to inactive metabolites.

Prednisone is rapidly converted by the liver to prednisolone. Since the 11-hydroxy steroids are the active species, in patients with liver disease, this product or other 11-hydroxy steroids such as methylprednisolone or dexamethasone may be administered directly.

Toxicity.   When hydrocortisone is used, a high-dose regimen used intermittently is preferred to chronic and prolonged daily administration so as to avoid the characteristic Cushingoid toxicities. A similar schedule may be valuable for the other derivatives also. The adverse effects of hydrocortisone include osteoporosis, fluid and electrolyte imbalance, hyperglycemia and glycosuria, infections, peptic ulceration, and behavioral change. Some of the derivatives of hydrocortisone have fewer side effects because of diminished mineralocorticoid activity for equivalent glucocorticoid or anticancer action. Nevertheless, these agents should be used with great care, especially in the elderly cachectic individual.

Table 5–10.   RELATIVE GLUCOCORTI-
COID AND MINERALOCORTICOID
ACTIVITIES OF CORTICOSTEROIDS

	GLUCO- CORTICOID ACTIVITY	MINERALO- CORTICOID ACTIVITY
Cortisol (hydro- cortisone XLV)	1	1
Cortisone (XLVI)	0.8	1
Prednisolone (XLVII)	4	0.8
Prednisone (XLVIII)	4	0.8
Methylpredni- solone (XLIX)	5	0.5
Triamcinolone (L)	5	0
Paramethasone (LI)	10	0
Betamethasone (LII)	25	0
Dexamethasone (LIII)	25	0

Newer Investigational Drugs

During the past few years several new drugs have been developed which are currently being evaluated in phase I and phase II studies.[49] Insufficient information is still available to provide more than a brief description of their features. The compounds listed here have been of special interest particularly in gynecologic cancer.

HEXAMETHYLMELAMINE

Hexamethylmelamine (LIV) is a synthetic compound related structurally to the alkylating agent, triethylenemelamine (TEM, VI). Unlike the latter drug, however, hexamethylmelamine does not behave chemically like an alkylating agent in vitro, and patients resistant to those drugs may still respond to hexamethylmelamine. Unlike alkylating agents, there is little likelihood that this compound can form a carbonium ion that would then react with a nucleophilic target. The drug also has no antifolate properties. At this time there is no indication as to the mechanism by which this drug produces its antitumor responses.[50]

Actions and uses.   Hexamethylmelamine alone or with melphalan is being evaluated in the treatment of women with stages 3 and 4 ovarian adenocarcinomas who have large residual disease

and in women with recurrent ovarian adenocarcinomas. Also usually in combination with other agents, it has been tried against advanced epidermoid cancer of the cervix, vagina, or vulva.

Pharmacokinetics.   The drug is well absorbed orally. Maximum plasma levels are reached about one to three hours after oral administration, mainly in the form of metabolites. The methyl groups are successively split off by the liver, leaving variously methylated melamine derivatives. The $t_{1/2}$ is about 12 hours. Most of the drug is recovered in the urine as the N-demethylated metabolites.

Toxicity.   Major adverse reactions are directed against the gastrointestinal tract. Most patients may exhibit nausea, vomiting, and anorexia, but tolerance to these effects may develop. Myelosuppression may also occur. Leukopenia is usually somewhat more pronounced than thrombocytopenia. Peripheral neuropathy and CNS toxicity have also been reported and are observed more after continuous daily treatment than intermittent therapy. Pyridoxine treatment may prevent the neurotoxicity. Alopecia and skin rash are also known to occur.

CIS-DIAMMINODICHLOROPLATINUM

The growth-inhibitory properties of platinum compounds were discovered by accident when a suspension of *Escherichiae coli* cells was exposed to electric current. The formation of long filamented bacteria was related to the dissolution of small quantities of platinum from the electrodes which eventually completely inhibited microbial cell division. Of a variety of platinum compounds,

LIV   Hexamethylmelamine

LV   Cis-diamminodichloroplatinum II

cis-diamminodichloroplatinum II (DDP) (LV) was found to possess the most favorable tumor-inhibitory properties in experimental animal systems, and is being studied in women. Remarkable structural specificity is required for antitumor effectiveness of the platinum compounds, and a cis planar relationship of the two chlorides is essential.

Actions and uses.   DDP has been shown to be effective against metastatic adenocarcinoma of the ovary and advanced epidermoid cancer of the cervix, vagina, and vulva.

Pharmacokinetics.   DDP is poorly absorbed after oral administration. When given intravenously to man, about 90 percent of the drug is removed from the circulation within the first hour. The values for $t_{1/2}$ (α and β) are about 45 minutes and 60 hours respectively. There is extensive protein binding, but there does not appear to be any selective uptake of the drug in any organ including the tumor. About 25 percent of the drug and metabolites is excreted in the urine within 24 hours, followed by another 25 percent by the end of the fourth day.[51]

Mechanism of action.   DDP produces a persistent and selective inhibition of DNA synthesis. The compound binds firmly to DNA and RNA, and one atom of Pt has been associated with two nucleotides. The exact nature of the ligand formation between Pt and purines is not clear, but it appears that adenine and/or guanine-Pt complexes play an important role in intra- and interstrand cross-linking.

There is a strong resemblance between the actions of Pt and those of alkylating agents. Indeed there is usually cross-resistance between these two classes of drugs, although there have been instances both in animals and in man where DDP has been effective in alkylating agent-resistant tumors. In general, the activity of DDP has been similar to that of cyclophosphamide, even though

combination of these two agents may still show synergism.

Toxicity.   Impairment of renal function and cumulative irreversible ototoxicity may be the dose-limiting toxicities of DDP, although lowering the drug dosages may retain the same antitumor effect with diminished toxicity. Nausea and vomiting occur frequently. DDP also produces some degree of anemia, leukopenia, and thrombocytopenia, although these effects usually are not dose limiting.

PIPERAZINEDIONE

Piperazinedione   (2,5-piperazinedione-3,6-bis-(5-chloro-2-piperidyl) dihydrochloride (NSC-135758)) (LVI), a newly isolated compound from the fermentation broth of *Streptomyces griseoluteus* cultures, has been found to have antitumor activity in experimental animals and is being tested for its clinical usefulness.

Actions and uses.   Piperazinedione is being tested in women who have histologically confirmed persistent or recurrent advanced local or metastatic

LVI   Piperazinedione

gynecologic cancer with documented disease progression (ovary and cervix).

Pharmacokinetics. Very preliminary data suggest that in women the drug disappears from the bloodstream with values for $t_{1/2}$ (α and β) of 0.5 and 3.0 hours, respectively. Radiolabeled drug is rapidly metabolized and total excretion is slow.

Mechanism of action. After a delay, the drug inhibits DNA synthesis and apparently acts as an alkylating agent. It is not purely cell cycle specific, although it exerts a major block during the G_2 phase. In animal systems, tumors resistant to cyclophosphamide may still retain sensitivity to piperazinedione.

Toxicity. Toxicity includes mainly leukopenia with granulocytopenia, thrombocytopenia, as well as occasional anemia, vomiting, sepsis, and fever.[52]

1-PROPANOL-3,3'-IMINODI-DIMETHANE SULFONATE (YOSHI 864)

1-Propanol-3,3'-iminodi-dimethane sulfonate, (LVII) a sulfonic ester of aminoglycol, is a new derivative similar to busulfan but differing, at least in experimental animals, in its antitumor spectrum.

LVII   1-Propanol-3,3'-iminodi-dimethane sulfonate

Actions and uses. Although its mechanism of action undoubtedly relies on the drug's actions as an alkylating agent, it has shown antitumor activity against animal tumors resistant to alkylating agents, including busulfan. In women it is being investigated against various advanced gynecologic cancers,[53] such as ovarian, cervix, and corpus.

Pharmacokinetics. Preliminary studies suggest a biphasis clearance from plasma with $t_{1/2}$ α and β of 7 minutes and 4.5 hours, respectively. Little of

the parent drug is excreted into the urine, but a urinary metabolite has alkylating properties.

Toxicity. Principal toxicity involves leukopenia and thrombocytopenia. Some gastrointestinal toxicity has been reported, and CNS depression may be dose limiting.

DIANHYDROGALACTITOL

The compound, 1,2: 5,6-dianhydrogalactitol (NSC 132,313) (LVIII) is a more recently introduced sugar derivative currently being investigated for its antitumor effectiveness in women, especially against advanced gynecologic cancers such as ovarian, cervix, and corpus. The compound is a derivative and perhaps even a metabolite of various dibromohexitols, such as dibromodulcitol and dibromomannitol.[54] Dihydrogalactitol is readily water soluble, chemically stable, and exerts pronounced biologic effects, compared to the other sugar derivatives.

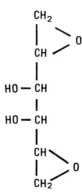

LVIII   1,2:5,6-dianhydrogalactitol

Actions and uses. This drug has been found useful against various experimental tumors, and appears to act like an alkylating agent, as judged by its cytologic effects and cross-resistance with other alkylating agents. The mechanism by which these compounds exert their effects undoubtedly involves cross-linking and inhibition of nucleic acid and protein synthesis. In animal systems, the drug readily crosses the blood-brain barrier. It is currently being studied in women with advanced or recurrent pelvic malignancies.

Toxicity. Toxicity is expressed mainly as thrombocytopenia, with depression of myeloid and lymphoid cells, gastrointestinal reactions and liver abnormalities.

CYTEMBENA

Sodium β-4-methoxybenzoyl-β-cis-bromoacrylate, or cytembena, (LIX) was found to be a cytostatic agent by researchers in Czechoslovakia. Since this compound differs from most other anticancer agents, it is hoped that a novel approach to tumor treatment may be developed.

LIX   Cytembena

Actions and uses.   In earlier European and South African studies, cytembena was reported to be valuable in the treatment of ovarian carcinoma and was believed to be superior to cyclophosphamide. It is too early to discuss recent clinical results from United States' studies,[55] particularly those relating to advanced cervical and corpus cancers.

Pharmacokinetics.   Cytembena is absorbed well after oral administration in animals. In the human the $t_{1/2}$ value of the β phase is about 14 hours. Urinary excretion is very slow, probably due to extensive tubular reabsorption, and only about 8 percent of the drug is recovered in urine.

Mechanism of action.   Several mechanisms have been proposed to explain the drug's actions. The compound inhibits purine biosynthesis and binds to formyltetrahydrofolate synthetase, which blocks the formation of N^{10}-formyltetrahydrofolate from formate and tetrahydrofolate. The drug also inhibits DNA polymerase, possibly via the formation of an active metabolite.

Toxicity.   In the earlier studies, principal toxicity included gastrointestinal effects and phlebitis. With higher dosages, the dose-limiting toxicity is "autonomic storm" consisting of hypertension, hyperperistalsis, diarrhea, paresthesias, and chest pain. This effect may be due to a norepinephrine-like response. No myelodepression was observed in any of the clinical trials. In patients with coronary artery disease, impaired renal function, or liver abnormalities, the drug is probably contraindicated.

PORFIROMYCIN

Porfiromycin (LX) is a tumor-inhibitory antibiotic isolated from *Streptomyces ardus* cultures which is the N-methyl derivative of mitomycin C, another naturally occurring alkylating agent (XXVIII).

LX   Porfiromycin

Actions and uses.   Porfiromycin has been tested for its tumor chemotherapeutic potential for many years,[56] but currently it is being reinvestigated for its potential usefulness in gynecologic malignancies, especially advanced epidermoid carcinoma of the cervix, vagina, or vulva. In addition, carcinoma of the ovary resistant to other alkylating agents may still respond to porfiromycin.

Mechanism of action.   Porfiromycin contains the three-membered ethylenimino ring, and in action and toxicity resembles nitrogen mustard–type alkylating agents. Like mitomycin, the compound is activated by reduction of its quinone ring, and reacts bifunctionally both at the ethylenimine group and the quinoid oxygen. The mechanism of interaction with nucleic acids is probably analogous to that of the other alkylating agents, and DNA guanine-porfiromycin complexes have been isolated.

Toxicity.   Toxicity to porfiromycin includes leukopenia, thrombocytopenia, and local tissue necrosis after extravasation. Some mild gastrointestinal toxicity has also been reported on occasion.

SEMISYNTHETIC PODOPHYLLOTOXIN DERIVATIVES

Two derivatives of podophyllotoxin, a natural product from the May apple plant, have been synthesized recently and are being evaluated for their carcinostatic potential. VM-26 (LXI), is epipodophyllotoxin, 4'-demethyl-9-(4,6-0-2-) the-

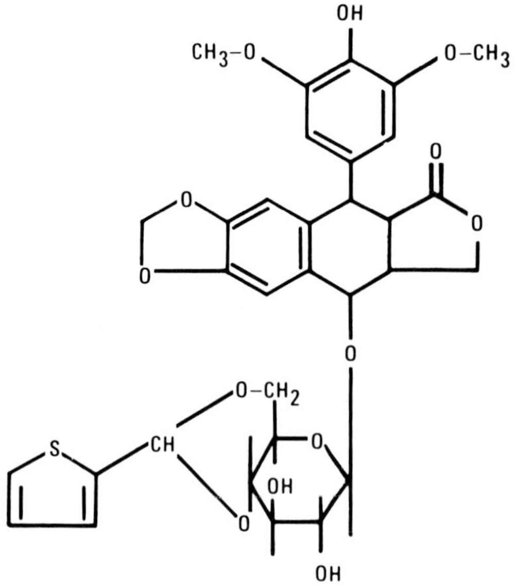

LXI   VM-26

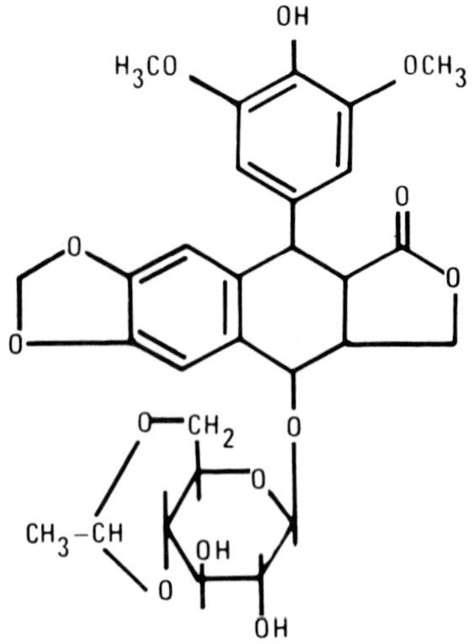

LXII   VP-16213

nylidene-β-D-glucopyranoside. VP-16213 (LXII) is 4'-demethyl-epipodophyllotoxin-β-D-ethylidene glucoside. Since these two derivatives appear to have virtually identical mechanisms of action as well as pharmacology, they will be considered together.

Actions and uses.   VM-26 has demonstrated some activity against brain tumors, lymphomas, leukemia, and bladder carcinomas. VP-16213 has been effective against lung tumors, lymphomas, and leukemia. These different antitumor spectra may rely on small differences in drug distribution. A number of advanced gynecologic cancers are being treated by these agents to evaluate their efficacy, such as cervical and ovarian cancer.

Pharmacokinetics.   Very little information is available on the disposition of these drugs in the human. Both drugs are extensively bound to serum proteins. In the rat there is little evidence

of selective drug concentration except in the organs of excretion. In the human about half the dose of VP-16213 appears in the urine. VM-26 penetrates the CNS somewhat better than VP-16213, which produces extremely low drug levels in the cerebrospinal fluid.

Mechanism of action.   Like the parent compound podophyllotoxin, the two newer derivatives arrest mitosis at metaphase, and act as spindle poisons. They differ, however, in that in addition, cells are gradually inhibited from entering prophase as well. For VM-26, this effect, which may result from inhibition of mitochondrial electron transport, is irreversible. At higher drug concentrations cells entering mitosis are lysed. The drugs inhibit DNA synthesis, and the G_2 and S phases are particularly sensitive to VP-16213.

Toxicity.   Major toxicity has included leukopenia, hypotension after rapid administration, alopecia, and occasionally gastrointestinal distress and thrombocytopenia.

THE FUTURE ROLE OF CANCER CHEMOTHERAPY

An exposition of the major drugs available for the chemotherapy of gynecologic cancer does not really provide an adequate assessment of the current status of the treatment of malignancies with drugs. However, these agents are now being used as the backbone for a multifaceted attack

against a group of fatal diseases that are still very poorly understood except in descriptive terms. Throughout these discussions, an effort has been made to pinpoint those developments that place the action of the drugs or their selective antitumor potential on a more rational basis. All too often this information is not available, or our working hypotheses may have been frozen into readily understandable but oversimplified and sometimes totally misleading dogmas, which may have discouraged newer and more constructive approaches.

Yet not all of the significant accomplishments in cancer chemotherapy have been rational and, as has happened so often in the treatment of any disease, progress relies heavily on the recognition and exploitation of a new finding which ultimately, perhaps decades later, receives a logical explanation.

The use of cancer chemotherapeutic agents in clinical practice now relies heavily on combinations of drugs. Combinations of two to five drugs may be used when we barely understand the optimal application of any of the various components. The aim, which is laudable, is to use agents effective against the particular disease, each with different mechanisms of action and targets of toxicity so that a selective antitumor effect will be enhanced and the emergence of resistance will be minimized. Chemotherapy is now being introduced also in conjunction with surgery and radiation modalities of cancer treatment, and new hope is rising for the success of adjuvant therapy. Immunotherapy, which has been developing for many years and still needs to become of practical value when the tumor population is large, is being added to the overall clinical protocols. The earlier diagnosis of tumors would permit chemotherapeutic intervention at a time when a cure is much more likely.

New efforts are being made to combat the toxicities created by the applications of anticancer agents: replacement of blood components depleted by bone marrow depression, protection against environmental or endogenous microbial flora ultimately responsible for nonresponsive infections, and more localized rather than systemic treatment to encourage the patient's own defense mechanisms to protect itself aginst the tumor and the adverse effect of the drugs.

The challenge of revised drug scheduling has provided remarkable advances in the effectiveness of presently available drugs and has greatly expanded their antitumor capabilities. In part, this reassessment has been possible because of our better understanding of the mechanisms of action and pharmacokinetics of the drugs, as well as the intricate behavior of the tumor cell. These are but some of the areas that have been guiding cancer chemotherapy and providing new hope for the future.

References

1. Zubrod CG: The development of drugs for the control of cancer. In Pharmacological Basis of Cancer Chemotherapy. 27th Annual Symposium on Cancer Research, University of Texas, Houston. Baltimore, Williams and Wilkins, 1975, pp 9–20

2. Hertz R: Eight years experience with the chemotherapy of choriocarcinoma and related trophoblastic tumors in women. In Holland JF, Hreshchyshyn MM (eds): Choriocarcinoma, UICC Monograph 3. Berlin, Springer, 1967, pp 66–71

3. Bonadonna G, Brusamolino E, Valagussa P, et al: Combination chemotherapy as an adjuvant treatment in operable breast cancer. N Engl J Med 294:405–410, 1976

4. Johnson RK, Goldin A: The clinical impact of screening and other experimental tumor studies. Ca Treat Rev 2:1–31, 1975

5. Freireich EJ, Gehan EA, Rall DP, Schmidt LH, Skipper HE: Quantitative comparison of toxicity of anticancer agents in mouse, rat, hamster, dog, monkey and man. Ca Chemother Rept 50:219–244, 1966

6. Skipper HE, Schabel FM, Jr, Wilcox WS: Experimental evaluation of potential anticancer agents. XIII. On the criteria and kinetics associated with "curability" of experimental leukemia. Ca Chemother Rept 35:1–111, 1964

7. Connors TA: What we know about cancer. In Harris RJC (ed): Chemother. London, Allen and Unwin, 1970, Chap 8

8. Griswold DP, Jr: Consideration of the subcutaneously implanted B16 melanoma as a screening model for potential anticancer agents. Ca Chemother Rep, Pt 2 3:315–324, 1972

9. Karnofsky DA, Clarkson BD: Cellular effects of anticancer drugs. Annu Rev Pharmacol 3:357–428, 1963

10. Henderson JF: Biochemical aspects of selective toxicity. In Sartorelli AC, Johns DG (eds): Antineoplastic and Immunosuppressive Agents I. New York, Springer, 1974, pp 341–351

11. Goldin A, Carter SK: Screening and evaluation of antitumor agents. In Holland JF, Frei E, III (eds): Cancer Medicine. Philadelphia, Lea and Febiger, 1973, pp 605–628

12. Zubrod CG: Chemical control of cancer. Proc Natl Acad Sci, U.S.A. 69:1042–1047, 1972

13. Zubrod CG: Agents of choice in neoplastic disease. In Sartorelli AC, Johns DG (eds): Antineoplastic and Immunosuppressive Agents I. New York, Springer, 1974, pp 1–11

14. Mandel HG: The physiological disposition of some anticancer agents. Pharmacol Rev 11:743–838, 1959

15. Pratt WB: Fundamentals of Chemotherapy. New York, Oxford, 1973, p 272

16. Brookes P: Reaction of alkylating agents with nucleic acids. In Plattner PA (ed): Chemotherapy of Cancer. Amsterdam, Elsevier, 1964, pp 32–43

17. Connors TA: Mechanism of action of 2-chloroethylamine derivatives, sulfur mustards, epoxides and aziridines. In Sartorelli AC, Johns DG (eds): Antineoplastic and Immunosuppressive Agents II. New York, Springer, 1975, pp 18–34

18. Goth R, Rajewsky MF: Persistence of O-6-ethylguanine in rat brain DNA: Correlation with nervous system-specific carcinogenesis by ethylnitrosourea. Proc Natl Acad Sci, U.S.A. 71:639–643, 1974

19. Connors TA, Cox PJ, Farmer PB, Foster AB, Jarman M: Some studies of the active intermediates formed in the microsomal metabolism of cyclophosphamide and isophosphamide. Biochem Pharmacol 23:115–129, 1974

20. Slavik M: Clinical studies with nitrosoureas in various solid tumors. Ca Treat Rept 60:795–800, 1976

21. Montgomery JA: Chemistry and structure activity studies of the nitrosoureas. Ca Treat Rept 60:651–664, 1976

22. Schein PS, Panasci L, Woolley PV, Anderson T: Pharmacology of chlorozotocin (NSC 178248), a new nitrosourea antitumor agent. Ca Treat Rept 60:801–805, 1976

23. Skibba JL, Beal DD, Ramirez G, Bryan GT: N-demethylation of the antineoplastic agent 4(5)-(3,3 dimethyl-1-triazene) imidazole-5(4) carboxamide by rats and man. Ca Res 30:147–150, 1970

24. Oliverio VT: Derivatives of triazenes and hydrazines. In Holland JF, Frei E, III (eds): Cancer Medicine, Philadelphia, Lea and Febiger, 1973, pp 806–817

25. Sirotnak FM, Donsbach RC: Differential cell permeability and the basis for selective activity of methotrexate during therapy of the L-1210 leukemia. Ca Res 33:1290–1294, 1973

26. Sirotnak FM, Donsbach RC: Further evidence for a basis of selective activity and relative responsiveness during antifolate therapy of murine tumors. Can Res 35:1737–1744, 1975

27. Kessel D, Hall TC: Retention of 6-mercaptopurine by intact cells as an index of drug responsiveness in human and murine leukemias. Ca Res 29:2116,–2119, 1969

28. LePage GA: Basic biochemical effects and mechanism of action of 6-thioguanine. Ca Res 23:1202–1206, 1963

29. Tidd DM, Paterson ARP: A biochemical mechanism for the delayed cytotoxic reaction of 6-mercaptopurine. Ca Res 34:738–746, 1974

30. Heidelberger C: Fluorinated pyrimidines. Prog Nucl Acid Res Molec Biol 4:1–50, 1965

31. Chadwick M, Rogers WI: The physiological disposition of 5-fluorouracil in mice bearing solid L-1210 lymphocytic leukemia. Ca Res 32:1045–1056, 1972

32. Kessel D, Hall TC, Wodinsky I: Nucleotide formation as a determinant of 5-fluorouracil response in mouse leukemias. Science 154:911–913, 1966

33. Mandel HG: The incorporation of 5-fluorouracil into RNA and its molecular consequences. Prog Molec Subcell Biol 1:82–135, 1969

34. Myers CE, Young RC, Chabner BA: Kinetic alterations induced by 5-fluorouracil in bone marrow, intestinal mucosa, and tumors. Ca Res 36:1653–1658, 1976

35. Chou TC, Hutchison DJ, Schmid FA, Philips FS: Metabolism and selective effects of 1β-D-arabinofuranosylcytosine in L-1210 and host tissues in vivo. Ca Res 35:225–236, 1975

36. Skipper HE, Schabel FM, Mellett LB, et al: Implications of biochemical, cytokinetic, pharmacologic and toxicologic relationships in the design of optimal therapeutic schedules. Ca Chemother Rept 54:431–450, 1970

37. Skipper HE, Schabel FM, Wilcox WS: Experimental evaluation of potential anticancer agents. XXI. Scheduling of arabinosylcytosine to take advantage of its S-phase specificity against leukemic cells. Ca Chemother Rept 51:125–165, 1967

38. Fishbein L, Flamm WG, Falk HL: Chemical mutagens. Environmental effects on biological systems. New York, Academic, 1970

39. Slavik M: Adriamycin (NSC-123127) activity in genitourinary and gynecologic malignancies. Ca Chemother Rept, Pt 3 6:297–303, 1975

40. Bachur NR: Adriamycin metabolism in man. In Hellmann K, Connors TA (eds): Chemotherapy, Vol. 7, Cancer Chemotherapy I. New York, Plenum, 1976, pp 105–111

41. Creasey WA: Vinca alkaloids and colchicine. In Sartorelli AC, Johns DG (eds): Antineoplastic and Immunosuppressive Agents II. New York, Springer, 1975, pp 670–694

42. Huggins C, Clark PJ: Quantitative studies of prostate secretion. II. The effect of castration and estrogen injection on normal and on the hyperplastic prostate glands of dogs. J Exp Med 72:747–761, 1940

43. Dao TL: Pharmacology and clinical utility of hormones in hormone-related neoplasms. In Sartorelli AC, Johns DG (eds): Antineoplastic and Immunosuppressive Agents II. New York, Springer 1975, pp 170–192

44. Carter SK, Slavik M: Chemotherapy of cancer. Annu Rev Pharmacol 14:157–183, 1974

45. Jensen EV, Jacobson HI: Fate of steroid estrogens in target tissues. In Biological Activities of Steroids in Relation to Cancer. New York, Academic, 1960, pp 161–178

46. Jensen EV: Estrogen receptors in hormone dependent breast cancers. Ca Res 35:3362–3364, 1975

47. Chan L, O'Malley BW: Mechanism of action of the sex steroid hormones. N Eng J Med 294:1322–1328, 1976

48. McGuire WL: Current status of estrogens in human breast cancer. Cancer 36:638–644, 1975

49. Carter SK, Slavik M: Investigational drugs under study by the United States National Cancer Institute. Ca Treat Rev 3:43–60, 1976

50. Legha SS, Slavik M, Carter SK: Hexamethylmelamine, an evaluation of its role in the therapy of cancer. Cancer 38:27–35, 1976

51. DeConti RC, Toftness BR, Lange RC, Creasey WA: Clinical and pharmacological studies with cis-diamminedichloro platinum (II). Ca Res 33:1310–1315, 1973

52. Folk RM, Peters AC, Pavkov KL, Swenberg JA: Preclinical toxicologic evaluation of 2,5-piperazinedione, 3,6(-bis-5-chloro-2-piperidyl)-dihydrochloride (NSC 135758) in dogs and monkeys. Ca Chemother Rept, Pt 3 5:37–41, 1974

53. Altman SJ, Fletcher WS, Andrews NC, Wilson WL, Pischer T: Yoshi-864 (NSC 102627) 1-propanol, 3, 3′-iminodi-dimethanesulfonate (Ester) hydrochloride: A phase I study. Cancer 35:1145–1147, 1975

54. Nemeth L, Institoris L, Somfai S, et al: Pharmacologic and antitumor effects of 1, 2: 5,6-dianhydrogalactitol (NSC 132313). Ca Chemother Rept 56:593–602, 1972

55. Frytak S, Moertel CG, Schutt AG, et al: A phase I study of cytembena. Cancer 37: 1248–1255, 1976

56. Carter SK: Porfiromycin (NSC 56410)-Clinical Brochure. Ca Chemother Rept, Pt 3 1:81–97, 1968

GENERAL REFERENCES ON CANCER CHEMOTHERAPY

Sartorelli AC, Johns DG (eds): Antineoplastic and Immunosuppressive Agents. New York, Springer, vol I, 1974; vol II, 1975

Holland JF, Frei E III, (eds): Cancer Medicine. Lea and Febiger, Philadelphia, 1973

Chabner BA, Myers CE, Coleman CN, Johns DG: The clinical pharmacology of antineoplastic agents. N Engl J Med 292:1107–1113, 1159–1168, 1975

Calabresi P, Parks RE, Jr: Chemotherapy of neoplastic diseases. In Goodman LS, Gilman A (eds): The Pharmacological Basis of Therapeutics, 5th ed. Macmillan, New York, 1975, pp 1248–1307

Chapter 6

Malignancy of the Vulva

ERNEST W. FRANKLIN, III, M.D.

Carcinoma of the vulva is a somewhat infrequent entity representing only 3 to 5 percent of malignancy in the female genital tract (Fig. 6-1); 95 percent of these lesions represent epidermoid carcinoma (Fig. 6-2), to which the majority of this chapter will be devoted, except where specific exceptions are noted. The disease is unique and intriguing in a number of aspects. When detected early and appropriate treatment is applied, the patient's chance for cure is often more favorable than for a number of other gynecologic malignancies. It is also a disease of some interest in terms of its epidemiology, particularly its association with other epidermoid neoplasia of the lower genital tract.[1] Epidemiology, the scrutiny of events affecting populations of individuals, has been most successful in the analysis of events surrounding the communicable diseases wherein medicine has made some of its most notable advances. Its contributions to the understanding of the possible pathogenesis of cervical cancer is also notable. Some understanding of the interaction between host (woman), agent, and the environment may provide a similar basis for improved understanding of the pathogenesis of epidermoid carcinoma.

EPIDEMIOLOGY

The Host

Epidermoid carcinoma of the vulva is primarily a disease of a population of advanced age, often of lower socioeconomic status and often occurring in association with multiple medical problems, including diabetes, hypertension, and obesity. These clinical characteristics of the elderly population are prominent in the mind of the clinician because of the obstacles that they present to the delivery of optimal treatment, but they are also possibly of some significance in the pathogenesis of the disease.

The majority of intraepithelial neoplasia of the vulva occurs in women during their fifth and sixth decades (Fig. 6-3).[1] Invasive carcinoma occurs over a wide range of age, with a median and average age of 63 years, some one-third of the patients being at least 70 years of age. Interestingly, review of the treatment of the latter patients reveals that some 35 percent of them will survive five or more years after appropriate treatment. It thus becomes increasingly important to understand the natural history of this disease and the prognostic factors associated in order to define an appropriate plan of therapy. It may be equally as important

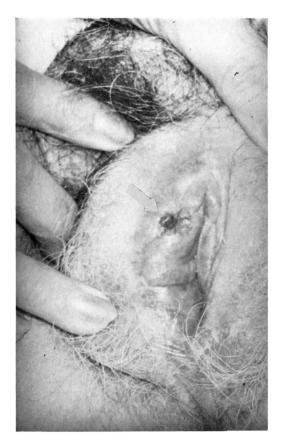

Figure 6–1. Cancer of right labium minus presenting as an ulcer.

to recognize when aggressive therapy is justified in a high-risk patient as it is to recognize when one may individualize treatment with less-aggressive therapy.

In a previous report[1] on the epidemiology of this disease among white patients comprising 71 percent of the patient population, the average age of 32 patients with carcinoma in situ was 15 years less than that of the average age of 63 years for those with invasive carcinoma. Conversely, among the 52 black patients within that series, the average age for both invasive and the intraepithelial carcinoma was 51 years. One may therefore postulate that different epidemiologic and pathogenic mechanisms may be operative in the black and white populations developing epidermoid carcinoma of the vulva.

A number of conditions have previously been suggested as predisposing an individual to carcinoma of the vulva, including chronic vulvar dystrophy, leukoplakia (a term too loosely defined to be of great value), syphillis, and chronic granulomatous disease. Bonney[2] and Tausig,[4] in independent retrospective analyses, concluded that 50

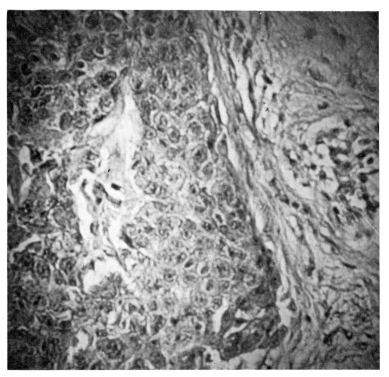

Figure 6–2. Epidermoid carcinoma of vulva. ×200.

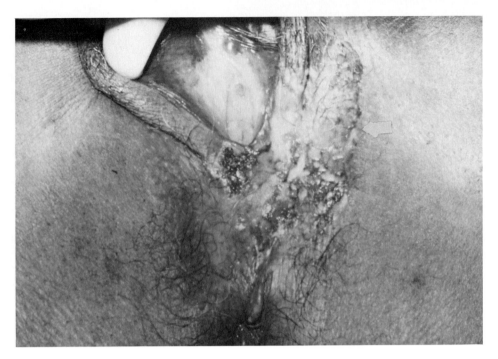

Figure 6–3. Carcinoma in situ of vulva.

percent of women with "leukoplakia," in which they included chronic vulvar dystrophies, would eventually develop epidermoid carcinoma within the subsequent 10 years of observation. They concluded that 50 percent of carcinoma was preceded by this condition. These conclusions are probably erroneous.[6] More accurate estimates of the risk based on prospective studies have suggested that cancer develops in only some 5 percent of patients with chronic vulvar dystrophy, rising to a high of 10 percent if atypical epithelial hyperplasia, now more appropriately referred to as dysplasia, is present.[5]

The Agent

To speak of a single agent as being of primary etiologic significance in epidermoid carcinoma of the vulva is undoubtedly premature and perhaps fallacious. Current knowledge centers about preexisting or coexisting conditions that by inference are suggested to be of etiologic significance in epidermoid carcinoma of the vulva. Emphasis has been placed on the frequency of syphillis and granulomatous venereal disease as conditions frequently preceding or possibly predisposing to the development of epidermoid carcinoma. Hay and Cole[7] reported on a series of black patients from

Jamaica in whom chronic granulomatous disease preceded epidermoid carcinoma of the vulva in 66 percent of cases. This conclusion has been confirmed by observation of cases within the United States, particularly in the black population, in which the stigmata of previous granulomatous disease including depigmentation and fenestration of the labia have been noted (Fig. 6–4).[8]

Of the 235 patients who were previously the subject of review by this author,[1] 29 were classified as luetic. Included among the luetics were two of the youngest patients in that series with invasive carcinoma, patients 23 and 25 years of age. Of the 24 luetic patients with invasive carcinoma, 17 had poorly differentiated lesions. This is in notable contrast to the distribution of histologic grade generally seen in invasive epidermoid carcinoma of the vulva, wherein the majority of the lesions are of low to intermediate grade, often with keratin pearl formation. Thus, by age distribution and histology, these patients are unique among the population having epidermoid carcinoma of the vulva. Unfortunately, as might be expected by their anaplastic histology, their prognosis is also markedly poorer than that of other patients with better differentiated lesions.

Equally as important as the benign conditions

that might define the patient population predisposed to carcinoma of the vulva is the frequency and character of associated neoplasia. The previous epidermiologic review of the records of 235 patients with preinvasive or invasive carcinoma revealed 20 percent with a second primary malignancy.[1] Of the 48 patients with second primary malignancy, there were 33 (15 percent) of the total population with prior, concurrent, or subsequent invasive or in situ carcinoma of the cervix. A recent review of this author's series of[52] patients with in situ lesions of the vulva reveal a 40 percent frequency of second primary malignancy of the cervix or vagina, a finding confirmed by other reports.[23]

Carcinoma on the vulva may be characterized by multifocal primary lesions some of which seem to be "induced" by adjacent lesions and are labeled "kissing" lesions of the labia, while others are spread over multiple areas of the vulva. It has also been observed that a broad area of anogenital skin encompassing the vulva, vagina, urethra, anus, and the skin of the intergluteal fold may be involved with intraepithelial or invasive epidermoid neoplasia at the time of initial diagnosis or during prolonged follow-up. It is therefore the thesis of this author that the anogenital epithelium is to be viewed as an unique epithelial organ system of common cloacal origin; it is probably subject to similar oncogenic agents whose venereal etiology is most suspect.

Current epidemiologic data dealing with the more common entity of carcinoma of the cervix associated the origin of this lesion with a venereal type of exposure including the herpes type II virus. If the postulate of a common etiologic agent operative over the entire anogenital organ system is valid, it should be possible to identify similar serologic evidence of herpes hominus and inclusions of herpetic deoxyribonucleic acid (DNA) within the vulvar epidermoid carcinoma.

The Environment

The environmental factors in oncogenesis have most notably included occupational exposure to carcinogenic substances, as in the case of scrotal carcinoma in chimney sweeps and bladder carcinoma among workers in the aniline dye industry. To date, no common environmental factor has been identified as being significant in the pathogenesis of vulvar carcinoma, and yet the behavior of the disease and the outcome of the therapy are significantly affected by delay in diagnosis and treatment. These are responsible for less than optimal results in treatment of the disease.

Notable is the fact that 60 percent of previously untreated patients have been found to be aware of a vulvar mass or "sore" for an average of 10 months prior to treatment[1] (Fig. 6–5). Vulvar bleeding and pain have been reported to be present in 31 percent and 16 percent of patients, respectively, for an average period of as long as six months. Equally distressing is the degree of physician delay noted among several series of patients reviewed, a delay that adversely affects the outcome of treatment; 25 percent of patients in the author's series had been under prior medical treatment without biopsy[1] (Fig. 6–6). Moreover, 30 percent of the patients with invasive carcinoma have experienced a physician delay in treatment of three or more months. Only a greater degree of suspicion and wider use of biopsy is required to affect earlier diagnosis with a significant im-

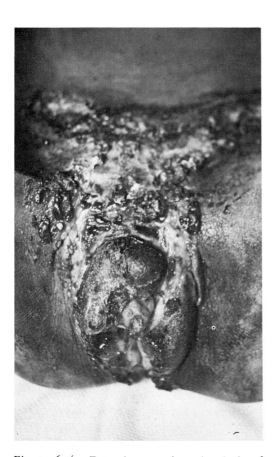

Figure 6–4.   Extensive granuloma inguinale of vulva and lower abdomen.

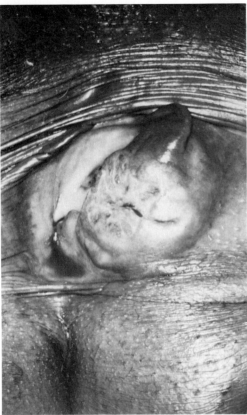

Figure 6–5. Large epidermoid cancer of left labium minus known by the woman to be present over 4 years.

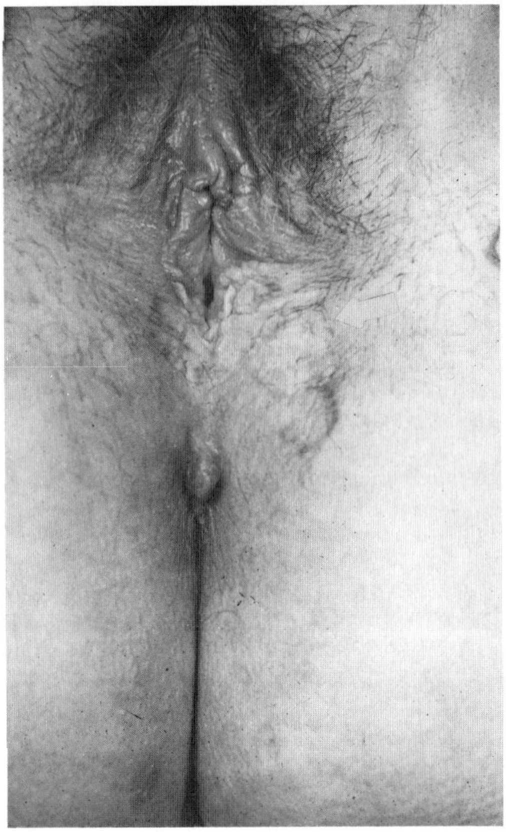

Figure 6–6. Invasive epidermoid cancer of vulva treated by physicians with various creams and applications for 6 months before diagnosis.

provement in overall survival rates for invasive carcinoma of the vulva.

Thus, review of epidemiologic data from several similar and dissimilar populations in whom the disease has been studied prompts several tentative postulations regarding the pathogenesis of the lesion. A most notable finding is the 15 to 40 percent incidence of second primary lesions within the cervix or vagina, primarily the former. With an epidemiologic association between the incidence of epidermoid carcinoma of the vulva and the cervix established, as well perhaps as that of the vagina and anus, the concept of an anogenital "organ system" as an entity susceptible to viral oncogenesis coupled with secondary initiating or accelerating factors is more feasible.

Should such data be forthcoming, it may be evident that a viral agent plays a primary role either in the alteration of DNA or cell membrane characteristics, such modifications proceeding with a certain probability to oncogenesis. Just as is

the case with cervical carcinoma, in which it has been suggested that certain periods of optimal susceptibility to oncogenesis exist, namely, puberty and the initial pregnancy, such a phase of optimal susceptability to initiation of viral oncogenesis may exist in the vulva. More important, however, may be the impact of accelerating or modifying factors such as granulomatous disease or a declining immunologic status of the host as has been observed with aging. Also of interest has been the increased frequency of intraepithelial neoplasia observed in several populations undergoing a change in immunologic status. Friedrich[9] has reported an histologically confirmed intraepithelial neoplasia diagnosed during pregnancy that regressed spontaneously in the postpartum period. Of interest to this author has been the increased frequency of such changes seen in patients during their second and third decades. Not only was the increased number of sexual partners experienced by the patients notable among this population, but also the finding of abnormal T-lymphocytes among a number of them, presumably as the result of smoking marijuana.

The associated venereal diseases, whether granulomatous, luetic, or condylomata accumenatum, may serve primarily as coexistant phenomenon, mere "venereal markers" because of the venereal etiology of the viral infection. It is possible, however, that these venereal lesions function as accelerating or modifying factors operative on a background in which viral oncogenesis has already been initiated or is present in a latent state awaiting activation. That the process of syphillis operates as more than a "venereal marker" and has some role in determining the rate of development and character of the lesion is suggested by the small group of patients previously described. Thus, syphillis, like granuloma-

tous venereal disease, may exercise a significant potentiating or accelerating influence in the pathogenesis of epidermoid carcinoma of the vulva.

While the foregoing are tenative conclusions awaiting further epidemiologic, serologic, and biochemical evaluation, the clinician must currently recognize the multifocal character of this disease occurring over the broad anogenital field. Although epidermoid carcinoma of the vulva is infrequent, the accessability of these lesions to early study and diagnosis should allow better understanding and treatment of the condition, particularly if the significant element of physician and patient delay can be avoided, thus initiating treatment at the stage of disease when optimal results can be expected.

INTRAEPITHELIAL CARCINOMA OF THE VULVA

As noted previously in the discussion of epidemiology of carcinoma of the vulva, intraepithelial carcinoma precedes invasive carcinoma by 10 years in the white population, whereas the average age of incidence for both invasive and intraepithelial carcinoma is the same in the black population. The lesion also seems to occur much less frequently in the black population. Problems in the definition of the "histologically acceptable" diagnosis of in situ carcinoma of the vulva arise, particularly after the previous use of podophyllin for condylomata accuminata. Despite a background of concern regarding the true histologic criteria for the diagnosis of these intraepithelial abnormalities, the nomenclature appropriate to their classification and the very real problem of the biologic potential of the lesion, it appears that in situ carcinoma of the vulva has increased in incidence.

Bowen,[10] in 1912, described two cases of indolent skin cancer with the characteristics that now bear his name, with subsequent description of similar lesions occurring over the vulva (Fig. 6–7). The symptoms and gross appearance of the lesion may vary considerably. As noted previously, intraepithelial and invasive carcinoma of the vulva are frequently associated with neoplasia of the cervix and vagina. It appears that this may be somewhat more frequent when the vulvar lesion has the characteristics of Bowen's disease.

In the planning of appropriate treatment of in situ carcinoma of the vulva, it is important to recognize that it is not merely the vulva that is at risk.

The lesion occurs as part of the disease process to which the entire anogenital epithelium including the cervix, vagina, vulva, perineum, anus, and intergluteal area are susceptible. On this basis, it is then inappropriate to recommend a total vulvectomy for a single focal intraepithelial lesion for the objective of removing the entire field at risk. The treatment should be planned on the basis of current documented pathology and not on the basis of potential future risk. This neoplastic process is quite indolent, and careful observation allows for individualized treatment of lesions as they occur. For the single lesion or a limited number of discrete lesions of the anogenital epithelium, appropriate treatment can consist of excision with wide margins. One is faced with the problem of intraepithelial abnormality surrounding the gross lesion. Careful evaluation of margins should be carried out to assure adequate excision.

In cases with extensive multiple lesions, or in which the in situ changes occur on the background of chronic vulvar dystrophy or other abnormal epithelium such as previously irradiated epithelium, multiple biopsies to rule out invasive carcinoma should be done. It is then possible to carry out a superficial vulvectomy to remove all of the diseased epithelium with replacement by a split thickness skin graft. The procedure may be carried out over a wide extent of the vulva with extension into the vagina and over the perineum and even tailored to approximate the anal verge. Such wide superficial vulvectomy may again be coupled with excision of isolated lesions. The

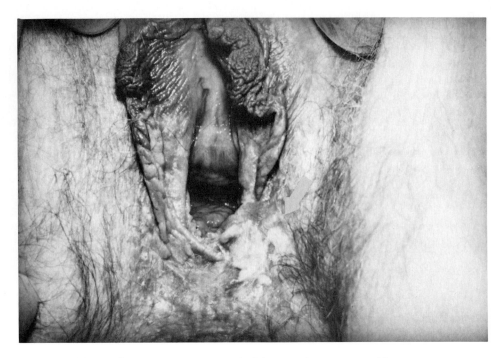

Figure 6–7.   Bowen's intraepithelial cancer in a 35-year-old woman.

functional status of patients following this procedure, including sensation and orgasm, justifies preservation of the underlying structures. For patients who have had a chronic vulvar irritation prior to surgery, coitus will be significantly improved. This approach plus careful follow-up is more appropriate than radical surgery for a rather indolent epithelial lesion.

Conservative therapy utilizing topical 5-fluorouracil was reported with considerable initial enthusiasm. Later reports have dampened the enthusiasm for this mode of therapy due to a significant recurrence rate, as well as a proportion of patients who fail to respond to the additional therapy. In addition, there is considerable morbidity entailed in the conscientious use of this modality of therapy.

Part of the indecision regarding the appropriate treatment for this lesion is due to the relatively indolent character of the lesion. While cases of invasive carcinoma of the vulva can be found associated with intraepithelial changes, documented cases of intraepithelial carcinoma noted to progress to invasion are infrequent. Even chromosomal studies of the in situ and invasive carcinoma have not demonstrated a clear correlation between chromosomal pattern and biologic behavior of intraepithelial carcinoma.

INVASIVE EPIDERMOID CARCINOMA

Appropriate therapy for invasive carcinoma of the vulva must emphasize an understanding of the natural history of the disease as reflected in definition of prognostic factors involved. A clinical staging of carcinoma of the vulva has been proposed and accepted for utilization by the International Federation of Obstetricians and Gynecologists (Tables 6–1 and 6–2). This classification emphasizes definition of the tumor by size and location, including the possible involvement of structures beyond the vulva, the clinical status of the inguinal nodes, and the presence or absence of distant metastases. When placed within the T, N, and M groupings by these criteria, stage I includes all lesions confined to the vulva with a maximum diameter of 2 cm or less and no suspicious groin nodes, stage II includes all lesions confined to the vulva with a diameter greater than 2 cm and no suspicious groin nodes, while stage III includes all lesions extending beyond the vulva without

Table 6–1.   CLINICAL STAGING OF CARCINOMA OF THE VULVA*

T: PRIMARY TUMOR

   T1 Tumor confined to the vulva—≤2 cm in larger diameter

   T2 Tumor confined to the vulva—>2 cm in diameter

   T3 Tumor of any size with adjacent spread to the urethra and/or vagina and/or perineum and/or anus

   T4 Tumor of any size infiltrating the bladder mucosa and/or the rectal mucosa or both, including the upper part of the urethral mucosa and/or fixed to the bone

N: REGIONAL LYMPH NODES

   N0 No nodes palpable

   N1 Nodes palpable in either groin, not enlarged, mobile (not clinically suspicious of neoplasm)

   N2 Nodes palpable either or both groins, enlarged, firm and mobile (clinically suspicious of neoplasm)

   N3 Fixed, confluent, or ulcerated nodes

M: DISTANT METASTASES

   M0   No clinical metastases

   M1A Palpable deep pelvic lymph nodes

   M1B Other distant metastases

*International Federation of Obstetricians and Gynecologists Classification, April 12, 1970.

grossly positive groin nodes as well as lesions of any size confined to the vulva with suspicious but not grossly positive groin nodes. Stage IV includes those lesions that are recognized to have a higher degree of failure, lesions extending beyond the vulva with grossly positive groin nodes, lesions involving the mucosa of the rectum, bladder, urethra, or the bone, plus all cases with distant metastases. Previous reports dealt with the validity of these criteria for staging and their applicability to clinical setting, and they have been found to be valid and satisfactory.[16] Use of these criteria has indicated a very impressive actuarial survival among stages I, II, and III of 60 to 70 percent.

Table 6–2.   CARCINOMA OF THE VULVA

STAGE 0		Carcinoma in situ, e.g., Bowen's disease, noninvasive Paget's disease
STAGE I	T1 N0 M0 T1 N1 M0	Tumor confined to the vulva, 2 cm or less in largest diameter. Nodes are not palpable or are palpable in either groin, not enlarged, mobile (not clinically suspicious of neoplasm)
STAGE II	T2 N0 M0 T2 N1 M0	Tumor confined to the vulva more than 2 cm in diameter. Nodes are not palpable, or are palpable in either groin, not enlarged, mobile (not clinically suspicious of neoplasm)
STAGE III	T3 N0 M0 T3 N1 M0 T3 N2 M0 T1 N2 M0 T2 N2 M0	Tumor of any size with 1) adjacent spread to the urethra and any or all of the vagina, the perineum, and the anus, and/or 2) nodes palpable in either or both groins (enlarged, firm and mobile, not fixed but clinically suspicious of neoplasm)
STAGE IV	T1 N3 M0 T2 N3 M0 T3 N3 M0 T4 N3 M0 T4 N0 M0 T4 N1 M0 T4 N2 M0 M1A M1B	Tumor of any size 1) infiltrating the bladder, mucosa, or the rectal mucosa, or both, including the upper part of the urethral mucosa, and/ or 2) fixed to the bone or other distant metastases

Prognostic Factors

An understanding of the prognostic factors and criteria for staging of epidermoid carcinoma is a basic requirement for planning of appropriate treatment if the patient is to have an optimal chance for cure. One must appreciate the character and behavior of the primary lesion, including its size, grade, depth of invasion, and extent. In addition, the planning of therapy must recognize not only the potential for regional lymphatic metastases but also the pathways that the metastases may take and factors that predispose the lesion to metastasize. Failure in treatment will ensue as frequently from failure to control the primary lesion or regional metastases as from distant metastases.

To evaluate prognostic factors indicative of success or failure in treatment, one must have some objective criteria against which to relate the validity of prognostic factors. Survival rates might be used, but they are too variable depending upon adequacy of therapy. Conversely, the frequency of metastatic lymphadenopathy does appear to be a very impressive and valid objective standard against which to relate these prognostic factors and is independent of adequacy of therapy. The status of the inguinal nodes does carry clear prognostic significance in epidermoid carcinoma of the vulva, for among patients with negative groin nodes, death due to disease will be infrequent.[11,21] Frequency of local recurrence will also vary somewhat with the adequacy of primary treatment but, like survival, is important in evaluating prognostic factors.

Using the presence or absence of inguinal node metastases as an objective parameter in the definition of prognosis, one can review the significance of histology and size of the lesion. It has long been recognized that the increasing size of the lesion is correlated with an increasing frequency of lymph node metastases and certainly may lead to problems with complete resection of the lesion. Similarly, the histologic grade of the lesion, even when corrected for variable size, does have an impact on the probability of metastasis to the groin nodes (Table 6–3) (Fig. 6–8). In addition to basic histologic grade and size of lesion, an entity recognized as superficially invasive epidermoid carcinoma of the vulva has also been defined, a lesion originally defined as extending less than 5 mm into the underlying stroma of the vulva. In the original report of these lesions,[16] no lymph node metastases were noted, a finding that was

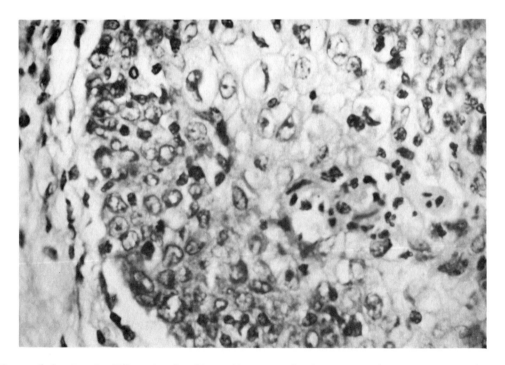

Figure 6–8. Poorly differentiated epidermoid cancer of vulva associated with inguinal and pelvic lymph node metastases.

Table 6-3. 117 PATIENTS WITH SIZE AND
HISTOLOGY OF LESION CORRELATED
WITH FREQUENCY OF NODE METASTASES*

| | MAXIMUM DIAMETER OF LESION | | | |
| | Nodes ≤2 cm | | Nodes >2 cm | |
HISTOLOGY	+	ELIGIBLE	+	ELIGIBLE
Superficial invasion	0	8	0	11
Grade I	0	6	4	12
Grade II	3	10	17	40
Grade III	4	7	18	38

*From Franklin EW, Rutledge FD: Obstet Gynec 37:892, 1971.

substantiated on further review and follow-up of these and additional cases. Subsequent to these two reports, there have been isolated cases reported in which superficial invasion was associated with lymph node metastasis. It appears that

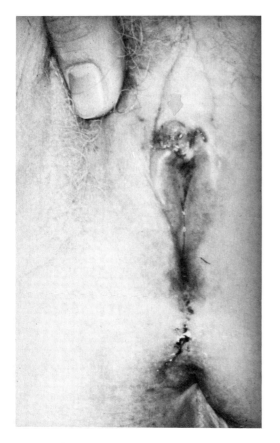

Figure 6-9. Primary epidermoid cancer of clitoris.

those cases of superficially invasive carcinoma metastatic to the groin nodes are associated with anaplastic tumors and clearly demonstrable invasion of vascular channels evident on the incisional biopsy from the primary lesion. Thus, histologic grade and the presence or absence of involvement of lymphatics are also of prognostic significance in planning of therapy.[12]

Increasing size of the lesion has been included as an important parameter in the International Federation of Gynecologists and Obstetricians (FIGO) staging for epidermoid carcinoma of the vulva and reflects the prognosis for the patient. What then of the relationship of the frequency of node metastasis and local recurrences when correlated with the extent of anatomic involvement by the primary lesion? Does involvement of the clitoris (Fig. 6-9), anus, and other sites beyond the vulva increase the frequency of lymph node metastases? A comparison of the T1 and T2 lesions confined to the vulva with T3 extending beyond indicates there is no increased frequency of node metastasis in the latter case.[11,27] Treatment failure with the lesion extending beyond the vulva is primarily related to an increased frequency of pelvic or vulvar recurrence relative to incomplete resection. Adequate excision of the primary lesion is the first step, then, in the planning of optimal therapy, including the planning of adequate margins beyond the neoplastic mass, with possible urinary or fecal diversion.

Treatment

Having planned for adequate excision of the primary lesion, the problem then is to determine the optimal management of the regional node metastases. The basic principles for cancer surgery in the carcinoma of the vulva were originally defined by Basset[13] in 1912, and have undergone subsequent modification, though always emphasizing an en bloc dissection between the primary mass and regional lymphatics.[3]

Details of studies of lymphatic pathways from the primary lesions have been published elsewhere. Based on clinical experience it appears that epidermoid carcinoma of the vulva follows a relatively predictable pattern of spread directly to the inguinal nodes, seeking aberrant pathways only when the inguinal nodes are obstructed by metastatic disease or other pathology. After the inguinal nodes, they then proceed to a second echelon of nodes within the pelvis. It is this characteristic of the disease that makes it emminently accessible to surgical extirpation by regional lymphadenectomy. While the anatomists can define specifically the fascial planes and lymph nodes, the surgeon must realize that he has to remove all of this en bloc within the groin area. Only if there is involvement within the groin area must he then consider pelvic node dissection for treatment of the patient with epidermoid carcinoma of the vulva.[11,14] It should be emphasized, however, that such predictable behavior allowing more concise planning of therapy is only possible in dealing with epidermoid carcinoma of the vulva and such conclusions may not be applicable to lesions such as sarcomas and melanomas.

The clinical evaluation of the status of the inguinal nodes has been subject to widespread misunderstanding and criticism due to variability in correlation of clinical impression and histologic status of the nodes. Among unsuspicious nodes, there has been a considerable variability from 12 to 43 percent in the frequency of metastatic

lymphadenopathy. Such variability can be explained on a statistical basis and is not simply variable clinical acumen. First, one must realize that there is a considerable variability in the frequency of positive nodes reported within any series, varying from 37 to 68 percent. This frequency of positive nodes is an uncontrolled variable merely reflecting the character of the population referred to each treatment center. A relatively constant 68 to 87 percent of the patients with suspicious nodes were found to have metastatic cancer. Also, a relatively consistent two-thirds to three-quarters of patients who have positive nodes will have palpable suspicious or clinically positive nodes prior to surgery. Conversely, one can then say that a relatively consistent 25 to 30 percent of the lymph node metastases are present in unsuspicious nodes. Thus, as the frequency of inguinal node metastasis increases (Table 6–4), one must recall that 25 to 30 percent of the metastasis will be present in unsuspicious nodes. These cases with occult metastases comprise an increasing proportion of the total population as the frequency of inguinal node metastasis within the series (an uncontrolled variable) increases. These occult metastases then represent an increasing proportion of patients with unsuspicious nodes.

Inguinal Lymphadenectomy

What can be concluded about the clinical status of the inguinal nodes? First, they do carry general prognostic significance, at least appropriate to staging if not to planning of individual treatment relative to the presence of inguinal node metastases. When the nodes are not palpable or are palable but unsuspicious, the nodes are frequently called "shotty," we will still find an ap-

Table 6–4. COLLECTIVE EXPERIENCE IN CLINICAL EVALUATION OF PRESENCE OF METASTATIC CANCER IN INGUINAL NODES

AUTHOR (REF)	NO. OF PATIENTS	FREQUENCY OF + NODES	NODES SUSPICIOUS		NODES UNSUSPICIOUS		NODES +	
			No.	%+	No.	%+	No.	% Palpable (Suspicious)
Way (21)	118	68	67	87	51	43	80	73
Green et al, (22)	69	51	34	68	34	34	35	66
Merrill, Ross (23)	82	37	25	76	57	14	28	75
Rutledge, Franklin (16)	151	37	48	70	93	12	46	76
Shingleton et al (24)	98	21	16	75	82	11	21	57
Morley (15)	205	37	80	34	54	19	83	64

proximately 11 percent risk of occult lymph node metastasis. When the nodes appear clinically suspicious, there will be a 70 percent frequency of lymph node metastasis, and when fixed or ulcerated, there will be a better than 90 percent frequency of lymph node metastasis.[11]

Secondly, the clinical status of the inguinal nodes does reflect the probability of pelvic lymph node metastasis. In a previous series among 85 patients who underwent iliac node dissection, 10 of 11 patients with positive pelvic nodes had clinically suspicious or positive inguinal nodes prior to surgery, while the remaining patient had a metastasis within the so-called "Cloquet's node" in the inguinal canal.[16] This information can then be utilized in selection of patients for whom pelvic lymphadenectomy is appropriate. It also confirms that lymphatic metastasis to the pelvis from epidermoid carcinoma of the vulva are rare in the absence of involvement of the inguinal nodes.

Thirdly, the clinical status of the inguinal nodes does predict the risk of local groin recurrence despite routine en bloc excision of skin and subcutaneous tissue overlying the inguinal area. In our previously reported series, among 40 patients with inguinal node metastases, 20 percent had thigh and groin recurrence.[16] All of the patients who experienced such recurrences had clinically suspicious or positive groin nodes prior to surgery. No patient with occult metastasis, i.e., metastases in a nonpalpable or unsuspicious node, experienced local recurrence. Indeed, among the patients having clinically suspicious or positive groin nodes prior to surgery, the local recurrence rate within the incision was 40 percent (Fig. 6–10). Some accommodation must then be made in planning of therapy for these patients.

The incision utilized in treatment of patients within that series emphasized excision of skin overlying the inguinal nodes with undermining of flaps superior and inferior to the inguinal nodes, often removing a skin flap in the groin of some 3 to 5 cm in width. It appears that lymphatic metastases seek collateral pathways through the cutaneous lymphatics when the inguinal nodes become obstructed with tumor, thus seeding themselves through the overlying skin with resultant local cutaneous recurrence. When an incision that emphasizes complete en bloc excision of all fat and overlying skin within the groin is utilized without undermining of peripheral skin flaps, the recurrence rate within the groin and thighs is reported to be markedly reduced.[14]

In the planning of appropriate therapy then,

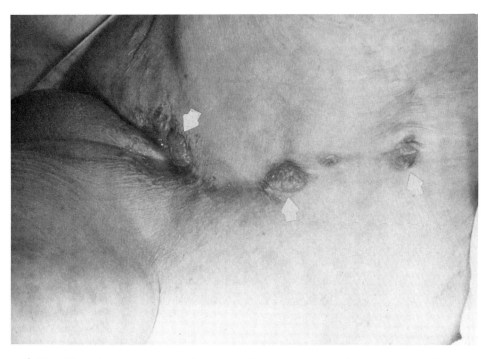

Figure 6–10. Multiple recurrences of invasive epidermoid cancer of vulva in areas of incision following operation.

one looks first to adequate treatment of the local lesion, and the probability of both local recurrence and regional spread is based on the size, histologic grade, and extent of the lesion (Fig. 6–11). Treatment of the groin node remains an intrinsic part of the treatment of carcinoma of the vulva and the histologic status of the nodes is a clear cut indicator of prognosis, as very few patients with negative inguinal nodes will succumb due to metastatic disease (Fig. 6–12).[11,21] Thus, while complete treatment of the local lesion and groin nodes is of fundamental importance, the management of possible pelvic lymph node metastases can be individualized. First, it can be demonstrated that direct metastases to the pelvis bypassing the inguinal nodes is rare. Indeed, in a collected series of some 500 cases from the literature,[15,17,21–24] the frequency of direct metastasis of epidermoid carcinoma to the pelvis is less than 3 percent. Mr. Stanley Way has stated that direct pelvic metastases bypassing the groins never occurs and attributes this small margin of error to failure of the pathologist to detect metastasis within the groin nodes.[14] Thus, the frequency of pelvic node metastasis reported within any series will be a reflection of the percentage of patients within the series who have inguinal node metastasis, an independent variable within any group of patients studied. Such incidence rates vary from 8.5 percent to 16.0 percent. With such a low frequency of involvement, one can immediately recognize that some individualization of therapy must be carried out. It is imperative that we try to recognize factors that characterize the patient at risk for pelvic node metastasis.

Pelvic Lymphadenectomy

What is the success rate in treatment of pelvic lymphadenopathy? While a great deal has been written about the possible role of radiation therapy in treatment of metastases to this area, there is no series that can provide adequate data regarding successful control of documented pelvic lymph node metastasis with radiation therapy. One would expect that the control rate would equal that obtained with cervical cancer. Again, however, one must be able to select the patient at risk for pelvic node metastasis. With surgery, the absolute survival rate after positive pelvic lymphadenectomy has been reported to vary from 12.5 to 25 percent.[11,15,21,22] Thus, if one can select the patient at risk for pelvic node metastasis, surgery and possibly radiation therapy do offer significant benefits after extended therapy. If one is only going to cure some 20 percent of the 16 percent of patients who may have pelvic node metastasis, it will be a very small percentage of the total population of patients who benefit from having a routine pelvic lymphadenectomy.

What can we therefore conclude regarding pelvic lymphadenectomy? First, that the status of the pelvic nodes does not carry the clear prognostic significance of the inguinal lymph nodes. Patients with no findings of metastatic disease at the time of pelvic lymphadenectomy may still succumb to metastasis, a finding not true of patients who have negative inguinal nodes.[11] Secondly, the patients with pelvic lymph node metastasis can be cured in approximately 15 to 20 percent of cases but only some 16 percent of cases will have the pelvic lymph node metastasis. Thus, only 3 to 4 percent of patients would benefit by cure from having pelvic lymphadenectomy carried out as a routine procedure in a high-risk population!

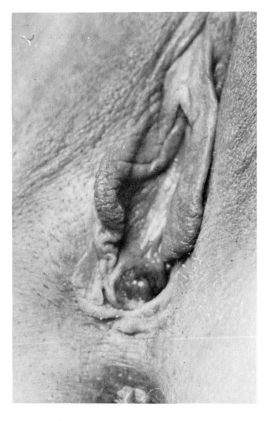

Figure 6–11. Clinical stage I (T1 NO MO) epidermoid cancer of posterior commissure of labia.

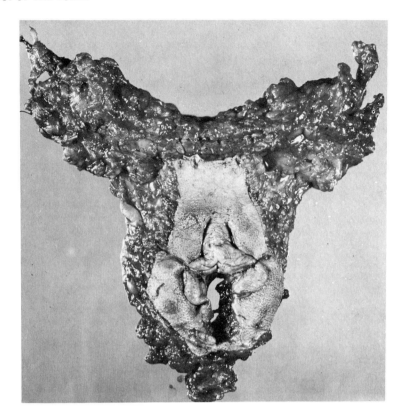

Figure 6–12. Radical vulvectomy with superficial and deep inguinal lymph node dissection of patient seen in Figure 11 following wide excisional biopsy. No nodes contained cancer.

What, then, are the determinants of pelvic lymph node metastasis? As we said earlier, the clinical status of the inguinal nodes is important in answering this question. In the author's previous series, 11 of 12 patients with pelvic lymphadenopathy had had clinically suspicious or positive inguinal nodes prior to surgery, while patients with occult inguinal node metastasis did not have pelvic node metastases. Secondly, there is the status of the so-called "Cloquet's node," which actually represents the lowest of iliac lymph nodes medial to the femoral artery. The data regarding the significance of this node is not substantial. In this author's previous series of 55 patients in whom the Cloquet's node is submitted independently for evaluation, only five patients had a positive Cloquet's node.[11] Two of these patients had positive pelvic nodes. Equally significant, of the 50 patients with negative Cloquet's nodes, no patient had evidence of pelvic node metastasis at surgery or in subsequent follow-up. It would therefore appear that one can select the patients at increased risk of pelvic lymph node metastasis on the basis of the presence or absence of inguinal node metastasis, the clinical status of the inguinal nodes prior to inguinal lymphadenectomy, and the presence or absence of metastases to Cloquet's nodes.

One can therefore conclude that in the planning of treatment of cancer of the vulva, it is equally important to recognize factors that necessitate complete and aggressive treatment in the high-risk patients, such as urinary or fecal diversion or pelvic lymphadenectomy, as it is to recognize the circumstances that justify less extensive treatment, vulvectomy, and groin dissection, with the more favorable lesion. Planning of treatment for epidermoid carcinoma of the vulva can be implemented on the basis of the FIGO classification with some latitude for individualization if the criteria for classification and the limitations of clinical judgement in staging are recognized. As with any clinical staging, one treats on the basis of clinical judgement regarding the extended behavior of disease and not strictly by the stage itself.

When the lesion is confined to the vulva without suspicious or positive groin nodes, whether a stage I lesion if of less than 2 cm diameter or a stage II lesion if greater than 2 cm in diameter, these are optimal lesions with similar survival rates. Indeed, some consideration may be given in the future for combining stage I and II within the FIGO classification. The corrected five-year survival rate for these patients will be approximately 90 to 95 percent. Use of survival rates that are corrected for intercurrent diseases is particularly important in evaluation of therapy among the patients having epidermoid carcinoma of the vulva, due to the advanced age of the majority of patients with multiple accompanying medical problems. The primary lesion must be treated by adequate local excision, which would consist of radical vulvectomy. When may vulvectomy alone be considered sufficient? As mentioned earlier, there have been published indications that the superficially invasive lesions, those penetrating no more than 3 to 5 mm below the surface, are very infrequently associated with metastasis in the absence of anaplastic histology or evidence of vascular invasion. The latter factors when present must be recognized as representing an increased risk of node metastasis and an indication for bilateral inguinal node dissection.

Treatment Without Lymphadenectomy

Any time the primary treatment of invasive carcinoma of the vulva is carried out without accompanying inguinal lymphadenectomy, it should be recognized that optimal therapy has not been accomplished. Such may indeed be justifiable for a small percentage of patients with concurrent major medical problems. This may prove satisfactory for such a high-risk population. Indeed, Morley[15] found that the absolute five-year survival rates for stage I patients treated by radical vulvectomy alone was 60 percent as compared to that of 85.5 percent for patients treated by radical vulvectomy with bilateral groin dissection. When one corrected for death due to intercurrent disease, however, the difference was only 81.3 and 88.3 percent respectively.

It has been argued that appropriate treatment would be to carry out a vulvectomy alone for the local lesion and then observe the inguinal nodes for sign of enlargement due to possible metastases. Such delay in waiting for "transit" or occult metastases to become clinically overt adversely affects the prognosis of the patient in a number of ways. First, there is a low risk of local (incisional) recurrence following an en bloc groin dissection even if occult metastases are present. In contrast, there will be a 20 percent risk of incisional (skin) recurrence despite wide en bloc resection if one waits until occult metastases become clinically overt (palpable). Secondly, the high curability (greater than 50 percent) present despite occult node metastases will be decreased to less than 50 percent after removal of clinically suspicious or positive nodes. Finally, it has been noted that there is a very low risk of pelvic and distant metastases with histologically negative groin nodes and even with clinically occult groin metastases. Pelvic node dissection may be deferred, especially if Cloquet's node is also negative. There is an increased risk of metastasis to the pelvic and distant sites if clinically suspicious or positive groin nodes are present. The necessity for pelvic node dissection or radiation is added, despite which recurrence may occur within the pelvis or at distant sites. In sum, one must always recognize the fallibility of clinical evaluation of the status of inguinal nodes for the individual patient, for clinically negative nodes may harbor occult metastases in a significant percentage of cases (10 to 12 percent).

Treatment of Stage III Cancer

With regard to stage III carcinoma of the vulva, those lesions extending beyond the vulva but without grossly positive nodes, i.e., without enlarged, fixed, or ulcerated groin nodes or lesions, or lesions of any size confined to the vulva with suspicious groin nodes, adequate treatment may still yield a 40 to 66 percent corrected five-year survival rate. In this more advanced stage of disease, there is an increased risk of failure due to extension beyond the vulva, which needs to be recognized and countered by aggressive local resection with urinary and fecal diversion if necessary and by use of skin graft to cover local defects. Among the stage III cancers of the vulva with clinically suspicious or positive groin nodes, the risk of local incisional recurrence will be more frequent. Wider resection must therefore be planned from the initiation of therapy and plans must be made to close a larger primary defect. Overall, one must recognize that 40 percent of the patients with groin node metastasis can be cured despite the presence of metastases.

When the nodes in the groin are extensive in size, matted, or fixed, it can be recognized that complete removal by primary surgery will be unsuccessful. If one carries out surgery and waits for the wound to heal before instituting postoperative irradiation, such healing may never occur. The groin may appear to undergo wound breakdown with subsequent granulation which proves to be recurrent malignancy on cytology or biopsy. It has therefore been our policy to initiate preoperative radiation in the presence of extensive groin metastasis that are confirmed on needle biopsy of the mass. Irradiation begins, often after a radical vulvectomy alone to remove the primary lesion, utilizing a dose of 5000 rads to a depth of .5 cm in the groins and to the midplane of the pelvis the portal is enlarged to include the pelvic nodes. Recognizing that radiation alone at this dose level will not erradicate large deposits of lymphatic metastases, adjunctive surgery is necessary. Primary closure and simple skin graft are doomed to failure due to the compromise of vasculature following surgery and irradiation. The most successful means of covering this defect with healthy skin and muscle undamaged by exposure to radiation therapy is the myocutaneous graft developed over the gracilis muscle and rotated to fill the large defect within the groin.[25]

Treatment of Stage IV Cancer

It is in the stage III and IV carcinoma of the vulva that treatment of the pelvic lymph nodes must be undertaken. With surgery alone, one can expect to control 15 to 25 percent of patients with pelvic lymph node metastasis. The precise yield after pelvic irradiation has yet to be accurately evaluated in terms of efficacy and indications, but it may well prove to be a satisfactory substitute for or adjunct to pelvic lymphadenectomy, as has been the case in cervical cancer. The greatest risk for pelvic metastases exists in the patient who has clinically suspicious or positive nodes prior to surgery. It is thus possible to identify prior to surgery the patient for whom one may wish to add adjunctive therapy within the pelvis. After inguinal lymphadenectomy, any nodes palpable within the specimen may be examined by frozen section to determine whether metastases are present. If so, one may proceed to pelvic lymphadenectomy during the same procedure. If no metastases are detected until the postoperative phase, one may then consider a second operation or adjunctive pelvic irradiation.

Stage IV carcinoma of the vulva will include the lesions at extremely high risk for local recurrence within the vulva, the pelvis, or the groins, as well as distant metastases. Local and regional control can best be accomplished by a combination of irradiation therapy and subsequent surgery with use of the gracilis myocutaneous flap to cover the surgical defect.[25] If such defects are not closed primarily at that time of the initial surgery, extensive and progressive necrosis will ensue.

Exenteration in Treatment of Vulvar Cancer

Note should also be made of the possible role of pelvic exenteration in treatment of carcinoma of the vulva, as we have frequently made reference to the possible necessity for sacrifice of bladder, urethra, or anus and rectum. Because the problem of local control of the disease is paramount in planning of therapy, one should recognize the possible success of this modality of therapy. Subtotal exenteration may find greater applicability under these circumstances than is the general case with the treatment of recurrent cervical cancer. The use of primary total or subtotal pelvic exenteration for the treatment of advanced malignancy has been reported to have a 50 to 75 percent success rate in control of disease.[16,17]

Radiation Therapy in Vulvar Cancer

Some comment should be made regarding the possible role of radiation therapy as a primary modality of therapy for invasive carcinoma of the vulva. The vulva, anus, and urethera have only limited tolerance to radiation therapy and such treatment requires meticulous local care and extended fractionation and delay in treatment. There would still be a high frequency resulting in atrophy and stricture (Fig. 6-13). Treatment by high-energy electrons to the vulva in association with radiation to the inguinal and pelvic lymph nodes has been reported with acceptable control of disease but with associated long-term complications as well, including severe complications of irradiation in the inguinal region (8 percent), cutaneous ulceration and scarring (24 percent), fistulas and abscess cavities, and obstruction of the urethra.[18]

A modified approach has also been reported in which radical vulvectomy was combined with radiation of the inguinal and pelvic nodes with Tx No squamous cell carcinoma of the vulva.[19] The authors in that series assumed that 20 to 30 percent of No patients would have involved groin nodes, a presumption that is invalid. The more

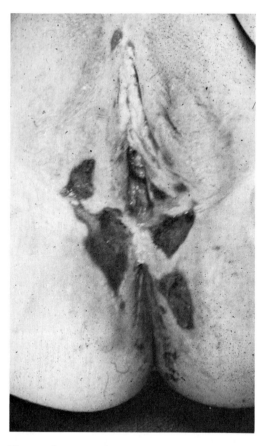

Figure 6–13. Diffuse atrophy and superficial ulcerations of vulva following irradiation therapy for vulvar cancer.

appropriate figure would be some 12 percent.[11] In describing their assumptions for planning of radiation therapy, the authors presumed both a rather low rate of control of disease in the absence of lymph node metastasis as well as a low rate of cure by surgery in the presence of positive nodes. The efficacy of radiation to the groins in controlling metastasis is unknown, as histologic status of the nodes prior to therapy could not be ascertained. A randomized prospective study with regard to the possible role of radiation therapy for treatment of occult metastases to the groins is perhaps indicated.

Recurrence

Factors predisposing to recurrence already have been noted. Recurrences following inadequate excision of the primary lesion can be controlled in approximately 50 percent of cases by further resection that should not be characterized by repeated timidity. Sacrifice of urethra or anus may be essential for preservation of life. Problems of disease with localized fixation to bone can best be managed by preoperative irradiation, resection, and closure of the defect with myocutaneous graft.

When the recurrence occurs within the groin incision or the surrounding skin, it is a more difficult problem to treat. The first hint of such a recurrence may be in delayed healing of the groin incision. Granular erythematous tissue in the groin may actually represent recurrent disease. In the groin incision that is showing delay in healing, a cytology and biopsy should be obtained to rule out recurrent disease. The first manifestation of recurrence within the skin flaps may be slightly elevated erythematous or darkened nodules, and such have been recognized occasionally to occur throughout the dermal lymphatics over the course of the lower limb. For localized recurrences, we feel that wide field of irradiation therapy is more adequate than surgical reexcision, for the probability of further metastasis within surrounding skin is high. Such cases are also at high risk of pelvic node metastasis and should receive adjunctive radiation therapy to that area as well.

More widespread dissemination can only be countered by chemotherapy and there appears to be no notable successful agent currently available, though regressions have been observed with use of methotrexate, Cytoxan, Adriamycin, and bleomycin with an occasional prolonged remission, although the overall response rate is low.

ADDITIONAL PROBLEMS IN TREATMENT OF MALIGNANCY OF THE VULVA

Beyond the epidermoid carcinoma of the vulva, there are a number of less frequent entities either metastatic or primary, the latter arising from among the accessory structures of the anogenital epithelium. The most common source of metastatic disease is from the cervix or endometrium followed by the kidney, urethra, ovary, and breast. The prognosis and treatment of these metastases will be reflective of the status of the treatment of the primary lesion, but is always adverse.

Carcinoma of the Bartholin's Glands

Among the accessory structures of the vulva in which malignancy may appear, the Bartholin's gland is notable. The infrequency of the reporting of this malignancy is partially due to the problem of differentiating this as a site of primary involvement when the lesion often presents in an advanced stage of local and regional dissemination. The age distribution of patients afflicted with disease suggests a slightly lower median age than epidermoid cancer, while the presenting complaints are usually nonspecific. These have suggested to the patient and physician a benign, cystic, or inflammatory lesion with resulting conservative therapy (Fig. 6–14). The diagnosis is usually made when the lesion fails to respond and incision and drainage or marsupialization is attempted. Even then, it is only with the development of some complication—poor healing, induration, infection, or distant metastases—that the original diagnosis may be made. With a background of such delay in diagnosis and institution of treatment, one can only expect an adverse prognosis. The lesion may be either adenocarcinoma, squamous carcinoma, adenoid cystic, or undifferentiated.

While the considerations pertinent to treatment of metastatic disease are similar to those with epidermoid carcinoma of the vulva, the treatment of the primary lesion may be complicated by its proximity to vital structures, with possible invasion into vagina, bone, anus, and rectum. Thus, diverting colostomy with preoperative irradiation and wide local resection followed by reconstructive surgery may be necessary for control of the primary lesion. Inguinal and probably pelvic lymphadenectomy are advisable.

Verrucous Carcinoma

This variant of squamous cell carcinoma occurs infrequently throughout the anogenital tract, possibly involving vulva, vagina, or cervix. The experience there has been similar to that relative to this lesion elsewhere in the body. The tumor

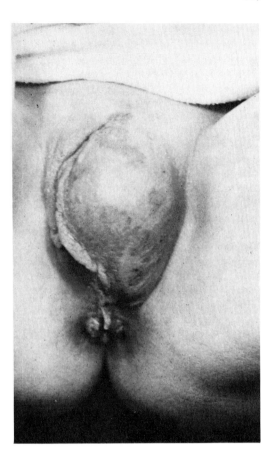

Figure 6–14. Carcinoma in situ of left Bartholin gland.

remains primarily locally aggressive and may extend deeply into the underlying tissues with penetration of bone. Only infrequently are lymph node metastases noted. Radiation therapy has been reported to have a low rate of control of the primary and metastatic lesion. Anaplastic transformation of the verrucous carcinoma after radiation therapy has also been reported with secondary lymph node metastasis. Primary surgical therapy is therefore appropriate. In circumstances in which the primary lesion has advanced to such a large size as to make complete primary resection with adequate clearance impossible, adjunctive chemotherapy or radiation could be considered.

Malignant Melanoma of the Vulva

As is true with the remainder of the anogenital epithelium, melanoma occurring within this area has characteristics akin to and different from similar lesions found elsewhere on the body. They represent only 0.5 to 5.0 percent of malignancy of the female genital organs, with less than 400 cases reported to date (Fig. 6–15). Their behavior is in notable contrast to the relatively predictable character of epidermoid lesions that predominate on the vulva and, when metastatic, spread in a rather predictable fashion to regional lymph nodes. The overall behavior of the melanoma gives it a prognosis for survival significantly less than that for epidermoid carcinoma, the five-year survival running approximately 35 percent.

Of particular interest is a system for description of prognosis in malignant melanoma based upon the specific level of the invasion as defined by Clark et al.[26] The applicability of this classification to melanomas of the vulva has recently been reviewed by Chung et al[20] with some accommodations made due to the variation in the character of subepithelial tissue of the clitoris and labia majus and minus from that of the skin elsewhere on the body. On this basis, it was possible to demonstrate a prognostic value to such classification,

but the conclusion of that study was that there was "little justification for performing less than a radical vulvectomy and node dissection for malignant melanoma of the vulva." This would seem to be the appropriate fundamental therapy until further studies substantiate the favorable prognosis for superficial melanomas. Conversely, the low survival rate currently obtained with radical surgery alone in these patients speaks heavily in favor for the necessity of adjunctive therapy to compliment surgery utilizing either chemotherapy or immunotherapy.

Paget's Disease of Anogenital Origin

Paget's disease represents changes within the epithelium within the anogenital area which are commonly extensive (Fig. 6–16). Debate continues regarding the origin and character of Paget's disease. With regard to clinical treatment, however, several recommendations can be made.

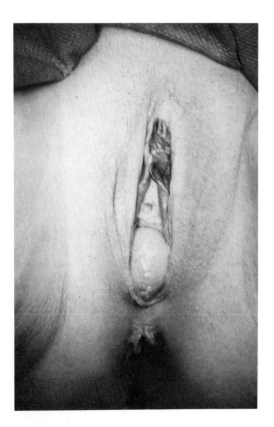

Figure 6–15. Malignant melanoma of clitoris.

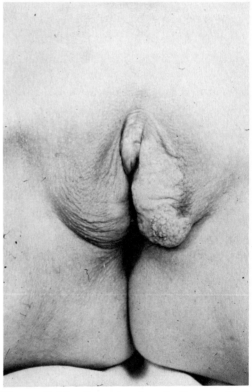

Figure 6–16. Extensive Paget's disease of left labium majus.

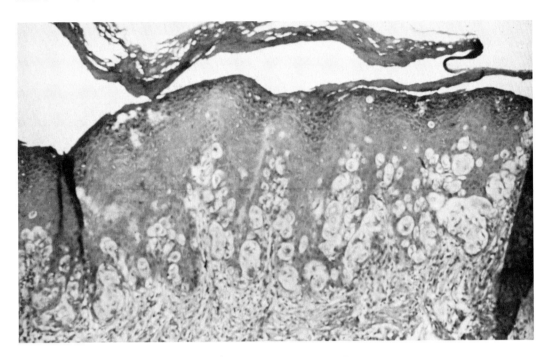

Figure 6–17.   Paget's disease of vulva.

First, it should be recognized that the lesions are commonly quite extensive with abnormalities in the epithelium surrounding the visible lesion, usually an erythematous macular process, to a considerable extent (Fig. 6–17). Thus, the first problem in therapy is to excise adequately the primary lesion. At the time of primary treatment extensive margins must be taken and checked by frozen section. The resultant defect is best covered by a split thickness skin graft. Knowledge of the availability of such techniques for coverage of the defect should embolden the surgeon to undertake adequate therapy. Having resolved the management of the local lesion, the problem then arises regarding possible metastasis. Metastases have been identified as being associated with underlying adenocarcinomas and also with areas of invasion that develop beneath undifferentiated portions of Paget's disease. Again, the fundamental therapy for the disease appears to be wide local excision of the primary, including radical vulvectomy in association with inguinal node dissection. For patients of advanced age with concomitant medical problems, it may be possible to carry out the radical vulvectomy alone and carefully evaluate the specimen for evidence of invasive carcinoma with careful follow-up of the inguinal nodes. It is not infrequent to see this disease among patients in whom surgery is not feasible. The use of radiation therapy to the primary lesion and to metastasis has been reported with equivocal results, while preliminary reports of the topical use of Bleomycin to local cutaneous recurrences has been reported to be successful.

References

1. Franklin EW, Rutledge FD: Epidemiology of epidermoid carcinoma of the vulva. Obstet Gynec 39:165, 1972
2. Bonney V: Connective tissue in carcinoma and certain inflammatory states that precede its onset. (Hunterian Lecture). Lancet 1:1465, 1908
3. Taussig FJ: Cancer of the vulva. Am J Obstet Gynec 40:764, 1949
4. Taussig FJ: Leukoplakia and cancer of the

vulva. Arch Dermat Syph 21:431, 1930

5. McAdams AJ, Kistner RW: The relationship of chronic vulvar disease, leukoplakia, and carcinoma in situ to carcinoma of the vulva. Cancer 11:740, 1958

6. Jeffcoate TNA: Chronic vulval dystrophies. Am J Obstet Gynec 95:61, 1966

7. Hay DM, Cole FM: Primary invasive carcinoma of the vulva in Jamaica. J Obstet Gynaec Br Common 76:821, 1969

8. Salztein SL, Woodruff JD, Novak ER: Postgranulomatous carcinoma of the vulva. Obstet Gynec 7:80, 1956

9. Friedrich EG, Jr: Reversible vulvar atypia. Obstet Gynec 39:173, 1972

10. Bowen JT: Cancer of the skin. J Cutan Dis 30:241, 1912

11. Franklin EW, Rutledge FD: Prognostic factors in epidermoid carcinoma of the vulva. Obstet Gynec 37:892, 1971

12. Parker RT, Duncan I, Rampone J, Creasman W: Operative management of early invasive epidermoid carcinoma of the vulva. Am J Obstet Gynec 123:349, 1975

13. Basset A: Traitement chirugical operatoire de l'epithelioma primitif du clitoris. Rev Chir 46:546, 1912

14. Way SA: Carcinoma of the Vulva. Guest lecture, Society of Gynecologic Oncologists, Key Biscayne, Florida, January, 1974

15. Morley GW: Infiltrative carcinoma of the vulva: results of surgical treatment. Am J Obstet Gynec 124:874, 1976

16. Rutledge F, Smith JP, Franklin EW: Carcinoma of the vulva. Am J Obstet Gynec 106:1117, 1970

17. Thornton WN, Flanagan WC: Pelvic exenteration in the treatment of advanced malignancy of the vulva. Am J Obstet Gynec 117:774, 1973

18. Frischbier HJ, Thomsen K: Treatment of cancer of the vulva with high energy electrons. Am J Obstet Gynec 111:431, 1971

19. Daly JW, Million RR: Radical vulvectomy combined with elective node irradiation for TxNo squamous carcinoma of the vulva. Cancer 34:161, 1974

20. Chung AF, Woodruff JN, Lewis JL: Malignant melanoma of the vulva, a report of 44 cases. Obstet Gynec 45:638, 1975

21. Way SA: Malignant Disease of the Female Genital Tract. Philadelphia, Blakiston, 1951

22. Green TH, Jr, Ulfelder H, Meigs JV: Epidermoid carcinoma of the vulva: an analysis of 238 cases. Part I. Etiology and diagnosis. Part II. Therapy and end results. Am J Obstet Gynec 75:848–864, 1958

23. Merrill JA, Ross NL: Cancer of the vulva. Cancer 14:13–20, 1961

24. Shingleton HM, Fowler WC, Palumbo L, Kock GG: Carcinoma of the vulva: influence of radical operation on cure rate. Obstet Gynec 35:106, 1970

25. Franklin EW, Bostwick J, Burrell MO, Powell JL: Reconstructive techniques in radical pelvic surgery. Am J Obstet Gynecol 129:285, 1977

26. Clark WH, From L, Bermardino EA: Histogenesis and biologic behavior of primary human malignant melanoma of the skin. Cancer Res 29:705, 1969

27. Piver MS, Xynos FP: Pelvic lymphadenectomy in women with carcinoma of the clitoris. Obstet Gynecol 49:592, 1977

Chapter 7

Radiation Therapy for Carcinoma of the Vulva

LUTHER W. BRADY, M.D.

Epidermoid cancer of the vulva is essentially a cutaneous disease, modified by its site in a specialized epithelium that is subjected to special environmental, hormonal, infectious, and functional factors. Vulvar cancer has a well-defined natural history and an at-risk population that is beginning to be identified. The disease, accounting for 3.5 percent of gynecologic cancer, constitutes the fourth most common primary malignancy of the genital tract.

Predominantly, carcinoma of the vulva occurs in elderly women, with the highest incidence in the seventh decade. Radical vulvectomy and bilateral inguinal node lymphadenectomy has in recent years become the standard method of treatment. Radiation therapy is not ordinarily employed as a primary method of therapy because of the poor tolerance of the vulvar tissue to external beam therapy. There is evidence, however, that radiation therapy may be as effective as surgery in controlling the potential for lymph node metastases.

Approximately 90 to 95 percent of malignancies of the vulva are squamous cell carcinomas.

The use of surgery to treat the primary lesion by means of radical vulvectomy, combined with radiation therapy to treat possible inguinal and pelvic lymph node metastases has been reported to be as effective as radical hysterectomy combined with bilateral radical vulvectomy and bilateral inguinal node dissection. This fact suggests that the primary area could be treated by surgery, with lymphatic drainage sites treated with radiation therapy, resulting in a marked reduction in morbidity to the patient. By utilizing radiation therapy to treat inguinal and pelvic lymph node metastases, the complications of wound infection, lymphedema, and prolonged hospitalization are markedly reduced.

There remain several controversies in the management of the patient with carcinoma of the vulva. First, what represents standard therapy and what is its basis? Are there prognostic and therapeutic values in the FIGO staging? Are there situations indicating departure from standard therapy?

Anatomic data relative to carcinoma of the vulva provide the basis for contemporary therapy. Extensive local resection is required for local control. The status of the regional lymph nodes appears pivotal in terms of curability as demonstrated by the collective experiences in Tables 7-1 and 7-2.[1-6] Age and associated infirmities have a significant impact on the ultimate outcome. Negative inguinal lymph nodes convey a better prognosis after definitive surgery than the data in Table 7-3[7] indicate. Way[4] has reported, for example, no cancer deaths among 44 patients with negative lymphadenectomy. Franklin and Rutledge[8] reported no deaths from cancer among 53 patients with negative lymphadenectomy.

Radical surgery for vulvar cancer is an estab-

Table 7–1. CARCINOMA OF THE VULVA:
SURVIVAL BY TREATMENT PLAN[1]

MODALITY	NO. PATIENTS TREATED	5-YR SURVIVAL No.	%
Radiation therapy	836	109	13.0
Simple vulvectomy	334	103	30.8
Vulvectomy plus radiation therapy	659	214	32.5
Radical vulvectomy and femoral lymphadenectomy	449	250	55.7
Radical vulvectomy and femoral and pelvic lymphadenec-tomy	440	278	63.2

Table 7–2. CARCINOMA OF THE VULVA:
SURVIVAL RATES FOR PATIENTS
WITH POSITIVE PELVIC NODES
(SURGICAL TREATMENT)

SERIES	NO. PATIENTS	5-YR SURVIVAL RATE (%)
Green et al (1958)[2]	16	12.5
Way (1957)[3]	9	22.2
Way (1960)[4]	8	37.5
Merrill & Ross (1961)[5]	3	33.3
Collins et al (1963)[6]	6	16.7
Total	42	21.4

lished technique. Local measures appear to save fewer patients than radical surgery, even in the presence of nodal metastases. Data from multiple authors suggest that the addition of radiation therapy to radical vulvectomy, when treatment is directed toward the pelvic and inguinal lymph nodes, or radical vulvectomy in conjunction with femoral and pelvic lymphadenectomy, may result in improved survival statistics (Tables 7–4 and 7–5).[9–19]

The survival results in stages III and IV reported by these authors demand the reevaluation of the surgical approach when this disease has spread near or beyond the range of radical vulvectomy. The use of radiation therapy for advanced cancer of the vulva deserves another clinical trial in view of the more effective techniques of modern irradiation. The use of the electron beam has special advantages because the depth of treatment can be controlled.

Treatment programs should be related to the

Table 7–3. CARCINOMA OF THE VULVA:
INFLUENCE OF REGIONAL NODAL[7]
INVOLVEMENT ON SURVIVAL

STATUS OF NODES	NO. PATIENTS	5-YR SURVIVAL No.	%
Negative	314	237	75.5
Positive	236	98	41.5

Table 7–4. RESULTS OF TREATMENT
FOR EPIDERMOID CANCER
OF THE VULVA[14]

STAGE	SURVIVAL (%)
0	100
I	100
II	83
III	36
IV	39
IVA	75
IVB	22
IVAB	0

Table 7–5. CARCINOMA OF THE VULVA: 5-YR SURVIVAL RATES (%)
FOR EACH TREATMENT REGIMEN

SERIES	RADIOTHERAPY ALONE	VULVECTOMY ALONE	VULVECTOMY & RADIOTHERAPY	RADICAL VULVECTOMY & LYMPHADENECTOMY
Smith & Pollock (1947)[9]	16.7	47.6	5.6	52.6
Huber (1953)[10]	19.2	39.4	—	36.4
Taussig (1940)[11]	4.8	8.3	—	58.5
Lunin (1949)[12]	20.0	25.0	—	100.0
Brandstetter and Krataeluvill (1961)[13]	10.3	17.6	—	58.3

Table 7-6. STUDY DESIGN GOG PROTOCOL FOR INVASIVE CARCINOMA OF VULVA

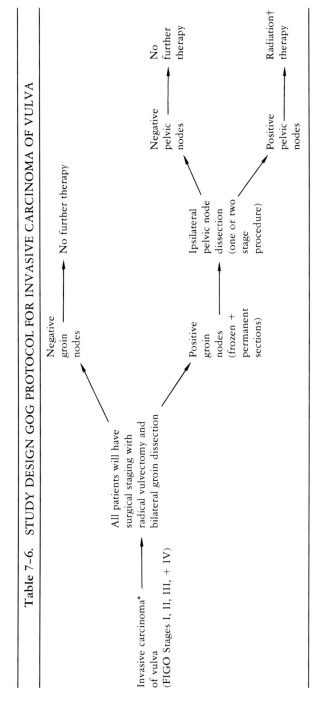

*All FIGO stages eligible for protocol where radical vulvectomy suffices for removal of all lesion, i.e., distal urethra.
†There will be two different radiation fields employed depending upon site of positive nodes, i.e., if distal pelvic nodes only positive (obrurator or external iliac) then field will not include para-aortic nodes; otherwise, if proximal nodes positive (common iliac), the para-aortic nodes will be treated.

FIGO staging (Tables 6-1 and 6-2). For those patients with invasive carcinoma of the vulva, in all stages, the patient should have surgical staging with radical vulvectomy and bilateral groin dissection. If inguinal lymph nodes are negative, no further treatment needs to be carried out except for careful, continued follow-up examinations. Individuals with positive inguinal lymph nodes should have either pelvic lymphadenectomy or radiation therapy directed toward the inguinal and pelvic nodes postoperatively. Radiation therapy should be carried out in such a way that 5000 to 6000 rads as a tumor dose minimum are delivered to the pelvic lymph node distribution in five to six elapsed weeks. A total of 5000 to 6000 rads should also be given to inguinofemoral lymph node distributions, using either a photon beam with bolus, or electron beam, with the treatment program being carried out in five to six weeks. The treatment volume should cover the whole pelvis, including the iliac, hypogastric, obturator, and deep inguinal nodes.

Critical T, N, M pretreatment staging for vulvar cancer, employing the FIGO system, deserves the support of the oncologist. Inherent in the system is the recognition of decreasing salvage based on local and regional spread.

Radical vulvectomy and inguinal node dissection should be performed in all operable cases. Pelvic lymphadenectomy should be included for N2 and N3 cases, and added later if not done when N0 and N1 cases are found to have regional metastatic disease. Histologic differentiation and depth of invasion are significant prognostic factors that should be taken into consideration in the treatment decision-making process. Local radiation therapy to the inguinal, pelvic, and femoral lymph nodes is an appropriate technique for postsurgical management. The Gynecologic Oncology Group is presently evaluating the various parameters to determine when postoperative radiation therapy should be employed. The protocol design is illustrated in Table 7-6.

The patient with vulvar cancer should be followed for the remainder of her life, with the physician continually searching for the disease in other locations. In 20 percent or more patients a second cancer, usually of the genital tract, will be found. Full treatment of these cancers is warranted. An active rehabilitation program, especially for the patients with advanced cancer, should be maintained and follow-up used for patient education and support.

References

1. Rutledge F, Boronow RC, Wharton JT: Carcinoma of the vulva in Gynecologic Oncology. New York, John Wiley and Sons, 1976

2. Green TH, Ulfelder H, Meigs JV: Epidermoid carcinoma of the vulva. Am J Obstet Gynecol 75:834, 1958

3. Way S: Carcinoma of the vulva. In Meigs JV, Sturgis SH (eds): Progress in Gynecology, vol. 3. New York, Grune and Stratton, 1957

4. Way S: Carcinoma of the vulva. Am J Obstet Gynecol 79:692, 1960

5. Merrill JA, Ross WL: Cancer of the vulva. Cancer 14:13, 1961

6. Collins CG, Collins SH, Barclay DL, Nelson EW: Cancer involving the vulva. Am J Obstet Gynecol 87:762, 1963

7. Plentl AA, Friedman EA: Lymphatic system of the female genitalia. Philadelphia, Saunders, 1971

8. Franklin EW, III, Rutledge F: Prognostic factors in epidermoid carcinoma of the vulva. Obstet Gynecol 37:892, 1971

9. Smith FR, Pollock RS: Carcinoma of the vulva. Surg Gynec Obstet 84:78, 1947

10. Huber J: Das primare carcinom der vulva. Strahlentherapie 29:61, 1953

11. Taussig FJ: Cancer of the vulva: An analysis of 155 cases. Am J Obstet Gynecol 40:764, 1940

12. Lunin AB: Carcinoma of the vulva. Am J Obstet Gynecol 57:742, 1949

13. Brandstetter F, Krataeluvill A: Ergebnisse der therapie biem vulva karzinom. Krebsaryt 16:16, 1961

14. Krupp PJ, Lee FY, Bohm JW, et al: Prognostic parameters and clinical staging criteria in epidermoid carcinoma of the vulva. Obstet Gynecol 46:84–88, 1975

15. Million R, Daly JW: Radical vulvectomy combined with elective node irradiation for

T-x, N-0 squamous cancer of the vulva. Cancer 34:161–165, 1974

16. Nobler MP: Efficacy of a perineal teletherapy portal in the management of vulvar and vaginal cancer. Radiology 103:393–397, 1972

17. Boronow RC: Therapeutic alternative to primary exenteration for advanced vulvovaginal cancer. Gynecol Oncol 1:233–255, 1973

18. Frischbier HJ, Thomsen K: Treatment of cancer of the vulva with high energy electrons. Am J Obstet Gynecol 111:431–435, 1971

19. Rutledge F, Smith JP, Franklin EW: Carcinoma of the vulva. Am J Obstet Gynecol 106:1117–1126, 1970

20. Kottmeier HL (ed): Annual Report on the results of carcinoma of the uterus, vagina and ovary, vol. 15. Stockholm, Sweden, 1973

Chapter 8

Vaginal Cancer

ROBERT C. PARK, M.D., COL, MC, USA
TIM H. PARMLEY, M.D.

The vagina is the fifth most frequent organ site for female genital tract malignancy. Although cancer of the vagina is relatively rare, it is not a new disease entity, being first described by Cruveilhier in 1826, before the Anatomical Society of Paris.[1] More often vaginal neoplasia is an extension of disease from the cervix, vulva, or endometrium, and in fact, tumors of these areas must be ruled out before a diagnosis of primary vaginal cancer can be entertained.

Primary cancer of the vagina is a rare disease accounting for only 1 to 2 percent of all gynecologic malignancies. From 1962 to 1975, at Walter Reed Army Medical Center, 1308 cases of invasive gynecologic malignancy were registered; 19 of these were primary vaginal cancers, for an incidence of 1.4 percent. The mean patient age at diagnosis was 58 with a range of 21 months to 91 years. However, 70 percent of patients were older than age 50 when the neoplasm was discovered.

The usual symptoms in patients with vaginal cancer are discharge, bleeding, and pain. Diagnosis is made by suspicion of the lesion, inspection, and biopsy (Fig. 8–1). Because the vaginal speculum obscures the lesion, 20 percent of tumors are missed at initial examination. Squamous cell type accounts for 85 to 90 percent of all vaginal tumors (Fig. 8–2). Adenocarcinoma, sarcoma, and melanoma make up the remaining 10 to 15 percent.[1–15]

Vaginal Embryology

An understanding of vaginal embryology helps to explain the source of the tissues that give rise to vaginal neoplasms and further defines the time of life during which they occur.[16–19]

Eight weeks from the maternal last menstrual period the paired Wolffian or mesonephric ducts of the female fetus have reached and opened into the urogenital sinus. The epithelium of the ducts is tall, pale, and columnar. In contrast, the urogenital sinus is lined by low, dark, cuboidal cells. The epithelium that lines the portion of the urogenital sinus that lies between the orifices of the two ducts resembles and is continuous with the epithelium of the ducts, i.e., it is pale and columnar rather than dark and cuboidal. This is either the result of modification of the sinus epithelium or incorporation of the Wolffian epithelium of the ducts into the wall of the sinus. If it is the latter, then this portion of the wall of the urogenital sinus is mesodermal and not endodermal. The point is obscure but critical, for it is from this pale epithelium that the squamous epithelium of the vagina develops. In this discussion it will be assumed that the vaginal squamous epithelium is mesodermal.

Between seven and eight weeks from the last menstrual period, near the top of the mesonephric body, the Mullerian or paramesonephric ducts begin as evaginations of the intraembryonic coe-

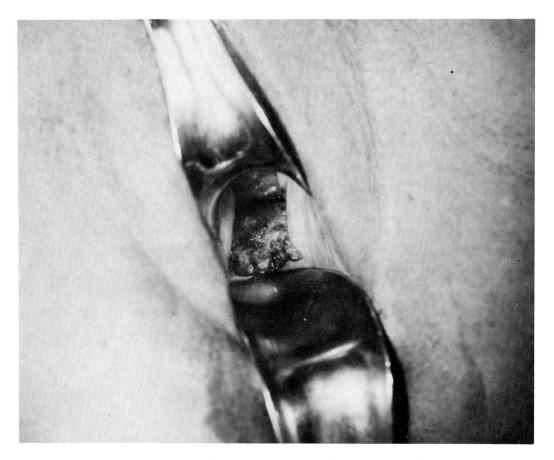

Figure 8–1. Squamous cancer of upper posterior wall of vagina separate from normal cervix.

lom. The tips of the developing ducts grow caudally closely applied to the wall of the mesonephric duct. At first lateral, the paramesonephric duct moves anterior and then medial to the Wolffian structure. The growing tip of the Mullerian ducts remain closely approximated to the wall of the mesonephric duct. At 10 weeks, the paired Mullerian ducts begin to fuse with each other, forming a single structure, and then reach the urogenital sinus. Between 10 and 11 weeks from the maternal last menstrual period the following relationships exist: The fused Mullerian ducts now constitute a single duct with a solid tip; the Wolffian ducts are still closely applied to the lateral walls of the single Mullerian duct; the tip of the latter abuts upon the urogenital sinus between the orifices of the two mesonephric ducts. This portion of the urogenital sinus is lined by tall, pale, columnar epithelium that is continuous, at their orifices, with the epithelium of the Wolffian ducts.

From this time until vaginal and cervical development is complete, at about 5 months, the following events take place: The Wolffian ducts begin to degenerate, and at the tip of the Mullerian duct the tall, pale, columnar epithelium lining the urogenital sinus begins to exhibit metaplastic proliferation. The result is a plaque or plate of squamous epithelium in the wall of the urogenital sinus. This is the vaginal plate. The vaginal plate proliferates until a column of squamous epithelium separates the sinus and the tip of the paramesonephric duct. The latter sits in a cup-shaped depression in the top of the column of squamous tissue. Degeneration in the tip of the Mullerian duct suggests that this structure regresses before the cranially extending vaginal plate. The squamous epithelium of the vaginal plate will give rise to the squamous epithelium of the vagina and the portio of the cervix. The most common type of vaginal cancer, epidermoid carcinoma is the result of malignant transformation

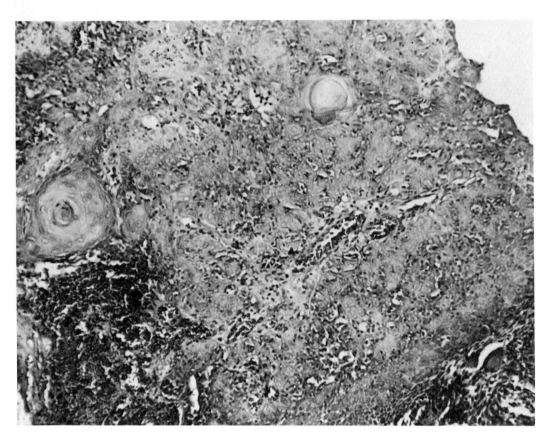

Figure 8–2.   Squamous cancer of vagina.

of this squamous epithelium in the adult woman.

The epithelium of the Mullerian duct will give rise to the columnar, mucus-secreting epithelium of the endocervix. The degree to which the Mullerian duct regresses consequently determines the level in the genital tract at which the squamocolumnar junction of the adult cervix will occur. It is, therefore, important to note that this regression of the Mullerian duct is regulated by a metaplastic transformation that takes place within the epithelium of the duct itself. The epithelial lining of the Mullerian duct is columnar and pseudostratified. Preceeding degeneration and regression, the most caudal portion of this epithelium is transformed into a three-cell-layered epithelium. This new lining is characterized by columnar cells at the base, cuboidal cells in the middle layer, and a flattened cell layer on the surface. It is only this transformed portion of the duct that regresses. The more cranial portion of the epithelium, which is not transformed, persists, and the portion of the duct that it lines does not regress. Consequently, the site of the most caudal exten-

sion of the columnar epithelium in the adult, the squamocolumnar junction, is determined by the level to which this metaplastic transformation extends.

Support for these assumptions is derived from the observation that high doses of estrogen will inhibit this transformation. When pregnant mice are given large doses of estrogen, the squamocolumnar junction in their female offspring is lower in the genital tract than the normal level.[16] Adenosis in the daughters of women treated with diethystilbestrol during pregnancy is the presumed clinical correlate in the human.[20]

It follows from these considerations that vaginal adenosis occurring spontaneously, or as the result of prenatal exposure to diethylstilbesterol, will be found most frequently in the upper vagina of young women. Clear cell adenocarcinoma of the vagina, which arises in conjunction with vaginal adenosis, obviously occurs in the same setting.

As the vaginal plate lengthens into a column of squamous epithelium separating the wall of the urogenital sinus from the tip of the Mullerian duct, not only does the epithelium of the duct become more cranially displaced but so also does the surrounding stroma of the duct wall. However, remnants of undifferentiated mesodermal stroma persist beneath the squamous epithelium of the upper vagina in neonatal females. In older children they may be found only as low as the cervix, and in adult women such stroma is usually totally confined to its adult position, i.e., the endometrial cavity. Therefore, tumors derived from this tissue, i.e., rhabdomyosarcomas or mixed mesodermal sarcomas, are not found in the vaginas of adult women but only in the vaginas of young children where their characteristic clinical presentation has earned them the name of "sarcoma botryoides."

The previous discussion has attempted to show how the development of the vagina explains the subsequent location of the tissues that give rise to the common vaginal cancers, and to offer an explanation for their observed age distribution. Sarcoma botryoides is a disease of the infant female, vaginal adenocarcinomas occur in young women, and epidermoid carcinoma is a disease of the adult. The only vaginal malignancy of note that has not been discussed is the melanoma. There is no adequate embryologic explanation for the presence of melanocytes in the vagina or cervix. Suffice it to say that benign nevi have been described in both the vagina and cervix and are the presumed source of malignant melanomas in these sites.

SQUAMOUS CARCINOMA

Most primary vaginal cancer (85 to 90 percent) is squamous cell type and is usually discovered in the adult female with a mean age of 60 at diagnosis (Fig. 8–2). Frequently the lesion is ulcerated and vaginal bleeding or discharge are often the presenting symptoms. When the tumor is in the mid or lower anterior vagina, urinary tract symptoms may also be present.[21] The tumor can be located anywhere in the vagina, although slightly more than 50 percent are in the upper third with a posterior location predominanting (Fig. 8–1). This leads to the speculation that accumulation of foreign material in the posterior fornix or chronic irritation, as with pessary use, may play an etiologic role. Although some cases reported in the older literature have been in patients wearing pessaries for prolapse, vaginal devices have never been proven as contributing factors. In addition, the presence of lower vaginal cancer, the second most frequent primary site, would be difficult to explain on the basis of chronic irritation or accumulation of foreign material.[1,3,6,7,11,13]

Diagnosis of invasive squamous vaginal lesions can usually be accomplished by speculum visualization and direct biopsy, a simple and safe outpatient procedure. Care must be taken to observe the entire vagina, as 20 percent of lesions are missed at first examination.[22,23] Vaginal cytology is frequently positive, however, it should never be a substitute for biopsy in the presence of an obvious lesion. To make a diagnosis of primary vaginal cancer, the lesion must be located in the vagina and not involve the cervix or vulva. In ad-

dition, no other primary tumor of similar cell type may be present in the genital tract.

Carcinoma in situ of the vagina is a recently recognized disease entity that is apparently increasing in frequency. In 1961, Scokel reported a single case and stated that one other had been recorded.[24] Since that time other reports have appeared, however, less than 200 cases are currently registered.[11,24–29] Eighty percent of these lesions are associated with other squamous neoplasias of the female genital tract with the cervix being the most frequent primary site.[27,30] Woodruff and co-workers suggest there are three possible origins for vaginal carcinoma in situ:[29] (1) In situ disease arising against the background of prior irradiation for another lesion in the adjacent area, (2) in situ disease resulting from incomplete surgery for the primary lesion, and (3) in situ disease representing examples of multicentric foci of neoplasia in the lower genital canal. Patients treated for cervical neoplasia, even when hysterectomy has been accomplished, should be followed periodically with examination and Pap smears for evidence of vaginal recurrence.

In situ lesions generally produce no symptoms and are most often suspected by the presence of abnormal vaginal cytology in a patient previously treated for genital tract neoplasia. Lugol's stain and colposcopy are helpful in locating the abnormal areas for directed biopsy confirmation. The majority of in situ lesions are in the upper vagina. It must be remembered, however, that the lesion is frequently multicentric, so careful examination of the entire vagina must be accomplished.

**Table 8–1.   CARCINOMA OF
THE VAGINA**

STAGE 0	Carcinoma in situ; intraepithelial carcinoma.
STAGE I	The carcinoma is limited to the vaginal wall.
STAGE II	The carcinoma has involved the subvaginal tissue but has not extended to the pelvic wall.
STAGE III	The carcinoma has extended to the pelvic wall.
STAGE IV	The carcinoma has extended beyond the true pelvis or has involved the mucosa of the bladder or rectum. Bullous edema as such does not permit a case to be allotted to stage IV.
STAGE IVA	Spread of the growth to adjacent organs.
STAGE IVB	Spread to distant organs.

Staging of vaginal cancer is clinical and it gives consideration to the involvement of neighboring structures (Table 8–1).

Treatment

As late as 1935, Taussig considered malignancy of the vagina to be extremely rare and universally fatal.[31] However, since that time numerous reports have shown a more optimistic outlook. Treatment planning for squamous vaginal cancer must consider lesion size, location, and potential spread patterns.

The vagina is a thin-walled structure situated in close proximity to the bladder and rectum. The vaginal mucosa and muscularis contain an anastomotic meshwork of lymphatics that combine laterally into larger drainage trunks. Lesions in the upper vagina, similarly to those of the cervix, spread to the lateral and deep pelvic lymph nodes. Midvaginal lesions spread anteriorly to the intrailiac and paravesical lymph nodes and posteriorly to the inferior gluteal, sacral, and rectal lymph nodes. Lower vaginal lesions, similar to those of the vulva, spread to inguinal lymph nodes in the femoral triangle. The incidence of nodal involvement has not been studied in this disease. However, it is felt that stage I lesions, 2 to 3 cm in diameter and smaller, have a low incidence of lymph node metastasis.[32]

Multicentric in situ lesions and most invasive lesions are best treated by irradiation as discussed in Chapter 9.[32,33] Many patients with vaginal cancer are older, medically unfit, and have tumors located such that primary exenterative surgery would be necessary to encompass the lesion. A primary radiotherapeutic approach in such patients would seem to produce the best chance for cure with the least treatment morbidity and mortality. A primary surgical approach is an acceptable alternative to irradiation, particularly in younger patients with upper vaginal tumors where radical hysterectomy, upper vaginectomy, and pelvic lymphadenectomy have also been shown to be curative.[34] An overall five-year survival rate of 30 to 40 percent is recorded in this disease.[2–4,7,9–11,13,14,32,35] However, cure rates for stage I and II lesions, particularly when located in the upper vagina, should approach 60 to 70 percent.[2,32]

In situ vaginal cancer presents an interesting therapeutic problem. Treatment by surgical excision, irradiation, and chemotherapy have all been employed, and therapy for each patient should be individualized.[11,22,27–29] Localized lesions delineated by Lugol's stain or colposcopy can be simply excised. Extensive or multicentric lesions are better treated by vaginectomy and grafting or irradiation.[11,27,32] Use of topical 5-fluorouracil (1 to 2 percent) has been reported by Woodruff et al.[29] They record cures in eight of nine patients treated with this agent and followed for six weeks to six years. The one therapeutic failure was in a patient with a hyperkaratotic lesion. Regardless of the treatment method employed, patients with a history of in situ vaginal cancer should be followed closely for evidence of persistent or recurrent genital tract neoplasia.

ADENOCARCINOMA

Adenocarcinoma accounts for 5 to 10 percent of all primary vaginal cancers.[3,4,7,9–11] From 1900 to 1970, only scattered reports of tumors with this cell type appeared in the world's literature and it was generally felt to be a disease entity developing in vaginal Mullerian duct rests. The age at diagnosis was found to be similar to that of squamous cell vaginal cancer. In 1970, Herbst and Scully[36] reported seven cases of adenocarcinoma occurring between the age of 15 and 22, a much younger age group than previously noted. Subsequently Herbst and his coworkers, through a detailed retrospective study, established the probable relationship between synthetic nonsteroidal estrogens taken during early pregnancy and development of adenocarcinoma of the vagina in female offspring.[20]

An adenocarcinoma of the vagina and cervix registry has been established and at latest report had recorded 250 cases of young female genital tract adenocarcinomas;[37,38] 70 percent of the registry cases give a positive or probable maternal history for nonsteroidal synthetic estrogens taken during pregnancy. Diethylstilbestrol has been the most frequent medication used, but Dienestrol and Hexestrol have been incriminated as well. The development of adenocarcinoma does not seem to be dose related, as one patient took 1.5 mg of diethylstilbesterol for only 12 days, however, it is critical that the drug was given during the first 18 weeks of pregnancy.

The age range at development of estrogen-related adenocarcinoma is 7 to 28, with most cases occurring postmenarche. The tumor presents as a polypoid growth predominantly in the upper and anterior vagina and symptoms, as with squamous cancers, are vaginal discharge and bleeding. A number of early cases have been asymptomatic and were diagnosed only at routine examination accomplished because of a history of maternal estrogen exposure. Diagnosis is usually established by direct visualization and biopsy, although vaginal cytology can be diagnostic when it is obtained directly from the lesion.[39] The usual morphology is a clear cell appearance with endometroid and mixed cell types being present in about 20 percent of the cases.[40]

TREATMENT

Treatment of vaginal adenocarcinoma must consider lesion size, location, and patient age. The spread pattern seems to be similar to that of squamous cancer with the unsubstantiated possibility that the tumor metastasizes earlier. Radical surgery and irradiation are both curative. Surgery has the advantage of ovarian preservation and identification of lymph node spread. Radical hysterectomy, upper vaginectomy, and pelvic lymphadenectomy are recommended for treatment of small upper vaginal lesions. Large lesions and mid to lower vaginal lesions are best treated by primary irradiation, as discussed in Chapter 9. Five-year cure rates are generally unknown at this time, as only a small number of cases has been observed for that length of time.[38] However, cure rates of up to 60 percent are to be expected.[37,38,40,46]

ADENOSIS

In nearly every instance of vaginal adenocarcinoma recorded, adenosis has also been present.[38,47,48] Adenosis of the vagina was first reported at autopsy by von Preuschenn in 1877. Bonnie and Glendenning in 1910 recognized the entity and proposed the term "adenomatosis vaginae" for this benign disease. In 1927, Plaut and Dreyfuss coined the term adenosis to describe the presence of areas of benign columnar epithelium in the vagina and the term has been used ever since.[37,38,47] The incidence of spontaneous adenosis is unknown, although Sandberg's study does indicate an occurrence rate of 40 percent in the postpubertal vagina.[49] Careful examination by Stafl and others, utilizing the colposcope, shows an adenosis incidence of 90 percent in the estrogen exposed female vagina.[47] Whether adenosis is a forerunner of adenocarcinoma is unknown at the present time, as no reports exist showing a malignant transformation from benign adenosis to adenocarcinoma. The incidence of adenocarcinoma developing in estrogen-exposed female offspring is only 1 in 1000.[38,45] With the large number of patients known to have adenosis, it would appear that if a malignant transformation does take place, it is indeed rare. It is known that adenosis tends to undergo metaplasia to squamous epithelium in the acid vaginal atmosphere.[50] Although malignant squamous change has not been noted, some investigators consider squamous cell disease of the vagina and cervix, as a sequelae of adenosis, a potentially greater hazard than adenocarcinoma.[47,51,52]

Usually adenosis is asymptomatic. Some patients, however, do complain of increased vaginal discharge when there is marked adenosis present.[40,47,50] The diagnosis is made by suspicion, inspection, and biopsy. The entire vagina must be surveyed as the lesion often is multicentric. Schiller staining is helpful in locating areas of adenosis, however, colposcopy is essential to adequately visualize and follow lesions. It is recommended that asymptomatic patients with a questionable or positive history of maternal estrogen exposure during early pregnancy have pelvic evaluation, including colposcopy, if possible shortly post menarche. Findings at that time will dictate the frequency of further examinations. Premenarchal children, if asymptomatic, need not be routinely examined, as the incidence of adenocarcinoma in this age group is extremely low.[47,50]

TREATMENT

Some controversy exists as to the proper treatment, if any, of vaginal adenosis. Sherman and others have recommended surgical excision.[53] No one to date, however, has demonstrated that adenosis is a premalignant lesion, therefore, most investigators recommend that if the adenosis is colposcopically benign, no specific treatment is necessary.[47,50] Acidifying gels or douches and topical progesterone may enhance the transformation from columnar to squamous epithelium.[54] However, these agents are not critical, as spontaneous transformation will occur. It is recommended that patients with known adenosis be followed colposcopically at six-month intervals until further information is gained. Areas of adenosis that appear to be undergoing abnormal transformation should be biopsied.

SARCOMA

Vaginal sarcoma is extremely rare, accounting for only 2 percent of all vaginal malignancies.[4,7,9-11,55] Leiomyosarcoma, reticulum cell, and stromal sarcoma have been reported. Leiomyosarcoma is the most frequent vaginal sarcoma and behaves in a manner similar to its corresponding cell type on the vulva.

Age range at diagnosis for patients with leiomyosarcoma is 50 to 70 and, as with other vaginal tumors, the primary symptom is bleeding. Surgical excision, adequate to completely remove the lesion, is the treatment of choice. Anterior, posterior, or total pelvic exenteration is indicated if the bladder or rectum is involved. Irradiation and chemotherapy have been used in this disease, but they have met with limited success. Five-year survival rates of 35 percent are reported.[55] It has been speculated that survival rates could be improved if the primary surgical approach were more aggressive.

SARCOMA BOTRYOIDES

The most common malignant tumor of the lower genital tract in female children is sarcoma botryoides.[56-59] This tumor is also recorded as mixed mesodermal sarcoma, rhabdomyosarcoma, and mesenchymal sarcoma. Tragically, this tumor arises in very young children, the mean age being 2 to 3 years with a range of 6 months to 16 years. These lesions are usually multicentric and are quite immature histologically, resembling embryonic mesenchymal tissue (Fig. 8-3). Rhabdomyoblasts frequently are present. The tumor presents as multicentric polypoid masses arising in the wall of the vagina. The most common symptom is vaginal bleeding. Frequently the patient is asymptomatic and presents only with a polypoid mass at the introitus (Fig. 8-4). Diagnosis is made by suspicion and biopsy. Any vaginal bleeding or blood-tinged discharge in the premenarchal female should be thoroughly investigated.

Pelvic exenteration has been the treatment of choice for sarcoma botryoides. Pelvic lymphadenectomy should also be accomplished, as nodes may be positive.[56,58,59] Hilgers, reviewing pelvic exenteration experience, records a 70 percent two-year survival rate in 8 patients with tumor confined to the vagina, and a 37 percent two-year survival rate in 13 patients with tumor spread from the vagina, but still surgically resectable.[56] He, as well as Piver and Kumor, propose combining irradiation and/or chemotherapy with surgical excision for treatment of this disease, particularly if tumor has spread from the vagina.[56,57,60] The efficacy of this therapeutic approach cannot be assessed at this time, as it is too recent to show survival improvement.

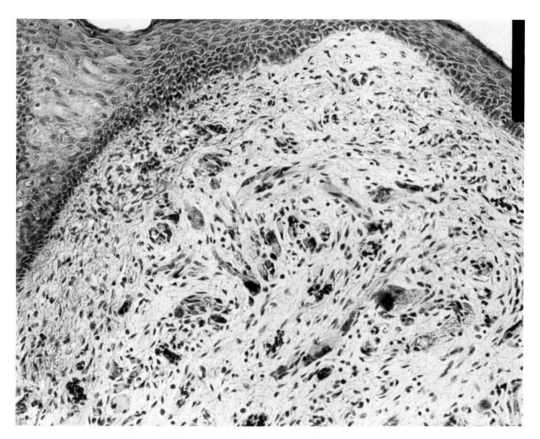

Figure 8–3. Sarcoma botyryoides of vagina in 3-year-old.

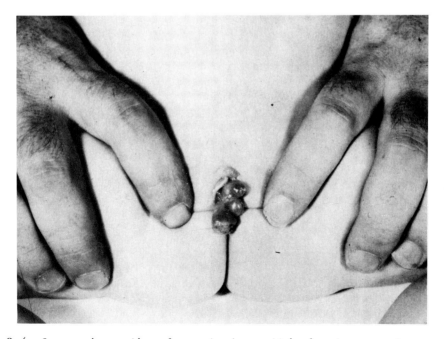

Figure 8–4. Sarcoma botyryoides of posterior lower third of vagina presenting as polypoid masses.

MELANOMA

Melanoma of the vagina, like vaginal sarcoma, is extremely rare, accounting for less than 2 percent of all vaginal malignancies.[4,7,9-11,61,62] The mean patient age at diagnosis is 55 with a range of 22 to 83. The tumor appears as a yellow to black lesion anywhere on the vaginal wall with a predilection for a lower anterior location. Bleeding and discharge are the usual symptoms and diagnosis is made by suspicion, visualization, and biopsy.

Treatment of vaginal melanoma is primarily surgical and should be based on the location and the extent of the disease.[61,63] Except in very superficial lesions, which might respond to vaginectomy alone, lymphatic drainage areas must be considered and should be removed. Mid to upper vaginal tumors may be treated by vaginectomy, radical hysterectomy, and pelvic lymphadenectomy. Lower vaginal lesions are best treated by vaginectomy, vulvectomy, and inguinal lymphadenectomy. Deeply invasive tumors require extended radical procedures including exenteration. Patients at risk for radical surgery may benefit from combinations of limited surgery and irradiation.

Survival rates for vaginal melanoma are very poor. Morrow and DiSaia, in an extensive review of female genital tract melanoma, found a five-year survival rate of only 5.1 percent.[62] Ultimate therapeutic success in this tumor may be with combinations of surgery, chemo- and immunotherapy.

METASTATIC AND RECURRENT VAGINAL CANCER

Vaginal cancer metastatic from a lesion of the endometrium, cervix, or vulva is more frequent than primary vaginal cancer. When these tumors are encountered, they should be treated similarly to the primary cancer. Irradiation, modifying the field size in order to cover the vaginal extension, is usually the treatment of choice for cervix and endometrial primaries. Extended vulvectomy with partial vaginectomy or pelvic exenteration is the preferred treatment for vaginal extension of a primary vulvar carcinoma.

Recurrent vaginal tumors are difficult to treat. Since most patients with primary vaginal cancer have received irradiation as initial treatment, extended radical surgery, as performed with cervical cancer recurrence, may be feasible. Those cases that recur after primary surgery may respond to irradiation. Chemotherapy has been used, but to date shows the same poor response seen with other squamous cell tumors.[64] A better chemotherapeutic response may be seen in recurrent adenocarcinoma and sarcoma.[65] However, there is insufficient data at present to confirm this observation. As with cervical tumors, survival rates following recurrence are poor. Therefore, the primary tumor should be given maximum initial therapy.

References

1. Palmer J, Bibock S: Primary cancer of the vagina. Am J Obstet Gynec 67:377, 1954
2. Dunn L, Napier J: Primary carcinoma of the vagina. Am J Obstet Gynec 96:1112, 1966
3. Frick C, Jacox H, Taylor H, Jr: Primary carcinoma of the vagina. Am J Obstet Gynec 101:695, 1968
4. Herbst A, Green T, Ulfelder H: Primary carcinoma of the vagina. Am J Obstet Gynec 106:210, 1970
5. Lang W, Menduke H, Golub L: The delay period in carcinoma of the vagina. Am J Obstet Gynec 80:341, 1960
6. Marcus S: Primary carcinoma of the vagina. Obstet Gynec 15:673, 1960
7. McGarrity K: Cancer of the vagina. Aust NZJ Obstet Gynec 7:170, 1967
8. Merrill J, Bender W: Primary carcinoma of the vagina. Obstet Gynec 11:3, 1958
9. Perez C, Arneson AN, Galakatos A, Samanth HK: Malignant tumors of the vagina. Cancer 31:36, 1973
10. Perticucci S: Diagnostic, prognostic, and therapeutic considerations in invasive carcinoma of the vagina. Obstet Gynec 40:843, 1972

11. Rutledge F: Cancer of the vagina. Am J Obstet Gynec 97:635, 1967

12. Smith F: Primary carcinoma of the vagina. Am J Obstet Gynec 69:525, 1955

13. Underwood P, Smith R: Carcinoma of the vagina. JAMA 217:46, 1971

14. Welton J, Kottmeier H: Primary carcinoma of the vagina. Acta Obstet Gynec Scand 41:22, 1962

15. Whitehouse W: Primary carcinoma of the vagina. J Obstet Gynec Brit Common 69: 481, 1962

16. Forsberg JG: Derivation and differentiation of the vaginal epithelium. Lund, Thesis, University of Bergan, Norway, 1963

17. Forsberg JG: Cervicovaginal epithelium: Its origin and development. Am J Obstet Gynec 115:1025, 1973

18. Koff AK: Development of the vagina in the human fetus. Contrib Embryol 24:59, 1933

19. Witschi E: Development and Differentiation of the Uterus. In Mack HC: Prenatal Life. Proceedings of the Third Annual Symposium on the Physiology and Pathology of Human Reproduction. Detroit, Wayne State Univ Press, 1970, pp 11-35

20. Herbst A, Ulfelder H, Poskanzer D: Adenocarcinoma of the vagina association of maternal stilbesterol therapy with tumor appearance in young women. N Engl J Med 284:878, 1971

21. Daw E: Primary carcinoma of the vagina. J Obstet Gynaecol Brit Common 78:853, 1971

22. Merchant S, Murad T, Dowling EA, Durant J: Diagnosis of vaginal carcinoma from cytologic material. Acta Cytol 18:494, 1974

23. Lewis BV, Chapman PA: Cytological diagnosis of a primary malignant melanoma of the vagina. Brit J Obstet Gynaecol 82:74, 1975

24. Scokel P, Collier F, Jones W, et al: Relation of carcinoma in situ of the vagina to the early diagnosis of vaginal cancer. Am J Obstet Gynec 82:397, 1961

25. Copenhover E, Salzmann F, Wright K: Carcinoma in situ of the vagina. Am J Obstet Gynec 89:962, 1964

26. Ferguson J, Maclure J: Intraepithelial carcinoma, dysplasia, and exfoliation of cancer cells in the vaginal mucosa. Am J Obstet Gynec 87:326, 1963

27. Gallup P, Morley G: Carcinoma in situ of the vagina. Obstet Gynec 46:334, 1975

28. Hummer W, Mussey E, Decker DD, Dockerty MB: Carcinoma in situ of the vagina. Am J Obstet Gynec 108:1109, 1970

29. Woodruff JD, Parmley T, Julian C: Topical 5-fluorouracil in the treatment of vaginal carcinoma in situ. Gynec Oncol 3:124, 1975

30. Gray L, Christophersen W: In situ and early invasive carcinoma of the vagina. Obstet Gynec 34:226, 1969

31. Taussig F: Early cancer of the vulva, vagina and female urethra—Five year results. Surg Gynec Obstet 60:477, 1935

32. Brown A, Fletcher G, Rutledge F: Irradiation of in situ and invasive squamous cell carcinoma of the vagina. Cancer 28:1278, 1971

33. Perez C, Arneson AN, Dehner LP, Galakatos A: Radiation therapy in carcinoma of the vagina. Obstet Gynec 44:862, 1974

34. Palumbo L, Shingleton HM, Fishburne JI, Pepper FD, Kock GG: Primary carcinoma of the vagina. South Med J 62:1048, 1969

35. Lewis G, Brady L: Carcinoma of the vagina. Clin Obstet Gynec 10:655, 1967

36. Herbst A, Scully R: Adenocarcinoma of the vagina in adolescence. Cancer 25:745, 1970

37. Herbst A, Kurman RJ, Scully RE, Poskanzer DC: Clear cell adenocarcinoma of the genital tract in young females—registry report. N Engl J Med 287:1259, 1972

38. Herbst A, Welch W, Scully R, et al: Registry of clear cell adenocarcinoma of the genital tract in young females. Unpublished report, Boston, 1975

39. Vooigs P, Ng A, Wentz B: The detection of vaginal adenosis and clear cell carcinoma. Acta Cytol 17:59, 1973

40. Yon J, Lutz MH, Gurtanner RE, Averette HE: Adenosis and adenocarcinoma of the vagina in young women: A review. Gynec Oncol 2:508, 1975

41. Gilson M, Dibona D, Knab D: Clear cell adenocarcinoma in young females. Obstet Gynec 41:494, 1973

42. Kanter H, Weinstein S, Kaye H: Clear cell adenocarcinoma in young women. Obstet Gynec 41:443, 1973

43. Nordqvist S, Fidler WJ, Woodruff JM, Lewis JL: Clear cell adenocarcinoma of the cervix and vagina. Cancer 37:858, 1976

44. Roth L, Hornbeck N: Clear cell adenocarcinoma of the cervix in young women. Cancer 34:1761, 1974

45. Ulfelder H: Stilbesterol adenosis and ade-

nocarcinoma. Am J Obstet Gynec 117:794, 1973

46. Wharton T, Rutledge FN, Gallager HS, Fletcher G: Treatment of clear cell adeno-carcinoma in young females. Obstet Gynec 45:365, 1975

47. Stafl A, Mattingly RF, Foley DV, Fetherston WC: Clinical diagnosis of vaginal adenosis. Obstet Gynec 43:118, 1974

48. Noller KL, Decker DG, Symmonds RE, Dockerty MB, Kurland LT: Clear-cell ade-nocarcinoma of the vagina and cervix: Sur-vival data. Am J Obstet Gynec 124:285, 1976

49. Sandberg E: The incidence and distribution of occult vaginal adenosis. Am J Obstet Gynec 101:322, 1968

50. Herbst A, Scully R, Robboy S: Vaginal adenosis and other diethylstilbesterol re-lated abnormalities. Clin Obstet Gynec 18: 185, 1975

51. Fetherston W: Squamous neoplasia of vagi-na related to DES syndrome. Am J Obstet Gynec 122:176, 1975

52. Veridiano N, Weiner E, Tancer M: Squa-mous cell carcinoma of the vagina associated with vaginal adenosis. Obstet Gynec 47: 689, 1976

53. Sherman A, Goldrath M, Berlin A, et al: Cervical-vaginal adenosis after in utero ex-posure to synthetic estrogens. Obstet Gy-nec 44:531, 1974

54. Herbst A, Robboy SJ, MacDonald GJ, Scully RE: Effects of local progesterone on

stilbesterol associated vaginal adenosis. Am J Obstet Gynec 118:607, 1974

55. Davos I, Abell M: Sarcomas of the vagina. Obstet Gynec 47:342, 1976

56. Hilgers R: Pelvic exenteration for vaginal embryonal rhabdomyosarcoma. Obstet Gynec 45: 175, 1975

57. Piver S, Barlow JJ, Wang JJ, Shah NK: Combined radical surgery, radiation therapy and chemotherapy in infants with vulvovag-inal embryonal rhabdomyosarcoma. Obstet Gynec 42:522, 1973

58. Rutledge F, Sullivan M: Sarcoma botry-oides. Ann NY Acad Sci 142:694, 1967

59. Smith J: Malignant gynecologic tumors in children. Am J Obstet Gynec 116:201, 1973

60. Kumar A, Wrenn EL, Fleming ID, Hustu HO, Pratt CB: Combined therapy to pre-vent complete pelvic exenteration for rhab-domyosarcoma of the vagina and uterus. Cancer 37:118, 1976

61. Fenn M, Abell M: Melanomas of vulva and vagina. Obstet Gynec 41:902, 1973

62. Morrow P, DiSaia P: Malignant melanoma of the female genitalia: A clinical review. Obstet Gynec Surv 31:233, 1976

63. Pomante R: Malignant melanoma-primary in the vagina. Gynec Oncol 3:15, 1975

64. Malkasian G: Chemotherapy of squamous cell carcinoma of the cervix, vagina, and vulva. Clin Obstet Gynec 11:367, 1968

65. Smith J: Chemotherapy in gynecologic can-cer. Clin Obstet Gynec 18:109, 1975

Chapter 9

Radiation Therapy for Carcinoma of the Vagina

LUTHER W. BRADY, M.D.

Primary malignant tumors of the vagina comprise 1 to 2 percent of all gynecologic malignancies. Squamous cell carcinoma predominates and, usually, occurs in the older age group with a mean age of 56 years. Adenocarcinomas are rarer and are most often found in young women in their early 20s. Frequently, there is a history of maternal stilbesterol ingestion in these patients, and the tumor is primarily described histologically as a clear cell cancer. Primary adenocarcinomas of the vagina also occur in older patients and can show the clear cell configuration. The vast majority of tumors involving the vagina occur as a consequence of metastases from other sites, namely, the cervix, corpus, colon, ovary, bladder, and urethra.

The proximity of these structures, namely, the bladder, rectum, ureter, and urethra increases the potential for complications from treatment. The thinness of the recto- and vesicovaginal septa poses the hazard of fistula and contamination. The vascularity of the same tissues adds the additional threat of hemorrhage.

The age of the patient at the time of onset of tumor does not significantly influence the long-term survival. The disease is rare in the black woman and almost totally absent in Jewish women.

A malignant lesion found in the vagina is most commonly metastatic from another site with the most common primary site being the cervix. Primary carcinoma of the vagina is usually located in the posterior upper third of the vagina, while metastatic lesions, particularly, from the endometrium are found not only in the upper vagina but also along the anterior vaginal vault and near the urethral meatus. The location of either a primary or secondary malignancy involving the vagina is critical in the treatment planning that must be employed. In general, involvement of the upper vaginal vault indicates that the pattern of spread will be similar to that seen in carcinoma of the cervix. Involvement of the lower third of the vaginal vault indicates that the tumor will resemble in its pattern of dissemination primary malignant tumors of the vulva. When the tumor occurs in the middle third, either or both patterns of involvement may be seen.

The average duration of symptoms prior to diagnosis is often long, approximately 7.4 months. Major symptoms include vaginal discharge and spotting, pain with urinary symptoms and inguinal masses. The preponderance of lesions are on the posterior of the vagina and offer the best prognosis.

EVALUATION AND STAGING

In the management of the patient with primary malignant tumors of the vagina, primary sites should be eliminated in the work-up. Studies should then be directed toward evaluation of the immediate structures in the pelvis, including the genitourinary tract, the colon and rectum, other genital structures, as well as studies to eliminate the potential prospect for disseminated disease. Speculum examination and biopsy are recommended for the establishment of histologic type as well as clinical extent (Table 8–1).

The most commonly described tumor grossly is a papillary friable, spongy lesion, histologically representing squamous cell carcinoma. It can be confused with disease of the cervix because of the similarity in microscopic appearance. The cervix, however, for a primary malignant tumor of the vagina should be clear of disease.

Grossly visible cancer of the vagina may be biopsied by a punch-type instrument or by knife excision of an adequate sample. The adjacent organs need thorough investigation as previously noted. Dilatation and curettage of the cervix along with surgical biopsy of the vagina are the initial requirements. Cystoscopy, intravenous pyelography, barium enema, proctosigmoidoscopy, and chest roentgenograms are basic pretherapy studies, along with biochemical evaluation and blood count. Other studies may be indicated on the basis of pathologic findings and the location of the vaginal lesion.

TREATMENT TECHNIQUES

A wide variety of approaches have been used to treat clear cell adenocarcinoma in the young individual.[1–4] Local excision, transvaginal radiation therapy, the implantation of radioactive needles, external radiation therapy, and intracavitary radiation therapy have been used singly or in combination. Vaginectomy alone, vaginectomy with radical hysterectomy, and exenteration have also been employed. Efforts have been directed toward preservation of the ovaries when management was by the surgical route. For the patients with radical surgery, reconstruction or replacement of the vagina has been suggested at a point following completion of treatment when all evidences of disease have been eradicated and no evidences of recurrence have been noted. Even though the radical surgical approach may avoid the side effects of radiation therapy, they often require the patient to live the remainder of her life with ostomies to replace her normal urinary and bowel functions. These functions may be preserved by the utilization of radiation therapy programs even though the ovarian function loss results but this can be replaced by hormones.

The 1975 Report of the Registry of Clear Cell Adenocarcinoma indicates that to date there are not enough patients to draw conclusions as to the five-year survival rates by the various treatment techniques employed. To date there have been 41 deaths and 22 patients with recurrent disease. Experience with chemotherapy is too limited at this time to suggest anything of value.

Radiation Therapy

The most widely applicable form of treatment for most primary vaginal malignancies is radiation therapy. This is especially true since many of the patients are elderly and in poor condition.[5–7]

The majority of patients with primary malignant tumors of the vagina can be successfully treated using radiation therapy techniques. Whether intracavitary, interstitial brachytherapy alone, or combined with external irradiation are employed depends on the extent and thickness of the tumor as well as parametrial extent.

The following principles for treatment have evolved over time and represent an appropriate approach to the radiation therapy management for patients with primary malignant tumors of the vagina (Table 9–1).

Carcinoma In Situ

Patients with carcinoma in situ have superficial tumors involving the vaginal mucosa. This tumor does not extend beyond the basement membrane of the squamous epithelium. An intracavitary application delivering between 6500 to 7000 rads to the mucosa is adequate to control all lesions. Because of the multicentric nature of this tumor, however, it is necessary to treat the entire vaginal vault. The control rate for patients with this lesion varies from 100 percent as reported by Prempree[7] (7/7) to 11 of 12 treated by Perez et al.[6] In

Table 9–1. CARCINOMA OF THE VAGINA
SUGGESTED RADIATION THERAPY
TREATMENT PLANS

Table 9–1. CARCINOMA OF THE VAGINA
SUGGESTED RADIATION THERAPY
TREATMENT PLANS

STAGE	EXTERNAL IRRADIATION	LOCAL
0	None	6,000–7,000 rads vaginal mucosa via vaginal cylinder
I (thin)	None	6,000–7,000 rads interstitial implant
I (thick)	4,000–5,000 rads whole pelvis in 4–5 wk	Interstitial implant 300–4,000 rads
IIA	5,000–6,000 rads whole pelvis in 5–6 wk	Interstitial implant 3,000–4,000 rads
IIB, III	5,000 rads in 5 wk, whole pelvis— 2,000 rads boost to vagina in 2 wk	Implant
IV	5,000 rads in 5 wk, whole pelvis and individualize	Implant

the Perez series, the patient with failure recurred distal to the area of treatment and was salvaged by anterior exenteration. This could have been avoided with more comprehensive intravaginal irradiation.

Higher doses of radiation are not required and may result in significant vaginal fibrosis and stenosis. Adequate dose distribution can be obtained using either a Bloedorn applicator, if the lesion is in the vaginal vault, or with a cylinder or Burnett vaginal applicator. This technique of management is simple, reproducible, and easily managed.

Stage I

Patients with stage I invasive lesions present generally with tumors that are 0.5 to 1 cm thick. They may be quite extensive involving rather large areas in the vaginal vault. The most superficial tumors are treated by intracavitary radium alone covering the entire vaginal vault. If the lesion is thicker, in addition to the intracavitary cylinder, a single plane implant should be used. This has the advantage of selectively increasing the depth dose without delivering excessive radiation to the vaginal mucosa. The majority of patients should receive 7000 rads calculated 0.5 cm beyond the plane of the implant, with the vaginal mucosa receiving an estimated dosage between 8000 and 10,000 rads.

Prempree reports five of six patients treated by this technique surviving without recurrent disease and Perez reports nine of nine patients treated by this method without recurrence. In those patients who were treated more aggressively, that is, a combination of intracavitary, interstitial therapy supplemented by external beam therapy, no local or pelvic failures were noted in the group of 19 patients. The whole pelvis in these patients received an additional 1000 to 2000 rads by external beam technique with a wedge midline block boosting the lateral pelvic wall dose to 4000 to 5000 rads in five to five and a half weeks. Megavoltage equipment is used in all external beam treatment plans.

Stage IIA

Patients with more advanced tumors, without extensive parametrial infiltration, are given a greater external radiation dosage to the whole pelvis, receiving 2000 to 4000 rads as a calculated tumor dose with an additional parametrial dose boosted to 5000 to 6000 rads to the lateral pelvic wall in about six weeks. This is supplemented by a combination of interstitial and intracavitary radium therapy.

Prempree reports 13 out of 21 patients cured by this aggressive radiation therapy technique and Perez reports 15 out of 35 patients cured by this technique.

Stages IIB, III, and IV

For stages IIB, III, and IV tumors, about 4000 rads are delivered to the whole pelvis with a total of 5500 to 6000 rads in five and a half to six weeks delivered to the parametrial areas in combination with interstitial and intracavitary radium therapy. The lateral parametrial portion of the tumors and the iliac lymph nodes in stages IIB, III, and IV should receive more than 5500 rads. Dosages below that level are inadequate and undoubtedly contribute to a high incidence of pelvic failure.

The data from Perez is summarized in Figure

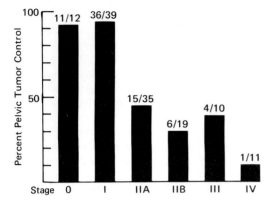

Figure 9–1. Carcinoma of the vagina (MIR 1950–1973); local and pelvic tumor control.[6]

9–1, with local and pelvic control in the patients treated according to the anatomic stage of the tumor. Over 95 percent of the patients with stage 0 or I showed no evidence of recurrent tumor. One patient with stage 0 failed distally to a single 20-mg source placed in the upper vaginal vault where a suboptimal treatment volume was treated. One of the three patients in the stage I group received interstitial colloidal gold and one was treated with external beam only where, again, inadequate therapy was carried out. In stage IIA,

the local pelvic control was disappointingly low, to a great extent because of the omission of external irradiation in a group of 16 patients where only four were cured. In stage IIB and stage III, pelvic control was achieved in only 30 to 40 percent of the patients, probably because of the large mass of tumor and the hypoxic radioresistant subpopulation of tumor cells. In only 1 of 11 patients (9 percent) with stage IV pelvic tumor was control accomplished.

Perez's data is summarized in Figure 9–2 illustrating a comparative analysis of local and pelvic control in all patients according to the type of therapy used. In stage 0 and stage I the addition of external beam irradiation did not prove significantly advantageous, probably because the entire tumor volume was included in the 6000 to 7000 rad dose delivered with the appropriate use of interstitial and intracavitary therapy dictated by the extent of the tumor. However, in stages IIA, IIB, and III, Perez found local control to be extremely poor unless external irradiation was given. Only 4 of the 16 patients with stage IIA (25 percent), 1 of 5 with stage IIB, none of 3 with stage III, and none of the 2 with stage IV were controlled with intracavitary or interstitial therapy alone. In contrast, 12 of 17 patients with stage IIA (70.5 percent), 5 of 14 with stage IIB (35.7 percent), and 4 of 7 with stage III (57 percent)

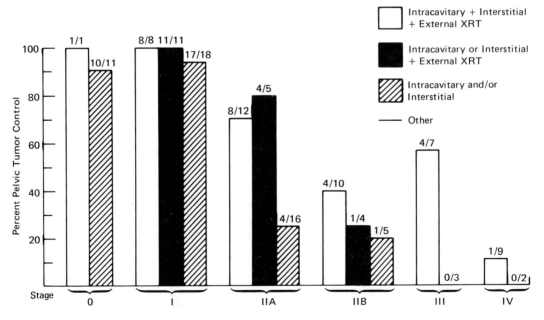

Figure 9–2. Epidermoid carcinoma of the vagina; tumor control in pelvis (3 years) and therapeutic modality.[6]

Table 9–2. CARCINOMA OF THE VAGINA
RADIATION THERAPY FOR
PRIMARY DISEASE[7]

STAGE	5-YR CURE (ABSOLUTE, %)
0	100 (7/7)
I	83.2 (5/6)
IIA	62 (13/21)
IIB	54.5 (6/11)
III	40 (8/20)
IV	0 (0/7)
Total	54 (39/72)

Table 9–3. CARCINOMA OF THE VAGINA
5-YR SURVIVAL OF PATIENTS WITH
INVASIVE SQUAMOUS CELL CARCINOMA
OF THE VAGINA[5] RADIATION THERAPY

STAGE	ABSOLUTE SURVIVAL (%)	INTER-CURRENT DISEASE OR LOST TO FOLLOW-UP	DETER-MINED SURVIVAL (%)
I	69 (11/16)	3	85 (11/13)
II	68 (13/19)	2	76 (13/17)
III	27 (4/15)	5	40 (4/10)
IV	(0/11)	2	(0/9)

experienced local and pelvic tumor control when external beam irradiation was an integral part of the therapy.

Prempree, in his report, evaluates 72 patients with the diagnosis of primary malignant tumors of the vagina. The histologic diagnosis was invasive squamous cell carcinoma in 92.5 percent of the patients, with 6 percent having adenocarcinomas, and 1.5 percent having malignant melanomas. The five-year data are summarized in Table 9–2. The overall absolute five-year cure rate for all stages combined was 54.0 percent. Comparable results and even better results in some stages (stage II and stage III) are thought to be due to proper integrated radiation therapy combining interstitial and intracavitary radium with external supervoltage radiation therapy.

The data from Brown et al confirm the value of radiation therapy in vaginal cancer (Table 9–3).[5]

COMPLICATIONS

The incidence of complications from this treatment program approach has been acceptable. In the early stages (0 and I), major complications were noted in two patients treated with interstitial colloidal gold by Perez prior to 1963. In five patients, vaginal fibrosis was observed by Perez, and five patients developed vaginal necrosis and one patient developed chronic radiation cystitis. All were treated conservatively and responded. In stage II there were six major complications (11 percent), rectal stricture in three patients, one patient with rectal vaginal fistula, and one with a severe hemorrhagic cystitis. Vaginal fibrosis or necrosis was noted in six patients and less severe radiation cystitis in one patient by Perez.

In stages III and IV, there were four major complications (19 percent), two patients with rectovaginal fistula, one rectal fibrosis, and one urethral stricture.

Complications occurred more frequently in the patients treated with a combination of brachytherapy and external beam irradiation as noted by Perez and Prempree. This may be related not only to the higher doses delivered, but also to the better survival.

SURGERY

Surgery for vaginal cancer has limited application because of the frequent advanced nature of the disease, the elderly status of the patient, and the frequent occurrence of medical complications. Local excision of noninvasive cancer has been mentioned as one form of surgery, and can be employed in almost all patients if they have a restricted disease process. On occasion, tumor extends anteriorly and/or posteriorly to involve the bladder or rectum. Under such circumstances, in suitably cleared medical candidates, total or partial exenteration may deserve consideration. For lesions in the middle or lower thirds of the vagina, inguinal node resection should be added to the surgical procedure. However, the generally poor prognosis for patients with vaginal carcinoma should limit the use of ultraradical surgery to relatively young individuals in good medical condition. Experience has yet to prove the value of surgery for patients with clear cell carcinoma.

Sarcoma botryoides is one of the lesions that has been treated by total pelvic exenteration with success, even in very young individuals. Elderly individuals with this form of malignancy usually are not suitable candidates for surgery. Irradiation has rarely proved to be of significant value for these lesions.

References

1. Wharton JT, Rutledge FN, Gallager HS, Fletcher G: The treatment of clear cell adenocarcinoma in young females. Obstet Gynecol 45:365–368, 1975
2. Greenwald P, Barlow JJ, Nasca PC, Burnett WS: Vaginal cancer after maternal treatment with synthetic estrogens. N Engl J Med 285:390–392, 1971
3. Herbst AL, Robboy SJ, Scully RE, Poskanzer DC: Clear cell adenocarcinoma of the vagina and cervix in girls: Analysis of 170 registry cases. Am J Obstet Gynecol 119:713–724, 1974
4. Robboy SJ, Herbst AL, Scully RE: Clear cell adenocarcinoma of the vagina and cervix in young females: Analysis of 37 tumors that persisted or recurred after primary therapy. Cancer 34:606–614, 1974
5. Brown GR, Fletcher GH, Rutledge FN: Irradiation of in-situ and invasive squamous cell carcinomas of the vagina. Cancer 28:1278–1283, 1971
6. Perez CA, Karba A, Purdy JA, Arneson AN: Dosimetric Consideration in Radiation Therapy of Carcinoma of the Vagina. Int J Rad Onc Suppl no. 1, October, 1976
7. Prempree T, Viravathana T, Slawson RG, Wizenberg MJ, Cuccia CA: Radiation management of primary carcinoma of the vagina. Int J Rad Onc Suppl no. 1, October, 1976

Chapter 10

Colposcopy

JOHN MARLOW, M.D.

HISTORY

Colposcopy began with the work of Dr. Hans Hinselmann of Germany. He was born on August 6, 1884, in Neumunster, Holstein, and completed his education in Keil, Germany, in 1908. From 1912 to 1925, he worked in Bonn, and following that became Director of Obstetrics and Gynecology at the General Hospital in Hamburg. There he became interested in developing a technique for the early diagnosis of carcinoma of the cervix. He correctly assumed that if the living tissue of the cervix could be visually inspected in sufficient detail, the very early stages of this cancer could be detected. He coined the term "colposcopy" and developed the first colposcope, which consisted of a front lamp (Von Eicken) and a magnifying glass elevated by books to the level of the vagina. Then he designed a binocular microscope of low magnification with illumination and an adjustable stand. This design is the basis of today's instrumentation. Dr. Hinselmann published his first clinical experiences in May of 1925. For the next 30 years until his death on April 18, 1959, he published on colposcopy and laid the foundation for this diagnostic method.

Colposcopy became the basic tool for the diagnosis of early cancer of the cervix in Germany and later in other European and English-speaking countries. Hinselmann's terminology was based on the surface topography as seen through the colposcope and much of it remains in use today.

However, the difficulty in translating the visual impression of the surface of the living tissue into corresponding pathologic histology delayed its acceptance into the English-speaking scientific communities.

Several other factors also contributed to the delay in acceptance of colposcopy in the United States. One was the introduction of cytology by Papanicolau and Trout in 1943, as an alternative effective screening tool for the diagnosis of early cancer of the cervix. Walter Schiller, a contemporary of Hinselmann in Vienna, experimenting with over 200 solutions in vivo, advocated the use of the iodine solution to detect early epidermoid cancer. Using his method, which he described in 1929, normal brown-staining squamous epithelium and noniodine staining areas could be identified. Unlike colposcopy, the inexpensive iodine test required no special equipment, was easily applied, and came into wide use throughout the United States. The iodine test, however, did not have the capacity for precise localization of the abnormal epithelium that colposcopy had. And the use of green filters on the colposcope, advocated by Kraatz in 1939, greatly enhanced inspection of blood vessels, thereby aiding localization of abnormalities even further.

The first American textbook on colposcopy was published in 1960, by Karl Bolten. An increasing interest in colposcopy in the United

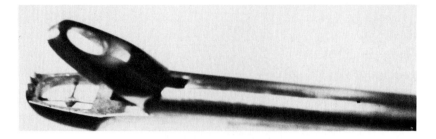

Figure 10–1. Cervical biopsy instrument (Whitner). Teeth on tip help to stabilize the instrument. The basket retains the biopsy specimen. Careful maintenance of the biopsy instrument is important to ensure that any abnormal lesion that is seen can be precisely sampled for histopathology.

States resulted in the foundation of the American Society of Colposcopy and Colpomicroscopy in 1964, with Warren R. Lang as its first president. Publications of Lang, Coppelson, Pixley, Reid, Stafl and Kolstad, Townsend, Schmitt, Wilbanks, Richart, Reagan, Gray and Ball, and others have stimulated the use of colposcopy as a complimentary diagnostic tool with cytology in America.

INDICATIONS

Colposcopy provides the physician with an opportunity to biopsy a cervical neoplastic lesion on the first office visit. If the lesion is visible, as 95 percent are, colposcopy can localize and outline its margins. A small lesion can be excised with a single directed biopsy (Fig. 10-1), while a larger lesion can require treatment extending into the fornix area of the vagina. The complications of cone biopsy from anesthesia, hemorrhage, stenosis, premature labor, abortion, and infertility can be reduced. The evaluation of repeated atypical cytology and the detection of carcinoma with false-negative cytology are examples of colposcopy complimenting cytology. Douching just prior to the examination has little effect on the diagnostic capability of colposcopy. Where cost is a concern, an office cervical biopsy is a fraction of the cost of a hospital conization. The endocervix may be difficult to examine with the colposcope (Fig. 10-2), although endocervical curetting is used to evaluate this area. The following are the indications for colposcopy.

1. Abnormal cytology
2. Macroscopic lesions of cervix, vagina, or vulva

3. Previous cancer of cervix, vagina, or vulva, treated with surgery or radiation
4. Abnormal genital discharge
5. Intermenstral or contact genital bleeding
6. Fetal DES exposure
7. Directed local treatment with cryosurgery, electrosurgery, or laser
8. Demonstration of living anatomy of visible external pelvis for students including use of television and videotape
9. Suspected cervical factors of infertility
10. Research concerning pathophysiology of cervix by mapping and colpophotography
11. Medicolegal inspection of hymen
12. Alternate to cone biopsy in patients
    a) Refusing cone biopsy
    b) Pregnant
    c) Very young
    d) At high risk for general anesthesia
    e) With bleeding or clotting abnormalities
    f) For economic concerns
13. Screening patients for cancer of the visible external pelvis where cytology services are not adequately available

TECHNIQUE

Colposcopy is performed prior to bimanual examination. The patient assumes a dorsal lithotomy position on an examining table with an adjustable height. The vaginal speculum is lubricated in warm tap water, inserted, and the cervix exposed. The exposure may be difficult due to a narrow

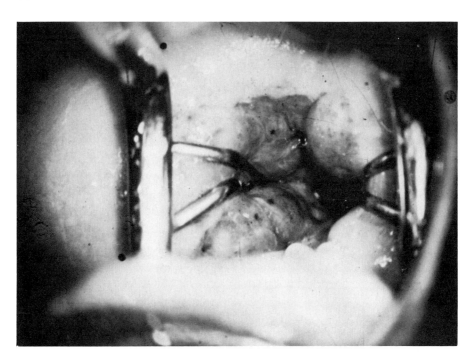

Figure 10–2. Endocervical speculum (10 power). Aides in evaluation of endocervix. Permits directed biopsy of lesion within canal.

hymen, a pelvic tumor, or relaxed vaginal walls. Rotating and manipulating the speculum and the use of a swab or forceps facilitates the exposure. The viewing angle of the colposcope should coincide with the long axis of the vagina. Elevating or lowering the patient's hips may be necessary to accomplish this. The use of a tubular speculum prevents the vaginal walls from obstructing the colposcopist's view. With adequate exposure, the cervix is scanned with a low-power magnification of 10 to 16. Cytology is taken to include samples from the endocervix.

A wet mount is taken if infection is suspected. Care is taken to include any suspicious area in the cytologic sampling. Surface discharge that prevents inspection of the cervix is removed gently with a swab, forceps, or normal saline. Next, the blood vessel architecture is inspected using a green or blue filter. These filters create a contrast between the vessels and their background. Acetic acid (3 percent) is applied in a soaked swab or by a squeeze-bottle stream. The acetic acid is mucolytic and accentuates atypical epithelium as well.

Columnar epithelium, when washed with dilute acetic acid, reveals a typical grape-like appearance. The acetic acid effect is transient and will vary according to the strength of the solution and

tissue reaction and lasts only two to three minutes. Applications of the acetic acid solution may be applied in succession for a complete examination. Glycogen staining with iodine, such as with Schiller's or Lugol's solution, is useful in defining squamous epithelium that is free of atypia. Other in vivo stains that have been used for colposcopy are (a) toluidine blue 1 percent, (b) solution of soda 10 percent, (c) alcohol 2 percent, (d) norepinephrine 1:1000, (e) acridine orange 1:1000, (f) salicylic alcohol .5 percent, (g) silver nitrate 3 to 10 percent, and (h) lactic acid.

Abnormal tissue is then biopsied as directed by the colposcopic findings. The location of the abnormal tissue is documented by photography and/or written in the chart (Fig. 10–3). If the atypical epithelium extends into the endocervical canal or that area is suspect, an endocervical curettage is performed. Hemostasis for cervical biopsies is accomplished by pressure over the biopsy site or by hemostatic compound such as Monsel's solution or silver nitrate. A topical antibiotic cream is inserted in the vagina to promote healing of the biopsy site. Following the colposcopy, a bimanual examination is performed. The patient is instructed to refrain from coitus for one week following the biopsy or until she is free of

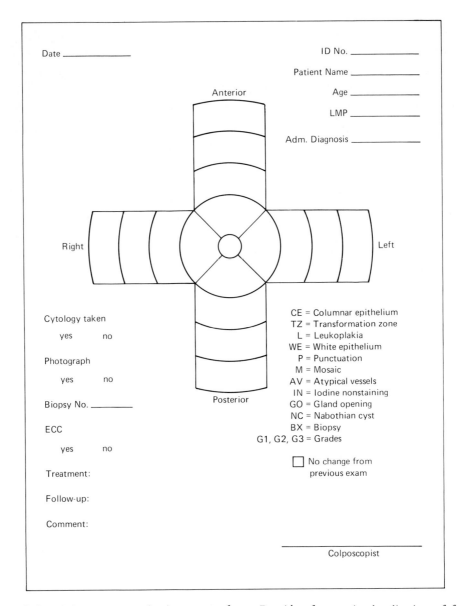

Date _____

ID No. _____

Patient Name _____

Age _____

LMP _____

Adm. Diagnosis _____

Anterior

Right

Left

Posterior

Cytology taken

  yes   no

Photograph

  yes   no

Biopsy No. _____

ECC

  yes   no

Treatment:

Follow-up:

Comment:

CE = Columnar epithelium
TZ = Transformation zone
L = Leukoplakia
WE = White epithelium
P = Punctuation
M = Mosaic
AV = Atypical vessels
IN = Iodine nonstaining
GO = Gland opening
NC = Nabothian cyst
BX = Biopsy
G1, G2, G3 = Grades

☐ No change from
   previous exam

_____
Colposcopist

Figure 10–3. Colposcopy examination report form. Provides for precise localization of findings, biopsies, and treatment.

pain or bleeding. The equipment used in colposcopy includes the following.

1. Colposcope
2. Examination table of adjustable height
3. Specula
   a) Vaginal—various sizes, including pediatric, normal, extra large, and tubular specula for use in pelvic relaxation and pregnancy
   b) Endocervical

4. Cytology collection equipment
   a) Swabs
   b) Spatula
   c) Aspirator
   d) Slides and cover slips
   e) Fixative
5. Solutions
   a) Normal saline
   b) Acetic acid 3 percent
   c) Iodine solution
   d) Toluidine 1 percent

6. Ring forceps
7. Cotton balls
8. Biopsy instruments
   a) Uterine sound
   b) Single-tooth tenaculum
   c) Cervical biopsy
   d) Endocervical and endometrial biopsy
   e) Specimen jars
   f) Hemostasis
      (1) Silver nitrate
      (2) Monsel's solution

   g) Forms
      (1) Consent
      (2) Identification labels
      (3) Histopathology request
9. Photographic equipment
   a) Immediate development
   b) 35 mm color film
10. Treatment
    a) Cryosurgery
    b) Electrosurgical
    c) Laser

TERMINOLOGY AND TOPOGRAPHY

The living tissue patterns visible in three dimensions through the colposcope are manifest by surface contour, vascular configurations, color, tissue reaction to specific solutions and the margins between benign and atypical tissue fields. The following outline presents a classification of these tissues.

1. Normal findings
   a) Original squamous epithelium (Fig. 10–4)
   b) Columnar epithelium (Fig. 10–5)
   c) Typical transformation zone (Fig. 10–6)

2. Abnormal findings
   a) Atypical transformation zone
   b) Leukoplakia
   c) White epithelium
   d) Punctation
   e) Mosaic structure (Fig. 10–7)
   f) Atypical vessels (Fig. 10–8 and 10–9)
3. Findings suspicious for carcinoma
4. Indecisive findings
5. Miscellaneous benign findings
   a) Vaginocervicitis
   b) True erosion
   c) Atrophy (estrogen deficient)

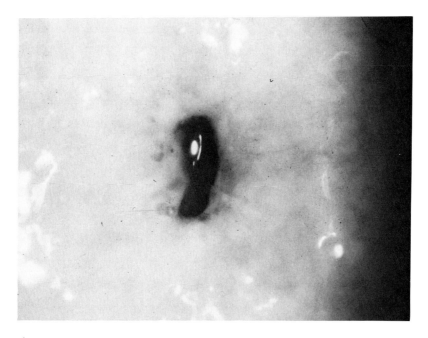

Figure 10–4. Normal cervix (16 power). Original squamous epithelium with smooth surface, no atypical changes visible.

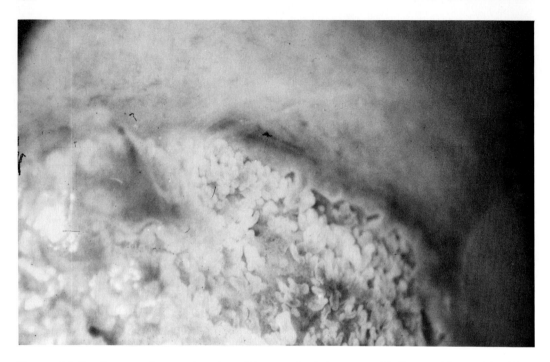

Figure 10–5. Squamocolumnar junction (25 power). Columnar epithelium evident with villous projections following 3 percent acetic acid application. A tongue of metaplasia is visible in the lower junction.

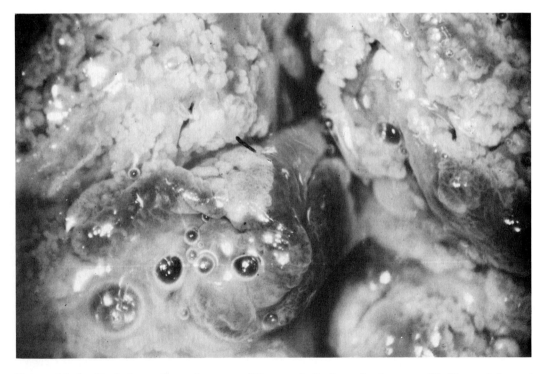

Figure 10–6. Typical transformation zone (25 power). Fusion of columnar villi. Deep clefts and clear mucous secretion at midcycle. Air bubbles within mucous also noted.

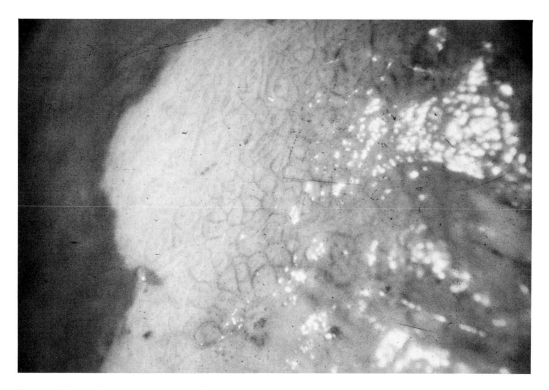

Figure 10–7. Mosaic structure (16 power). Atypical epithelial changes on biopsy of carcinoma in situ. The cobblestone effect is produced by surface blood vessels. Note the margin between normal squamous epithelium and the mosaicism.

d) Condylomata and papilloma
e) Radiation effect
f) Endometriosis

g) Angiomata
h) DES syndrome

NORMAL FINDINGS

Original Squamous Epithelium

Normal squamous epithelium has a smooth surface, is pink, and resistant to trauma (Fig. 10–4). The thickness of the epithelium corresponds to the endogenous estrogen. Premenarche or post menopausal epithelium will manifest the subepithelial stromal blood vessels because of the thin superficial cell layer. Glycogen is present and will be stained brown with iodine.

Columnar Epithelium

This mucous-secreting epithelium is red or salmon colored due to the closeness of the vascularity to the surface. Macroscopically, it may appear suspicious and an unnecessary biopsy taken. Under colposcopic view, the columnar epithelium is easily recognized. The distinct pattern of grape-like villi or tufts following acetic acid application provides an easy identification. Surface ridges reflect the cervical stroma. Columnar epithelium is delicate and may bleed easily with contact. Mucous secretions and central capillaries are visible (Fig. 10–5). Pregnancy causes the cervix to enlarge and the villi to become hypertrophied. Columnar epithelium does not stain with iodine. The squamocolumnar junction is usually asymmetrical, irregular, and extends to the vaginal fornix in 4 percent of patients.

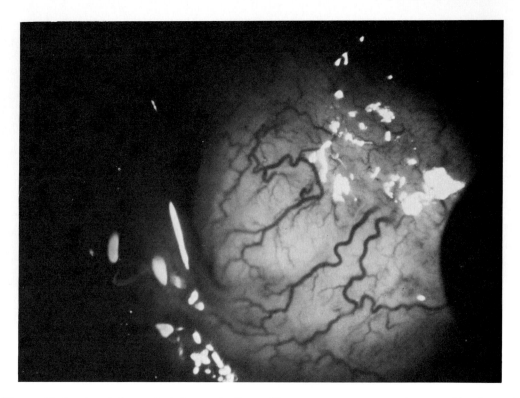

Figure 10–8. Atypical vessels (16 power). Green filter accentuates contrast between blood vessels and background stroma. A 16-year-old on oral contraceptives with vascular hyperplasia.

Typical Transformation Zone

Under certain stimulation, such as low Ph, infection, or trauma, the columnar epithelium is transformed through a metaplastic phase to squamous epithelium. This transformation or "T" zone is important because it is the most common site for cervical intraepithelial neoplasia. It is visible as an intermingling of squamous epithelium metaplasia and columnar epithelium corresponding to the maturity of the transformation process. The be-

ginning of the transformation zone is marked by gland openings or arborized vascular patterns at the site of the original squamocolumnar junction (Fig. 10–6). Early, the villi fuse, which is evident on the more exposed contours. These fusions ultimately result in a smooth surface. The transformation to squamous epithelium tends to be most advanced near the original squamous columnar junction and least advanced at the new squamocolumnar junction.

ABNORMAL FINDINGS

Atypical Transformation Zone

The optical properties of this zone are determined by the epithelial thickness, nuclear density, amount of surface keratin, and vascular configuration. Coppelson and Pixley have developed a sys-

tem of grading atypical transformation zone as follows:

Grade I.   Flat, white epithelium with or without a regular pattern of fine caliber vessels

Grade II.   Flat, white epithelium with or without irregular pattern of coarse caliber vessels

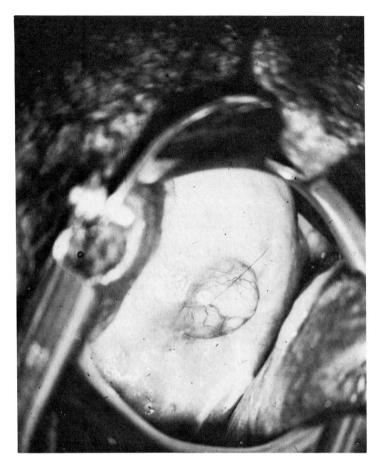

Figure 10–9. Nabothian cyst (6 power). The accentuation of the overlying benign blood vessel pattern is common.

Grade III. Very white epithelium with an irregular pattern of coarse caliber, coiled, or bizarre blanching vessels, usually wide intercapillary distance, and an irregular surface contour.

Leukoplakia

Leukoplakia refers to a white plaque visible without magnification and without the application of acetic acid. Histologically, the surface usually shows hyperkeratosis and is firmly adherent. It may also be removed revealing bare (ground) punctate stromal vessels. Leukoplakia is usually elevated from surrounding surface, has a sharp border, and does not stain with iodine or toluidine. Leukoplakia is not a constant precursor to cancer.

White Epithelium

In contrast, white epithelium becomes visible only following the application of acetic acid. The term "acetic acid staining" may avoid confusion with leukoplakia but has not gained general acceptance. This tissue reaction represents intraepithelial neoplasis in 6 to 14 percent of cases. As with columnar epithelium, the acetic acid effect is transient and may last only a few minutes.

Punctation

Punctation describes a zone of red dots that represent stromal papillae and blood vessel loops. The surface is usually smooth and does not stain with iodine.

Mosaic Structure

A mosaic structure is a cobblestone, cross-hatched, honeycomb field. Elevation of punctation may be referred to as papillary punctation. Surface vessels outline the mosaic pattern. The polygonal structures vary in size and may be fine (small) or coarsely (large) mosaic. Their outlines are usually sharp and noniodine staining. The margin between the mosaic and surrounding epithelium may be diffuse or sharp. The latter indicates a potential neoplastic field (Fig. 10-7).

Atypical Vessels

Malignant epithelium with its increased metabolic need is accompanied by an increased growth of blood vessels. This vascular hypertrophy is not symmetrical with progressively smaller blood vessels. In contrast to the benign arborized or tree-like branching (Figs. 10-8 and 10-9), the vessels in invasive cancer make sharp angulations, and corkscrew or hairpin turns. The distance between vessels is increased and an asymmetrical, bizarre pattern is formed.

FINDINGS SUSPICIOUS FOR CARCINOMA

Advanced invasive epidermoid carcinoma of the exophytic type may be easily suspect without the colposcope. Less obvious macroscopic appearances precede this stage and are manifest colposcopically with an irregular surface contour, abnormal vessel patterns, as described in the preceding paragraph, and an umbilicated border. Directed biopsy provides the clinician with the most rapid diagnosis possible.

Indecisive Findings

The entire transformation zone must be visible to be certain that atypical findings are not present. In older women, or in those with previous conization and cervical narrowing, the "T" zone may not be seen and the colposcopic findings must be described indecisive. An important landmark here is the new squamocolumnar junction or inner border of the transformation zone.

MISCELLANEOUS BENIGN FINDINGS

Vaginocervicitis

Vaginocervicitis is a diffuse hyperemia of stippled double capillary vessels similar to punctation. Unlike punctation, it extends beyond the transformation zone.

True Erosion

True erosion is an area mechanically denuded of epithelium usually as a result of trauma. The surface layer may be folded upon itself or only the cervical stroma visible from abrasion with a retained foreign object such as a pessary.

Atrophy

Atrophied or estrogen-deprived epithelium is typically smooth, thin and easily traumatized resulting in subepithelial hemorrhages. Blood vessels are more readily visible through the thin epithelium. A similar pattern less vulnerable to trauma is seen in the premenarche period.

Condylomata and Papilloma

Condylomata and papilloma are exophytic found often multifocal inside and outside at the transformation zone. Kolstad has described curbed hairpin-like capillaries with the ascending and descending parts of the long loops characteristically close together.

Endometriosis

Endometriosis, although rarely visible through the colposcope, may be seen. A focal hemorrhagic bleb more commonly on the cervix may be the presenting evidence.

Angiomata

Angiomata tend to be more common in postmenopausal patients. The vascular patterns are usually multifocal and of uniform vessel caliber.

DES Syndrome

Diethylstilbesterol (DES), which was synthesized in 1936, was administered to large numbers of women in the 1950s as a treatment and preventative for habitual and threatened abortions. In a few rare cases, young women born following fetal exposure with DES were found to have adenocarcinoma of the cervix and vagina. The typical findings are cervical and vaginal ridges, hoods, cock's comb, adenosis, and eversion. The screening of these patients is difficult. Exfoliative cytology may be negative even with the presence of adenocarcinoma. The iodine test is not precise in the localization of pathologic changes. Colposcopy provides an additional diagnostic tool. Directed biopsies may be taken to histologically follow these patients whose changes may involve the entire vagina.

Bibliography

Bolten KA, Jacques WE: Introduction to Colposcopy. New York, Grune and Stratton, 1960

Coppleson M, Pixley E, Reid B: Colposcopy, a Scientific Approach to the Cervix in Health and Disease, vol. 1. Springfield, Ill., Charles C Thomas, 1971

Coppleson M, Ried B: Preclinical Carcinoma of the Cervix: Its Origin, Nature and Management. New York, Pergamon, 1967

Gray LA: Dysplasia, Carcinoma In Situ and Microinvasive Carcinoma of the Cervix Uteri. Springfield, Ill, Charles C Thomas, 1964

Hinselmann H: Verbesserung der Inspektionsmöglichkeit von Vulva, Vagina und Portio. Münchener medizinische Wochenschrift 77: 1733, 1925

Hinselmann H: Zur Kenntnis der praekanzerosen Veränderungen der Portio. Zentralblatt fur Gynakologie 51:901, 1927

Hinselmann H, Schmitt A: Colposcopy. Girardet, Wuppertal-Elberfeld, 1954

Jordan JA, Singer A: The Cervix. Philadelphia, W.B. Saunders, 1976

Kolstad P, Stafl A: Atlas of Colposcopy. Oslo, Universitetsforlaget, 1972

Lang WR, Rakoff AE: Colposcopy and cytology: comparative value in the diagnosis of cervical atypism and malignancy. Obstet Gynecol 8: 312, 1956

Scott JW: Stereocolposcopic Atlas of the Uterine Cervix. Kendall, Florida, Zephyr, 1971

Schiller W: Hodpinselung und Abschabung des Portioepithels—Zentralblatt für Gynokologie, 1929

Chapter 11

Cervical Cancer

HUGH R. K. BARBER, M.D.

Cancer of the uterine cervix is a disease of the inner city. Although it is the most common cancer of the gynecologic system, cancer of the ovary is the leading cause of death from gynecologic cancer. Population-based data from the state of Connecticut show a reversal in the frequency of invasive versus in situ carcinomas of the cervix from the time periods 1955 through 1959 and 1965 through 1969. In the early period, two-thirds of the cancers were invasive while in the latest period two-thirds of the cancers were diagnosed while in situ. Among cancers diagnosed in 1969 and reported by the Third National Cancer Survey, the same relationship of two in situ cancers for each invasive cancer exists. Since the absolute number of invasive cancers has decreased only slightly over the time periods covered by this report, it would seem that extensive cytologic screening accounts for the reported increase of in situ cancers. The use of the Papanicolaou smear has dramatically lowered the incidence of invasive carcinoma of the uterine cervix.

When the age distribution for patients with cervical cancer is considered, a distinct difference is noted between in situ and invasive diagnoses. Only 9 percent of women with invasive cancers are under age 35 at diagnosis. In contrast, data from Connecticut and the Third National Cancer Survey, both for cases diagnosed in 1969, show that 53 percent of the in situ carcinomas are in women under 35 years of age.

There has been no significant improvement over the past quarter of a century in the number of women surviving five years after the treatment of invasive cervical cancer. About one-half of these cancers continue to be diagnosed as localized disease and one-third as regional disease.

Age has an influence on whether the disease is localized or not. The survival rates are generally favorable for one-third of all patients who were under the age of 45 at the time of diagnosis of cervical cancer; 65 percent of these cancers were diagnosed as localized disease. There is a steady decline in the proportion of localized disease as the age of the patient increases, so that among the one-fourth of all patients who were 65 years of age or older, only 38 percent had localized disease and about one-fifth had distant metastases at the time of diagnosis. The shift to a higher stage of disease with increasing age is reflected in the survival rates which decrease steadily as age increases. Stage for stage of disease the age gradient is less significant. The big difference is that the older patients have a more advanced stage of disease. The observed median survival time by age in a 1955 to 1964 series shows that the median survival for all ages is 7.3 years, under 35 years is >10 years, 35 to 44 years is >10 years, 45 to 54 is 10 years, 55 to 64 years is 6.0 years, and over 65 years is 2.5 years.[1]

ETIOLOGY AND EPIDEMIOLOGY

The goal of cancer etiology—the study of the causes of cancer—is cancer prevention. Three types of agents have been shown to cause cancers: chemicals, radiation, and viruses. Of these, two—chemicals and radiation—clearly cause cancer in man, and the third, viruses, are, on the basis of present knowledge, highly suspect.[2]

Cancer epidemiology seeks to correlate differences in the incidence of different types of cancer with differences in the external or internal environments of the persons developing these cancers as has already been established e.g., between cigarette smoking and lung cancer, sexual intercourse and cancer of the cervix. The results so far of epidemiologic research strongly suggest that variations in exposure to environmental agents and in social practices are largely responsible for variations in the incidence of cancers among different groups of people. Therefore, if such environmental exposures and social practices could be identified and eliminated, the majority of cancers in man might be prevented. Because of the complexity of the relationship between man and his environment and the long latent period of cancer development, the identification of particular cancer-inducing factors is extremely difficult, but there is currently no other area of cancer research that holds more promise for cancer prevention.

Both the etiology and epidemiology of cancer of the cervix have been studied in great detail and certain findings have been repeatedly reported. Cervical cancer is found more often in women of low socioeconomic status, married women, especially those marrying at an early age, women with early age of first coitus, women who are prostitutes, women having coitus with uncircumcised partners—especially those practicing poor hygiene—and women who are infected with herpesvirus type 2.

Cancer of the cervix is seldom seen in Jewish women or Moslems. It is high in Hindu women. The circumcision of Jewish and Moslem men has been suggested to have some relation to this low incidence of cervical cancer. However, among the Parsees, who are scrupulously clean, cancer of the cervix is rare, even though the men are not circumcised. Among nuns, virgins, orthodox Jewish women, and Navajo Indians cervical cancer is rare.[16] The stress and mores of modern society are almost certainly major factors in the genesis of this disease, but the precise mechanism is unknown.

It is accepted that cervical cancer has a direct relationship to sexual activity, but circumcision of the male sex partner in itself is not a preventive measure. Cleanliness seems to play a role in prevention of cancer of the cervix. The question has been raised whether it should be included as a venereal disease. The relationship between sexual activity and cervical cancer led investigators to speculate on the possibility of a venereally transmitted viral etiology for this neoplasm. Genital herpesvirus (HVS type 2) fits the carcinogenic model. It is venereally transmitted and relatively prevalent around the world. Direct evidence favoring the herpes virus hypothesis in human cervical cancer has been adduced during the past several years from several research groups.[3]

There is increasing evidence that there is an association between herpesvirus type 2 and carcinoma of the cervix. The herpesvirus type 2 is chemically and serologically distinct from the herpes type 1 that occurs in the mouth. Type 1 viruses are commonly associated with lesions of the mouth, lips, and keratoconjunctivitis. It is transmitted by the ororespiratory route. Type 2 viruses are isolated from genital lesions and are transmitted sexually. Despite the general impression that all genital herpes infections are caused by the type 2 virus, approximately 13 percent are caused by the type 1 strain. Published data report that antibodies to herpesvirus type 2 do not appear in the population before puberty. Antibodies to type 2 herpesviruses are rarely found among chaste women but are commonly found among prostitutes.

There are several reports on the occurrence of herpesvirus type 2 antibodies in women with invasive cancer as compared to matched control groups.[4-6] In one study, 72 percent of Negro women with cervical cancer had antibodies to the virus, while antibodies were found in only 22 percent of control women. There is clearly an association between herpesvirus type 2 and carcinoma of the cervix. Herpesvirus type 2 has been shown to have oncogenic potential in animal studies. The antigens from this virus have been found in the cells of cervical cancers and the virus has also been isolated from cells obtained from cancer in situ of the cervix.

Aurelian has presented data recently that is superior to that previously reported. Studies in the past testing for antibodies in the serum to herpesvirus 2 found that not all patients with cancer have antibodies to herpesvirus 2 while many patients without cervical cancer do have antibodies. Aurelian exposed human epidermoid cervical cancer cells to herpesvirus type 2 for four hours following which an antigen was found and called AG-4.[7] Antibodies to this antigen can be detected in the serum of patients with cervical cancer by complement fixation tests. They were not identifiable in the serum of matched controls. Furthermore, the antibodies to AG-4 disappear from the serum of cancer patients after treatment that has been considered to be successful. In addition, there seems to be a progressively positive correlation between the presence of antibodies to AG-4 and atypia, in situ carcinoma, and invasive cancer. The evidence is highly suggestive but not conclusive that the association between the virus and the cancer may be an etiologic one.[8]

LIFE HISTORY

There is a difference of opinion about the etiology and epidemiology of cancer of the cervix. Three types of agents have been shown to cause cancer: carcinogens, radiation, and viruses. The first two clearly cause cancer in man. Although viruses are only highly suspect in humans, recent reports indicate that herpesvirus 2 may be an etiologic factor. Once irreversible cellular changes indicate a malignant process, the progression of growth through various stages of development from dysplasia to in situ to invasive cancer has been generally accepted. Richart has reported this as a continuum of the same process, has supported the concept of a single clone of cells for the origin of the cancer, and calls the spectrum cervical intraepithelial neoplasia (CIN).[9] He states that CIN usually begins as a single-cell lesion at the squamocolumnar junction, more commonly on the anterior than on the posterior lip and rather infrequently at the lateral angles. In the beginning, it is well differentiated histologically as a mild dysplasia. As the lesion develops it replaces contiguous adjacent epithelium in the transformation zone of the exposed portion of the cervix and then later by extension into the endocervix with displacement of the columnar epithelium. As it extends to the transformation zone and to the endocervix, it becomes less well differentiated, with the least amount of change at the periphery and the greatest amount in the interior or endocervical portion of the growth. This may be a property of the cancer cell or of the tissue chalones. With growth there is a loss of specialized differentiated cell functions with an increased mitotic rate documented by tritiated thymidine uptake studies. In the earliest detectable lesions, the abnormal cells contain abnormal numbers of chromosomes and this aneuploidy persists throughout the spectrum of CIN, producing a heterogenous genetic makeup. Eventually,

one group of cells prove dominant and produce invasive cancer. In the beginning, the lesion is unifocal and probably unicellular. The field theory of cancer is not applicable to cervical cancer. The progression rates are not uniform and are higher in the later stages of the continuum than in its earlier stages.[10]

All the accumulated objective data, both in direct clinical follow-up studies and in laboratory experiments, are consistent with regard to the spectrum of intraepithelial neoplasia as a continuum. Richart reports that there is no objective evidence to support the arbitrary division of CIN into two diseases—dysplasia and in situ—and to base therapy upon such a division.

Mass screening programs have been undertaken to detect this neoplasia as carcinoma in situ, where the cure rate is virtually 100 percent.[11] Ongoing programs, such as those in British Columbia, Louisville, and Toledo, have shown a decrease in invasive cancers. Boyes, in British Columbia, was able to examine approximately one-third of the women aged 20 years and over and treated stage 0 cervical lesions. Clinical carcinoma of the cervix was reduced by 30.6 percent between 1955 and 1960, its incidence falling from 28.4 per 100,000 to 19.7 per 100,000, and by 1963 it was 15 per 100,000. Boyes[12] suggested that probably the correct incidence of invasion developing in patients with stage 0 lesions of the cervix is 60 percent with a time interval of 13 to 20 years, but emphasized that the data available are insufficient to guarantee this assessment being statistically reliable. It is important to know that in the first screening, the prevalence rate (invasive cancers present and those developing invasive) is being evaluated. Repeat screening of the same population will detect those patients developing the earliest changes in the CIN continuum (the incidence rates).[13-15]

CAUSES OF DEATH FROM CANCER OF THE CERVIX

In understanding the natural history of cancer of the cervix, it is important to know the cause of death.[16] Uremia, infection, and hemorrhage contribute to the mortality in most series. Although these are the most common, increasing numbers are dying from distant metastases. In a Memorial Hospital study of patients dying from cervical cancer or its complications, 50 percent had no disease beyond the pelvis. Other studies have served to confirm this observation.[17]

AGE

The peak incidence for carcinoma in situ of the cervix (Fig. 11-1 and 11-2) is between 30 and 40 years of age, while for invasive cancer it is between 40 and 50 years. However, cancer of the cervix may occur at any age, and following the so-called sexual revolution, an increasing number

of cases are being detected in women 20 years of age and under.

SYMPTOMS

Bleeding and/or a watery, bloody discharge are the most common symptoms associated with cancer of the cervix. The bleeding is bright red and lawless and not predictable as to time, amount, or duration. It is more frequent after intercourse or any vaginal manipulation. There may not be any symptoms present. A high index of suspicion on the part of the physician and routine pelvic examinations are important in the detection of cancer of the cervix (Fig. 11-3). Pain, swelling of the legs, weight loss, and marked anemia are associated with a very advanced lesion. In this day and age with the potential to eradicate cancer of the cervix available to us, it is intoler-

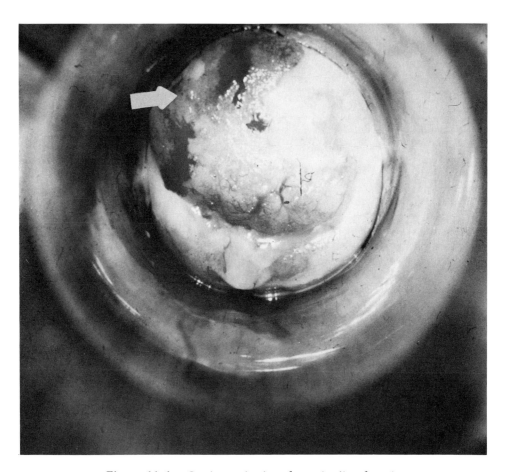

Figure 11–1.   Carcinoma in situ of anterior lip of cervix.

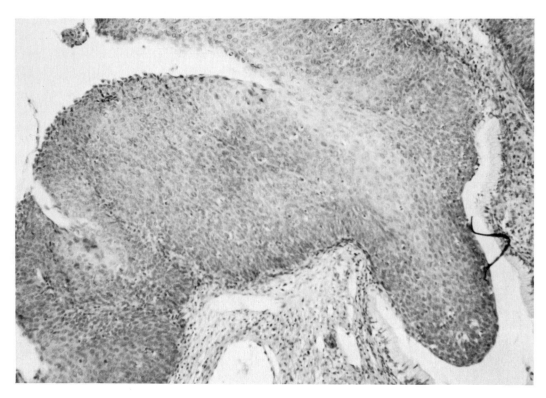

Figure 11–2.   Carcinoma in situ.

able and unacceptable to have the diagnosis made in this advanced stage of the disease.

DIFFERENTIAL DIAGNOSIS

An accurate diagnosis is essential before definitive treatment is instituted. The Pap smear is a screening method and may give a false-negative reading in the presence of a gross cancer of the cervix. The final arbiter for the diagnosis is histologic confirmation of cancer. However, a differential diagnosis should include chancres, tuberculosis, granuloma inguinale, lymphogranuloma venereum, condyloma accuminata, and radium eschars. A point to emphasize is that other lesions may be present concurrently with cancer of the cervix. This argues strongly for biopsy proof of disease. A surgical conization of the cervix is required to make the diagnosis for many carcinomas in situ and invasive lesions and all microinvasive disease. Direct biopsy of the cervix to confirm a clinically invasive lesion can be done in a physician's office (Figs. 11–4 and 11–5). Coordination of cytopathology and colposcopy will markedly reduce the need for cold-knife conization of the cervix.

INTERNATIONAL CLASSIFICATION (CLINICAL)[18] CERVICAL CANCER

There have been many classifications proposed for staging cancer of the cervix. None have been completely satisfactory. Recently, the League of Nations Classification has been updated and is presented as follows.

Stage 0	Carcinoma in situ, intraepithelial carcinoma.
Stage I	Carcinoma confined to the cervix (extension to the corpus should be disregarded).
Stage Ia	Microinvasive carcinoma (early stromal invasion).
Stage Ib	All other cases of stage I. Occult cancer should be marked "occ."
Stage II	The carcinoma extends beyond the

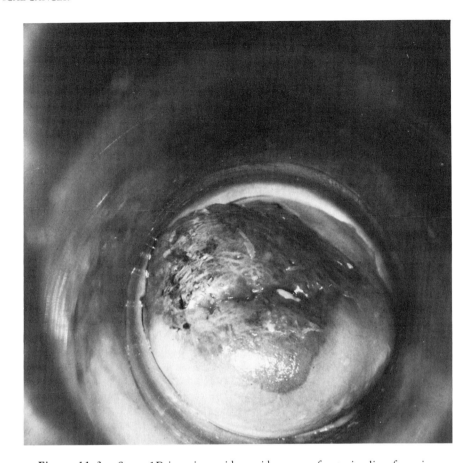

Figure 11–3. Stage 1B invasive epidermoid cancer of anterior lip of cervix.

cervix but has not extended to the pelvic wall. The carcinoma involves the vagina, but not the lower third.

Stage IIa   No obvious parametrial involvement.

Stage IIb   Obvious parametrial involvement.

Stage III   The carcinoma has extended to the pelvic wall. On rectal examination there is no cancer-free space between the tumor and the pelvic wall. The tumor involves the lower third of the vagina. All cases with hydronephrosis or nonfunctioning kidney.

Stage IIIa   No extension to the pelvic wall.

Stage IIIb   Extension to the pelvic wall and/or hydronephrosis or nonfunctioning kidney.

Stage IV   The carcinoma has extended beyond the true pelvis or has clinically involved the mucosa of the bladder or rectum. A bullous edema does not classify as stage IV.

Stage IVa   Spread of the growth to adjacent organs.

Stage IVb   Spread to distant organs.

QUALIFICATIONS IN STAGING CANCER OF THE CERVIX

Stage IA (microinvasive carcinoma) represents those cases of epithelial abnormalities in which histologic evidence of early stromal invasion is unambiguous. The diagnosis is based on microscopic examination of tissue removed by biopsy, conization, portio amputation, or removal of the uterus. Cases of early stromal invasion should thus be allotted to Stage IA.

The remainder of Stage I cases should be allotted to Stage IB. As a rule, these cases can be diagnosed by routine clinical examination.

Occult cancer is a histologically invasive cancer that cannot be diagnosed by routine clinical examination. As a rule, it is diagnosed on a cone, the amputated portio, or on the removed uterus.

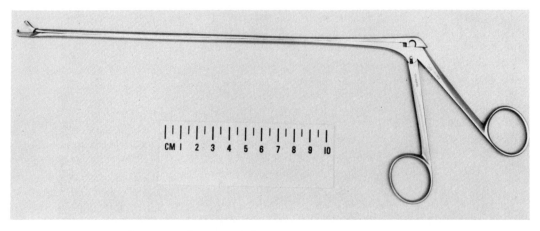

Figure 11–4.   Cervical biopsy instrument (Kevorkian).

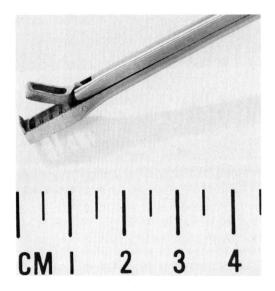

Figure 11–5. Open jaws of instrument (Fig. 11–4) allows a maximum biopsy of 5 to 8 mm (length), 3 mm (width), and 2 to 3 mm (deep) of cervix.

Such cancers should be included in Stage IB and should be marked "Stage IB, occ." Stage I cases can thus be indicated in the following ways:

Stage IA   Carcinoma in situ with early stromal invasion diagnosed on tissue removed by biopsy, conization, or portio amputation, or on the removed uterus
Stage IB   Clinically invasive carcinoma confined to the cervix
Stage IB occ.   Histologically invasive carcinoma of the cervix which could not be detected at routine clinical examination but which was diagnosed on a large biopsy, a cone, the amputated portio, or the removed uterus.

As a rule, it is impossible to estimate clinically whether a cancer of the cervix has extended to the corpus or not. Extension to the corpus should therefore be disregarded.

A patient with a growth fixed to the pelvic wall by a short and indurated but not nodular parametrium should be allotted to Stage IIB. It is impossible, at clinical examination, to decide whether a smooth and indurated parametrium is truly cancerous or only inflammatory. Therefore, the case should be placed in Stage III only if the parametrium is nodular on the pelvic wall or if the growth itself extends to the pelvic wall.

The presence of hydronephrosis or nonfunctioning kidney due to stenosis of the ureter by cancer permits a case to be allotted to Stage III even if, according to the other findings, the case should be allotted to Stage I or Stage II.

The presence of bullous edema, as such should not permit a case to be allotted to Stage IV. Ridges and furrows into the bladder wall should be interpreted as signs of submucous involvement of the bladder if they remained fixed to the growth at palposcopy (i.e., examination from the vagina or the rectum during cystoscopy). Finding malignant cells in cytologic washings from the urinary bladder requires further examination and a biopsy from the wall of the bladder.

The above is strictly a clinical classification and a change in classification is not to be made after therapy is initiated.

There is an error of at least 10 to 15 percent between the clinical staging and the extent of disease found at surgery.

Cases of stage 0 should not be included in any therapeutic statistics.

SURGICAL PATHOLOGIC CLASSIFICATION

Meigs and Brunschwig[19] suggested an additional classification that is employed by those engaged in a surgical program to treat cancer of the cervix and is based on the gross and microscopic findings. It permits comparison between programs even continents apart with very little error in the staging. The classification is as follows.

Class 0   Carcinoma in situ, microcarcinoma.
Class A   Carcinoma limited to the cervix.
Class Ao   After positive biopsy of infiltrating carcinoma, no tumor in the cervix in the surgical specimen.
Class B   Carcinoma extends from the cervix to involve the vagina, except the lower third; the carcinoma extends into the corpus; the carcinoma may involve the upper vagina and corpus; vaginal or uterine extension, or both; may be by direct or metastatic spread.
Class C   The carcinoma has involved paracervical or paravaginal tissue, or both, by direct extension or by lymphatic vessels, or in nodes within such tissues or direct extension, or both, into the lower third of the vagina.
Class D   Lymph vessel and node involvement beyond paracervical and paravaginal regions; this includes all lymphatic vessels or nodes, or both, in the true pelvis, except as described in class C; metastases to the ovary or tube.
Class E   The carcinoma has penetrated to the serosa, musculature, or mucosa of the bladder, colon, rectum, or some combination of these.
Class F   The carcinoma involves the pelvic wall (fascia, muscle, bone, or sacral plexus, or some combination).

Combinations are used, for example, DC, node at the periphery of the pelvis and parametrial or paracervical extension; CN, parametrial or paracervical extension as well as a positive node in the parametrial or paracervical area. D is reserved for positive nodes at the periphery of the pelvis.

PR   Preoperative irradiation
R   Curative irradiation followed by failure
S   Surgical attempt at cure prior to recurrence
RS   Irradiation and surgery employed curatively but require further surgery for persistence or recurrence of disease

Carcinoma of the cervical stump is classified in the same manner as cervical cancer with the uterus intact.

Adenocarcinoma of the cervix is classified in the same manner as epidermoid cancer.

Although the classification is long, it supplies a real need, permitting a study of the natural history of disease as well as serving to anticipate prognosis.

Prefixes have been added to describe previous therapies, e.g., PR for preoperative radium administered as part of planned therapy and R for radium that has been used but failed to cure. The prefix S is used when previous surgery failed to cure, and RS when both methods have been used unsuccessfully.

The above classifications are very useful in reporting end results of treatment and estimating prognosis, and each patient should receive the benefit of a careful staging of the disease and should be properly recorded before the work-up is considered complete.

THERAPY

Prior to 1895, there were few attempts at definitive therapy for cancer of the cervix, either by vaginal or abdominal hysterectomy, and the only therapy offered was by application of chemical caustics, cauterization, or amputation of the cervix. This limited therapy gave predictably poor results. In 1895, John G. Clark[24] introduced a more radical procedure and by the early part of the twentieth century, Wertheim reported approximately 500 cases with encouraging results. Abbe, in 1903, introduced radium into chemical practice and showed that cancer of the cervix was a radiocurable lesion with a low mortality and low immediate morbidity. It became the treatment chosen, and overnight, sentiment swung to radium as the preferred therapy. Joe V. Meigs was disappointed with the result of radium therapy in stages I and II and reintroduced a surgical program. He combined the Wertheim hysterectomy with the Taussig node dissection and introduced the radical hysterectomy and pelvic node dissection. Although he selected his cases for surgery during the early years of his program, it proved that surgery could be carried out with a low morbidity and mortality. Brunschwig expanded the scope of the operation and operated upon "all comers," with selection held to a minimum, and confirmed the possibility of low morbidity and mortality. This set off a controversy over the better form of treatment, radiation or surgery, and has provided one of the most interesting chapters in the history of gynecology.[20] The question from 1939 until the early 1960s had been, which is the more effective primary treatment, surgery or radiation? By 1960, it became evident that surgery and radiation had both exhausted their potential for further improvement. Therefore, it was necessary to explore "other" combinations or select patients for these two most effective therapeutic weapons. Increasing realization of the need for teamwork by radiotherapists and surgically oriented gynecologists in exploring the potential of existing techniques, and possibly the development of new ones, gave promise for improving the survival rates. The new orientation has changed the emphasis from which is better, surgery or radiation, to the more enlightened attitude of which is *better for a given patient*—surgery or radiation. In turning from treating the cancer to treating the patient, the philosophy has swung from standardization to individualized therapy.

THERAPY

The fine points of therapy will be discussed in detail after the outline for the overall treatment in each stage of the disease is presented.

Stage Ia   a)   Early stomal invasion. In general, this lesion is to be treated as invasive cancer. In cases in which the invasion is indefinite or only 1 to 2 mm in depth, does not cover a wide area, and in which there is no vascular or lymphatic involvement, the treatment is then the same as that suggested for carcinoma in situ.

                b)   Occult cancer (carcinoma hidden in the cervix). In general, the treatment is radical hysterectomy and bilateral pelvic node dissection, *or* radiation therapy.

                c)   Post-surgical. The management is best individualized and will consist of a combination of radical surgery including bilateral pelvic lymphadenectomy and radiation therapy, *or* primary radiation therapy.

Stage Ib   Radical hysterectomy and bilateral pelvic lymphadenectomy (Fig. 11–6). Radiation therapy in those patients in whom surgical therapy is not to be performed because of age or general health.

Stage IIa   The same treatment as for Stage Ib.

Stage IIb   Primary radiation therapy.

Stage IIIa   Same as for stage IIb.

Stage IIIb   Same as for stage IIb.

Stage IV   a)   Primary radiation therapy. This therapy may require preradiation diversion of the fecal and/or urinary stream.

                b)   Primary pelvic exenteration may be selected for those patients with central disease that extends into the bladder and in whom it is possible that the disease can be totally removed.

Microinvasion I_a. There is a great debate about whether this should be managed as an in situ lesion or as an invasive lesion. There is agreement that it is a surgical rather than a radiation disease. Frick proposed a Stage Ia to include carcinomas up to 5 mm in size. Most have their own definition of microinvasion and as yet there is no classification acceptable to all. Microinvasion has a predominant histologic picture of carcinoma in situ but has in addition a focus of invasion and is confined to the most superficial stroma. Microinvasion is found in about 6 to 10 percent of those patients presenting as carcinoma in situ. A review of the literature reports only a handful of patients in which there was involvement of submucosal

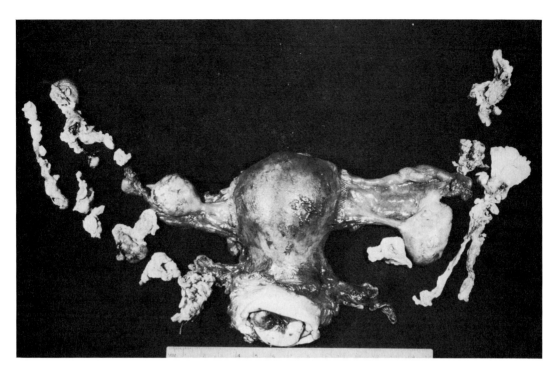

Figure 11–6. Radical hysterectomy and pelvic node dissection of same patient seen in Figure 11–3. Lymph nodes (32) were negative for cancer.

lymphatics or lymph nodes. The survival rates in patients with microinvasion treated by total hysterectomy and a cuff of vagina have been excellent. The infinitesimal risk of node metastases is adequately balanced by small mortality associated with radical hysterectomy. If, on serial or step biopsies, there is lymphatic involvement or the invasion is more than 5 mm in depth, the patient should be treated as stage I cancer of the cervix. My own preference for treating microinvasion is a classical Wertheim (hysterectomy, a cuff of paravaginal, paracervical area and the upper quarter of the vagina). The ovaries are managed according to the age of the patient.

Occult carcinoma. An apparently normal-appearing cervix that proves to have invasive carcinoma is not necessarily a "microcarcinoma." The designation of "occult carcinoma" should not be confused with this group. A sizeable lesion may be hidden within the endocervical canal and these should be termed "occult" carcinomas. Cases of occult cancer may be found in a cone or in the specimen from a large-wedge biopsy performed in cases of carcinoma in situ or dysplasia. Obviously, they are invasive and should be treated

with the appropriate radical operation or planned cancericidal radiation therapy.

Invasive cancer, stages I_b, II_a, II_b, III, and IV. There are only two methods of treatment that give predictable opportunity for cure in the treatment of invasive cancer of the cervix, i.e., radiation or surgery or a combination of radiation and surgery. Radiation has been the treatment of choice for the country as a whole. However, there has been a change in attitude in the last few years reflected in a review of the 14th Annual Report collected by Kottmeier.[25] During the years 1934 to 1938, 4 percent of the patients were operated upon in 20 percent of the institutions reporting, while in 1953 to 1957, 33 percent of the patients were operated upon in 74 percent of the institutions listed. In the 14th Annual Report, only 11 of the 124 institutions reported have no operated cases, while at 5 institutions, the operation percentage in stage I exceeded 90 percent. It demonstrates clearly a change in philosophy from treating the disease to treating the patient and a swing away from standardization to individualizing treatment. Whatever treatment is chosen, it should be based on a knowledge of the natural

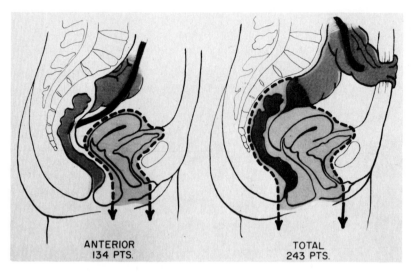

ANTERIOR
134 PTS.

TOTAL
243 PTS.

Figure 11–7.   Pelvic exenteration for cervical cancer.

history of the disease as well as an understanding of the treatment chosen and its complications.[21] It is to be emphasized that poor radiation is no better than poor surgery and is fraught with the same high morbidity and mortality.

SURGERY

When Meigs reintroduced radical surgery for cancer of the cervix in 1939, an additional modality of therapy became available.[26] In the past, cancer of the cervix, had been regarded as a surgical problem on the Gynecologic Service of the Memorial-James Ewing Hospitals. This approach has been modified in the last five years. In order to follow a surgical program, it was necessary to employ 10 operations. To speak in terms of one operation immediately implies a degree of selection and the implication must be assumed that those patients in whom the procedure cannot be carried out are beyond the possibilities of treatment. In the Memorial series, selection is held to a minimum within the overall framework of employing surgery as the treatment of choice, but there is selection in the type of operation selected for a given patient. In pursuing a surgical program, it was necessary to carry out a pelvic exenteration* in about 15 percent of the cases and in no other series is this reported (Fig. 11–7). It

serves to indicate that selection has been held to a minimum.

The philosophy of the Gynecologic Service at the Memorial Hospital prior to 1967 was to tailor the procedure to the status of the patient and the extent of disease rather than to carry out a standard procedure in each instance. Our interests have been more in the potentialities of the overall surgical attack rather than in a single type of operation (Fig. 11–8). This approach permits the opportunity for a surgical attack in the greatest number of patients. It has been accepted by the Brunschwig school that the best form of treatment for cancer of the cervix in a given case is surgery. However, the universal application of this approach by all doctors to all cases of cancer of the cervix is not realistic, i.e., there are not enough trained doctors or hospitals with adequate facilities to carry out a program of radical surgery. Recognizing this, it is self-evident that radiation therapy, for the present, is the treatment chosen for the country as a whole. From a review of the surgical program, it is now evident that selection of patients for the different forms of treatment is not only justified but indicated. The rationale and indications for radical surgery are set forth as follows:[22]

---

*Essentially, there are three types: anterior, posterior, and total exenteration. Total pelvic exenteration is a synthesis of three major procedures (1) radical hysterectomy with bilateral pelvic node excision and bilat-

eral salpingo-oophorectomy, (2) total cystectomy, and (3) combined abdominoperineal resection of the rectum. The anterior exenteration is the removal of the above structures with preservation of the rectum while the posterior exenteration is the removal of the above structures with preservation of the bladder.

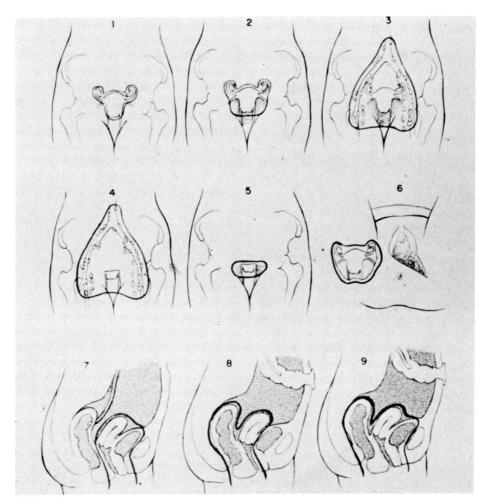

Figure 11–8. Different operations for cancer of the cervix: 1. Hysterectomy; 2. classic Wertheim; 3. radical hysterectomy and pelvic node dissection; 4. radical stump excision and pelvic node dissection; 5. radical stump excision; 6. radical vaginal hysterectomy (Schauta); 7. anterior pelvic exenteration; 8. posterior pelvic exenteration; 9. total pelvic exenteration.

1. Young women
2. Pregnancy
3. Stages I, IIa, selected stage IV, and endocervical cancer
4. An atrophic, conical, inelastic vagina
5. Fear of irradiation
6. No local recurrence in the cervix
7. No new cancers develop in the uterus or cervix
8. Relative radioresistance in cancer
9. Less bowel damage
10. Removal of nodal metastases
11. Pelvic infections (PID, salpingitis)
12. Simultaneous ovarian pathology
13. Simultaneous uterine pathology
14. No waiting period
15. Obesity
16. Inadequate facilities for irradiation
17. Evaluate extent of disease
18. Less expensive for the patient
19. Previous irradiation
20. Recurrence after irradiation

ADENOCARCINOMA OF THE CERVIX

Adenocarcinoma constitutes about five percent of cancer of the cervix. The average age is slightly higher than in squamous cancer. On the other hand, cancers of the cervix occurring at an early age (20 years and under) are almost universally adenocarcinoma. The same diagnostic measures are carried out as for squamous cancer. There has been divided opinion about whether adenocarcinoma responds to radiation as well as squamous carcinoma. After a review of the literature, it is concluded that the treatment is the same as for squamous cancer. If surgery is chosen as the method of treatment, it must be radical, and if irradiation is selected, it must be well planned and carried to a cancericidal dose. Since confusion sometimes exists as to whether the lesion is primarily endocervical or an extension of a corpus cancer, accurate diagnosis is important. It is important to distinguish this lesion from that termed carcinoma corporis et collis, which is applied when the site of the growth is in the uterus and the cancer is present in both the corpus and in the cervix. This makes it difficult to place the case in either of the two groups, carcinoma of the corpus or carcinoma of the cervix. These cases should be treated as carcinoma of the cervix rather than corpus carcinoma. The attack should include radical hysterectomy and node dissection, or complete cancericidal doses of radiation both with radium and external therapy, plus hysterectomy and an extended vaginal cuff.

ENDOCERVICAL CANCER

Carcinoma involving the endocervix involves the corpus more often than is commonly realized. It is this observation that has resulted in the addition of hysterectomy to the basic radiation therapy. Patients with a cervical carcinoma spreading into the corpus will in most cases be diagnosed correctly only after hysterectomy. Myometrial invasion is an obvious source of clinically recurrent cancer if hysterectomy is not performed.

CERVICAL STUMP

Cancer in the stump constitutes about 4 percent of all cancers of the cervix. If it is found within two years of the subtotal hysterectomy, it is probable that it was present at the time of hysterectomy. It is obvious that total hysterectomy will serve to prevent the development of stump cancer. Stump cancer can be treated by either surgery or irradiation. A review of the literature reveals that the survival rate from either modality of treatment is essentially the same as if the uterus were present with only a very slight increase in morbidity. However, in pursuing a surgical program, we have found that approximately 15 percent required some type of pelvic exenteration to encompass the disease.

RECURRENT OR PERSISTENT CANCER OF THE CERVIX

During the past three decades, two important advances have been made in detecting and treating cancer of the cervix: (1) the cytologic screening test adapted to early detection of malignant changes in the cervix by Papanicolaou, and (2) the treatment as well as the rehabilitation of the patients with advanced cancer by Brunschwig. The latter also demonstrated that following radiation therapy, failure, or recurrence, an appreciable salvage of these patients is possible by appropriate surgery if extrapelvic metastases have not occurred. The problem of persistent or recurrent cancer of the cervix after an attempt at cure by some modality, usually irradiation, is a serious problem and one that taxes the ingenuity of the responsible physician and the resources of the hospital. The fact remains that the majority of patients with cancer of the cervix given primary treatment are still dying of their disease. It is important to convince the patient with recurrence that you have something left to be tried which will help them and they should never be abandoned. Treatment, either palliative or curative, should be offered only if there is no inordinate increase in the morbidity and mortality.

Early diagnosis in recurrent cancer is equally important for salvaging the patient as it is for the treatment of untreated cancer of the cervix. Any new symptoms or signs, as well as the development of uterine asymmetry or nodularity and pyelogram changes, should be suspect.

The treatment is best by a surgical approach. Reradiation has little to offer in terms of cure and is accompanied by a high complication rate and augmentation of symptoms. A point to be emphasized in the surgical treatment of recurrence is that not all patients require pelvic exenteration to encompass their disease. Approximately 20 percent can be managed by less than a pelvic exenteration. For those requiring a pelvic exenteration, the five-year survival rate is 20 percent and it jumps to 43 percent among those treatable by less than a pelvic exenteration. The surgical mortality among the nonexenteration group was 2.5 percent, a rate especially to be cited since in this group the five-year salvage was 43 percent.

The indications for pelvic exenteration in advanced cancer of the cervix, new case or recurrent, the type of operation depending on the judgment of the surgeon and the extent of disease are (1) actual invasion of bladder and/or rectum by cancer of the cervix, (2) such close extension to the bladder and/or rectum that separation of one or both would lead to problematic removal of all neoplasms so that sacrifice of one or both adjacent organs is consistent with wide resection of cancer, and (3) spread into the paravaginal and/or paracervical area beyond the ureter but still within the pelvis and not approaching the side wall of the pelvis.

The contraindications have been extensively reviewed elsewhere.[23] The main ones are (1) metastases outside the pelvis, (2) swelling and/or sciatic type of pain in one or both legs, (3) psychosis, and (4) when, at exploratory laparotomy, it is determined that a plane of separation cannot be developed between the cancerous pelvic mass and the sides of the pelvis so that if exenteration were carried out, neoplastic tissue, of necessity, would be left behind.

The results of pelvic exenteration accepting all-comers and achieving a resectability rate of 45 percent is 22 percent five-year survival. The surgical mortality defined as death within 30 days of operation, regardless of cause, is approximately 10 percent.

The five-year survival rate for pelvic exenteration for advanced cancer of the cervix among several categories of patients achieved are as follows: (1) previously untreated cases with negative nodes, 36 percent; (2) radiation failures with negative nodes, 20 percent; (3) previously untreated patients with positive nodes, 14 percent; and (4) radiation failures with positive pelvic nodes, 5.8 percent.

Pelvic exenterations, complete or partial, are difficult operations and the postoperative care presupposes thorough training in abdominopelvic surgery in the broadest sense. Perhaps one of the greatest deterrents to a more widespread execution of these operations is a spirit of defeatism and a lack of appreciation of what can be achieved. The most serious and unfortunate factor is the habit of procrastination until such time that opportunities for benefit to the patient are greatly reduced even to nil, when indeed, the situation becomes hopeless.

Persistent cancer of the cervix is defined here as gross evidence of disease with positive biopsy within a minimum of six months after initial radiation therapy. Recurrent cancer of the cervix is defined as negative clinical findings six months or more after radiation or other therapy followed by eventual return of positive clinical findings and positive biopsy.

In the treatment of recurrent cervical cancer, it can be stated that since 50 percent of patients die with disease confined to the pelvis, there is logic for carrying out a surgical attack. The pelvic exenteration is now established as a method of attack on recurrent cancer of the cervix. Unless the disease has spread outside the pelvis, the patient should be given the benefit of an exploratory laparotomy and the decision of resectability can be made at that time. The surgical morbidity and mortality depend upon the conditions encountered in each patient, such as the extent of secondary infection, previous radiation, and tissue reaction, as well as the status of the urinary tract.

References

1. End Results in Cancer. Rept No. 4, U.S. Department of Health, Education and Welfare, Public Health Service, National Institutes of Health, National Cancer Institute, Bethesda, Md., 1972, p 104

2. Stallworthy J, Bourne G: Recent Advances in Obstetrics and Gynecology, 11th ed. Boston, Little, Brown, 1966, p 338

3. Nahmias AJ, Naib ZM, Josey WE, Franklin E, Jenkins R: Prospective studies of the association of genital herpes simplex infection and cervical anaplasia. Ca Res 33:1491–1497, 1973

4. Rawls WE, Kaufman RH, Gardner HL: Relation of herpesvirus type 2 to carcinoma of the cervix. Clin Obstet Gynec 15:919, 1972

5. Kaufman RH, Rawls WE: Herpes genitalis and its relationship to cervical cancer. Ca 24:258–65, 1974

6. Gall SA, Haines HG: Cervical carcinoma antigen and the relationship to HSV-2. Gynecol Oncol 2:451, 1974

7. Aurelian L, Schumann B, Marcus RL, Davis HJ: Antibody to HSV-2 induced tumor specific antigens in serums from patients with cervical cancer. Science 181:161, 1973

8. Kessler II, Aurelian L: Uterine cervix can-

cer. In Schottenfeld D (ed): Cancer Epidemiology and Prevention. Springfield, Ill., Charles C Thomas, 1975, Chap. 14

9. Richart RM: Cervical intraepithelial neoplasia. In Sommers, SC (ed): Genital and Mammary Pathology Decennial 1966–1975. New York, Appleton, 1975, p 1

10. Richart RM: A theory of cervical carcinogenesis. Obstet Gynec 24:874, 1969

11. Gellman DD: Cervical cancer screening programs. Canad Med Assoc J 114:1003, 1976

12. Boyes DA: The British Columbia screening program. Obstet Gynec 24:1005, 1969

13. Christopherson WM, Parker JE: Control of cervix cancer in women of low income in a community. Cancer 24:64, 1969

14. Bryans FE, Boyes DA, Boyd JR, Fidler HK: The cytology program in British Columbia. Management of preclinical carcinoma of the cervix. Canad Med Ass J 90: 62, 1974

15. Hammond EC, Burns EL, Seidman H, Percy C: Detection of uterine cancer. High and low risk groups. Cancer 22:1096, 1968

16. Graham JB, Sotto LSJ, Poloncek FP: Carcinoma of the cervix. Philadelphia, Saunders, 1962

17. Brunschwig A, Pierce VK: Necropsy findings in patients with carcinoma of the cervix. Implications for treatment. Am J Obstet Gynec 56:1134, 1948

18. Nelson JH, Averette HE, Richart RM: Detection, diagnostic evaluation, treatment of dysplasia and early carcinoma of the cervix. Ca 25:134, 1975

19. Meigs JV, Brunschwig A: Proposed classification for cases of cancer of the cervix treated by surgery. Am J Obstet Gynec 66:413, 1952

20. Barber HRK: Results of surgical treatment of cancer of the cervix at the Memorial-James Ewing Hospital. In Marcus S, Marcus C (eds): Advances in Obstetrics and Gynecology. Baltimore, Williams and Wilkins, 1967, chap. 45, p 622

21. Rutledge F: Surgery versus x-ray for treatment in cancer of the cervix. In Reid DE, Barton TC (eds): Controversy in Obstetrics and Gynecology. Philadelphia, Saunders, 1969, p 397

22. Barber HRK: When should you operate in cancer of the cervix? Res Staff Physician, June 1970

23. Barber HRK: Relative prognostic significance of preoperative and operative findings in pelvic exenteration. Surg Clin N Amer 49:431, 1969

24. Clark JG: A more radical method of performing hysterectomy for cancer of the uterus. Johns Hopkins Hosp Bull 6:120, 1895

25. Kottmeier HL: Annual report on the results of treatment in carcinoma of the uterus and vagina. Boktrycheriet PA (ed). Stockholm, Norstedt and Söner, Vol 14, 1967

26. Meigs JV: Wertheim operation for carcinoma of the cervix. Am J Obstet Gynec 49:542-553, 1945

Chapter 12

Radiotherapy Treatment of Cervical Cancer

LUTHER W. BRADY, M.D.

The turn of the century witnessed the almost simultaneous successful development of a curative surgical approach (Wertheim's radical hysterectomy, 1900)[34] as well as a curative radiotherapeutic technique (Margaret Cleaves' radium application, 1903)[8] for the treatment of carcinoma of the uterine cervix. The high operative mortality associated with major surgery prior to the era of antibiotics and modern anesthesia limited the application of radical surgery to only a few gynecologists and for carefully selected cases. These limitations afforded the opportunity to develop radium techniques and to prove the efficacy of radiation therapy in the treatment of carcinoma of the cervix. Limitations of intracavitary radium were shortly recognized, and as early as 1924 supplementary external beam x-ray treatment to the lateral pelvic wall was introduced for the first time at the Radiumhemmet in Stockholm.

During the years that followed World War II, both surgical and radiotherapeutic techniques were revolutionized. On the surgical front the risk of primary mortality was minimized by antibiotics, better anesthesia, and better understanding of surgical physiology. This revived the interest in radical hysterectomy as an alternative to radiotherapy for early carcinoma of the cervix and introduced pelvic exenterative procedures for advanced but salvageable cases.[5,21] On the radiotherapeutic front, physical and biologic improvements in the treatment were refined by the

availability of kilocurie Co60 teletherapy units, megavoltage x-ray machines, and sophisticated radiotherapeutic technology.

In 1978 approximately 20,000 new cases of invasive carcinoma of the cervix will be diagnosed, and there will be 7400 deaths due to persistence or recurrence of the tumor.[1] Also during this year, over 40,000 new cases of in situ carcinoma of the cervix will be diagnosed.

Even though well-established programs for the treatment of carcinoma of the cervix have existed for many years, new evidence recently accumulated indicates that more data are needed concerning the route of spread and the extent of the disease at the time of initial presentation. Currently under way is a project under the aegis of the Gynecologic Oncology Group to evaluate the pattern of lymph node involvement in patients with carcinoma of the cervix utilizing pretreatment surgical exploration (Tables 12-1–12-3).[2–4,11,14,20,32]

Relationship between stage and the potential probability of involvement of pelvic and para-aortic lymph nodes is important in the planning of treatment programs for the management of carcinoma of the cervix (Tables 4 and 5). The extension of radiation therapy treatment fields to include para-aortic lymph node involvement requires change not only in treatment techniques but also in the manner of the delivery, to include para-aortic nodes and is associated with increasing

Table 12–1.   INCIDENCE OF POSITIVE
PELVIC NODES

STAGE	NO. OF PATIENTS WITH POSITIVE PELVIC NODES	PERCENT	NO. OF PATIENTS STUDIED
I	204	18	1134
II	319	29	1096
III	286	42	676

From Brady: *Cancer* 38:553, 1976.

complications from the radiation therapy. Both Taylor et al and Piver have reported the high risk involved in para-aortic irradiation.[2,6,23,28]

However, appropriate treatment-planning techniques and variations in the fractions deliv-ered daily to the para-aortic lymph nodes in relation to the fractions delivered daily to the pelvic structures suggest the possibility of improving the patient's ability to tolerate the radiation therapy, thereby increasing the potential for survival.

RESOURCES FOR MANAGEMENT

The best results in the treatment of cervical cancer may be anticipated when treatment is carried out by physicians who are well acquainted with pelvic anatomy, the malignancy's characteristic, and modalities of the treatment being employed, whether by surgery or irradiation. Over 50 years of experience indicates that radiation remains the most generally applicable method for tumor control of frankly invasive cancer of the cervix. Current trends toward early discovery of cervical cancer through cytologic screening is increasing the importance of surgery in early diseases (in situ carcinoma and microinvasive carcinoma). These data also indicate the need for selection of proper treatment for a wide variety of lesions. Extreme care must be exercised to choose the appropriate approach to each problem, for both under- and overtreatment are equally undesirable. Irradiation, for example, remains an extremely important means for tumor control, but its use must be tempered by its known potential for causing crippling or fatal sequelae. Radical surgery, on the other hand, has the potential for greater harm than benefit if misapplied. A Wertheim operation used for a noninvasive cancer is an illustration of the inappropriate application of that technique.

The primary objective of the physician in the management of the patient with carcinoma of the cervix must be to achieve a balance between a maximum potential for cure and a minimum incidence of complications.

Table 12–2.   STAGING DATA DERIVED FROM PRETREATMENT EXPLORATORY
LAPAROTOMY FOR SQUAMOUS CELL CARCINOMA OF THE CERVIX

STAGE	NO. OF PATIENTS WITH CLINICAL STAGE	SURGICAL STAGE AGREEING WITH CLINICAL STAGE	POSITIVE PERIAORTIC NODES	STAGING DIFFERENCE (%)
IB	145	107	7	26
IIA	20	11	2	45
IIIA	3	1	{4	66
IIIB	16	3		94
IVA	3	1	2	66
Total	207	123		

From Brady: *Cancer* 36:661, 1975.

Table 12–3. INCIDENCE OF POSITIVE PERIAORTIC LYMPH NODES (LYMPHANGIOGRAM OR SURGERY)

STAGE	NO. OF PATIENTS WITH POSITIVE PERIAORTIC NODES	PERCENT	NO. OF PATIENTS STUDIED
IB	10	9.3	107
IIA	11	12.8	86
IIB	9	23.7	38
III	18	18.2	99
IVA	3	42.9	7

Summary of data from Averette et al.,[2] Ucmakli and Bonney,[32] Fletcher and Rutledge,[14] Littman et al.,[20] and Douglas and Sweeney.[11]

Table 12–4. CARCINOMA OF THE CERVIX, STAGE II-B: METASTASES TO PERIAORTIC NODES

AUTHORS	NO. OF PATIENTS	NO. WITH POSITIVE NODES	PERCENT
Averette et al.[2]	19	2	11.0
Buchsbaum et al.[6]	12	1	8.0
Nelson et al.[23]	31	5	16.0
Piver and Barlow[28]	19	1	5.2

Table 12–5. CARCINOMA OF THE CERVIX, STAGE III: METASTASES TO PERIAORTIC NODES

AUTHORS	NO. OF PATIENTS	NO. WITH POSITIVE NODES	PERCENT
Averette et al.[2]	19	8	41
Buchsbaum et al.[6]	20	7	35
Nelson et al.[23]	28	13	46
Piver and Barlow[28]	32	12	32

The wide spectrum of cervical malignancy involvement and the great variety of approaches to the treatment of these lesions has made it impossible for any one physician to be an expert in all the phases of management for cervix cancer. It is therefore mandatory that various specialists who deal with cervical cancer work together as a team in order to accomplish the thorough care of the patients. This team should consist of at least a cytopathologist, a pathologist, a radiation oncologist, a radiation therapy physicist, and a gynecologist skilled in the management of gynecologic malignancies. The latter individual today is referred to as a gynecologic oncologist. In addition, the team should include as the needs arise, a urologist, proctologist, or general surgeon who will increase the effectiveness of the group. Membership and functions of the team should be well coordinated so that every step from the initial discovery of the cancer to the final follow-up operates smoothly. A program of success in the management of cancer of the cervix requires a multidisciplinary approach by this team, experienced and trained in cancer management, with a sufficient continuing case load that will insure continued capability.

Within the environment for treatment of the patient with cancer of the cervix must be available a broad range of therapeutic equipment properly serviced and maintained by well-trained ancillary personnel. There must be available various forms of radium or radium substitutes for intracavitary and interstitial use, as well as a wide variety of intracavitary applicators. Megavoltage devices for external beam therapy must be available. A well-integrated treatment planning team must be available with computer dosimetry and mould room facilities. Surgery requires well-equipped operating rooms, personnel for operating teams, intensive care units, and effective laboratories with blood banks capable of supplying the needs of the most extensive types of operations.

Finally, the attitudes expressed by those individuals who make decisions and lead the treatment team must demonstrate a balance of aggressiveness and restraint that is appropriate to each situation presented by the individual patient. Extremes of philosophy are as dangerous as ignorance of proper therapy or a lack of required equipment. Knowledge, skill, and equipment must be blended with attitudes to provide the optimum environment for cancer management, especially in the field of cancer of the cervix.

PATIENT WORK-UP

The principles of population screening for cervical cancer detection should be accepted without question by the staff involved in cancer management. The cytologic screening examination should be accepted as routine procedure for individuals where the medical status permits its performance—excluding terminal medical or surgical cases.

Borderline findings must be evaluated thoroughly, recognizing that strongly positive cytologic results place the burden upon the clinician to demonstrate whether the cancer is definitely present. Unsatisfactory smears should have an incidence of less than 5 percent. All positive and suspicious cases should be reviewed by the cytopathologist with a policy of systematic review for negative smears. The cytopathologist should routinely correlate suspicious and routine smears with biopsy and operative findings.

A tissue diagnosis of cancer of the cervix—with no exceptions—is mandatory in every new case. Knife cone biopsy with dilatation and curettage should be the diagnostic procedure when suspicious or positive smears are encountered in the absence of a clinically obvious lesion. In the patient with a gross malignancy, directed biopsy should be considered acceptable only when microscopic examination reveals more than microscopic invasion. An extensive cone biopsy, which might be considered adequate for carcinoma in situ, is unnecessary for gross malignancy, since a cone in such a circumstance could interfere with the placement of radium sources in the treatment program. In the situation of gross malignancy, examination under general or local anesthesia with dilatation and curettage should be performed in addition to the directed biopsy in order properly to determine the clinical stage of the malignancy. Specific attention should be directed toward evaluation of the potential for extention of the disease to involve the endometrial cavity. The cone biopsy should include the squamocolumnar junction since most cancers arise in this area. Multiple sections of the cone biopsy should be taken so that the entire specimen is embedded in paraffin, therefore making the entire area available for study by serial sections when indicated. If the cone biopsy is to serve as the therapeutic modality, in lieu of hysterectomy, it should be oriented and tagged in such a way that the pathologist can evaluate the cut edges and the free margins.

There is definite value in obtaining endocervical curettings as well as endometrial curettings. These should be submitted, appropriately labeled for the pathologist. Perez et al[27] have demonstrated the major impact of endometrial extension on survival.

The pathologist should have a clearly conceived definition of dysplasia, carcinoma in situ, microinvasive cancer, and gross invasion. In addition, the pathologist must exhibit a willingness to be thorough in searching tissues to determine the extent of a given lesion.

Diagnostic findings should be related to general policies of management that are subject to modification by a number of factors. Noninvasive and microinvasive carcinomas generally should lead to hysterectomy. Modification may be made in the presence of pregnancy or after the expressed desire for pregnancy. The age of the patient and the medical status remain the other major considerations. Invasive cancer will generally be managed by radiation therapy. Recurrent disease from noninvasive to extensive disease will require the ability to vary treatment from none to total exenteration. In the case either of a primary new lesion or of a recurrence there must be a basic foundation of thorough tissue examination.

Initial discovery of cervical cancer may tend to draw attention to the pelvic region with resultant neglect to the rest of the patient. As in every other illness, a thorough history and physical examination are basic requirements along with considerations relative to the complete medical, economic, and social status.

The institution must offer the minimum laboratory studies, including a complete blood count, serologic test for syphilis, fasting and two-hour postprandial blood sugars, biochemical profile, and complete urinalyses. The department of diagnostic radiology must provide facilities for roentgenograms of the chest, spine, and pelvis, and for intravenous urogram and barium enema. These studies are imperative in all cases with invasive cancer (microinvasion or gross invasion) both for the "baseline" appearance of the vital contiguous tracts and for comparison with future studies as well as to establish the presence or absence of lesions in these locations. For the same reasons, proctosigmoidoscopy and cystoscopy are necessary to eliminate clinically the possibility that the bowel or the bladder have been invaded by the cervical cancer or the presence of other pathology. Other special tests or examinations may be required, depending on the findings of these initial studies; these include liver function studies, liver scans, electrocardiograms, retrograde pyelograms and complete gastrointestinal examinations, and bone scans. During recent years, the value of lymphangiography in the evaluation of the patients has assumed an important place in the management of cervical cancer as well as pretreatment surgical exploration with biopsies of pelvic and para-aortic lymph nodes. In 1971 intravenous urography findings were included in clinical staging by FIGO (Table 12-6), but lymphangiography, computed tomography (whole body), and pretreatment surgical staging are not used in clinical staging. Planning for treatment should use these data when they are available.

Treatment the patient finally receives will result from careful selection and planning based upon the following considerations:

1. Appraisal of the findings from medical evaluation, laboratory studies, radiographic studies, and clinical staging;
2. Equipment and facilities available in the particular institution or community;
3. The knowledge, skill, and attitudes (philosophy) of those who do the selection and planning of treatment. Variations of therapy under widely different circumstances makes it impossible to define standard programs, and treatment may vary from none to radical radiotherapy or surgery. Gynecologic cancers are best treated where a functioning team exists; thus the cancer patient should be referred to the proper environment.

There are multiple factors influencing the prognosis in carcinoma of the cervix:

1. Clinical stage and extent of tumor;
2. Anatomic variation within stage, e.g., barrel-shaped cervix, endometrial extension, etc.;
3. Gross tumor characteristics, e.g., exophytic, infiltrating, or ulcerating tumor;
4. Histologic variations, e.g., small cell, clear cell, etc.;
5. General status of the patient, e.g., hypertension, anemia, tumor necrosis, tuboovarian inflammatory disease, colon or bladder pathology, regional ileitis, and diabetes mellitus with blood vessel degeneration;
6. Management, facilities, and expertise.

Selection of proper treatment will depend upon medical status of the patient and extent of the malignant disease. Patients with terminal medical conditions may remain untreated. In some instances, local excision, cauterization, arterial ligation, transvaginal radiation therapy, intracavitary radium placement, or limited fields of external radiotherapy may provide control for untoward signs or symptoms without an attempt at eradication of the tumor. For patients whose medical status is unfavorable but not terminal, other problems of therapy selection are encountered.

In general, the institution qualified to carry out all aspects of treatment for cervical cancer must have a broad array of radiation therapy equipment including not only megavoltage devices, e.g., ^{60}Co teletherapy, a 6 mv linear accelerator, and betatron or 4 mv linear accelerator, but also a broad array of radium sources or radium substitutes, radium instruments, and applicators. Intracavitary and interstitial radioactive sources should be available for management.

In general, radiation therapy techniques remain the most applicable method for tumor control in invasive cervical cancer, but the following situations are in general better managed by surgical techniques:

1. Stage 0 or noninvasive carcinoma;
2. Microinvasive carcinoma;
3. Pregnancy complicating Stage I or Stage IIA cancer (in some instances, such as in early pregnancy, radiation techniques might be an alternative to surgery);
4. Stage I and Stage II-A cases with previous extensive pelvic surgery or widespread adhesions resulting from chronic pelvic inflammatory disease;
5. Stage I or Stage II-A cases with a potentially malignant adnexal mass (if the mass is benign, radiation therapy techniques might be an alternative to surgery);
6. Patients refusing radiotherapy or not complying with the prolonged course of the treatment required by radiation;
7. Patients with Stage IV lesions involving the rectum or bladder, but with no parametrial involvement;
8. Patients with persistent or recurrent malignancy following adequate courses of radiotherapy.

When surgery is elected, it should be a mutual decision among the team dealing with the prob-

---

Table 12–6. CARCINOMA OF THE CERVIX UTERI

Stage 0	Carcinoma in situ, intraepithelial carcinoma.
Stage I	The carcinoma is strictly confined to the cervix (extension to the corpus should be disregarded).
Stage I-A	Microinvasive carcinoma (early stromal invasion).
Stage I-B	All other cases of Stage I; occult cancer should be marked "occ."
Stage II	The carcinoma extends beyond the cervix but has not extended to the pelvic wall. The carcinoma involves the vagina, but not as far as the lower third.
Stage II-A	No obvious parametrial involvement.
Stage II-B	Obvious parametrial involvement.
Stage III	The carcinoma has extended to the pelvic wall. On rectal examination, there is no cancer-free space between the tumor and the pelvic wall. The tumor involves the lower third of the vagina. All cases with a hydronephrosis or nonfunctioning kidney are included.
Stage III-A	No extension to the pelvic wall.
Stage III-B	Extension to the pelvic wall and/or hydronephrosis or nonfunctioning kidney.
Stage IV	The carcinoma has extended beyond the true pelvis or has clinically involved the mucosa of the bladder or rectum. A bullous edema as such does not permit a case to be allotted to Stage IV.
Stage IV-A	Spread of the growth to adjacent organs.
Stage IV-B	Spread to distant organs.

Stage I-A represents those cases of epithelial abnormalities in which histologic evidence of early stromal invasion is unambiguous. The diagnosis is based on microscopic examination of tissue removed by biopsy, conization, portio amputation, or removal of the uterus. Cases of early stromal invasion should thus be allotted to Stage I-A.

The remainder of Stage I cases should be allotted to Stage I-B. As a rule, these cases can be diagnosed by routine clinical examination.

Occult cancer is a histologically invasive cancer that cannot be diagnosed by routine clinical examination. As a rule, it is diagnosed on a cone, the amputated portion, or on the removed uterus. Such cancers should be included in Stage I-B and should be marked "Stage I-B, occ."

Stage I cases can thus be indicated in the following ways:

Stage I-A	Carcinoma in situ with early stromal invasion diagnosed on tissue removed by biopsy, conization, or portio amputation, or on the removed uterus.
Stage I-B	Clinically invasive carcinoma confined to the cervix.
Stage I-B, occ.	Histologically invasive carcinoma of the cervix that could not be detected at routine clinical examination but was diagnosed on a large biopsy, a cone, the amputated portio, or the removed uterus.

A patient with a growth fixed to the pelvic wall by a short and indurated but not nodular parame-

trium should be allotted to Stage II-B. It is impossible, on clinical examination, to decide whether a smooth and indurated parametrium is truly cancerous or only inflammatory. Therefore, the case should be placed in Stage III only if the parametrium is nodular on the pelvic wall or if the growth itself extends to the pelvic wall.

The presence of hydronephrosis or nonfunctioning kidney due to stenosis of the ureter by cancer permits a case to be allotted to Stage III even if, according to the other findings, the case should be allotted to Stage I or Stage II.

The presence of bullous edema, as such, should not permit a case to be allotted to Stage IV. Ridges and furrows into the bladder wall should be interpreted as signs of submucous involvement of the bladder if they remained fixed to the growth at palposcopy (i.e., examination from the vagina or the rectum during cystoscopy). Finding malignant cells in cytologic washings from the urinary bladder requires further examination and a biopsy from the wall of the bladder.

The TNM system of describing the findings should be applied when surgical, pathologic, and cytologic information is additionally available, but without changing the original clinical staging.

T — Primary Tumor

TIS	Preinvasive carcinoma (carcinoma in situ). [FIGO Stage 0]
T1	Carcinoma confined to the cervix. Extension to the corpus should be disregarded.
T1a	Preclinical invasive carcinoma (i.e., cases that can be diagnosed only histologically). [FIGO Stage I-A]

lem. In conjunction with the gynecologic oncologist, the radiation oncologist and radiation physicist should devise treatment plans for the patient, utilizing the optimum radiation therapy techniques available. During the course of radiotherapy, the patient should be seen on a regular basis, preferably every week, and jointly with the gynecologic oncologist and radiation oncologist, so that modifications of treatment may be made if necessary. All members of the team should understand the values underlying the radiation therapy program, the goals set for the patient, and the potential possibility for complications. If the placement of radium or radium substitute is required as a part of the planned program of treatment, it should be done as a cooperative effort between the radiation oncologist and gynecologic oncologist (Table 12-7), with consultation from the physics staff in terms of calculation of dose distribution within the pelvis. The institution should be prepared to have the necessary radiographic studies done so that the calculation of dose distribution within the pelvis can be accomplished. These films should be right-angle films taken in the anterior–posterior and lateral positions of the pelvis, with contrast material in the bladder and rectum and with the cervix marked with a metallic clip. From these films and the magnification factor and dose distributions through the pelvis can be calculated, allowing for more intelligent integration of the external-beam radiation dose with the radium dosage. In general, a combination of external-beam and intracavitary radiation offers the greatest opportu-

T1b	Clinical invasive carcinoma. [FIGO Stage I-B]			
T2	Carcinoma extending beyond the cervix but not reaching the pelvic wall, *or* carcinoma involving the vagina but not the lower third.			
T2a	The carcinoma has not infiltrated the parametrium. [FIGO Stage II-A]			
T2b	The carcinoma has infiltrated the parametrium. [FIGO Stage II-B]			
T3	Carcinoma involving either the lower third of the vagina *or* reaching the pelvic wall (there is no free space between the tumor and the pelvic wall). [FIGO Stages III-A and III-B] (Note: The presence of a hydronephrosis or a nonfunctioning kidney due to stenosis of the ureter by growth allots the case to T3, even if according to the other findings the case should be allotted to a lesser category.)			
T4	Carcinoma involving the mucosa of the bladder or the rectum or extending beyond the true pelvis (the presence of bullous edema is not sufficient evidence to classify the tumor as T4). [FIGO Stage IV] (Note: Enlargement of the uterus alone does not constitute grounds for assignment to T4.)			
T4a	Carcinoma involving the bladder or the rectum only and histologically proved.			
T4b	Carcinoma extending beyond the true pelvis.			

N — Regional Lymph Nodes

NX	When it is not possible to assess the regional lymph nodes, the symbol NX is used, permitting eventual addition of histologic information, thus: NX− or NX+.
N0	No deformity of regional nodes as shown by available diagnostic methods.
N1	Regional nodes deformed as shown by available diagnostic methods.
N2	There is a fixed palpable mass on the pelvic wall with a free space between this and the tumor.

M — Distant Metastases

M0	No evidence of distant metastases.
M1	Distant metastases present, including nodes above the bifurcation of the common iliac arteries.

Stage Grouping

The categories N0 and N1 are not taken into account in stage grouping.

Stage "0"	T1S		
Stage I-A	T1a	NX	M0
Stage I-B	T1b	NX	M0
Stage II-A	T2a	NX	M0
Stage II-B	T2b	NX	M0
Stage III	T3	NX	M0
	T1b	N2	M0
	T2a	N2	M0
	T2b	N2	M0
Stage IV-A	T4	NX	M0
	T4	N2	M0
Stage IV-B			Any M1

Table 12–7. COMPARISON OF
PHYSICAL PARAMETERS OF
VARIOUS RADIONUCLIDES USED
IN BRACHYTHERAPY IN
CARCINOMA OF THE CERVIX

RADIO-NUCLIDE	HALF-LIFE (YRS)	ENERGY (MeV)	HVL IN MM OF LEAD	K FACTOR (R/HR AT 1 CM)
Ra	1620	0.8	8	8.25
^{60}Co	5.27	1.2	12	13.4
^{137}Cs	30	0.66	6	3.3

Table 12–8. COMPARISON OF 5-YEAR
SURVIVAL RATES OF THE SEQUENCE
OF RADIUM PLUS EXTERNAL
PELVIC IRRADIATION WITH THAT
OF EXTERNAL PELVIC IRRADIATION
PLUS RADIUM

SEQUENCE	NO. OF PATIENTS	5-YEAR SURVIVAL RATE (%)
Radium followed by external pelvic irradiation	116	35.3
External pelvic irradiation followed by radium	105	45.7

*From Patterson and Russell: *Clin Radiol* 13:313,
1962.

nity to obtain adequate tissue dosage within the
pelvis with minimal likelihood of injurious sequelae. Treatment administration should be managed
by the team dealing with the patient's problem
throughout the entire period of treatment itself.

Programs in radiation therapy are devised so
that external-beam radiation therapy precedes radium placement. External pelvic irradiation followed by radium placement reduces tumor bulk
and volume, diminishes infection, and assists in
returning a displaced uterus to its normal posi-

tion. Data from Patterson et al[24] indicate that
five-year survival rates in patients with Stage III
cervix carcinoma are improved when external-
beam radiotherapy is followed by the radium
placement (Table 12-8).

TREATMENT

The choice of treatment in carcinoma of the cervix is best decided after careful individual appraisal. For best results, a long-term view must be
agreed upon initially, and careful follow-up by the
same team is obligatory. At present, surgery, radiotherapy, and combinations of these two modalities have been successfully employed (Table
12-9).[10,13] Facilities, experience, and interest of
the personnel involved determine to a great extent the type of therapy to be employed. Generally, the choice of treatment is determined
by the staging.

From the point of view of radiotherapy, a combination of external and internal radiation is most
frequently practiced. Many different internal
applicators exist, but the essential common feature is to calculate dosage to Point A (paracervical
area) and to Point B (representing the pelvic
sidewall).[23] The general dosages employed are
7000 to 8000 rads to Point A, combining both
techniques, and 5000 to 6000 rads to Point B,
delivered in a period of 5 to 7 weeks.

Only limited success has been reported by the
utilization of various chemotherapeutic agents.

Recent reports with bleomycin in combination
with methotrexate[9] and with hydroxyurea[16] have
shown significant promise. The data from bleomycin and methotrexate have been on recurrent
carcinomas of the cervix; hydroxyurea has been
utilized in conjunction with radiotherapy as primary management.

Stage 0 (Carcinoma in Situ) and Stage I-A

Treatment for preinvasive carcinoma or carcinoma in situ and microinvasive cervical cancer is
best carried out utilizing surgery as the treatment
of choice, consisting of a hysterectomy and including a margin of the upper vaginal cuff in
women with carcinoma in situ. Removal of the
ovaries is elected depending on a number of individual factors, such as the age of the patient and
the menstrual history. When it is desired to retain
the child-bearing function, a wide-cone biopsy is
done as definitive treatment for carcinoma in situ,
but under these circumstances careful monitoring

Table 12–9. COMPARISON OF PRIMARY
SURGERY AND DEFINITIVE
RADIATION THERAPY

STAGE	PRIMARY SURGERY (%)	DEFINITIVE RADIATION THERAPY (%)
I	86.3	91.5
II-A	75.0	83.5
II-B	58.9	66.5
Other Stages	34.1	—
III-A	—	45.0
III-B	—	36.0
IV	—	14.0

From Currie: *J Obstet Gynaecol Brit Commonw* 78:385, 1971; Fletcher: *Textbook of Radiotherapy, 2nd ed,* Philadelphia, Lea & Febiger, 1973.

of the status of the cervix should be carried out.

In patients with carcinoma in situ where operation is not possible because of medical reasons or because of the patient's reluctance to have surgery, one or two intracavitary and cervical applications for 7000 to 8000 mg hours will give local control in over 97 percent of the patients treated.

After histologic definition of microinvasive (Stage IA) cervical cancer, a primary surgical approach is preferred.

Stages I-B and II-A

In most institutions, radiation therapy is the most frequently utilized treatment technique for carcinoma of the cervix in these stages. Surgery can be employed in selected cases with comparable survival figures. Postoperative radiation therapy should be employed in those individuals following radical surgery where tumor is found at the resected border, where there are positive lymph nodes in the specimen, where there is ovarian involvement or a more advanced lesion identified, or where residual tumor is left in the pelvis. Postoperative radiation therapy following radical surgery increases the complication rate from the treatment program. Radiation therapy for Stages I-B and II-A involve treatment techniques as follows:

1. The maximum dose is delivered to the tumor with a minimum dose to the normal tissue within the tolerance of the patient;

2. Radium with a combined intrauterine and vaginal application is used as a supplement to the external beam program;
3. External irradiation is basically the mainstay to deliver adequate dosage to the parametrial tissues and to the pelvic lymph nodes;
4. Large, bulky tumors may preclude a satisfactory application and are best treated with external beam therapy with the radium application ensuing after shrinkage has been obtained.

The principle of complete treatment to the maximum tolerable limits is usually advocated whether radiation therapy or surgery is used because a second course of treatment for recurrence is more often unsuccessful and greatly increases morbidity.

The external-beam radiation-therapy program precedes in most instances radium placement. The technique may involve a four-field summated technique, rotational techniques, a three-field summated technique, or two fields with energy levels using the betatron. The treatment program may be set up with or without wedges or with differential loading. It is preferable that the treatment set-up be on an isocentric technique and that all fields be treated each day. A calculated tumor-dose minimum of 5000 rads in 5 weeks is delivered to the pelvis, preferably by a four-field summated technique using megavoltage devices with a homogeneity factor approaching 1.0. The treatment program is carried out with five fractions per week with 200 rads tumor-dose minimum per fraction, 1000 rads per week over a period of 5 elapsed weeks. Following or near completion of the external-beam radiation therapy, a radium application is carried out using one of the multiple devices but with preference for the Fletcher–Suit afterloading device. A tumor dose of 3000 rads is delivered to Point A (2 cm cephalad from the upper vaginal fornix and 2 cm from the midline in the plane of the uterus as described by Tod). From this placement, Point B, representing the pelvic lymph nodes as the sidewall, will receive about 1000 rads. Point B is defined as 2 cm cephalad from the vaginal fornix and 5 cm from the midline of the pelvis. Within this context, the maximum dosage to the bladder and rectum should not exceed 2500 to 2800 rads.

Patients with Stages I-B and II-A with a barrel-shaped cervix or with endometrial extension should be treated by external-beam radiation therapy, receiving 2000 rads to the pelvis as a tumor-dose minimum in 2 weeks and a boost of 3000 rads to the regional lymph nodes in the parametrium delivered in 3 weeks. Placement of radium in the cervix should be carried out following this, delivering about 2000 rads to Point A. This would then be followed by extrafascial hysterectomy without lymphadenectomy in 4 to 6 weeks.

Stages II-B and III-B

Patients with Stage II-B and Stage III-B should be treated by administration of a 5000-rad tumor dose minimum using a four-field summated technique in 5 weeks. This would be delivered so that the homogeneity factor approaches 1. The patient would then receive a radium placement delivering 3000 rads to Point A and about 1000 rads to Point B, using the Fletcher–Suit afterloading device. In patients with Stage III-B lesions, the pelvic lymph nodes may be boosted by an additional 1000 rads through parametrial fields bilaterally in 1 week.

Stage III-A

Patients with Stage III-A lesions should receive the treatment as described for Stages II-B and III-B, but because of the extension of the tumor to the distal vaginal vault, a local radium needle implantation is necessary to insure adequate tumor dose distribution into that volume. This is done using a Patterson and Parker technique, radium needles being inserted in a circumferential fashion to the vagina with a central radium core, the ends of the implant being crossed by needles in the vulva. An additional 3000 to 3500 rads would be given as tumor-dose minimum to that volume.

Stage IV-A

Patients with Stage IV-A lesions, with the tumor extending to the bladder or to the rectum without parametrial extension, would be treated by pelvic exenteration, anterior, posterior, or total. In other patients with Stage IV-A lesions, the pelvis will be treated through a four-field summated technique delivering 5000 rads to the pelvis as a tumor dose minimum, with a homogeneity factor

approaching 1. This treatment would be followed by a 1000-rad boost to the pelvic lymph node and parametrial areas in one week. Subsequently, the patient would have a radium placement using the Fletcher–Suit device delivering 3000 rads to Point A and about 1000 rads to Point B.

Palliative radiation therapy may be employed for control of the pelvic disease in patients who have extrapelvic dissemination. This may be accomplished by delivering 5000 rads as a tumor-dose minimum to the pelvis using a four-field summated technique in five weeks, with a radium placement in order to insure local control of the disease. The intent from such a major treatment program is to control vaginal bleeding, infection, and discharge. Where these are not controlled, the patient is uncomfortable and becomes a major medical-management situation.

In general the treatment programs are designed to deliver about 8000 rads to the paracervical tissues, 5500 to 6000 rads to the electively treated pelvic lymph nodes in Stages I-B II-A, or 6000 to 7000 rads to the pelvic nodes in more advanced lesions where there is a high probability of lymph node metastases such as would be seen in Stages II-B, III, and IV-A.

External radiation therapy should be delivered utilizing a high-energy beam. Parallel, opposed anterior–posterior portals can be used with a 22 mv betatron. This is not possible, however, in patients who are over 22 cm in anterior and posterior diameter using energies of 4MV or less. Otherwise, with lower energies, the four-field box technique is preferred. The external radiation-therapy program should be carefully integrated with the intracavitary radium program.

Special care should be taken in the type of intracavitary applicators that are used. The dose distribution around the tandem and ovoids, and modifications in dose distribution that are produced by the geometric position of the applicators in relation to the cervix, the vaginal vault, and the pelvic organs is of major importance.

The limiting organs in the treatment of carcinoma of the cervix are the rectum, where the radiation dose should be less than 6500 rads, the bladder, where the maximum dose should be less than 7000 rads, and the paracervical tissues, where the maximum dose should not exceed 8000 rads. The dose given to the pubis or the femoral heads should be considered in the integrated treatment program. Isodose distributions are critical, both for the external beam and for the intracavitary insertions in order to achieve optimal dose distributions.

Endometrial Extension of Cervix Cancer

Extension of the squamous cell carcinoma of the cervix to involve the uterine cavity significantly influences the end results, as has been pointed out by Perez et al.[27] Where this is identified in the pretreatment work-up, special treatment plans must be devised in order to insure that there is adequate dose distribution throughout the entire uterus. In large measure, this can be accomplished by sequentially utilizing intracavitary uterine multiple sources along with the conventional cervix applicators. Treatment plans devised using such a program would allow for a 5000-rad tumor dose minimum to be delivered to the pelvis through a four-field summated technique in 5 weeks, to be followed by the uterine intracavitary multiple capsule radium placement delivering 3000 rads to the serosal surface of the uterus. This would be followed by a Fletcher–Suit afterloading device delivering 2000 rads to Point A and about 700 rads to Point B. Data from Antoniades indicates a 75 to 80 percent survival in those individuals treated using this technique.

Carcinoma of the Cervical Stump

When subtotal hysterectomy has been performed for a benign condition, carcinoma arising in the residual cervical stump presents special problems. If more than two years have elapsed since the subtotal hysterectomy, it is assumed that surgery was not performed in the presence of carcinoma. On the other hand, if the surgery has been performed in less than two years, we assume that the subtotal hysterectomy was performed in the presence of carcinoma of the cervix and therefore consider them to be coincident cases. This latter situation contributes to make the prognosis worse, as has been borne out by published studies of coincident cases.

The same clinical stages are used in classifying carcinoma of the cervical stump as are used for other carcinomas of the cervix, and the same pretreatment evaluation of the patient should be carried out.

The treatment of such problems is more com-

Table 12–10. COMPARISON OF 5-YEAR SURVIVAL RATES, TREATING CANCER OF THE CERVIX, THE INTACT UTERUS, AND THE CERVICAL STUMP

STAGE	INTACT UTERUS (N=1705) (%)	CERVICAL STUMP (N=189) (%)
I	91.5	97.0
II-A	83.5	93.0
II-B	66.5	67.0
III-A	45.0	61.0
III-B	36.0	32.0
IV	14.0	0

From Fletcher: *Am J Roentgenol* 111:225, 1971.

plex because it is not possible to utilize the uterine tandem of the usual length; more emphasis must be placed on vaginal radium and external irradiation. Often it is possible to identify a cervical canal, and by careful probing, tandems of sufficient length can be inserted. Otherwise, the compromise in the vaginal radium placement cannot be compared to the adequate tandem and ovoid placement. For these reasons, the dose delivered to the parametrium by the radium would be less.

Treatment techniques recommended in our institution include whole-pelvis irradiation, delivering 5000 rads as a tumor-dose minimum, with a homogeneity factor approaching 1 in five weeks, using a four-field summated technique. In the advanced stages, the parametrial areas would be boosted by an additional 1000 rads delivered in one week. This would then be followed by a radium placement delivering 3000 rads to Point A utilizing the Fletcher–Suit application. However, careful attention must be given to the dose distribution from the radium placement to avoid exceeding the maximum allowable tolerance of the bladder and rectum.

The five-year survival rates for patients treated with carcinoma of the true cervical stump are approximately the same as for the usual carcinoma of the cervix (Table 12-10).[12]

With the emphasis on total hysterectomy in most institutions, carcinoma of the cervical stump is disappearing. This policy of hysterectomy is fully justified in light of the low morbidity and mortality after hysterectomy. Steps are also necessary to eliminate coincident cases. With such a situation identified, prompt treatment programs are necessary with full cancericidal dosages to be given.

Recurrent Cancer of the Cervix

In spite of the fact that squamous cell carcinomas of the cervix represent one of the most curable malignancies, treatment is unsuccessful in nearly one-half of all cases. Persistent or recurrent carcinoma of the cervix, which are the consequence of treatment failure, creates a difficult situation that represents a major challenge in gynecologic oncology.

Since most treatment failures occur in the more advanced stages of the disease, the preceding treatment program would have been by radiation therapy (Table 12-11).[25] Few treatment failures are anticipated after primary surgical therapy because the modality is largely reserved for cases in which the tumor is confined to the cervix. Treatment failure after primary surgical therapy is usually managed by a definitive radiation therapy program.

Pretreatment evaluation of the patient should be carried out with the same degree of skill and care as with a new patient presenting with the diagnosis. This pretreatment evaluation should include tissue biopsies, cytology obtained from the vaginal vault and cervix, radiographic studies including intravenous urography, chest roentgenograms, radiographs of the axial skeleton, lymphangiography, radionuclide scans including bone, liver, and brain, and, on occasion, exploratory laparotomy for periaortic lymph node biopsy.

Recurrences should be managed after careful evaluation and separation of those in which there is a possibility of cure from those in which palliative treatment is the only treatment available. Potentially curable lesions include isolated central pelvic recurrences, isolated single-lung metastasis, and lower vaginal extensions. Isolated central recurrence is the most commonly encountered potential curable type. Surgical management must be tailored to the patient's needs and in almost all cases of central recurrence following definitive radiotherapy, ultraradical surgery is necessary.

On occasion the recurrence will be in the lower-third of the vagina, isolated in character and particularly in the suburethral area. In general, a metastasis in this location indicates the presence of widespread disease. Local irradiation is the treatment of choice, with emphasis on the potential prospects of inguinal-node metastases secondary to these lesions. Such incidence is high. Treatment of this type of recurrence should include therapy to the inguinal nodes even though there is no evidence of metastatic disease in other locations.

Metastatic carcinoma to the lung is viewed with extreme pessimism but when the lesion is limited in character and easily excised, the absence of other metastatic lesions directs excision of the metastasis. Five-year survivals in such situations have been reported in the range of 15 to 30 percent. The addition of long-term intermittent chemotherapy with methotrexate and bleomycin increases the cure potential.

The great majority of recurrences are suitable for palliative management only. Radiation therapy alone or in combination with chemotherapy give rise to significant levels of local control and symptomatic relief. The recurrence of disease in

Table 12–11. STATUS OF DISEASE IN PATIENTS DEAD UP TO 5 YEARS*

STAGE	NO. OF PTS.	PTS. WITH CENTRAL ACTIVE DISEASE ALONE OR AT OTHER SITES	DISEASE WITHIN IRRADIATED VOLUME OR COMPLICATION	DISTANT METASTASES AND INTERCURRENT DISEASE ONLY	NO. DATA
I	407	1.5% (12)	4.2% (17)	24	2
II-A	327		8.0% (29)	28	6
II-B	291	5.0% (15)	18.9% (55)	34	9
III-A	324	7.5% (24)	33.6% (109)	44	8
III-B	275	17.0% (49)	48.0% (132)	21	12
IV	81	39.0% (32)	72.8% (59)	5	—
Total	1705	132	401	156	37

From Paunier et al.: *Radiology* 88:555, 1967.
*(Patients treated with megavoltage external irradiation September 1954 to December 1963)

multiple sites may be managed by local radiotherapy with or without systemic chemotherapy. Some of the more effective agents available at this time are bleomycin and methotrexate in combination or hydroxyurea alone.

Data from Prasasvinichai and Glassburn[31] indicate the validity of careful work-up in the patient with recurrence of carcinoma of the cervix and the fact that definitive programs for disease limited to the pelvis can be associated with significant five-year survivals.

Periaortic Disease

Extension of disease to periaortic lymph nodes is often a cause of failure in patients with carcinoma of the cervix following definitive pelvic irradiation. Regional failure occurs where it is not possible to destroy metastatic cancer in the regional lymph nodes and central failure where it is not possible to control the disease in the cervix. The areas of failure giving rise to primary concern are those related to geographic misses, where the tumor extends outside the pelvis, or regional failure, where the disease remains in the pelvic lymph nodes. These two areas were shown to be significant in an analysis of failure sites in 148 patients who had exploratory celiotomy and pelvic lymphadnectomy following full course radiation therapy by Fletcher and Rutledge (Table 12-12).[35] Further studies suggested that those patients with residual cancer in the pelvic lymph nodes following irradiation had extensive involvement prior to the initiation of treatment. Thus, the volume of cancer in lymph nodes evolves as a critical factor in determining curability.

Exploratory celiotomy performed before the onset of the radiation therapy program would provide histologic proof of the extent of the metastatic cancer in lymph nodes as well as in other areas within the abdomen.

When disease is found to involve the common iliac and periaortic lymph nodes, the treatment fields must be changed in order adequately to encompass those lymph-node groups in the volume being irradiated. When tumor is found in the external iliac nodes, the treatment fields should be extended to cover the common iliac nodes. This field extends to the lower level of L-4 and provides a margin of safety above the highest identified tumor involvement. When positive common iliac or periaortic lymph nodes are found, the treatment fields must be extended to the level of T-12 in order adequately to encompass all the potential sites of the tumor in the nodal areas.

In patients with established disease in the common iliac and periaortic lymph nodes, dosages in the range of 4800 to 5000 rads can be delivered to the periaortic lymph nodes without significantly increasing the complications as a consequence of the treatment program.

Utilizing a 6-mv linear accelerator, anterior posterior fields are utilized encompassing the pelvis and periaortic lymph nodes to the level of T-12. The target axis distance utilized is in the range of 160 to 180 cm. Bilateral pelvic lateral fields are used. The dose distributions are summated in such a fashion that 140 to 150 rads are delivered to the midplane of the periaortic lymph nodes through the pan-handle fields, and 200 rads are delivered as tumor dose minimum to the pelvis. Homogeneity of distribution is excellent. At the completion of pelvic program of irradiation, the handle of the pan-handle is continued in such

Table 12–12. RESULTS OF PARA-AORTIC IRRADIATION

	ALIVE		DEAD			
STAGE	NED*	Cancer	Cancer	Complications	NOT EVALUATED†	TOTAL
I-B	13	1	3	4	0	21
II-A	6	1	2	1	0	10
II-B	15	4	11	7	3	40
III-A	16	3	4	3	7	33
III-B	2	0	2	0	4	8
IV	1	0	0	0	0	1
Total	53	9	22	15	14	113

From Wharton, in Rutledge et al. (eds): *Gynecologic Oncology.* New York, Wiley, 1976.
*No evidence of disease.
†Less than 6 months follow-up.

a way to bring that dose to 4800 to 5000 rads. The time in which the treatment is delivered is five weeks to the pelvis and about 6½ to seven weeks to the periaortic lymph nodes.

Intracavitary radium is used as a part of the treatment program in the pelvis, depending upon the volume and the extent of the tumor. When this technique is utilized, the incidence of short-term and long-term complications is acceptable.

Preirradiation exploratory celiotomy as a special procedure is used to evaluate the extent of cancer spread. It is not without serious complications. The surgical dissection in the pelvis must be kept to an absolute minimum, as must the surgical dissection of the periaortic lymph nodes (it is more appropriate to remove the individual suspicious nodes selectively). By keeping the surgical intervention to a minimum or by using extraperitoneal approach to do the lymph node biopsies, the complication rate can be decreased dramatically. The data from Rotman,[30] Key and Park,[18] and Perez et al.[26] indicate the validity of such an approach by the significant increase in the survival in individuals who have disease extending beyond the ordinary conventional treatment volumes.

GENERAL CARE

Before any type of treatment is employed, the general physical and emotional health of the patient should be evaluated. Anemias should be corrected to 12 g of hemoglobin and 35 percent hematocrit. Infection should be appropriately treated and general well-being should be assured. Family and professional emotional support are necessary. Hypertension should be reduced. Metabolic abnormalities such as diabetes should be controlled at all times.

Radiation complications include bladder and rectal ulceration, fistula formation, and fractures and necroses. The occurrence of these complications is unusual and should be less than 5 to 6 percent of the total series with current techniques. They are often associated with the stage of the disease occurring most commonly in patients with advanced tumor.

HYPERBARIC OXYGEN IN CARCINOMA OF THE CERVIX

Hyperbaric oxygen has been used with clinical radiation therapy for nearly 25 years, since its introduction by Churchill-Davidson.[7] The modern hyperbaric chamber has been available since 1960.

The rationale for the use of hyperbaric oxygen

Table 12–13.   TREATMENT USING RADIATION THERAPY AND HYPERBARIC OXYGEN

STAGE	TREATMENT	NO. OF PATIENTS	% SURVIVAL, 1 YEAR	% SURVIVAL, 3 YEARS
III	HPO	59	80	53
	Air	69	74	47
IV	HPO	23	56	16
	Air	12	33	10
Pelvic Failure				
III	HPO	59	19	27
	Air	69	22	49
IV	HPO	23	43	53
	Air	12	58	80

Patients treated in hyperbaric oxygen show a significant reduction in pelvic failure in stages III and IV and small but sustained improvement in survival. From Halnan, in *Proceedings of the XI International Cancer Congress,* Florence, 1974.

is simple. Hypoxic cell populations have diminished radiosensitivity. They are present in most tumors and account for partial failure of local tumor control. Utilization of the hyperbaric oxygen chamber is a practical method to increase the oxygen saturation in these hypoxic cells. Modern microelectrode techniques have confirmed that oxygen tension within the tumor can be increased when the tumor is under hyperbaric oxygen pressure.

The data achieved by Halnan[17] in the treatment of carcinoma of the cervix support the concept as a valid and important clinical research effort (Table 12-13). The Radiation Therapy Oncology Group data[29] confirm the reports from Halnan in the treatment of carcinoma of the cervix, Stage II-B, Stage III, and Stage IV-A. The preliminary data from the Radiation Therapy Oncology Group indicate a high rate of local control with a minimum of complications in those patients treated within the hyperbaric chamber. However, the techniques require meticulous radiation therapy techniques, adequate saturation time of 15 to 20 minutes within the hyperbaric oxygen chamber before the radiation therapy program is initiated, and a small number of large factions (between 6 and 10), and all fields must be treated at each session.

Even though previous investigators have felt that the benefits were probably not sufficiently great to stand on their own, proper clinical trials must be performed in order to evaluate effectively the potentials of this treatment program.[15]

FOLLOW-UP

For an institution to be qualified to manage the problems relative to cervical malignancy, facilities should be available for adequate follow-up examination, where all members of the team may see the patient at each subsequent follow-up examination. In general, the patient should be seen at monthly intervals during the first year, every two months during the second year, every three months during the third year, every four months during the fourth year, and every six months thereafter. In general, the gynecologic oncologist and radiation oncologist share the major responsibility for this follow-up. Follow-up examinations should include complete history and physical examination, including pelvic examination. Pap smears are performed at every examination, beginning three months following completion of the radiation therapy. Roentgenograms of the chest are obtained on a yearly basis, and other studies as indicated by the patient's history and physical examination.

The development of hydronephrosis, unilateral lower-extremity edema, or pelvic pain extending into the lower extremities indicate the high probability of recurrence of the malignant tumor. Patients under those circumstances should be worked up appropriately and decisions made as to the need for surgical intervention to establish the diagnosis and for management.

Special problems may occur in patients who have had prior treatment for cervical malignancy, whether by surgery or by radiation techniques. The presence of a well-coordinated, well-functioning team in the management of the disease will bring to these problems the sophistication and skill necessary to deal with them promptly and adequately. Patients with carcinoma of the cervix have an increased incidence for a second primary tumor, and these are most commonly malignant tumors of the lung, thyroid, rectum, and multiple myeloma.

Finally, it is difficult to maintain adequate skills when dealing with cervical malignancy unless 20 to 25 new patients are seen annually, with adequate opportunity for all members of the team to maintain their skills and abilities to deal with the various problems of management.

The primary objective of treatment is to achieve a balance between a maximum potential for cure and a minimum incidence of complication. The spread of five-year survival for cervical cancer among the 100 institutions reporting to the International Federation of Gynaecology and Obstetrics (FIGO) is the following: in the Stage I carcinomas of the cervix, the minimal acceptable end result would be 75 to 80 percent for five-year survival without disease; in Stage II, 45 to 55 percent five-year survival without disease; in Stage III, 20 to 30 percent five-year survival without disease; and for Stage IV, 2 to 15 percent five-year survival without recurrent disease.

Minimum end results must be achieved with a maximum potential for complication being no greater than 10 percent severe complications that result in death or necessitate operative intervention. Survival figures are reported in terms of crude survival and are related to a well-functioning follow-up system where no more than 5 percent of the patients are lost to follow-up.

References

1. American Cancer Society Facts and Figures, 1978
2. Averette HE, Dudan RC, Ford JH Jr: Exploration celiotomy for surgical staging of cervical cancer. Am J Obstet Gynecol 113: 1090, 1972
3. Brady LW: Future prospects of radiotherapy in gynecologic oncology. Cancer 38:553, 1976
4. Brady LW: Advances in the management of gynecologic cancer—radiation therapy. Cancer 36:661, 1975
5. Brunschwig A: The surgical treatment of cancer of the cervix Stage I and II. Am J Roentgenol Radium Ther Nucl Med. 102: 147, 1968
6. Buchsbaum HJ, Keetal WC, Latourette HB: The use of radioisotopes as adjunct therapy of localized ovarian cancer. Semin Oncol 2:247, 1975
7. Churchill-Davidson I, Metters JS, Foster CA, Bates TD: The management of cervical lymph node metastases by hyperbaric oxygen and radiotherapy. Clin Radiol 24: 498, 1973
8. Cleaves M: Radium: with a preliminary note on radium rays in the treatment of cancer. J Adv Ther 21:667, 1903
9. Conroy JF, Lewis GC, Brady LW, et al.: Low dose Bleomycin and Methotrexate in cervical cancer. Cancer 37:660, 1976
10. Currie DW: Operative treatment of carcinoma of the cervix. J Obstet Gynaecol Brit Commonw 78:385, 1971
11. Douglas RG, Sweeney WJ III: Treatment of carcinoma of cervix with combined radiation and extensive surgery. Am J Obstet Gynecol 84:981, 1962
12. Fletcher GH: Cancer of the uterine cervix. Am J Roentgenol 111:225, 1971
13. Fletcher GH: Textbook of Radiotherapy, 2nd ed. Philadelphia, Lea & Febiger, 1973
14. Fletcher GH, Rutledge FN: Extended field technique in management of cancers of the uterine cervix. Am J Roentgenol Radium Ther Nucl Med 114:116, 1972
15. Glassburn JR, Brady LW, Plenk H: Hyperbaric oxygen in radiation therapy. Cancer 39:751, 1977
16. Gynecologic Oncology Report, 1977
17. Halnan KE: Recent trials of radiotherapy in hyperbaric oxygen. In Proceedings of the XI International Cancer Congress, Florence, 1974
18. Keys H, Park RC: Treatment of patients with cancer of the cervix and nodal metastases. Int J Radiat Biol 1:1091, 1976
19. Lewis GC, Brady LW, Lee J, Kramer S: Improving results for treatment of endometrial cancer. Phila Med 71:103, 1975
20. Littman P, Davis LM, La Panto P: Evaluation of nodal metastasis in patients with cervical carcinoma. Cancer 31:1307, 1973
21. Meigs JV, Liu W: Surgical and pathologic classification for cancer of the cervix. Surg Gynecol Obstet 100:555, 1955
22. Moss WT: Radiation Oncology—Rationale, Technique, Results. St. Louis, Mosby, 1973
23. Nelson JH Jr, Macasack MA, Lu T, et al.: Incidence and significance of para-aortic lymph node metastases in late invasive carcinoma of the cervix. Am J Obstet Gynecol 118:749, 1974
24. Patterson R, Russell M: Cancer of the cervix uteri. Clin Radiol 13:313, 1962
25. Paunier JP, Delclos L, Fletcher GH: Causes, time of death, and sites of failures in squamous cell carcinoma of the uterine cervix on intact uterus. Radiology 88:555, 1967
26. Perez C, Askin F, Baglan R, and Weiss D: Effect of irradiation on mixed mesodermal tumors of the uterus. Int J Radiat Biol (to be published)
27. Perez C, Zivnuska F, Askin F, et al.: Prognostic significance of endometrial extension from primary carcinoma of the uterine cervix. Cancer 35:1493, 1975
28. Piver MS, Barlow JJ: Para-aortic lymphadenectomy in staging patients with advanced local cervical cancer. Obstet Gynecol 43: 544, 1974
29. Radiation Therapy Oncology Group: Report, June 1977
30. Rotman M: Personal communication.
31. Prasasvinichai S, Glassburn JR: Personal communication.
32. Ucmakli A, Bonney WA Jr: Exploratory laparotomy as routine pretreatment investigation in cancer of the cervix. Radiology 104:371, 1972
33. UICC/American Joint Committee for Can-

cer Staging: Classification and staging of malignant tumors in the female pelvis. ACOG Technical Bulletin, no. 47, June 1977

34. Wertheim E: Radical abdominal operation in carcinoma of the cervix uteri. Surg Gynecol Obstet 4:1, 1907

35. Wharton JT: Pretreatment evaluation and therapy selection for patients with invasive carcinoma of the cervix. In Rutledge F, Boronow RC, Wharton JT (eds): Gynecologic Oncology. New York, Wiley, 1976

Appendix:

A Summary of Procedures for the Reduction of Morbidity and Mortality from Cervical Cancer

LARRY McGOWAN, M.D.

SCREENING EXAMINATION

Visualization of the Cervix

Visualization of the cervix with good illumination is the essential first step in a screening examination and is too often neglected. Good visualization can reveal a gross, exophytic lesion on the cervix which may no longer be shedding well preserved neoplastic cells and may result in an unsatisfactory or even a negative Pap smear.

Collection of the Cytologic Sample

Poorly collected specimens are the most common cause for a false-negative report from the laboratory or for one labeled "unsatisfactory." Two specimens should be collected: (1) a firm ectocervical scrape including the region of the squamocolumnar junction at the cervical os, and (2) a swab of the endocervical mucosa. These should be transferred to separate halves of one slide or to two separate slides and marked accordingly. They should be fixed in 95 percent ethyl alcohol and sent to the laboratory. Vaginal pool samples are not recommended for the detection of cervical cancer, but may be of some value in postmenopausal women for the detection of endometrial cancer.

Bimanual Pelvic Exam

Bimanual pelvic palpation, vaginal and rectal, should be an integral part of the examination, but is, unfortunately, often omitted in large-scale screening programs, at health fairs, or at public screening clinics.

PROCESSING AND INTERPRETATION OF CYTOLOGIC SPECIMENS

The slides should be stained by the Papanicolau procedure (hematoxylin and eosin or acridine orange are not recommended).

The laboratory personnel should be adequately trained. Each cytotechnologist should not have to examine more slides per day than he or she can examine thoroughly in a working period. In general, the American Society of Cytology suggests that a reasonable work load should be, on the average, 80 to 100 slides per day per cytotechnologist.

The laboratory should handle at least 10,000

234

gynecologic cases per year. It should meet the requirements of the American Society of Cytology, or the American College of Pathologists, or the Center for Disease Control, and should comply with state laws.

The laboratory should have a good quality control program. The accuracy of Pap smears varies greatly according to the training, experience, and interest of those taking the samples and of those in the laboratory who process and interpret the slides. False-negative cytosmears have varied from 5 percent to as much as 30 percent. This points to the necessity for education about quality control measures.

Record keeping should be impeccable and all cytosmear slides should be kept at least five years. Abnormal slides should be retained for the lifetime of the patient. A continuing correlation between cytologic interpretation and histologic confirmation is mandatory.

DIAGNOSTIC WORK-UP

Most physicians can and should perform visually directed cervical biopsies for suspected malignant lesions.

All obstetricians and gynecologists should be capable of carrying out diagnostic procedures for cancer and basic surgical operations including conization for cervical cancer. They should share in the follow-up and rehabilitation or terminal care of the women with invasive disease.

If the laboratory interprets a Pap smear as severe dysphasia, in situ or invasive cancer, the patient should undergo a diagnostic work-up as promptly as possible. This involves:

Biopsy of an obvious cervical lesion.
Biopsy of an area that does not take an iodine (Lugol's solution) stain.
If a biopsy shows invasive cancer, the patient should be referred to a gynecologic oncologist for treatment planning and definitive treatment.
If no lesion can be seen for direct biopsy and an expert colposcopist is not available, a diagnostic conization should be performed.

If no abnormal area is found on direct visualization and if an experienced colposcopist is available, a colposcopic examination of the cervix and vagina should be performed.
If an abnormal area can be seen in its entirety by colposcopy, a colposcopy-directed biopsy and an endocervical curettage should be performed.
If no lesion can be seen by colposcopy or if a lesion extends into the endocervix, the patient should undergo a diagnostic conization of the cervix (including curettage of the endometrium).
If carcinoma in situ is diagnosed by direct biopsy and an expert colposcopist is not available, a diagnostic conization should be performed.
If microinvasive cancer is found by biopsy (direct visualization or colposcopy), a diagnostic conization of the cervix must be carried out to determine the extent of the lesion.
If the diagnostic work-up does not provide an explanation for the presence of dysphasic or malignant cells, continued medical surveillance is necessary until an explanation is found.

COMMUNICATION BETWEEN LABORATORY AND CLINICIAN

There should be good communication between the clinician and the cytopathologist and pathologist so that the clinician can personally discuss any questionable findings and so that the cytopathologist and pathologist can obtain the information necessary for correlation of cytology, colposcopy, and biopsy findings.

Thus there is a great advantage in having both cytology and pathology examinations performed in close proximity to the examining physician instead of sending specimens to a distant laboratory.

The laboratory personnel should be provided with pertinent background information on each specimen, including the patient's age, major physical findings referable to the pelvis, menstrual status, current medication at the time the samples were taken, and the sites from which they came.

Cytology laboratory reports should be transmitted to the clinician in descriptive and clearly understandable form, and not by numerical ranking.

Pathology reports should also be descriptive and should follow standard nomenclature.

TREATMENT

If the biopsy shows only dysplasia, efforts should be made to determine the cause, and appropriate treatment methods should be utilized. The patient should be kept under periodic surveillance.

If carcinoma in situ is diagnosed, the treatment must be individualized according to the judgement of the physician who must consider the extent of the disease, the age of the patient, and the need for preservation of the uterus for child bearing.

If the biopsy or conization specimen shows invasive cancer (including microinvasive), treatment planning should be undertaken promptly and treatment individualized to the patient.

The physician responsible for treatment planning, treatment, follow-up, and rehabilitation or terminal care of the woman with invasive cervical cancer is the gynecologic oncologist.

In general, this will require a team effort of the cytopathologist, pathologist, diagnostic radiologist, radiation oncologist, expert in nuclear medicine, urologist, medical oncologist, and others as needed, under the coordination of the gynecologic oncologist.

FOLLOW-UP

Every woman who has had a cervical cytosmear interpreted as dysphasia, carcinoma in situ, or invasive cancer must be followed to make certain that she is seen by a physician and receives appropriate diagnostic work-up and treatment.

Each woman who has been treated for cervical cancer must be followed with periodic pelvic examinations and Pap smears for the rest of her life to detect and treat any possible recurrence. Since the vaginal vault or wall may be involved,

Pap smears are still valuable after hysterectomy.

Effective follow-up of cervical cancer patients requires efficient record systems or registries, usually maintained by the hospital where the patient receives treatment.

Records of Pap smear screening should be maintained for at least five years.

Abnormal slides should be retained for the lifetime of the patient.

FREQUENCY OF SCREENING

There is reason for flexibility on this subject. An annual Pap smear, which might be considered an optimum schedule, may not be feasible in some situations for logistic or budgetary reasons. A possible compromise providing good protection at minimum cost would appear to be the following procedure: have three entirely normal Pap smears taken one year apart beginning at age 21 or the age of beginning sexual activity, then every three years to age 35, then every three to five years thereafter. Screening frequency should be increased if any pelvic abnormalities are found or if the patient is taking oral contraceptives or estrogen therapy.

The obtaining of an annual cervical cytosmear can be part of a general examination for cancer which would include breast and pelvic exams.

Although the number of new cases of cervical cancer in frequently screened women may be small, continued medical surveillance of postmenopausal women for endometrial cancer is mandatory. As the Pap smear will only detect 10 to 50 percent of endometrial cancers, endometrial cytologic and/or tissue aspiration should be performed yearly in perimenopausal and postmenopausal women who are at increased risk for the development of endometrial cancer.

References

1. Management of abnormal cytology by colposcopy and/or conization. ACOG Tech Bull. Number 38, May, 1976

2. Christopherson WM, Lundin FE, Mendez WM, Parker JE: Cervical cancer control. Cancer 38:1357, 1976

3. Moss AJ, Wilder MH: Use of selected medical procedures associated with preventive care. Vital and Health Statistics. Series 10, No. 110, March 1977
4. Report of the Committee on Terminology. New nomenclature for colposcopy. Obstet Gynecol 48:123, 1976
5. Rylander E: Negative smears in women developing invasive cervical cancer. Acta Obstet Gynecol Scand 56:115, 1977
6. Shingelton HM, Gore H, Austin JM: Outpatient evaluation of patients with atypical Papanicolaou smears: contribution of endocervical curettage. Am J Obstet Gynecol 126:122, 1976
7. Cervical cancer screening programs. Can Med Assoc J 114:1003, 1976
8. Workshop on Cervical Cancer Screening. Interagency Coordinating Committee on Cancer Control & Rehabilitation. Department of Health, Education, and Welfare. Bethesda, Md., September 29, 1976

Chapter 13

Endometrial Cancer

LARRY McGOWAN, M.D.

Endometrial cancer has had a facade of benignity assigned to it by many, a nonchalant association with postmenopausal uterine bleeding, and a misconception as to the validity of the Pap smear to detect endometrial cancer. Also, there has been a lack of appreciation that the disease should be staged accurately and treatment individualized.

True figures as to the incidence of endometrial cancer and changing trends are difficult to determine.[1] The reasons for that are many mortality figures for uterine cancer do not delineate primary cervical from primary endometrial cancer, the inclusion of dysplastic lesions of the endometrium with invasive ones, and the lack of pathologic confirmation for some regional studies associating exogenous hormones with increased numbers of endometrial cancers. Lyon and Gardner state the number of hysterectomies performed in the United States increased about 60 percent between 1965 and 1973, far in excess of population growth. This has altered the population at risk for uterine malignancies, and many published incidence rates do not correct for this

effect. They assume no effect of hysterectomy on endometrial cancer rates prior to 1950 and determined a 20 to 30 percent rise in endometrial cancer incidence since that time.[2] The American Cancer Society has estimated that there will be approximately 28,000 new cases of endometrial cancer and 3300 deaths due to the disease in 1978.[3] Cancer of the corpus is the predominant genital malignancy in white women over age 50. Cramer and Cutler observed an age-adjusted rate for invasive corpus cancer in whites to be 21.6, significantly higher than the 12.2 for blacks.[4] In situ carcinomas of the corpus occur an average of 7.4 years earlier than invasive malignancies of the corpus. Of newly diagnosed invasive cancers of the female genital organs, approximately 38 percent originate in the corpus. Cancers of the corpus are relatively infrequent until age 40 but increase rapidly, reaching a peak at 65 to 74 and declining thereafter. Women with adenoacanthoma of the corpus are 2.6 years younger than those with adenocarcinoma of the endometrium (58.1 vs 60.7 years).[4]

ETIOLOGY

The possible role of a prolonged period of abnormal, unopposed estrogenic stimulation in the genesis of endometrial carcinoma has long been suspected but is difficult to prove conclusively.

The levels of estradiol 17B-dehydrogenase activity has been found by Gurpide and Tseng to be more than 10 times higher in secretory human endometrium than in proliferative tissue. The total amount of estradiol receptor levels was found by them to be drastically reduced during the luteal phase.[5] Progesterone may regulate estradiol receptor levels in human endometrium as well as reduce intracellular estradiol concentrations.

Siiteri et al in their extensive studies have demonstrated the exclusive production of estrone by anovulatory women having a high risk for development of endometrial cancer which led them to the formulation of the "estrone hypothesis."[6] Their hypothesis suggests that unopposed exposure of target tissues, endometrium, to estrone may be a causal factor in the development of cancer. They had noted estrogen binding to nor-mal and abnormal endometrial cytoplasmic and nuclear receptors. Estrone binds to cytoplasmic receptors, and the resulting complex was transferred into the nucleus suggesting that estrone is an active estrogen in human endometrium.[7]

Rao and Wiest from their studies believe that progesterone exerts its normal physiologic action on the uterine endometrium by an initial interaction with a cytoplasmic protein component with receptor-like properties, and that as a consequence of this interaction, the hormone-induced changes in endometrial functions take place.[8] Progesterone by its absence may be a factor in the production of endometrial cancer.

THE WOMAN AT RISK

The personal risk factors for endometrial cancer according to MacMahon may be divided into three groups: (1) variations of normal anatomy or physiology (obesity, nulliparity, late menopause), (2) the presence of frank abnormality or disease (diabetes mellitus, hypertension, Stein-Leventhal syndrome, cancer of other sites), and (3) exposure to known external causes of disease (radiation exposure, estrogen).[9,10]

Obesity

Obesity seems to be frequently associated with the endometrial cancer patient particularly in the

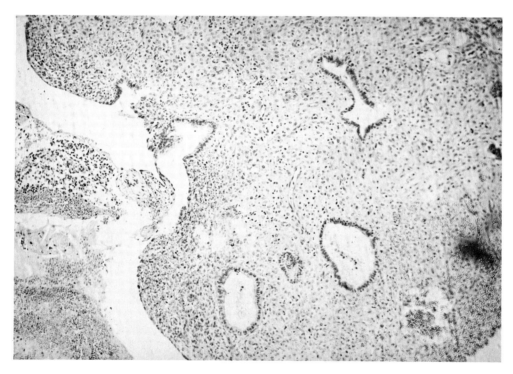

Figure 13–1. Endometrium with deciduoid reaction in a 23-year-old woman who is 5 ft. 3 in. tall, 275 pounds, nulliparous, hypertensive, has elevated blood sugar, and has metrorrhagia. ×160.

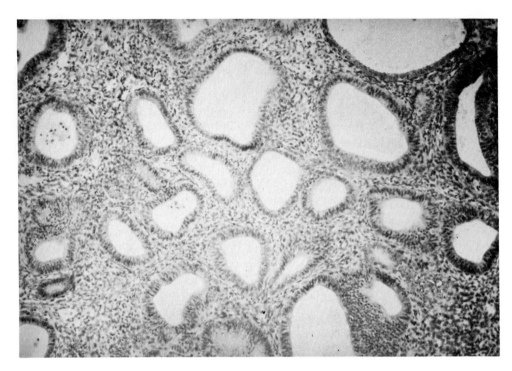

Figure 13-2. Atypical adenomatous hyperplasia of the endometrium in the same woman as in Figure 13-1, six years later. She has menometrorrhagia. ×160.

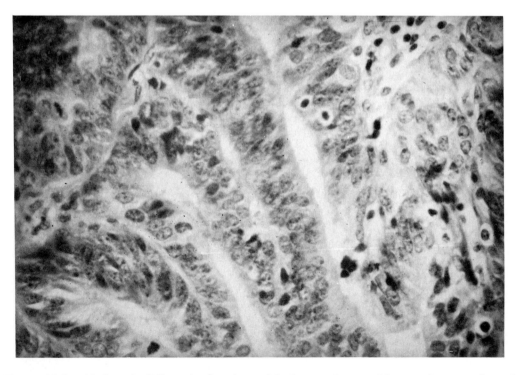

Figure 13-3. Moderately differentiated endometrial adenocarcinoma with extension to endocervix in same woman as in Figures 13-1 and 13-2 obtained one year following Figure 13-2. ×640.

postmenopausal years. As endometrial cancer may be caused by different etiologic factors, it is not unusual that all patients do not have the same clinical features. Extreme obesity is a strong risk factor for endometrial cancer (Figs. 13-1 to 13-3). However, it would be expected only approximately one-half of women with endometrial cancer are in the extreme overweight category.

Nulliparity

Although women with endometrial carcinoma are notably less fertile, nulliparous women have a rate for development of the disease perhaps twice as high as for those women with one child and more than three times as high for those with five or more children (Figs. 13-1 to 13-3). Utilization of nulliparity as the sole identification factor would only be associated with approximately 50 percent of women with endometrial cancer in Mac-Mahon's study.[9]

Late Menopause

The average age of menopause among women with endometrial cancer is commonly higher than in normal women. There is approximately a two times greater risk of endometrial cancer among women whose menopause occurs after the age of 50 to those whose menopause occurs prior to age 49.

Diabetes Mellitus

Brown, utilizing an oral glucose tolerance test, with analysis of blood glucose demonstrated a carbohydrate intolerance in women with endometrial cancer as compared to the controls. The degree of intolerance was modified by obesity.[11] A high frequency of diabetes, whether diagnosed by history or by abnormal glucose tolerance test at the time of diagnosis of the endometrial cancer is reported consistently in the literature. It seems most likely that diabetes is associated with increased risk of endometrial cancer (Figs. 13-1 to 13-3). Some have placed the relative risk at slightly better than two for the development of endometrial cancer in a woman with a history of diabetes.[9]

Hypertension

High blood pressure has not been as consistently a characteristic of endometrial cancer as the previous four factors discussed. One would not be surprised to find elevated blood pressure in women with endometrial carcinoma considering their usual postmenopausal age group, being fre-

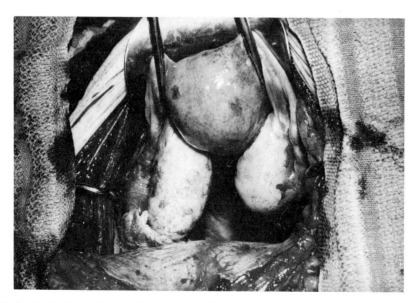

Figure 13–4. Stein-Leventhal syndrome in a 34-year-old woman with oligomenorrhea, male-type hirsutism, and a well-differentiated adenoacanthoma (stage IA, G1) of the endometrium. Enlarged and smooth ovaries are seen posterior to a normal-size uterus.

quently overweight, and having carbohydrate intolerance (Figs. 13-1 to 13-3).

Sclerocystic Ovaries

The Stein-Leventhal syndrome is an uncommon disorder usually associated with anovulation, menstrual irregularities, infertility, a tendency toward being overweight, and abnormal body hair development (Figs. 13-4 and 13-5). Chamlian and Taylor, in their study of young women with endometrial hyperplasia and Stein-Leventhal syndrome, have recorded the progression to adenocarcinoma. Of all cases of endometrial carcinoma, no more than 3 to 5 percent occur before the age of 40. It does stress the importance of following women with sclerocystic disease very carefully and those who have a significant degree of endometrial hyperplasia attempting to induce ovulation, and in married couples, pregnancy, as this management has the highest chance of preventing progression of endometrial hyperplasia to adenocarcinoma.[12]

The extremely uncommon association between a functioning granulosa-theca cell tumor of the ovary and endometrial cancer has been documented but with extreme rarity.

Cancers of Other Sites

Incidence data from the Third National Cancer Survey was used to study geographic variations in the occurrence of several cancers. There were high correlations between breast, corpus, and ovary[13] (Fig. 13-6). Also, the association of cancer of the endometrium and bowel has been reported. These results could be from demographic and personal factors that are common to women with the three diseases or from common etiologic agents.

Radiation Exposure

Exposure to large doses of radiation in the course of medical therapy is the best documented of the exogenous risk factors for endometrial cancer. The same association with radiation exposure and sarcoma of the uterus has been noted.

Exogenous Estrogens

Exogenous estrogens, notably conjugated estrogens, may be associated with the development of endometrial cancer (Figs. 13-6 and 13-7). Users

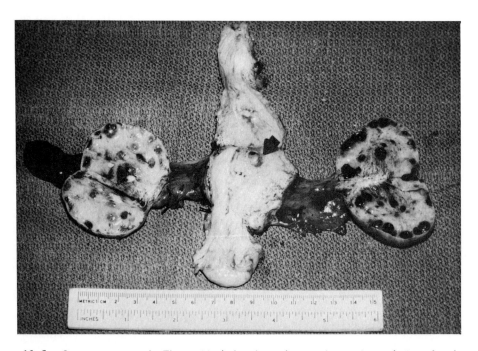

Figure 13-5. Same woman as in Figure 13-4 showing sclerocystic ovaries and site of endometrial cancer. There was no myometrial invasion.

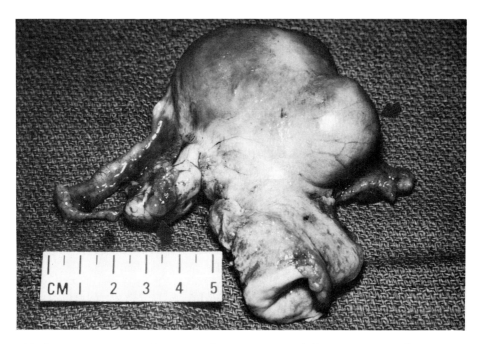

Figure 13–6. Posterior view of uterus and ovaries removed from a 71-year-old woman who had been on Premarin 2.5 mg and other oral estrogens for 12 years. She had irregular uterine bleeding for many of these years and was told by her physician to increase the estrogens. She had numerous normal Pap smears. The uterus contained a well-differentiated adenocarcinoma of the endometrium (stage IA, G1). A subserous myoma is seen on the right and a serous papillary cystadenoma of borderline malignancy (carcinoma of low malignant potential) in the ovary to the left.

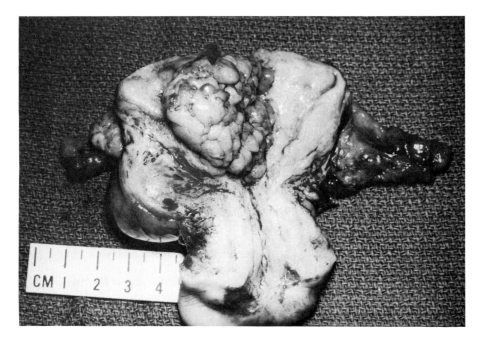

Figure 13–7. Opened uterus of Figure 13-6 demonstrating an exophytic endometrial cancer that invaded one third of the myometrial wall.

of other forms of systemic estrogens show similar elevations in relative risk. Gray et al have observed the relative risk of endometrial cancer to be related to duration of use, progressing from no evidence of risk in their study patients among those using the hormone for less than 5 years to an 11.5-fold greater risk for those using it for 10 years or more. They noted, as have others, that risk is also related to the strength of the medication. The relative risk for users of the 1.25 mg conjugated estrogens was 12.7 as compared to a two- to fourfold greater risk among users of lesser strength tablets in their study.[14]

Some areas of the country, particularly on the west coast of the United States, have experienced a significant increase in the incidence rates of endometrial carcinoma after years of relative stability. In other areas of the country in which there has been a low rate of use of conjugated estrogens there has not been an appreciable impact on the incidence of endometrial cancer.[15]

For those women who do have vasomotor symptoms of the menopause, cyclic administration of the lowest effective dose of estrogen for the shortest period of time with appropriate monitoring for endometrial cancer is advised. Women in whom atrophic vaginitis is a problem can be treated with intravaginal estrogenic creams. The effectiveness of estrogens in delaying osteoporosis is under review, but current information as to the positive impact on osteoporosis of a proper diet and exercise program should not be overlooked. There is no satisfactory evidence that coronary artery disease in postmenopausal women is prevented or delayed by estrogen replacement.[16]

Sequential oral contraceptives were withdrawn from the United States market in 1976, as there was a strong suggestion that the sequentials were associated with a greater risk of endometrial cancer than the combination oral contraceptives.[17-21] Also, the sequential oral contraceptives had a decreased effectiveness and had a greater risk of thromboembolism than the combination products.[19]

Patients with gonadal dysgenesis (Turner's syndrome) may develop endometrial carcinoma after prolonged unopposed treatment with stilbesterol and after long-term combined estrogen-progestogen therapy.[22,23]

STAGING

The results of treatment modalities have been difficult to evaluate in endometrial cancer, because in the past, there has been a lack of uniformity in clinical classification. In 1971, the International Federation of Gynaecology and Obstetrics published their classification and staging of malignant tumors in the female pelvis which was accepted by the American College of Obstetricians and Gynecologists (see Table 13-1).

The clinical classification takes into consideration uterine size as one index of tumor growth. Corpus cancer tends to grow locally for long periods of time and expands the uterus commonly with its exophytic intraluminal growth (Fig. 13-7). The determination of uterine cavity length at the time of fractional curettage of the uterus is part of the staging process. Uterine size may be altered by parity, menopausal status, and benign growths such as leiomyomata (Fig. 13-6). The presence or absence of malignant tissue in the endocervical canal as obtained by fractional curettage should be precisely carried out. Care must be exercised during the curetting of the endocervical mucosa so as to obtain a specimen solely from that area and not from the lower part of the corpus or from tissue hanging into the isthmus from a primary corpus lesion. In addition, an estimate as to the location and size of the lesion within the endometrial cavity should be attempted.

One of the virulence factors for endometrial cancer is its degree of histologic dedifferentiation and this microscopic criterion must be recognized. The poorer differentiated cancers of the endometrium are related with deeper myometrial involvement and consequently greater chance of dissemination of disease outside of the uterus (Figs. 13-8 and 13-9). Not included in the staging classification is the depth of myometrial penetration by tumor which is determined by examining the uterus following hysterectomy. The gross uterine specimen should be inspected to locate the primary site of the tumor (Figs. 13-7 and 13-9). Endocervical, fundal, or cornua involvement carries special significance as to the possibility of lymph node involvement from pathways that vary according to the site of origin of the disease in the uterus.

Endometrial cancer may spread by direct extension to nearby structures through the wall of the uterus, as well as transcervically, transtubally, or possibly by spillage at the time of operation. Lymphatic spread is the primary method for the

Table 13–1. CLASSIFICATION AND STAGING OF CARCINOMA OF THE CORPUS UTERI

STAGE 0. Carcinoma in situ. Histologic findings suspicious of malignancy. Cases of Stage 0 should not be included in any therapeutic statistics.

STAGE I. The carcinoma is confined to the corpus.

STAGE Ia. The length of the uterine cavity is 8 cm or less.

STAGE Ib. The length of the uterine cavity is more than 8 cm.

The Stage I cases should be subgrouped with regard to the histologic type of the adenocarcinoma as follows:

G1. Highly differentiated adenomatous carcinoma.
G2. Differentiated adenomatous carcinoma with partly solid areas.

G3. Predominantly solid or entirely undifferentiated carcinoma.

STAGE II. The carcinoma has involved the corpus and the cervix, but has not extended outside the uterus.

STAGE III. The carcinoma has extended outside the uterus but not outside the true pelvis.

STAGE IV. The carcinoma has extended outside the true pelvis or has obviously involved the mucosa of the bladder or rectum. A bullous edema as such does not permit allotment of a case to Stage IV.

STAGE IVa. Spread of the growth to adjacent organs.

STAGE IVb. Spread to distant organs.

disease to extend outside the uterus but venous dissemination does occur (Fig. 13–10) and is of somewhat lesser significance. Plentl and Friedman state that "in general lymph flow from the uterine fundus travels upward in the direction of the adnexa and the infundibulopelvic ligament, while that from the lower and the middle portions of the corpus tends to move caudally in the direction of the base of the broad ligament toward the lateral pelvic wall."[25] The corpus uteri is drained by

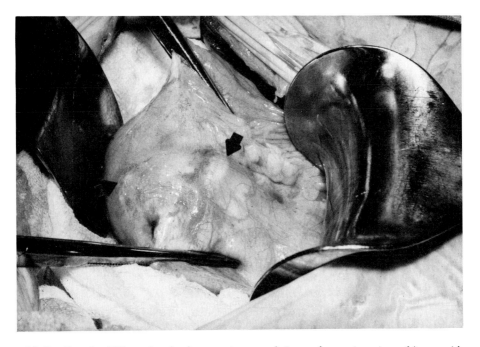

Figure 13–8. Poorly differentiated adenocarcinoma of the endometrium in a 64-year-old woman (stage IA, G3). The cancer has gone through the myometrium to the serosal surface in several areas.

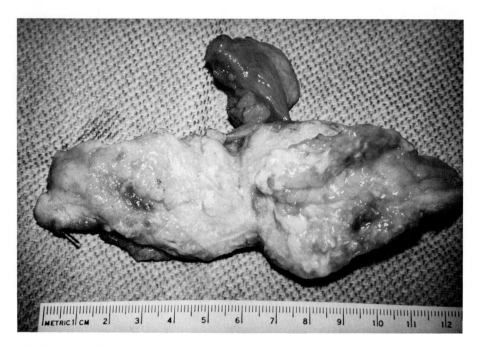

Figure 13–9. Opened uterus of Figure 13-8 exhibiting extensive endometrial involvement in a normal-size uterus.

four well-established channels. Their existence has been verified by all investigators in the field according to Plentl and Friedman. They include (1) channels draining the fundus uteri in company with the ovarian vessels to the aortic nodes (Figs. 13–11 to 13–14), (2) efferents utilizing the folds of the broad ligament, terminating in the interiliac nodes, (3) anastomotic channels along the mesosalpinx and fallopian tube, and (4) smaller lymphatics along the round ligament directed to-

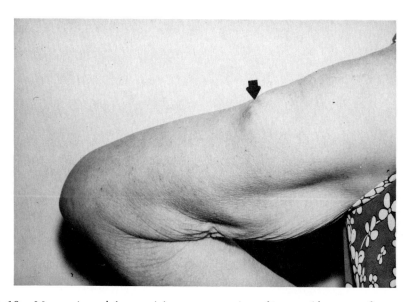

Figure 13–10. Metastatic nodules to right upper arm in a 61-year-old woman from a moderately differentiated endometrial adenocarcinoma (stage IA, G2) that had penetrated 80 percent of the myometrium.

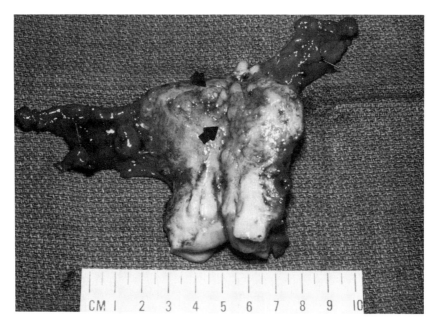

Figure 13–11. A normal-size uterus with a poorly differentiated adenocarcinoma of the endometrium. The main complaint of this 59-year-old postmenopausal woman was painless uterine bleeding.

ward the femoral regions. The primary regional nodes draining the corpus uteri are the aortic, the interiliac, and the femoral nodes. The first two may be regarded as the primary pathways.[25]

The clinical significance of the drainage channels and anastomosis of the corpus uteri is that by way of ovarian and tubal lymphatics, the primary efferent lymph easily reaches nodes outside of the pelvis (Figs. 13-11 to 13-14).[26]

The importance of these pathways of distribu-

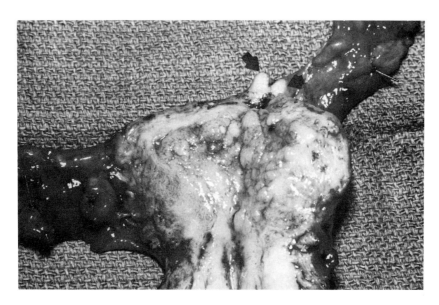

Figure 13–12. The same uterus as Figure 13-11 showing involvement of the left cornua with 20 percent myometrial invasion by cancer. The intramural and isthmic (arrows) portion of the left fallopian tube contains an extension of the endometrial cancer.

248

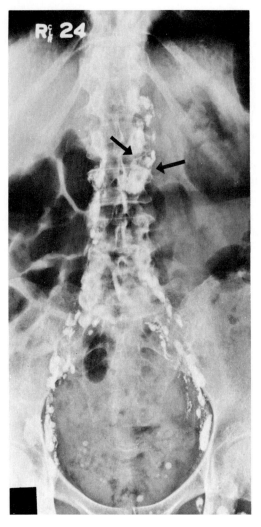

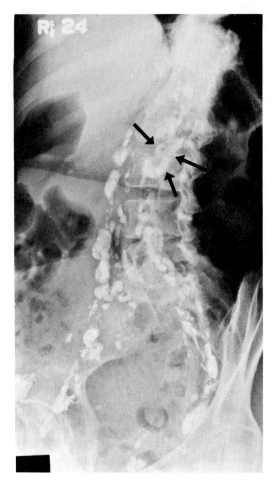

Figure 13-14. A left oblique 24-hour film of the same woman in Figures 13-11 to 13-13 displays metastatic disease seen as peripheral filling defects in slightly enlarged left para-aortic nodes at the level of L3.

Figure 13-13. A preoperative lymphangiogram was obtained on the woman in Figures 13-11 and 13-12. A roentgenogram obtained 24 hours after injection of the dye exhibits metastatic disease, seen as a defect in the left para-aortic lymph nodes (arrows).

tion of neoplasm is illustrated in Muelenaere's study of women dying after treatment of endometrial carcinoma. Women who had persistent malignant disease at the time of their death fell into four groups: (1) death due to tumor in the pelvis, 25 percent, (2) death due to spread of tumor to the abdominal cavity, 44 percent, (3) death due to hematogenous spread of tumor, 21 percent, and (4) death due to unrelated causes in the presence of nonlethal metastases, 10 percent. The deaths occurred despite the original clinical stage of endometrial carcinoma was thought to be stage I, disease confined to the corpus, in 73 percent of women.[27]

DIAGNOSIS

Endometrial carcinoma is essentially a disease of the menopausal and postmenopausal age groups. Postmenopausal uterine bleeding or perimenopausal abnormal bleeding are the almost universal complaints. A woman with postmenopausal uterine bleeding has endometrial cancer until proved otherwise (Figs. 13-7, 13-8, and 13-11). Procope, in a study of women with postmenopausal genital bleeding that occurred at least one year from their last menstruation, found the bleeding was due to a malignant process in the uterus in 28 percent of women. Atrophic endometrium was the cause of bleeding in 20.5 percent of the women, hormonal reaction in the endometrium in 18.5 percent, an endometrial or cervical polyp in 17.2 percent, cervicitis with erosion in 12.1 percent, and senile vaginitis in 1.3 percent.[28] Pyometria, an intrauterine collection of pus caused by interference with natural drainage of the uterus, was associated with coincident carcinoma in 15 percent of women in Whiteley and Hamlett's study. In 35 percent of their women with pyometria, it was caused by previous gynecologic surgery or radiotherapy.[29]

A postmenopausal woman with uterine bleeding should have a pelvic examination under anesthesia, the length of the uterine cavity determined, and fractional curettage of the uterus performed because of the high association with endometrial cancer in this type of patient. Asymptomatic women, particularly those at high risk for developing endometrial cancer, as well as those perimenopausal women with minimal irregular bleeding, should have their endometrial cavity studied. Earlier diagnosis of endometrial cancer in these types of patients is best accomplished by the use of a combination of cytologic and histologic techniques. Which technique is best for an individual patient will depend upon such factors as accuracy of pelvic examination as to size and position of the uterus, degree of cervical stenosis, the diameter of the cannula used to obtain endometrial samples, availability of experienced cytopathology personnel to interpret cytologic specimens, and awareness by physicians and patients alike that endometrial cancer can be detected early.

Endometrial cancer and its precursors exfoliate cells into the uterine cavity. The use of a small-diameter, flexible endometrial cannula for aspirating endometrial cells is the most simple, safe, inexpensive and reliable method for physicians to use in their offices to routinely screen asymptomatic women at high risk for endometrial cancer (Fig. 13-15). An accuracy of at least 85 to 90 percent for detection of endometrial carcinoma should be expected. The precision of determining the presence of precursors of adenocarcinoma of the corpus with the cytologic techniques is yet to be defined. The goal of detecting cytologic abnormalities years before histologic proof of endometrial cancer may not be universally attainable today. However, the detection of endometrial cancer cytologically before symptoms appear and consequently at an earlier stage of growth is possible. A practical advantage that the cannula used for endometrial cytologic aspirations has is that it is smaller in diameter than any currently available instrument being used to obtain histologic sampling of endometrial tissue.[30]

Histologic sampling of endometrial tissue can not only detect endometrial cancer in its early stages but also its precursors. These procedures may be carried out on an outpatient basis by use of a number of instruments. The oldest and still one of the most widely used histologic sampling methods is the endometrial aspiration biopsy (Fig.

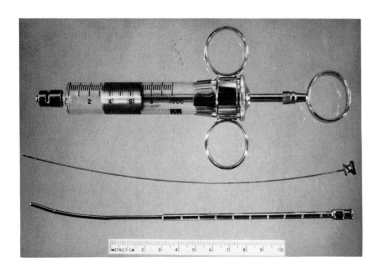

Figure 13–15. A Kleegman flexible endometrial cannula (outside diameter 2.4 mm) with stylet. A three-ring, B-D glass-barrelled aspiration syringe with metal plunger and sana-lok tip which attaches to the cannula to aspirate the cytologic specimen.

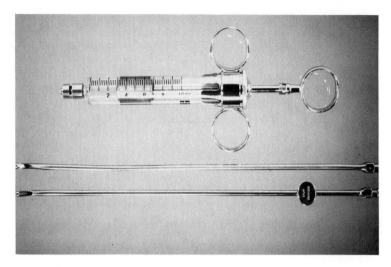

Figure 13–16. A Randall and a Novak endometrial biopsy instrument. The syringe aids in the suction curettage.

13-16).[31] This method utilizes one of several metal or plastic cannulas or curettes ranging in length from 15 to 20 cm and varying in diameter from 5 to 6 mm. For over 25 years, the range of accuracy for detection of endometrial cancer by office biopsy has been 75 to 90 percent. More recently, the concept of suction curettage has been applied in an attempt to make an early diagnosis of endometrial cancer.[32,33] One of these instruments, the Vabra aspirator, is a disposable suc-

tion curette for the endometrium which can be used in the office or outpatient clinic. The instrument has a steel tube 210 mm long and 3.004 mm in diameter. The tip is slightly curved with an opening 1.5 cm × 16 mm (Fig. 13-17). Walters and his group were able to complete the aspiration curettage in 89 percent of women in whom the procedure was attempted. The diagnosis was correct in 95.5 percent of the patients, as confirmed by conventional hospital curettage.[32] They

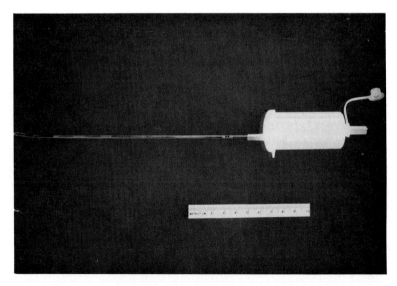

Figure 13–17. A Vabra disposable curette and aspiration cannula attached to a plastic chamber to collect the aspirate. The chamber is fitted with a filter to prevent the tissue from being withdrawn while the pump is exerting 50 to 60 cm Hg of vacuum.

believe the Vabra suction curettage should not be accepted as a definitive procedure in an enlarged uterus over eight weeks in size (whether fibroids are present or not), when scanty material is obtained and there is any question that the fundus has been completely and adequately explored, cervical stenosis prevents using the procedure, and during pregnancy. In addition, if bleeding continues and no satisfactory diagnosis is obtained on aspiration, a polyp may be present which may be too large for removal with the aspiration curette. In this situation, sharp curettage is indicated.[32]

If the procedures for cytologic or histologic screening for cancer can not be performed, inadequate samples are obtained, or the patient continues to be symptomatic a pelvic examination under anesthesia, determination of uterine size and a fractional curettage of the uterus must be performed. Endometrial cancer must be properly staged with the clinical classification based on physical findings and histologic confirmation of the disease.

Cytologic specimens obtained by cervical scraping, from the posterior vaginal fornix, or by cervical aspiration have an accuracy of less than 50 percent for detecting asymptomatic endometrial cancer (Fig. 13-6).

A patent cervical canal is necessary for endometrial cells to reach either the cervix or posterior vaginal pool. In older patients with vaginal atrophy and cervical stenosis, malignant endometrial cells may not appear in the vaginal pool. The cervical canal must be sounded prior to cytologic sampling in examination of older women. Endocervical aspiration is more accurate than posterior vaginal pool aspiration, with cervical scraping yielding the lowest accuracy of detecting endometrial cancer. The cells spontaneously desquamate to these three locations inconsistently and may be in a degenerative condition that only permits inaccurate interpretation.

More women with endometrial cancer will be found on cervical-vaginal cytosmears if the age of the patient and date of last menstral flow are correlated with the finding of not only malignant but benign endometrial cells in postmenopausal women or in the latter half of the menstral cycle for women over age 45.

With increased interest in establishing the earlier diagnosis of carcinoma, hysteroscopy and hysterography are being utilized to define tumor volume, location, and site of origin of the neoplasm. The ultimate value of these techniques will be determined when five-year follow-up statistics are available for comparison with presently available data on patients treated without these aids.[34,35]

PROGNOSIS

The prognosis for carcinoma of the endometrium depends upon the age of the patient, the general medical problems, stage of the tumor at the time of diagnosis, histologic dedifferentiation of the tumor, volume of tumor producing increased uterine size, and depth and location of myometrial penetration by tumor.[36-38]

Endometrial carcinoma seems to have a much worse prognosis as related to five-year survival after diagnosis in the older patient. The younger women are more apt to have a less advanced stage of their disease (Figs. 13-4 and 13-5) than individuals past 60 years (Figs. 13-8, 13-10 to 13-13).

If women with endometrial carcinoma also happen to be obese or hypertensive, these factors may have the same influence on decreasing the longevity of these patients as they would on individuals not harboring endometrial cancer. They could have a definite deleterious influence on prognosis by modifying the treatment in utiliza-

tion to less effective modalities of eradicating the disease and hence result in a poor survival.

Frick and associates clearly document that the stage of disease at the time of diagnosis influences prognosis with over a 70 percent five-year survival for disease confined to the corpus, 36 percent survival with cervical involvement, and 3 percent survival with widespread or stage IV disease.[36]

Another characteristic associated with virulence of endometrial cancer is the volume of tumor. This is crudely evaluated by clinical pelvic examination to approximate uterine size as well as the determination of depth of the uterine cavity. The uterus may be enlarged for reasons other than tumor bulk, such as with leiomyomas (Fig. 13-6), and for this reason is not as reliable a prognostic indicator as is grading or staging.

The majority of endometrial carcinomas are grade I or well-differentiated tumors and are confined to the corpus or stage I disease. Disregarding stage of lesion, grade I endometrial carcinomas can be expected to have an almost 80 percent five-year survival in contrast to grade III tumors composed of totally anaplastic cells, with no evidence of glandular patterns being associated with a poorer prognosis (30 percent five-year salvage). It appears that at the time of diagnosis, individuals with well-differentiated tumors are more apt to have their tumors in an earlier stage (Figs. 13-4 and 13-5).

The prognosis of the patient is adversely effected by the depth of myometrial penetration by tumor, which unfortunately cannot be accurately estimated prior to surgical excision of the uterus (Figs. 13-8 and 13-9). The usefulness of this factor to assay the virulence of the tumor is at times obscured by treatment regimens involving preoperative irradiation. The five-year survival in

Fricks' study of women who had no disease in the hysterectomy specimen due to either curettage or preoperative radium was 91.6 percent and for women who had deep penetration, over two-thirds of the uterus, the survival rate was one-half (45.2 percent) of that with no disease in the specimen.[36] Grades 2 and 3 endometrial cancers are more apt to occur in lesions with deeper myometrial penetration of tumor (Figs. 13-11 to 13-14).

Each of these prognostic factors provides an index of probability that the endometrial cancer has spread beyond the uterus. The risk of metastases significantly increases with extensive myometrial invasion, loss of histologic differentiation, and extension to the isthmus of the cervix or the intramural part of the fallopian tube.

TREATMENT

The successful treatment of carcinoma of the endometrium is, of course, better accomplished when the disease is discovered in its earliest stages, or preferable during its precursor stage of growth (Fig. 13-2). The foundation for proper treatment planning and consequently, appropriate treatment is based upon integrated application of the prognostic variables to the particular woman with endometrial cancer.

The object of treatment is to reduce morbidity as low as possible for that particular woman with endometrial carcinoma and to cure her of her disease. Any therapeutic regimen must recognize that most of these women with disease are over the age of 50 and commonly have medical disorders such as diabetes, hypertension, and other degenerative disorders normally found in this age group, all of which can take their toll before the disease does so. Not only from the standpoint of reduction of morbidity but from a cost-effectiveness standpoint, a woman with endometrial cancer should not be overtreated. She should also not be undertreated because the death process resulting from endometrial cancer can be an extended one.

During treatment planning the laboratory investigation should at the minimum include a complete blood count with differential and platelet count, urea nitrogen, creatinine, bilirubin, alkaline phosphatase, lactic dehydrogenase (LDH), and glutamic-oxaloacetic acid transaminase (SGOT). A clean midstream voided urine for urinalysis and microscopic examination

should also be included with optional procedures, such as cystoscopy and sigmoidoscopy, being done on an individual basis. Roentgenographic studies of the chest, kidneys, ureters and bladder, colon and sigmoid should also be included. For lesions known to be moderately to poorly differentiated with suspected fundal or cornual uterine involvement or known endocervical involvement, lymphangiography is currently more commonly being utilized before definitive therapy to better evaluate lymph node metastases in the pelvis and para-aortic region (Figs. 13-11 to 13-14).

Stage I

Stage IA, Grade I

A uterus that is small or normal in size with a well-differentiated endometrial adenocarcinoma not involving the cervix can be treated by primary hysterectomy and bilateral salpingo-oophorectomy. If pathologic inspection of the uterus determines that the disease is in fact confined in a small- to normal-size uterus, is well differentiated with no endocervical or cervical involvement, and there is no more than one-third of the myometrium penetrated with disease, no further therapy seems indicated (Figs. 13-4 and 13-5).[39]

Since clinical stage I patients are usually subjected to hysterectomy at some time during their treatment, initial hysterectomy with surgical and pathologic staging may permit more concise evaluation of the various prognostic parameters and serve as a guide for therapeutic decision.[40]

Stage IA, Grade II and Grade III and Stage IB, All Grades

The conventional treatment for endometrial adenocarcinoma that is less than a well-differentiated tumor has been the utilization of preoperative or postoperative radium or external pelvic irradiation and hysterectomy.[41-43] The time interval from the end of radiation to hysterectomy has been shortened and usually takes place no more than two weeks following radiation, so as to permit a better pathologic examination of the uterus.[42]

These poorer differentiated lesions are commonly associated with deep myometrial penetration of disease, and if over two-thirds of the myometrium is involved, will require pelvic radiation therapy and radiation therapy to the para-aortic node area, if the deep penetration of disease is located in the fundal or cornual area of the uterus (Figs. 13-11 to 13-14).

It becomes increasingly clinically evident that of all the prognostic variables for endometrial cancer, the depth of penetration of the disease into the myometrium is one of the most if not the most significant factor associated with increased probability of metastatic disease to pelvic and para-aortic lymph nodes. The determination of the depth of involvement and its location in the uterus is made more difficult and at times impossible by the use of preoperative intracavitary and vaginal radium or external pelvic radiation therapy. Current clinical investigation is being carried out on the use of primary abdominal hysterectomy, bilateral salpingo-oophorectomy, and selective pelvic and para-aortic lymphadenectomy for women with stage I and early stage II endometrial cancer. Patients with stage I endometrial cancer and stage II occult (microscopic evidence of cervical involvement but no gross clinical involvement) and all grades of differentiation who are found on pathologic examination of the uterus to have 50 percent myometrial involvement or positive pelvic and/or para-aortic lymph nodes will undergo external radiation therapy (Figs. 13-8 and 13-9). The benefits of primary surgical and pathologic staging of endometrial cancer are that many patients who have in the past been routinely given preoperative radium or external radiation therapy may in reality not need such therapy, as

the disease is only superficial in the endometrium with no nodal involvement (Figs. 13-6 and 13-7). Also for those women with specific areas of deep myometrial involvement, pelvic irradiation may commonly be inadequate and para-aortic radiation required (Figs 13-11 to 13-14).

Stage II

Approximately 6 to 15 percent of all cases of endometrial carcinoma will be of stage II, with at least a 22 percent incidence of positive lymph nodes.[44,45] The greater volume of tumor (corpus

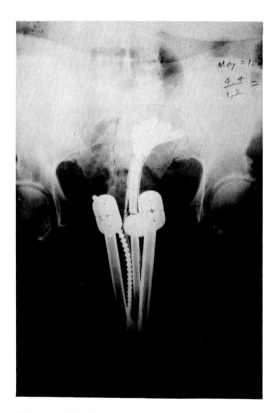

Figure 13-18. A 71-year-old woman with moderately differentiated adenocarcinoma of the endometrium and cervix (stage II) in whom 10 medium-size Heyman intrauterine radium capsules and Fletcher-Suit uterine tandem and vaginal ovoids are in place. The tandem and ovoids contain radium. The chain that is located in the rectum and the radiopaque dye in the bulb of the catheter at the trigone of the bladder are seen. The latter two are used as markers to calculate the quantity of radiation to the rectum and bladder respectively.

and cervix) in stage II probably accounts for some of the increased risk of lymphatic penetration of tumor. Primary surgical treatment should include a radical abdominal hysterectomy and pelvic lymphadenectomy with selective para-aortic lymph node sampling. Another treatment regimen would include the use of intracavitary and vaginal radium (Fig. 13–18) plus external radiation therapy to the pelvis followed by hysterectomy.[44,45] Deep penetration of disease into the fundal or cornual area of the uterus or positive para-aortic nodes suggests the need of para-aortic irradiation.

Stage III

Approximately 10 percent of all women with endometrial carcinoma have stage III (the carcinoma has extended outside the uterus but not outside the true pelvis) disease at the time of diagnosis.

Antoniades et al have identified three main patterns of tumor extension in stage III disease: (1) lateral into the parametrium and the pelvic wall which has the poorest prognosis and comprises more than 50 percent of all cases, (2) downward into the vagina or the vagina and the cervix, and (3) to the ovaries. Ovarian extension has the best prognosis when treated by abdominal hysterectomy and bilateral salpingo-oophorectomy followed by postoperative radiotherapy. Extension to the vagina or to the vagina and the cervix can be treated successfully by a combination of external beam and local radium placements.[46]

Stage IV

Endometrial cancer that has extended outside the true pelvis or has obviously involved the mucosa of the bladder or rectum makes up approximately 3 percent of all stages. Treatment must be individualized but is usually treated with external radiation therapy. Also in this stage of disease usually following radiation therapy, progestational therapy may be utilized. An oral active synthetic progestin, megestrol acetate, is being evaluated for this stage of disease with melphalan and 5-fluorouracil or megestrol acetate combined with adriamycin, cytoxan, and 5-fluorouracil.[47,48]

Residual or Recurrent Disease

Hydroxyprogesterone caproate may be utilized in the dosage of approximately 1 gm a week intramuscularly for those women with progressing advanced adenocarcinoma of the uterine corpus no longer responding to established anticancer measures.[48,49] The best responders are those women with slowly growing tumors that have had a prolonged interval between initial treatment and recurrence.[50] Also, an oral synthetic, progestin megestrol acetate, may be administered in these types of patients.[47] For nonresponders to the single-agent progestins, the three- to four-drug regimen as mentioned for treatment in stage IV disease may be considered.

SURVIVAL

Most women with endometrial carcinoma today are thought to be in an early clinical stage of a slowly growing disease, and as such are treated by hysterectomy and bilateral salpingo-oophorectomy with or without accompanying irradiation therapy. Yet even today, if all stages of endometrial carcinoma are considered, one out of five women will die from the disease. A very significant proportion of endometrial carcinomas are small in size, well-differentiated lesions with minimal to no penetration into the myometrium (stage IA, GI) and will be associated with over a 90 percent five-year survival free of disease.[39]

If a patient with endometrial cancer survives to the seventh year following treatment without clinical evidence of recurrence, she is unlikely to die of uterine cancer or its sequelae. Monson et al further have observed the conventional five-year survival rate as a reasonable measure of the likelihood of cure of endometrial cancer, since deaths prior to the fifth anniversary encompass approximately 92 percent of the total deaths likely to occur as a result of the cancer.[51]

In stage II endometrial adenocarcinoma, both gross and occult cervical involvement have a relatively bad prognosis and require aggressive therapy, with a survival of 36 to 55 percent at five years.[36,44,45] Stage III endometrial carcinoma has a 25 to 44 percent five-year survival,[36,46] and stage IV, 0 to 3 percent five-year survival.[36]

The survival for histologic types of carcinoma of the endometrium other than adenocarcinoma varies somewhat. Kurman and Scully noted the clinical profile of women with clear cell carcinoma of the endometrium closely parallels that of women with the usual types of carcinoma of the endometrium. The actuarial survival for all stages is about 55 percent at five years, which is somewhat lower than that of adenocarcinoma of the endometrium in general.[52] Silverberg et al observed that the ability of a well-differentiated endometrial carcinoma to form histologically benign squamous elements (adenoacanthoma) seems to improve a prognosis that is already relatively favorable. They found an actuarial five-year survival of 82.9 percent for adenoacanthomas. They also established that the poorly differentiated (i.e., histologically malignant) squamous elements in mixed adenosquamous carcinoma of the endometrium are a function of poorly differentiated glandular elements and are associated with an unfavorable prognosis resulting in approximately a 35 percent actuarial five-year survival.[53] Julian et al, in their study of "mixed" cancers of the endometrium, discovered little prognostic difference between very poorly differentiated endo-

metrial cancer, adenoepidermoid carcinoma, or adenosquamous carcinoma of the endometrium. In their series, they have the same distribution of five-year survival rates and the same degree of myometrial extension, and seem to respond in the same way to therapy.[54]

Although not necessarily contributing to an enhanced survival, there has been an unquestioned reduction to almost a complete absence of vaginal recurrences following preoperative radiation and hysterectomy in early disease.

The successful treatment of endometrial carcinoma is dependent upon the close cooperation of the already identified health care delivery team members and bringing together the known generalities of endometrial carcinoma to the needs of the specific patient. It cannot be overstressed that earlier diagnosis is associated with better survival and this means more frequent sampling of the endometrium (Figs. 13–15 to 13–17) of those women at risk for developing endometrial cancer. Endometrial cancer is a surface lesion (Figs. 13–5, 13–7, 13–9, and 13–11) in the accessible uterine cavity and amenable to early diagnosis.

References

1. Cramer DW, Cutler SJ, Christine B: Trends in the incidence of endometrial cancer in the United States. Gynec Oncol 2:130, 1974

2. Lyon JL, Gardner JW: The rising frequency of hysterectomy: Its effect on uterine cancer rates. Am J Epidemiol 104:439, 1977

3. Cancer Facts and Figures. American Cancer Society, 1978

4. Cramer DW, Cutler SJ: Incidence and histopathology of malignancies of the female genital organs in the United States. Am J Obstet & Gynec 118:443, 1974

5. Gurpide E, Tseng L: Factors controlling intracellular levels of estrogens in human endometrium. Gynec Oncol 2:221, 1974

6. Siiteri PK, Schwarz BE, MacDonald PC: Estrogen receptors and the estrone hypothesis in relation to endometrial and breast cancer. Gynec Oncol 2:228, 1974

7. MacDonald PC, Siiteri PK: The relationship between the extraglandular production of estrone and the occurrence of endometrial neoplasia. Gynec Oncol 2:259, 1974

8. Rao BR, Wiest WG: Receptors for progesterone. Gynec Oncol 2:239, 1974

9. MacMahon B: Risk factors for endometrial cancer. Gynec Oncol 2:122, 1974

10. Gusberg SB: The individual at high risk for endometrial carcinoma. Am J Obstet Gynec 126:535, 1976

11. Brown R: Carbohydrate metabolism in patients with endometrial carcinoma. J Obstet Gynaec Brit Common 81:940, 1974

12. Chamlian DL, Taylor HB: Endometrial hyperplasia in young women. Obstet Gynec 36:659, 1970

13. Winkelstein W, Sacks ST, Ernster VL, Selvin S. Correlations of incidence rates for selected cancers in the nine areas of the third national cancer survery. Am J Epidemiol 105:407, 1977

14. Gray LA, Christopherson WM, Hoover RN: Estrogens and endometrial carcinoma. Obstet Gynec 49:385, 1977

15. McDonald TW, Annegers JF, O'Fallon WM, et al: Exogenous estrogen and endometrial carcinoma: Case-control and inci-

dence study. Am J Obstet Gynec 127:572, 1977

16. Estrogens and endometrial cancer. FDA Drug Bulletin 6:18, 1976
17. Lyon FA: The development of adenocarcinoma of the endometrium in young women receiving long-term sequential oral contraception. Am J Obstet Gynec 123:299, 1975
18. Silverberg SG, Makowski EL, Roche WD: Endometrial carcinoma in women under 40 years of age. Cancer 39:592, 1977
19. Sequential oral contraceptives removed from the market. FDA Drug Bulletin. 6:26, 1976
20. Kelley HW, Miles PA, Buster JE, Scragg WH: Adenocarcinoma of the endometrium in women taking sequential oral contraceptives. Obstet Gynec 47:200, 1976
21. Cohen CJ, Deppe G: Endometrial carcinoma and oral contraceptives agents. Obstet Gynec 49:390, 1977
22. Roberts G, Wells AL: Oestrogen-induced endometrial carcinoma in a patient with gonadal dysgenesis. Brit J Obstet Gynaecol 82:417, 1975
23. McCarroll AM, Montgomery DA, Harley JM, McKeown EF, MacHenry JC: Endometrial carcinoma after cyclical Oestrogen-progestogen therapy for Turner's syndrome. Brit J Obstet Gynaecol 82:421, 1975
24. International Federation of Gynaecology and Obstetrics classification and staging of malignant tumors in the female pelvis. Internat J Gynaecol Obstet 9:172, 1971
25. Plentl AA, Friedman EA: Lymphatic System of the Female Genitalia. Saunders, Philadelphia, 1971
26. Henriksen E: The lymphatic dissemination in endometrial carcinoma. Am J Obstet Gynec 123:570, 1975
27. Muelenaere GF: The distribution of neoplasm in patients dying after treatment of endometrial carcinoma. Brit J Obstet Gynaecol 83:576, 1976
28. Procope B: Aetiology of postmenopausal bleeding. Acta Obstet Gynec Scand 50: 311, 1971
29. Whiteley PF, Hamlett JD: Pyometra—A reappraisal. Am J Obstet Gynec 109:108, 1971
30. McGowan L: Cytologic methods for the detection of endometrial cancer. Gynec Oncol 2:272, 1974

31. Creasman WT, Weed JC: Screening techniques in endometrial cancer. Cancer 38: 436, 1976
32. Walters D, Robinson D, Park RC, Patow WE: Diagnostic outpatient aspiration curettage. Obstet Gynec 46:160, 1975
33. Cohen CJ, Gusberg SB, Koffler D: Histologic screening for endometrial cancer. Gynec Oncol 2:279, 1974
34. Anderson B, Marchant DJ, Munzenrider JE, Moore JP, Mitchell GW: Routine noninvasive hysterography in the evaluation and treatment of endometrial carcinoma. 4:354, 1976
35. Wallace S, Jing BS, Medellin H: Endometrial carcinoma: Radiologic assistance in diagnosis, staging, and management. Gynec Oncol 2:287, 1974
36. Frick HC, Munnell EW, Richart RM, Berger AP, Lawry MF: Carcinoma of the endometrium. Am J Obstet Gynec 115: 663, 1973
37. Boronow RC: Endometrial cancer—Not a benign disease. Obstet Gynec 47:630, 1976
38. Nolan JF, Morrow CP, Anson J: Factors influencing prognosis. Gynecol Oncol 2: 300, 1974
39. Keller D, Kempson RL, Levine G, McLennan C: Management of the patient with early endometrial carcinoma. Cancer 33: 1108, 1974
40. Lewis GC, Mortel R, Slack NH: Endometrial cancer. Cancer 39:959, 1977
41. Onsrud M, Kolstad P, Normann T: Postoperative external pelvic irradiation in carcinoma of the corpus stage I: A controlled clinical trial. Gynec Oncol 4:222, 1976
42. Underwood PB, Lutz MH, Kreutner A, Miller MC, Johnson RB: Carcinoma of the endometrium: Radiation followed immediately by operation. Am J Obstet Gynec 128:86, 1977
43. Gusberg SB: The evolution of modern treatment of corpus cancer. Cancer 38: 603, 1976
44. Antoniades J, Mortel R, Lewis GC, et al: The management of carcinoma involving the cervix and body of the uterus. Obstet Gynec 42:208, 1973
45. Homesley HD, Boronow RC, Lewis JL: Stage II endometrial adenocarcinoma. Obstet Gynec 49:604, 1977
46. Antoniades J, Brady LW, Lewis GC: The management of stage III carcinoma of the

endometrium. Cancer 38:1838, 1976

47. Wait RB: Megestrol acetate in the management of advanced endometrial carcinoma. Obstet Gynec 41:129, 1973

48. Joelsson I (ed): The effect of gestagens in the treatment of carcinoma of the uterine corpus. Acta Obstet Gynec Scand 19s:1, 1972

49. Moe N: Short-term progestogen treatment of endometrial carcinoma. Acta Obstet Gynec Scand 51:55, 1972

50. Kohorn EI: Gestagens and endometrial carcinoma. Gynec Oncol 4:398, 1976

51. Monson RR, MacMahon B, Austin JH: When may endometrial cancer be considered cured? Cancer 30:419, 1972

52. Kurman RJ, Scully RE: Clear cell carcinoma of the endometrium. Cancer 37:872, 1976

53. Silverberg SG, Bolin MG, DeGiorgi LS: Adenoacanthoma and mixed adenosquamous carcinoma of the endometrium. Cancer 30:1307, 1972

54. Julian CG, Daikoku NH, Gillespie A: Adenoepidermoid and adenosquamous carcinoma of the uterus. Am J Obstet Gynec 128:106, 1977

Chapter 14

Radiotherapy Treatment of Endometrial Cancer

JOHN G. MAIER, M.D., Ph.D.

Adenocarcinoma of the lining cells of the uterus is the most common gynecologic malignancy seen in the United States today. About two-thirds of patients are postmenopausal, with the remaining patients being in the climacteric years. Patients with this disease are characterized by obesity, hypertension, diabetes mellitus, and low fertility.

They present with vaginal bleeding following menopause or give a past history of irregular bleeding with periods of amenorrhea and late menarche. There may be a history of endometrial or cervical polyps, endometrial hyperplasia, or endometrial cancer in the family.

NATURAL HISTORY AND ROUTES OF SPREAD

Clinical investigations show that about 70 percent of women developing adenocarcinoma of the endometrium will have such tumors confined to the body of the uterus (International Federation of Gynecologists and Obstetricians [FIGO] stage I) on initial presentation (Table 13–1). Another 15 percent will have extension into the endocervix with so-called Corpus et Colli lesion (FIGO, stage II). The importance of fractional dilatation and curettage for proper staging has been stressed. In 10 percent of patients, there will be extension outside the uterus to include the parametrium and vagina, but remaining within the pelvis (FIGO, stage III). Only 5 percent of patients will present clinically with tumor extending beyond the pelvis or with involvement of the mucosa of the bladder or rectum.

The true incidence of lymphatic metastases is not entirely clear. Metastases to pelvic structures such as ovaries, fallopian tubes, and peritoneal surfaces of the pelvic cavity have been reported as 7 percent by Fletcher.[1] In only 1 of 66 lymphadenectomies were nodes found to contain cancer in the pelvis, whereas 6 patients had positive lumbar para-aortic nodes. LeFevre[2] reviewed the literature and found that of 246 patients with endometrial cancer subject to lymph node dissection, 48 (20 percent) showed node metastases and these involved the obturator, hypogastric, and iliac nodes. Barber and Brunschwig[3] reported positive nodes in 14 percent of 93 patients undergoing lymphadenectomy. More recently, Boronow et al[4] reported a series of 74 patients undergoing pelvic lymphadenectomy and lumbar para-aortic nodal sampling. There were 10 patients, or 13.5 percent with metastatic pelvic nodes. In these 10 patients, 6 also had positive para-aortic nodal metastases. For stage I grade I lesions, only 3 percent had metastatic pelvic nodes and in grade 2 lesions, 11 percent had metastatic pelvic nodes.

The relatively high incidence of involvement of the lumbar para-aortic nodes as compared to involvement of the regional lymphatics in the M.D. Anderson series[1] can be explained on the basis of primary lymphatics of the corpus, particularly the fundus and cornual regions, draining upward via the infundibulopelvic ligament. Thus, the first group of nodes encountered are the common iliac, lumbar, and para-aortic clusters. Involvement of pelvic structures can be explained by tumor invading the myometrium and spreading through the serosa and/or through the fallopian tubes to the abdominal cavity. With involvement of the lower uterine segment or endocervix, lymphatic drainage becomes similar to primary carcinoma of the cervix with involvement of pelvic lymph nodes to include the obturator, hypogastric, and iliac nodes. Morrow et al[5] reported a 10.6 percent incidence of pelvic lymph node metastases in a combined series of 369 patients with FIGO stage I corpus cancer. In stage II, the incidence was 36.5 percent in 85 patients studied.

TREATMENT

The traditional treatment of corpus cancer by hysterectomy has been relatively successful and met with little challenge until the early reports from the Radiumhemmet by Heyman[6,7] and later by Kottmeier.[8,9] Almost 50 years ago, Heyman[6] reported a 60 percent five-year survival for the technically operable (medically inoperable) group of patients with corpus cancer who were treated by radiotherapy, and an absolute survival of 43.5 percent for all patients treated by radiotherapy. More recently Landgren et al[10] reported a 68 percent five-year survival for stage I and II medically inoperable patients treated primarily by radiotherapy. A comparative study of these two modalities of treatment with comparable patients has yet to be carried out. However, the success of each of these methods of treatment has led to the concept that a combination of both would lead to improvement. In considering the appropriate treatment for corpus cancer, certain factors must be taken into consideration as follows.

1. Operability
    a) Medical inoperability
    b) Medical factors limiting radical surgery
    c) Technical inoperability due to extent of disease
2. Extension of tumor beyond endometrium
    a) Myometrial or serosal extension
    b) Endocervical involvement
    c) Parametrial invasion
    d) Pelvic lymph node metastases
    e) Para-aortic lymph node metastases
    f) Local invasion of bladder or rectum
    g) Distant metastases
3. Histologic grading
4. Uterine enlargement

First, a consideration will be given to those patients in which surgery is feasible.

Treatment for Medically and Technically Operable Patients

For several decades, it seemed clear that patients treated by hysterectomy faired better than those treated by *radium alone* and hysterectomy was the treatment of choice for endometrial adenocarcinoma confined to the body of the uterus. No increase in salvage rate has been evident when radical hysterectomy combined with pelvic lymphadenectomy has been employed in an unselective manner for stage I disease.[11] Furthermore, these patients are older, more obese, and more subject to a variety of medical problems. Such medical and geriatric considerations increase the risk of radical surgery.

What then is the role of radiotherapy in stage I disease? In answer to this, one might ask another question. What are the results by surgery alone and does adjunctive radiotherapy improve those results? Unfortunately, the answer to this latter question is not too clear. No series is available where parallel cases with regard to myometrial invasion, uterine size, and histologic grade have been randomized prospectively to receive surgery with or without adjunctive radiotherapy. The evidence for the value of adjunctive radiotherapy is somewhat indirect. After hysterectomy alone, the incidence of vaginal persistance or recurrent tumor has been summarized by Moss et al[12] to be between 10 to 15 percent. In 740 patients undergoing surgery alone, there were 87 such recurrences, whereas in 755 patients having preoperative irradiation, there were only 16 recurrences. Once a recurrence has developed, the chance of cure is only 20 to 25 percent by irradiation and seldom if ever by surgery. In spite of the apparant limited nature of some vaginal recurrences, most are usually one manifestation of widespread disease.

Perhaps an even more compelling reason for combining irradiation with surgery is the fact that the cure rate in stage I disease limited to the uterus is not 100 percent. In 3025 stage I patients reported by Kottmeier[9] in the Annual Report in 1973, the five-year survival rate was only 70 percent. In a more recent contemporary summary by Boronow et al,[13] the survival was 76 percent for 1860 patients with stage I disease. The results in individual series ranged from 71 to 86 percent. In a recent publication by Landgren et al,[10] the actuarial survival in a series of 86 medically inoperable stage I patients treated by radiotherapy alone was 78 percent.

Another point of interest is the local microscopic sterilization of tumor in the uterus by preoperative radium or external irradiation which has been reported in between 40 and 70 percent of resected uteri.[14] A time lapse of three to six weeks is needed following irradiation to observe such results. Uteri resected before this time lapse following irradiation may still show seemingly viable tumor cells that have not had adequate time to divide and die.

Based on the above discussion, the following treatment plans are recommended for the various clinical situations:

FIGO Stage IA G1(Normal-size uterus—cavity 8 cm or less on sounding, tumor well differentiated) (Table 13–1)

Surgery alone in form of abdominal hysterectomy and bilateral salpingo-oophorectomy with removal of wide vaginal cuff is recommended. Under these circumstances, the incidence of vaginal recurrences is low and either pre- or postoperative irradiation has not been shown to improve survival.

FIGO Stage IA G2, IB G1, or G2 (Uterus normal size, moderately differentiated [IA G2] tissue, or enlarged uterus [IB G1] either well or moderately well differentiated histology IB G2)

Preoperative vaginal and uterine radium or preoperative whole pelvic irradiation is recommended. This is to be followed by abdominal hysterectomy and bilateral salpingo-oophorectomy with removal of wide vaginal cuff in two to six weeks after completion of irradiation. There is no clear cut superiority of either radium or external irradiation from the data available for analysis. Both

are effective in reducing the vaginal recurrence rate. Radium can be administered more rapidly over three to four days, whereas external irradiation requires five to six weeks. Some institutions have done subsequent surgery in three to seven days following intracavitary radium application with minimal complications. In general, radium applications show a higher rate of local sterilization of the endometrial cancer on subsequent histologic examination than external irradiation.[15,16] However, the dose to the lateral pelvic lymph nodes is minimal and external irradiation can be expected to sterilize occult cell metastases in lymph nodes in a certain number of patients.

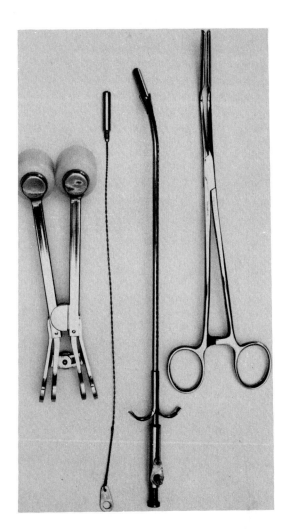

Figure 14–1. Heymans capsules with inserters and Fletcher-Suit afterloading vaginal ovoids.

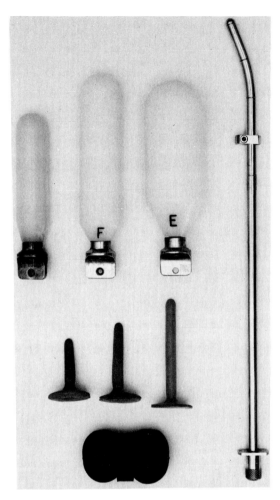

Figure 14–2. Burnett vaginal applicator (top ×3), afterloading Fletcher-Suit uterine tandem (right), Manchester tandems (×3) and ovoids (bottom).

In utilizing radium or radium substitutes, Heymans[7] capsules are preferred for packing the uterus as shown in Figures 14–1 and 14–2. In most instances, the number 2 capsule has been employed with 10 mg of radium or equivalent with [137]Cesium. As a rule of thumb, a minimum of five number 2 capsules must be loaded with the last capsule being located in the endocervical canal. Fletcher-Suit afterloading vaginal ovoids are placed in the lateral fornices. In most instances, only one application is performed and the radium in the uterus is given 4000 to 6000 mg hr. The radium in the vaginal ovoids remains in position

to give a dose of 5000 to 7000 rad at the lateral surface of the ovoids. Vaginal cylinders or other devices to irradiate the lower vagina have not been employed in our institution since recurrences in the vagina in our clinical experience have been located in the vaginal apex or upper one-half of the residual vagina. If two applications are planned, only 2500 to 3000 mg hr to the uterus and 4000 rad surface dose to the lateral vaginal wall are administered per application. The two applications are separated by a three-week interval. Although we have occasionally utilized two applications for patients with enlarged uteri to reduce the bulk of the tumor by fractionating the dose, in most instances only one application is employed and subsequent surgery not delayed. Since the larger uteri are associated with an increased incidence of lymph node metastases, it would seem that external irradiation is preferable. When employing external irradiation, a minimum dose of 5000 rad is administered in five to six weeks with supervoltage therapy. A four-field box technique is quite satisfactory for ^{60}Co teletherapy or 4-6MV Linear Accelerator therapy. A composite isodose curve is shown for 4MV and 10MV photons in Figures 14–3 and 14–4. A daily fraction of 180 to 200 rad at the midplane of the pelvis is administered five times each week. The superior margin of the pelvic field is the superior aspect of the fifth lumbar vertebra. The lower margin is the mid- or lower portion of the obturator foramina. The lateral margins include at least 1 cm margin of the bony pelvic inlet. For the average-sized patient, the anterior field will measure 16 × 16 cm and the lateral field 10 × 16 cm. It is preferable to treat all four fields daily.

FIGO Stage IA or IB G3 (Either normal or enlarged uterus with predominantly solid or entirely undifferentiated carcinoma)

For anaplastic or undifferentiated grade 3 adenocarcinoma, external irradiation preoperatively is recommended because of the increased incidence of pelvic and lumbar para-aortic nodal metastases. Boronow, et al[4] reported a 38 percent incidence of metastatic pelvic lymph nodes in stage I grade 3 lesions. Lymphangiograms are recommended. A minimal dose of 5000 rad in five to six weeks is given to the midplane of the pelvis as described above. Vaginal and uterine radium in addition to external irradiation is optional, but if employed, the external beam dose must be reduced accordingly.

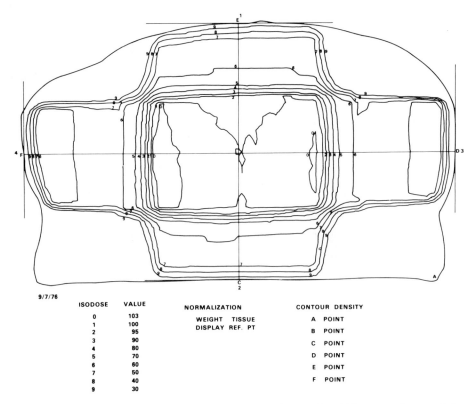

9/7/76

ISODOSE	VALUE	NORMALIZATION	CONTOUR DENSITY	
0	103		A	POINT
1	100	WEIGHT TISSUE		
2	95	DISPLAY REF. PT	B	POINT
3	90			
4	80		C	POINT
5	70		D	POINT
6	60			
7	50		E	POINT
8	40			
9	30		F	POINT

Figure 14–3. Four-field pelvic composite isodose distribution for 4MV x-ray beam of linear accelerator.

FIGO Stage II (Endocervical involvement)

When there is either subclinical microscopic involvement of the cervix or gross clinical extension, the likelihood of pelvic lymph node metastases increases substantially. However, the true incidence of this happening is far from being clearly established. Nevertheless, any form of treatment must take this into account. There are three feasible alternatives to treatment that include primary treatment by irradiation, primary treatment by radical hysterectomy with pelvic lymphadenectomy, and a combination of preoperative irradiation with abdominal hysterectomy and bilateral salpingo-oophorectomy. The data in the literature does not indicate a clear choice of one over the other. At the present time the Gynecologic Oncology Group, which is a National Multidisciplinary Cooperative Group, is doing a randomized prospective study in an effort to determine which of these three methods is most appropriate. However, it will be some time before this study is completed. When irradiation is given alone, the protocol calls for 5000 rad to the pelvis plus intracavitary irradiation with tan-

dem and ovoids, sequentially, with a dose of 3500 rad specified to point A (a point in the pelvis located 2 cm superiorly and 2 cm laterally to the external os). When abdominal hysterectomy and bilateral salpingo-oophorectomy is employed following irradiation, the external beam dose to the midline of the pelvis is blocked after 4000 rad.

Treatment for Medically Operable but Technically Inoperable Patients

FIGO Stage III (Tumor has extended outside the uterus, but not outside the pelvis)

Patients with stage III disease should be treated primarily by irradiation and are considered technically inoperable. In most instances, external irradiation to the pelvis followed by intracavitary irradiation is preferred. When radium is not feasible because of mechanical reasons, field size reductions are recommended after 5000 rad from 15-×-15-cm fields to 12-×-12-cm fields and again after 6000 rad to a 10-×-10-cm field. Seldom is it

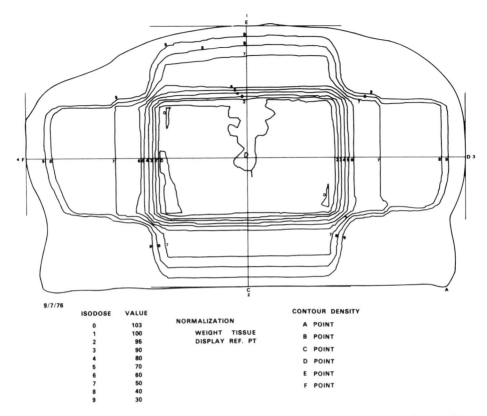

Figure 14–4. Four-field pelvic composite isodose distribution for 10MV x-ray beam of linear accelerator.

advisable to carry the total dose beyond 7000 rad in seven to eight weeks even with reduced volumes. Landgren et al[10] have reported a 26 percent actuarial survival at 5 and 10 years in stage III lesions. In many cases, external irradiation seem to be very effective in controlling parametrial or pelvic wall disease, whereas external irradiation or external irradiation in combination with diminished doses from radium fails to control central disease. There is a tendency to use external irradiation when the disease mass is large, but it appears that intracavitary radium applications remain superior to high doses of external irradiation in sterilizing uterine and vaginal disease. When external irradiation is required to treat peripheral pelvic disease, it should be supplemented with one or more radium applications if at all feasible.

FIGO Stage IV (Tumor has extended outside the true pelvis or has obviously involved the mucosa of the bladder or rectum) (Table 13–1)

Even when tumor has extended into the bladder or rectum, a few patients may be salvaged by aggressive irradiation with an acceptable complication rate. Patients are treated as in stage III to normal tissue tolerance doses. Progestins may be helpful in about one-third of patients and may be used in conjunction with irradiation. Relatively little information is available regarding utilization of other chemotherapeutic agents.

Treatment for Medically Inoperable Patients

The decision as to medical operability is somewhat arbitrary and varies somewhat in different institutions. The common criteria for inoperability in patients with endometrial carcinoma include significant obesity, severe hypertension, cardiac disease, severe diabetes mellitus, and advancing age. The efficacy of primary treatment by irradiation in patients with endometrial carcinoma was firmly established by Heyman in 1947,[7] in a series of patients who were technically operable but medically inoperable. In this series of 279 such patients, a 48 percent absolute five-year survival rate was obtained at the Radiumhemmet. Although the radium techniques had been well established at the time, there was some limitation on dose that could be given by external beam irradiation since this was the orthovoltage era and supervoltage equipment had not yet been developed. In a more recent report Landgren et al[10] at the M.D. Anderson Hospital reported results in 150 medically inoperable patients with endometrial carcinoma treated primarily with radiotherapy. They obtained 78 percent five-year survival for 86 stage I patients, a 60 percent five-year survival for 38 stage II patients, and a 26 percent five-year survival for 26 stage III and IV patients.

Radiotherapy treatment techniques as previously described for stage II operable disease are recommended for the medically inoperable group of patients. When anesthesia is not possible precluding intracavitary radium the external beam technique as described for stage III disease can be utilized.

Treatment of Recurrent Endometrial Cancer

The incidence of recurrent vaginal or pelvic cancer following primary treatment for carcinoma of the endometrium has been markedly reduced following combination therapy with irradiation and surgery. An isolated vaginal recurrence alone is unusual without associated pelvic disease or distant metastases either to lung, abdomen, or bone. The treatment of an apparent isolated vaginal recurrence depends on the extent and location of the recurrence. When no previous radiotherapy has been administered, primary treatment with external irradiation in combination with vaginal radium (Fig. 14–2) is preferred. When a vaginal recurrence has taken place, the probability of pelvic lymph node metastasis is high. Therefore, external whole pelvic irradiation as described previously is administered to doses of 4000 to 5000 rad. A more localized boost dose is then given to the site of recurrence. This can be done with reduced external beam fields or with intracavitary or interstitial radium application. It is seldom wise to exceed 5000 to 5500 rad to full pelvic fields following hysterectomy because of subsequent positioning of the small bowel in the pelvis. It is also rare to exceed this dose level by external beam irradiation to the lower third of the vagina or labia because of normal tissue tolerance. Intracavitary or interstitial radium can be applied to the vaginal recurrences to bring the total dose up to 7000 to 8000 rad. Tolerance levels of the rectum and bladder must be considered under these circumstances and it is rare to exceed 7000 rad to these structures.

At times, small central disease may be better treated by surgery, particularly if previous irradiation has been given. Barber and Brunschwig[3] cured 5 of 36 patients for vaginal recurrence in which pelvic exenteration was possible; 11 patients had positive metastatic lymph nodes to the pelvis, and only 1 such patient was cured. There was a 61 percent complication rate with such surgery and 10 of these patients required a second operation. Available data from the literature indicate a salvage cure rate of less than 20 percent[14] for recurrent vaginal tumor either by subsequent surgery or radiotherapy.

Several synthetic progestational agents have been used in the management of recurrent endometrial cancer. These include hydroxyprogesterone caproate (Delalutin—E.R. Squibb) and medroxyprogesterone (Provera, Depo-provera—Upjohn). The basis of such treatment is the production of endometrial cell atrophy by continuous heavy dosage of this compound. Objective remissions of 30 to 50 percent have been reported for short periods of time, but it is unknown whether such agents will enhance the response to irradiation for recurrent disease.

References

1. Rutledge FN, Delclos L: Adenocarcinoma of the uterus. In Fletcher GH (ed): Textbook of Radiotherapy, 2nd ed. Philadelphia, Lea & Febiger, 1973 pp 665–681
2. LeFevre H: Radical surgery in the treatment of carcinoma of the body of the uterus. In Meigs JV, Sturgis HS (eds): Progress in Gynecology. New York, Grune & Stratton, 1957
3. Barber HRK, Brunschwig A: Treatment and results of recurrent cancer of corpus uteri in patients receiving anterior and total

exenteration: 1947–1963. Cancer 22:949–955, 1968

4. Boronow RC, DiSaia PJ, Creasman W: Gynecologic Oncology Group Minutes, June 1975. Los Angeles, California, P-M 72

5. Morrow CP, DiSaia PJ, Townsend DE: Current management of endometrial cancer. Obst Gynec 42:399–405, 1973

6. Heyman J: Radiological or operative treatment of cancer of the uterus. Acta Radiol 8:363–366, 1927

7. Heyman J: Radiotherapeutic treatment of cancer corpus uteri. Brit J Radiol 20:85–91, 1947

8. Kottmeier HL: Carcinoma of corpus uteri: diagnosis and therapy. Am J Obst & Gynec 78:1127–1140, 1959

9. Kottmeier HL (ed): Annual report on the results of treatment in carcinoma of the uterus, vagina and ovary. Vol. 15. Stockholm, Sweden, International Federation of Gynecology and Obstetrics, 1973

10. Landgren RC, Fletcher GH, Delclos L, Wharton JT: Irradiation of endometrial cancer in patients with medical contraindications to surgery or with unresectable lesions. Ann J Roentgenol Rad Ther & Nuc Med 126:148–154, 1976

11. Ingersoll FM, Meigs JV: Lymph node dissection for carcinoma of the endometrium. Proceedings of the Second National Cancer Conference. New York, American Cancer Society, Inc., 1954

12. Moss WT, Brand WN, Battifora H: Radiation Oncology Rationale, Technique, Results, 4th ed. St Louis, Mosby, 1973 pp 454–469

13. Boronow RC: Endometrial cancer and endometrial hyperplasia. In Rutledge F, Boronow RC, Wharton JT (eds): Gynecologic Oncology. New York, Wiley, 1976 pp 97–129

14. Badib AO, Kurohara SS, Vongtama VU, Webster JH: Evaluation of primary radiation therapy in Stage I, Group 2, endometrial carcinoma. Radiology 93:417–421, 1969

15. Chau PM: Technique and evaluation of preoperative radium therapy in adenocarcinoma of the uterine corpus. In Anderson Hospital Report: Carcinoma of the uterine cervix, endometrium and ovary. Chicago, Year Book, 1962

16. Strickland P: Carcinoma corporis uteri: a radical intracavitary treatment. Brit J Radiol 16:112–118, 1965

Chapter 15

Sarcoma of the Uterus

LARRY McGOWAN, M.D.

Uterine sarcomas are difficult to diagnose early, necessitate detailed pathologic study, and are commonly associated with a poor survival. Reliable statistics as to the frequency of sarcoma in relation to other malignant neoplasms of the uterus are not available, but it is estimated that uterine sarcomas together account for less than 1 percent of malignant uterine neoplasms. Cramer and Cutler observed that sarcomas of the corpus appear at younger ages than adenocarcinoma of the corpus (56.5 vs 60.7 years). They also noted for cancer of the corpus a proportionately greater number of sarcomas in blacks and fewer adenocarcinomas than in whites.[1]

The occurence of uterine sarcomas following radiation therapy to the pelvis is well documented in the literature. Today when the association of the two occurs, it does so usually 5 to 10 years following primary irradiation therapy for squamous cell carcinoma of the cervix. Although the linkage of the two conditions is rare, it does stress the need for prolonged follow-up examinations of all patients treated for squamous cell carcinoma of the cervix.[2]

CLASSIFICATION AND NOMENCLATURE

The close working relationship between the clinician and the pathologist is required for the proper identification of uterine sarcomas. Numerous classifications of uterine sarcomas have been proposed. The classification as suggested by Kempson is commonly used (Table 15-1).[3]

An unquestioned reduction in the number of smooth muscle tumors diagnosed as leiomyosarcomas has occurred since Norris has continually stressed the importance of the number of mitoses in the tumor to indicate its aggressiveness. An interested pathologist who will take the necessary time to meticulously study these sarcomas, particularly those borderline lesions, is imperative if

therapy and the interpretation of results of such therapies is to be meaningful.

In Kempson's classification, sarcomas are divided into three major types: pure, mixed, and malignant mixed Mullerian tumors. They are further subdivided as to whether the malignant cells are morphologically recognizable as forming tissue normally present in the uterus (homologous) or whether the tumor cells have differentiated into tissues not found in the normal uterus such as bone, cartilage, or striated muscle (heterologous). Pure sarcomas contain only a single type of recognizable sarcomatous tissue, whereas mixed sarcomas contain tumor cells that are differentiated

Table 15–1. CLASSIFICATION OF UTERINE SARCOMAS

I. *PURE SARCOMAS*
- A. Pure homologous
  1. Leiomyosarcoma
  2. Stromal sarcoma
  3. Low grade endometrial sarcoma (Endolymphatic stromal myosis)
  4. Angiosarcoma
  5. Fibrosarcoma
- B. Pure heterologous
  1. Rhabdomyosarcoma (including sarcoma botryoides)
  2. Chondrosarcoma
  3. Osteosarcoma
  4. Liposarcoma

II. *MIXED SARCOMAS*
- A. Mixed homologous
- B. Mixed heterologous

Mixed heterologous sarcomas with or without homologous elements

III. *MALIGNANT MIXED MULLERIAN TUMORS (MIXED MESODERMAL TUMORS)*
- A. Malignant mixed Mullerian tumor, homologous type
  Carcinoma plus leiomyosarcoma, stromal sarcoma or fibrosarcoma, or mixtures of these sarcomas
- B. Malignant mixed Mullerian tumor, heterologous type
  Carcinoma plus heterologous sarcoma with or without homologous sarcoma

IV. *SARCOMA, UNCLASSIFIED*

V. *MALIGNANT LYMPHOMA*

into two or more separate types of sarcoma without epithelial elements. The mixed elements may be homologous, heterologous, or mixed homologous and heterologous.[3]

Leiomyosarcomas constitute the majority of uterine sarcomas.[4] The average yearly incidence rate for leiomyosarcoma is approximately 0.5 per 100,000 women 20 years old and older.[4,5]

DIAGNOSIS

The clinician's concern with uterine sarcomas is how to make the diagnosis earlier in order to enhance survival (Fig. 15–1). The disease is infrequent and many times inaccessible in its early stages to the usual cervical and endometrial cancer screening and diagnostic aids. Vaginal dis-

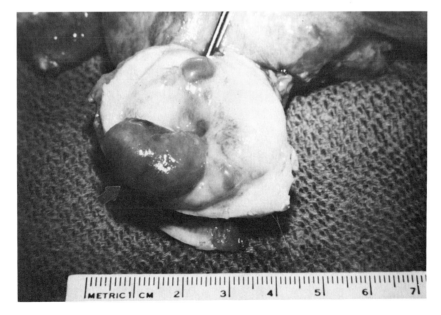

Figure 15–1. Leiomyosarcoma of the cervix.

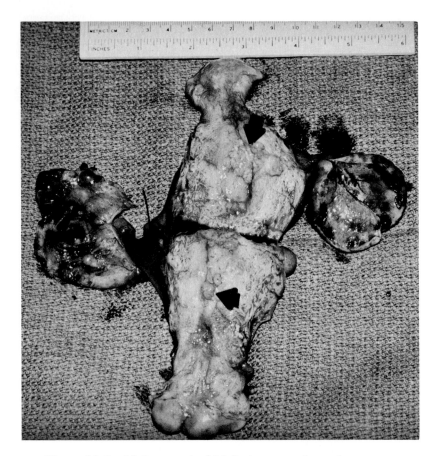

Figure 15–2. Malignant mixed Mullerian tumor, heterologous type.

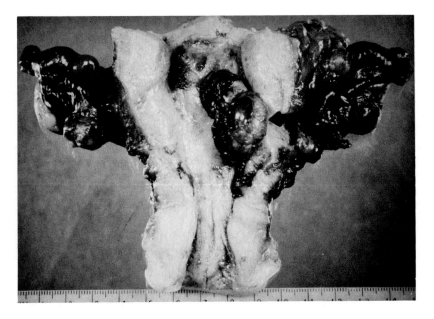

Figure 15–3. Malignant mixed Mullerian tumor, homologous type.

charge and irregular bleeding are the most common symptoms in women with uterine sarcomas (Fig. 15-2). Lower abdominal pain coupled with an enlarging lower abdomen also may be present.[4,6]

Women with stromal sarcomas have a mean age of 45 to 48 years, those with leiomyosarcomas have a mean age of 55 to 57 years, and those with malignant mixed Mullerian tumors have a mean age of 62 to 65 years.[4-7]

A polypoid mass within the uterus and commonly protruding from the cervical os in a woman with an enlarged uterus is a common clinical observation with malignant mixed Mullerian tumors (Fig. 15-3).[6,7]

PROGNOSIS

The prognosis of leiomyosarcoma depends on the extent of the tumor at the time of operation and the amount of mitotic activity. Christopherson, et al substantiate that mitotic counts accurately separate leiomyosarcomas from cellular leiomyomas. In their study, no patients with fewer than five mitoses per 10 high-power field (HPF) died of disease.[5]

Malignant mixed Mullerian tumors have a prognosis directly related to the extent of the tumor at the time of operation. Survival is extremely uncommon in any patient with a malignant mixed Mullerian tumor of either homologous or heterologous type who has extrauterine tumor extension at the time of operation.[4] Extension of tumor through more than one-half the thickness of the myometrium is also usually associated with the demise of the patient. Further study is awaited as to the significance of the presence or absence of specific cell types in malignant mixed mesodermal tumors and their relationship to ultimate survival.[6,7]

Endolymphatic stromal myosis (low-grade endometrial stromal sarcoma) may infiltrate the myometrium, has less than 10 mitoses in 10 HPF, and can metastasize. It may persist or recur in the pelvis and its vascular and lymphatic invasion may be massive, giving rise to distinctive gross and microscopic patterns. Recurrences are usually slow to develop. Stromal sarcoma is an infiltrating tumor with more than 10 mitoses in 10 HPF and prognosis is dependent upon the extent of the lesion at the time of operation.[3]

TREATMENT

A postmenopausal woman with uterine bleeding as well as a perimenopausal woman with irregular uterine bleeding should undergo a diagnostic curettage as these are common complaints of women with uterine sarcomas. A perimenopausal or postmenopausal woman with a suspected leiomyoma of the uterus noted to be enlarging should undergo hysterectomy after a normal diagnostic curettage. A diagnosis of sarcoma of the uterus must be suspected in this type of patient as well as one with an enlarging uterus during this period of life.

The treatment of uterine sarcomas is abdominal hysterectomy and usually bilateral salpingo-oophorectomy.[4,8,9] Pelvic irradiation as an adjuvant to surgery in leiomyosarcoma appears not to increase survival.[10,11]

Certain types of sarcomas respond better to a primary surgical approach than the usual uterine sarcomas.[12-14] Homologous mixed Mullerian tumors (carcinosarcomas) confined to an endometrial polyp presents as an early tumor permitting surgical extirpation of the uterus to be linked with a better survival than usually expected with sarcomas.[12] In addition, the low-grade endometrial sarcomas (endolymphatic stromal myosis) tends to be a less aggressive lesion, with pelvic and vaginal recurrences appearing many years after initial surgery. For that reason Krieger and Gusberg have advocated radical abdominal hysterectomy and pelvic lymphadenectomy for stage I and certain stage II lesions where operation would not involve cutting across tumor or leaving tumor behind.[13]

Chemotherapy is of increasing importance following primary surgery for uterine sarcomas. Sarcomas confined to the uterus with no residual disease noted at operation but with invasion through at least one-half of the myometrium are candidates for adriamycin 60 mg/sq meter of body surface administered intravenously every three weeks for approximately eight cycles. For those women with extrauterine disease or recurrent uterine sarcomas, adriamycin 60 mg/sq meter of body surface with or without dimethyl triazeno imidazole carboxamide (DTIC) 250 mg/sq meter of body surface on day one with adriamycin plus four more days, and one or both repeated every three weeks is the treatment of choice. This therapy is continued for approximately eight cy-cles or until a total total dose of adriamycin of 550 mg/sq meter of body surface is administered. Women who do not respond to this treatment may be given a combination of vincristine, dac-tinomycin, and cyclophosphamide.

SURVIVAL

The overall survival for uterine sarcomas is ap-proximately 20 to 30 percent.[4-7,9] In leiomyo-sarcomas, there is a clearly increasing mortality with increasing number of mitoses. If detailed mi-croscopic study of smooth muscle tumors reveals fewer than five mitoses per 10 HPF, it is rare for a patient to die from the tumor. Low-grade endometrial sarcoma (endolymphatic stromal myosis) is associated with a 75 to 80 percent 5-year survival, although metastases and death can occur over 20 years following initial diagnosis.[13]

Meaningful survival figures for leiomyosar-comas must clearly exclude the bizarre and cellu-lar leiomyomas.[5] Other related, generally benign uterine neoplasms must be histologically de-lineated from sarcomas.[15,16] It is hoped that cooperative clinical studies that allow the study of sufficient numbers of defined uterine sarcomas will substantiate the clinical impression that chemotherapy positively influences the course of the disease.

References

1. Cramer DW, Cutler SJ: Incidence and his-topathology of malignancies of the female genital organs in the United States. Am J Obstet Gynec 118:443, 1974
2. Fehr PE, Prem K: Malignancy of the uterine corpus following irradiation therapy for squamous cell carcinoma of the cervix. Am J Obstet Gynec 119:685, 1974
3. Kempson RL: Sarcomas and related neo-plasm in The Uterus. Norris HJ, Hertig AT, Abell MR (eds). Baltimore, Md, Wil-liams and Wilkins, 1973, p 298–319
4. Saksela E, Lampinen V, Procope B: Malig-nant mesenchymal tumors of the uterine corpus. Am J Obstet Gynec 120:452, 1974
5. Christopherson WM, Williamson EO, Gray LA: Leiomyosarcoma of the uterus. Cancer 29:1512, 1972
6. Williamson EO, Christopherson WM: Ma-lignant mixed Mullerian tumors of the uter-us. Cancer 29:585, 1972
7. Hayes D: Mixed Mullerian tumour of the corpus uteri. J Obstet Gynaec Brit Com-mon 81:160, 1974
8. Abell MR, Ramirez JA: Sarcomas and car-cinosarcomas of the uterine cervix. Cancer 31:1176, 1973
9. Mortel R, Koss LG, Lewis JL, D'Urso JR: Mesodermal mixed tumors of the uterine corpus. Obstet Gynec 43:248, 1974
10. Gilbert HA, Kagan AR, Lagasse L, Jacobs MR, Tawa K: The value of radiation therapy in uterine sarcoma. Obstet Gynec 45:84, 1975
11. Belgrad R, Elbadewi N, Rubin P: Uterine sarcoma. Radiology 114:181, 1975
12. Kahner S, Ferenczy A, Richart RM: Ho-mologous mixed Mullerian tumors (carcino-sarcoma) confined to endometrial polyps. Am J Obstet Gynec 121:278, 1975
13. Krieger PD, Gusberg SB: Endolymphatic stromal myosis—a grade I endometrial sar-coma. Gynec Oncol 1:299, 1973
14. Clement PB, Scully RE: Mullerian adeno-sarcoma of the uterus. Cancer 34:1138, 1974
15. Kurman RJ, Norris HJ: Mesenchymal tu-mors of the uterus. VI. Epithelioid smooth muscle tumors including leiomyoblastoma and clear-cell leiomyoma. Cancer 37:1853, 1976
16. Norris HJ, Parmley T: Mesenchymal tu-mors of the uterus. V Intravenous leiomy-omatosis. Cancer 36:2164, 1976

Chapter 16

Radiotherapy Treatment of Sarcoma of the Corpus

JOHN G. MAIER, M.D., Ph.D.

The role of radiotherapy in the treatment of uterine sarcoma is difficult to ascertain. This is due in part to the rarity of these tumors, since they make up less than 3 percent of patients with uterine cancer. Most series reported in the literature regarding treatment and results are retrospective analyses in which a multiplicity of treatment methods have been employed.[1,2,3] Surgery for early disease is unquestioned with radiotherapy being employed prior to or after surgery. Both external beam irradiation as well as intracavitary radium individually or together have been utilized. More recently, chemotherapy particularly with adriamycin has had some success.[4] Many series combine all the varieties of sarcoma of the uterus together, with no attempt to subdivide the various histologic varieties and the specific treatment rendered accordingly. Very often little attention is paid to prognostic factors, such as stage, uterine size, depth of myometrial invasion, or tumor grading with counting of mitotic activity. Only by separating out of these various factors along with grouping of histologic varieties can we appreciate the results by different treatment methods and choose the best treatment method.

PATHOLOGY

Four main histologic categories of uterine sarcomas are reported in most series. These include leiomyosarcoma, mixed mesodermal sarcoma, carcinosarcoma, and endometrial stromal sarcoma. The frequency of these four varieties are fairly equally divided in most series. All except leiomyosarcoma occur at about the same age as patients with endometrial carcinoma, whereas patients with leiomyosarcoma tend to develop the tumor at an earlier age. Endolymphatic stromal myosis and cellular myomas are more benign lesions and should not be included with uterine sarcomas. Norris and Taylor[5,6,7] have utilized a number of 10 mitoses per 10 high power microscopic field to distinguish the endometrial stromal sarcomas from endolymphatic stromal myosis. Kempson and Bari[8] and Silverberg[9] have reported malignancies with counts per high power field less than 10 among the uterine sarcomas. Certainly this feature is helpful in distinguishing malignancy but not the final answer.

TREATMENT

For stage I or II disease, there is little question that abdominal hysterectomy and bilateral salpingo-oophrectomy is required for uterine sarcomas. Radiotherapy can be administered as an adjunct either prior to or after surgery. Preoperative irradiation has been more popular for both biologic and technical reasons. In contrast to endometrial carcinoma, acceptable guidelines for external beam irradiation or intracavitary radium application have not been well established for uterine sarcomas. No data is available for specific radiosensitivity of the four histologic varieties. Recommended dosage of either external beam or intracavitary radium or combinations is somewhat based on normal tissue tolerance either with or without surgery. Table 16-1 depicts recommended guidelines to radiotherapy for uterine sarcomas. Most authors agree that radiotherapy is of value for mixed mesodermal sarcomas, endometrial stromal sarcomas, and carcinosarcomas. However, the value in leiomyosarcoma is questionable. In 1969, Edwards[2] reported a 52 percent survival in 29 patients at M.D. Anderson Hospital with localized uterine sarcoma treated with preoperative irradiation and surgery, as compared to 30 percent in 21 patients treated by surgery alone. The improved survival was true in all histologic varieties except leiomyosarcoma. However, Wharton[10] has indicated that preoperative irradiation is still the treatment policy at M.D. Anderson Hospital for leiomyosarcoma in 1976, except for small, well-circumscribed sar-

Table 16–1.   GUIDELINE TO RADIOTHERAPY FOR UTERINE SARCOMA

CLINICAL STATUS	TREATMENT TO UTERUS AND/OR PELVIS	TREATMENT TO VAGINA
Preoperative: Total abdominal hysterectomy and bilateral oophorectomy 4–6 weeks after completion of irradiation.	5000–6000 rad in 5–7 weeks whole pelvic irradiation	Pelvic irradiation includes vagina
	or	Vaginal ovoids 4000–5000 rad surface dose
	4000 rad in 4–5 weeks whole pelvis plus Heymans capsules 2500 mg hr and/or uterine tandem for small volume uterus or	Vaginal ovoids 4000 rad surface dose ×2 applications
	Heymans capsules 2500–3000 mg hr ×2 applications at 3-week interval	
Postoperative: Initiate irradiation 7–10 days after total abdominal hysterectomy and bilateral salpingo-oophorectomy	5000 rad in 5–6 weeks whole pelvic irradiation	Vaginal ovoids 3000 rad surface dose
	or	
	5000 rad whole pelvis followed by 1000–2000 rad boost to reduced fields for gross residual tumor. Treatment time 6–8 weeks	
Medically or technically inoperable	4000–5000 rad in 4–6 weeks whole pelvis irradiation plus one or two Heymans capsules and/or uterine tandem depending on uterine size	Vaginal ovoids 4000 rad surface dose
	or	
	7000 rad in 7–8 weeks whole pelvis. Reduce fields after 5000 rad & 6000 rad	

comas with a low mitotic index discovered in a postoperative specimen. There is little evidence that radical hysterectomy or pelvic lymphadenectomy improves results.

Belgrade et al[1] combined results in four institutions and found a two-year survival was improved by pre- or postoperative irradiation for all types except leiomyosarcoma. However, a follow-up time period of five years appears necessary to evaluate results. Vongtoma et al[3] reported a 62 percent two-year survival in 104 patients with uterine sarcoma, which fell to 42 percent at five years. In 31 patients receiving either preoperative or postoperative irradiation, the five-year survival was 53 percent compared to 40 percent for patients having surgery alone. The best results were found in patients having endometrial stromal sarcomas with a five-year survival of 62 percent in 25 patients in this category.

Additional support for the value of adjunctive irradiation is the reduction in amount of tumor remaining in the excised uterus and sterilization in 10 of 29 resected uteri following preoperative irradiation in the M.D. Anderson Hospital series.[2] Of possibly equal importance is the fact that local treatment failures (i.e., pelvic recurrence) were less than half for the irradiated group than for those having surgery alone (26 vs 57 percent) in the series from Roswell Park Memorial Institute.[3]

Treatment for recurrent pelvic tumor or metastatic disease can be given with primary irradiation and/or chemotherapy. The VAC regimen has been used more frequently with vincristine, cytoxan, and actinomycin D. More recently, adriamycin has been shown to be effective and has produced favorable responses in patients with sarcomas.[4,11] Very little data is available for combined treatment with irradiation and adriamycin for advanced disease. However, there is evidence that adriamycin sensitizes cancerous tissue to the destructive effects of irradiation by preventing repair of broken nucleic acid helices.[4]

References

1. Belgrade R, Elbadawi N, Rubin P: Uterine sarcoma. Radiol 144:181–188, 1975
2. Edwards CL: Undifferentiated tumors. In : Cancer of the Uterus and Ovary. Chicago, Year Book, 1969, pp 84–94
3. Vongtoma V, Karlen JR, Piver S, Tsukada Y, Moore RH: Treatment, results and prognostic factors in stage I and II sarcomas of the corpus uteri. Am J Roentgenol Rad Ther & Nucl Med 126:139–147, 1976
4. Watring WG, Byfield JE, Lagasse LD, et al: Combination adriamycin and radiation therapy in gynecologic cancer. Gynec Oncol 2:518–526, 1974
5. Norris HJ, Taylor HB: Clinical and pathological study of 53 endometrial stromal tumors. Cancer 19:755–766, 1966
6. Norris HJ, Taylor HB: Clinical and pathological study of 31 carcinosarcomas of the uterus. Cancer 19:1459–1465, 1966
7. Taylor HB, Norris HJ: Diagnosis and prognosis of leiomyosarcoma of uterus. AMA Arch Path 82:40–44, 1966
8. Kempson RL, Bari W: Uterine sarcomas: Classification, diagnosis and prognosis. Hum Pathol 3:331–349, 1970
9. Silverberg SG: Leiomyosarcoma of the uterus. Obstet Gynec 38:614–628, 1971
10. Wharton JT: Sarcomas of the uterus, In Rutledge FN, Boronow RC, Wharton JT (eds): Gynecologic Oncology. New York, Wiley, 1976, pp 131–138
11. O'Bryan RM, Luce JK, Talley RW, et al: Phase II evaluation of adriamycin in human neoplasia. Cancer 32:1–8, 1973

Chapter 17

Fallopian Tube Cancer

ROBERT C. PARK, M.D., COL, MC, USA
TIM H. PARMLEY, M.D.

The fallopian tube, though frequently the site of non-neoplastic tumor formation, such as tubal pregnancy and hydrosalpinx, is the least likely female genital organ to develop primary malignancy. Most often fallopian tube cancer is an extension of the more frequently encountered neoplasias of the ovary or endometrium, and tumors of these organs must be ruled out before primary fallopian tube cancer can be diagnosed. Renoud in 1847 and Orthmann in 1888 published the first descriptions of this disease, and to date approximately 900 cases have been described in the English speaking literature.[1-17]

Primary fallopian tube cancer is extremely rare, accounting for only 0.16 to 1 percent of all gynecologic malignancies.[1,2,6-8] At Walter Reed Army Medical Center from 1962 to 1975, three primary tubal cancers were recorded in 1308 invasive gynecologic malignancies, for an incidence of 0.23 percent. The mean patient age at diagnosis is 52 with a range of 18 to 80. The usual patient, however, is 45 to 60 years old.[4,7,10,11] Symptoms are variable, although abnormal bleeding, pain, or leukorrhea are frequently present.[2,5,10,11]

Tubal cancers are predominantly adenocarcinomas, histologically similar to epithelial ovarian tumors. Rarely are mixed mesodermal, malignant teratoma, and choriocarcinoma seen.[18-20]

FALLOPIAN TUBE EMBRYOLOGY

An understanding of tubal embryology helps to explain the source of the tissues that give rise to these neoplasms. Eight weeks from the maternal last menstrual period the paired Wolffian or mesonephric ducts of the female fetus have reached and opened into the urogenital sinus. Between seven and eight weeks from the last menstrual period (12-to-14-mm embryo), near the top of the mesonephric body, the Mullerian or paramesonephric ducts begin as evaginations of the intraembryonic coelom. The mesothelial cells of the coelomic epithelium begin to proliferate and become cuboidal or columnar. The coelomic epithelium is thrown into folds producing a series of longitudinal grooves immediately above and lateral to the developing gonad and adrenal. One of these grooves deepens and becomes the tip of the developing paramesonephric duct. It then grows caudally into the mesoderm. Some of the adjacent grooves will also deepen and later their lumens will join with the lumen of the primary groove, the folds between them becoming the fimbria of the adult tube. Occasionally they fail to join the primary duct, and either accessory tubal structures or cystic remnants, the Hydatids of Morgagni, are formed. Occasionally incomplete fusion with the primary duct is achieved, and the adult tube will have an accessory lumen.

At first lateral, the paramesonephric duct moves anteriorly and then medial to the Wolffian structure. The growing tip of the paramesonephric duct remains closely approximated to the wall of the mesonephric duct. At 10 weeks, the

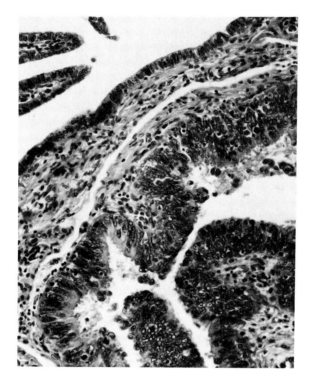

Figure 17–1. In situ cancer.

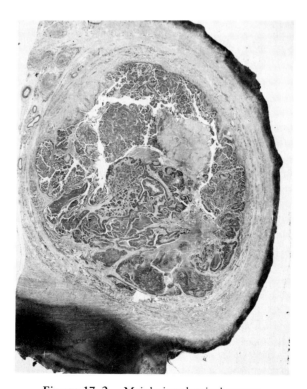

Figure 17–2. Mainly intraluminal cancer.

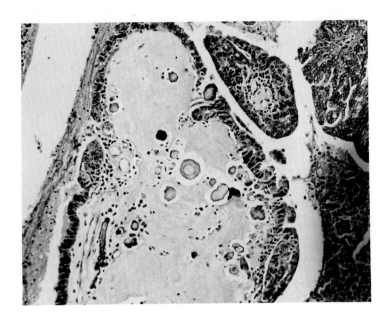

Figure 17–3.   Psammoma bodies in tubal cancer.

paired Mullerian structures begin to fuse with each other. Forming a single duct, they reach the urogenital sinus. The fused portions of the Mullerian duct will become the uterine body and cervix.

It is important to realize that the epithelium of the Mullerian duct is only a locally differentiated portion of the coelomic epithelium. This same epithelium in the adult will line the peritoneal cavity and constitute the surface of the ovary. Also, it is this epithelium that lines ovarian inclusion cysts. The epithelium of the Mullerian duct

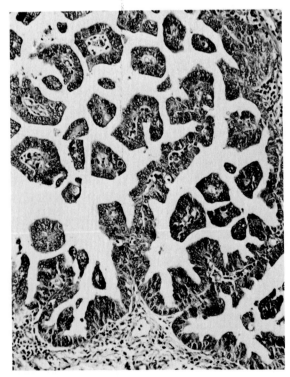

Figure 17–4.   Papillary form of tubal cancer.

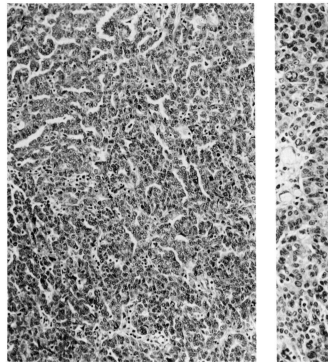

Figure 17–5. Papillary alveolar tubal cancer.

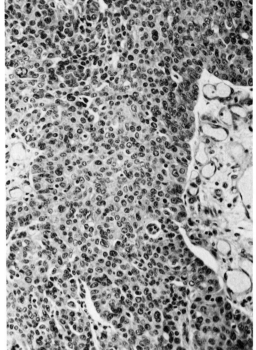

Figure 17–6. Solid type of tubal cancer.

proper will become the ciliated epithelium of the oviduct, the glandular epithelium of the endometrium, and the mucous-secreting epithelium of the endocervix with its tendency to squamous metaplasia. Similarly, the undifferentiated mesodermal stroma that lies beneath the coelomic epithelium is identical to that which lies beneath the diffcrentiated Mullerian duct epithelium at all levels.[21-25]

It follows then that malignant neoplasms of the fallopian tube epithelium will be histologically similar to those seen at other levels in the upper genital tract. It also is seen that when on those rare occasions neoplasms of the tube arise from the underlying stroma, they resemble the stromal tumors, i.e., mixed mesodermal tumors, seen in the ovary, endometrium, and cervix.

Beginning as an in situ malignancy (Fig. 17–1), epithelial tubal cancers characteristically fill and distend the lumen of the tube before they invade its wall (Fig. 17–2). As in ovarian cancers psammoma bodies may be seen (Fig. 17–3). Papillary (Fig. 17–4), papillary alveolar (Fig. 17–5), and solid (Fig. 17–6) patterns have been described. When papillary fronds of malignant epithelium agglutinate, the resulting gland-like spaces give an alveolar pattern, and with increasing cellular proliferations solid sheets of epithelium may result. All of these patterns may be seen in the same tumor (Figs. 17–2 to 17–6).

ADENOCARCINOMA

The usual primary tumor of the fallopian tube is an adenocarcinoma. The mean age at diagnosis is 52 and 50 percent of the patients are nulliparous (Fig. 17–7). A history of pelvic inflammatory disease is frequent.[2,11] Preoperative diagnosis is suspected in less than 5 percent of instances, as the disease is quite rare and symptoms are inconsist-ent.[2,4,5,11,14] Primary symptoms are abnormal bleeding, pain, and leukorrhea. The occasional preoperative diagnosis is usually made in the patient who presents with the typical bright yellow discharge "hemohydrops tubae profluens" first described by Latzko in 1915.[5] This is a syndrome of colicky pain relieved by a gush of watery yel-

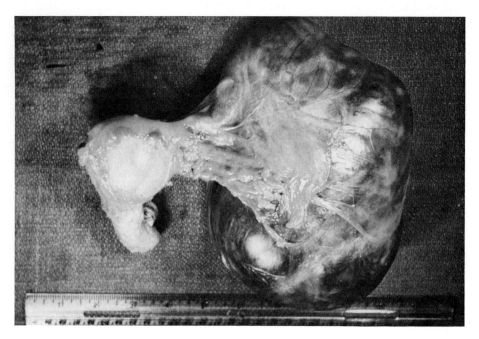

Figure 17–7.   Large left fallopian tubal cancer.

low fluid from the vagina. However, this distinctive symptom is present in very few cases.[10,11] In every instance the affected tube has been enlarged and the diagnosis should be suspected in any patients with abnormal bleeding or discharge where an enlarged adnexae is present and etiology is not evident.[7,11] In addition, any postmenopausal patient with bleeding not of uterine origin or symptoms similar to pelvic inflammatory disease should be suspect for tubal carcinoma.

The definitive diagnosis of fallopian tube cancer is histologic and should contain the following features:[2] (1) Grossly the main tumor is in the tube; (2) the ovaries and uterus are normal; and

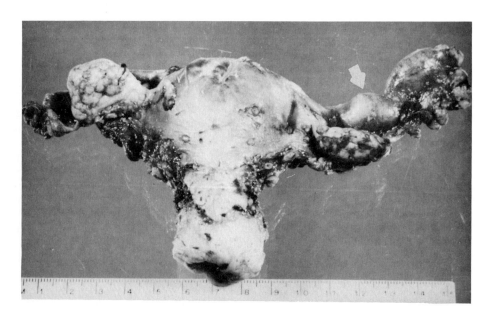

Figure 17–8.   Small nodular cancer in midportion of left tube separate from ovary.

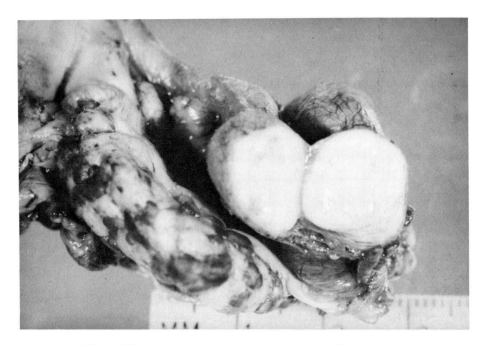

Figure 17–9. Bisection of tubal cancer seen in Figure 17–8.

(3) microscopic exam should show that (a) chiefly the mucosa is involved, (b) a papillary pattern should be noted, (c) transition between benign and malignant epithelium should be demonstrated, and (d) cells should resemble endosalpinx.

There is no recognized staging system for fallopian tube carcinoma. Several have been proposed, but none has been officially recognized.[2,9] An acceptable alternative is to use the FIGO staging system for ovarian carcinoma (Chap. 19).

Treatment

The treatment of choice for fallopian tube cancer is en bloc tumor removal to include the uterus, opposite tube, and ovaries (Figs. 17–8 and 17–9). This tumor spreads similarly to ovarian cancer, and the operative treatment of both is to remove as much gross disease as possible. Careful intra-abdominal exploration need be accomplished, and suspected metastatic areas including lymph nodes should be biopsied. Twenty percent of these tumors are found to be bilateral.

Traditionally, postoperative treatment has been irradiation as covered in Chapter 18. If bulk tumor remains, however, chemotherapy is probably more appropriate. Alkalyating agents, 5-fluorouracil and progesterone are known to be active against this disease.[2,3,11] However, no studies to date show any agent to be superior. Drugs known to be effective against epithelial ovarian tumors should also be effective against fallopian tube tumors. The overall five-year survival for patients with fallopian tube carcinoma is 20 to 30 percent with a survival of 50 to 60 percent when tumor is confined to one tube.[2-4,6,7,9-11] Since survival is so poor, all patients with tubal carcinoma should probably receive either irradiation or chemotherapy postoperatively.

CHORIOCARCINOMA, SARCOMA AND MALIGNANT DERMOID TUMORS

Choriocarcinoma, mixed mesodermal sarcoma, and malignant dermoid tumors of the fallopian tube have been reported.[18-20,26,27] Surgical extirpation followed by irradiation or chemotherapy is indicated in the latter two cell types. Choriocarcinoma has always followed tubal pregnancy and is best treated by chemotherapy as in gestational trophoblastic diseases of other sites. Human chorionic gonadotrophin monitoring is valuable to help determine the therapeutic end point.

References

1. Adams G: Carcinoma of the fallopian tube—Report of two cases. Nebr Med J 58:306, 1973
2. Dodson M, Ford J, Jr, Averette H: Clinical aspects of fallopian tube carcinoma. Obstet Gynec 36:935, 1970
3. Boutselis J, Thompson J: Clinical aspects of primary carcinoma of the fallopian tube. Am J Obstet Gynec 111:98, 1971
4. Crist T, Palumbo L, Shingleton H: Primary carcinoma of the fallopian tube. South Med J 61:311, 1968
5. Glenn J: Adenocarcinoma of the fallopian tube. Am J Obstet Gynec 120:200, 1974
6. Hanton E, Malkasian G, Dahlin D, et al: Primary carcinoma of the fallopian tube. Am J Obstet Gynec 94:832, 1966
7. Momtazee S, Kempson R: Primary adeno-carcinoma of the fallopian tube. Obstet Gynec 32:649, 1968
8. Pauerstein C, Woodruff JD: Cellular patterns in proliferative and anaplastic disease of fallopian tube. Am J Obstet Gynec 96:486, 1966
9. Schiller H, Silverberg S: Staging and prognosis in primary carcinoma of the fallopian tube. Cancer 28:389, 1971
10. Sedlis A: Primary carcinoma of the fallopian tube. Obstet Gynec Surv 16:209, 1961
11. Turunen A: Diagnosis and treatment of primary tubal carcinoma. Internat J Gynec Obstet 7:294, 1969
12. Chalmers JA, Marshall AT: Carcinoma of the fallopian tube. Brit J Obstet Gynaec 83:580, 1976
13. Kinzel GE: Primary carcinoma of the fallopian tube. Am J Obstet Gynec 125:816, 1976
14. Benson PA: Cytologic diagnosis in primary carcinoma of fallopian tube. Acta Cytolol 18:429, 1976
15. Phelps HM, Chapman KE: Role of radiation therapy in treatment of primary carcinoma of the uterine tube. Obstet Gynec 43:669, 1974
16. Picha E, Weghaupt K: Twenty cases of primary carcinoma of the fallopian tube seen between 1950 and 1963. Zentralblatt Fur Gynakologie 92:596, 1970
17. Fogh I: Primary carcinoma of the fallopian tube. Cancer 23:1332, 1969
18. Segal S, Adoni A, Schenker J: Choriocarcinoma of the fallopian tube. Gynec Onco 3:40, 1975
19. Sweet R, Selinger H, McKay D: Malignant teratoma of the uterine tube. Obstet Gynec 45:553, 1975
20. Wu J, Tanner W, Fardal P: Malignant mixed mullerian tumor of the uterine tube. Obstet Gynec 41:707, 1973
21. Faulconer RJ: Observations on the origin of the mullerian groove in human embryos. Contrib Embryol 34:15, 1951
22. Gruenwald P: Common traits in development and structure of the organs originating from the coelomic wall. J Morph 70:353, 1942
23. Hunter RH: Observations on the development of the human female genital tract. Contrib Embryol 22:91, 1930
24. Streeter GL: Developmental horizons in human embryos. Contrib Embryol 32:133, 1948
25. Witschi E: Embryology of the uterus. Ann NY Acad Sci 75:412, 1959
26. Blaikley JB: Sarcoma of the fallopian tube. J Obstet Gynec Brit Common 80:759, 1973
27. Acosta AA, Kaplan AL, Kaufman RH: Mixed mullerian tumors of the oviduct. Obstet Gynec 44:84, 1974

Chapter 18

Radiotherapy in Carcinoma of the Fallopian Tube

JOHN G. MAIER, M.D., Ph.D.

The role of radiotherapy in the treatment of primary carcinoma of the fallopian tube is difficult to ascertain because of the rarity of such tumors and the nonuniformity of treatment rendered. Hu et al[1] collected 466 cases from the literature and added 12 personal cases. They found the incidence of primary fallopian tube cancer to be 0.3 percent of all gynecologic malignancy. Jones[2] reported that only 10 of 780 cases reported in the literature through 1965 had a correct preoperative diagnosis. Obviously, preoperative irradiation is seldom considered.

CLINICAL FINDINGS

Patients with primary fallopian tube cancer may present with a triad of vaginal bleeding, pelvic pain and cramps, and a tubal or pelvic mass. The vaginal bleeding may be either intermenstrual or postmenopausal with the average about 50 years. Sedlis[3] reported a bilateral incidence of 26 percent in a review of the literature. Unilateral tumors were equally divided between the right and left sides. Most tumors are located in the middle or outer two-thirds of the fallopian tube. Spread of the tumor is usually by direct extension. Spread tends to be earlier when the tubes are patent. When the fimbriated end is sealed, spread tends to occur later. Thus, infection may be an actual barrier to spread. However, the incidence of fallopian tubal tumors is higher with associated chronic infections. Slightly more than half of the patients are nulliparous. Clinical staging prior to surgery is seldom of value. Hysterosalpingograms and culdoscopy are not helpful since the gross and radiographic appearance of chronic salpingitis and hydrosalpinx are similar to carcinoma of the tube. Surgical staging at the time of laparotomy has proven of value. The staging system of Erez et al[4] has been most widely used and is described as follows:

Stage I. The tumor is limited to the tube without invasion of the serosa.

Stage II. The tumor has extended to the serosa or has invaded adjacent pelvic organs.

Stage III. The tumor has extended beyond the pelvis, but is still confined within the abdominal cavity.

Stage IV. Extra-abdominal metastases.

TREATMENT

There is little question that surgery is the primary treatment for fallopian tube adenocarcinoma. For early stages (I and II), a bilateral salpingo-oophorectomy and total abdominal hysterectomy can be curative in 60 to 70 percent of patients. No value has been shown for an additional pelvic lymphadenectomy. The value of postoperative irradiation has been questioned by Momtazee and Kempson.[5] Such treatment did not appear to be of value in a collected series of 30 patients from five separate reports. Most of the patients were either stage I or early stage II and no value of postoperative irradiation could be anticipated for tumor that was completely resected. Ross et al[6] reported a 40 percent five-year survival in a series of patients given postoperative irradiation com-pared to a five percent year survival for surgery alone. Engstrom[7] reported a similar 38 percent five-year survival when postoperative irradiation was administered versus 15 percent when no ir-radiation was administered.

Details as to dosage and equipment employed are somewhat scanty in such reports in the litera-ture. However, midplane pelvic doses of 5000 rad in five to six weeks given postoperatively ap-pears appropriate for stage II disease as described in Chapter 20 for ovarian cancer. Bulky abdomi-nal tumor metastases would appear to be more appropriately treated by systemic chemotherapy. Minimal abdominal metastases may respond to moving strip or abdominal bath techniques as de-scribed for ovarian malignancies.

References

1. Hu CY, Faymor ML, Hertig AT: Primary carcinoma of the fallopian tube. Am J Obstet Gynec 79:24, 1960
2. Jones OV: Primary carcinoma of the uterine tube. Obstet Gynec 26:122, 1965
3. Sedlis A: Primary carcinoma of fallopian tube. Obstet Gynec Surv 16:209, 1961
4. Erez S, Kaplan AL, Wall JA: Clinical staging of carcinoma of the uterine tube. Obstet Gynec 30:547, 1967
5. Momtazee S, Kempson RL: Primary adeno-carcinoma of the fallopian tube. Obstet Gynec 32:659, 1968
6. Ross WM, Ward CV, Lindsay C: Primary car-cinoma of the fallopian tube. Am J Obstet Gynec 83:425, 1962
7. Engstrom L: Primary carcinoma of fallopian tube. Acta Obstet Gynec Scandinav 36:289, 1957

Chapter 19

Ovarian Cancer

LARRY McGOWAN, M.D.

Ovarian cancer is the fourth leading cause of cancer deaths in American women. It follows breast, large intestine, and lung cancers, in that order. It makes up approximately 5 percent of all cancers in women and contributes to about 6 percent of their cancer deaths.[1] Although ovarian cancer composes 25 percent of all invasive genital cancers,[2] it kills more women than cervix and endometrial cancer together today. There are approximately 14 new cases of ovarian cancer each year per 100,000 women of all ages.[2]

The overall five-year survival for ovarian cancer is approximately 30 to 35 percent and this figure has not changed in the past 30 years.[3-7] Poor survival is partly attributable to late diagnosis and that is based on our current inability to define the woman at risk for developing ovarian cancer. We also do not know the etiologic factors associated with ovarian cancer and cannot prevent the disease.

ETIOLOGY

The etiology of ovarian cancer is not known, but there is a suggestion that those of epithelial histogenetic origin may be related to the hormone excretion of the pituitary-gonad axis. Fraumeni and associates have observed a relative infertility in nuns and single women to be a common characteristic of women with ovarian cancer[8] and Joly et al have noted the protective effect of early pregnancy for cancers of the ovary.[9]

It is of interest that in the domestic fowl, with its frequent egg production, ovarian carcinoma is the most common tumor of unknown etiology in the hen.[10] Furthermore, in the hen only the left ovary and oviduct are functional. The right organs remain vestigial and cancer free.[11] Manipulation of older hens' egg production by presenting addi-

tional or less light over natural sources increases or decreases egg production and the incidence of ovarian cancer respectively (Fig. 19-1). This probably occurs by pituitary stimulation.

Fathalla comments that in women, ovulatory cycles are almost continuous from puberty to the menopause. As pregnancy infrequently results, there is incessant ovulation. The hypothesis that the extravagant and mostly purposeless ovulations in women may play a contributing role in neoplasia of the surface epithelium of the ovary is interesting.[12,13] The impact of this hypothesis on the incidence of ovarian cancer with the widespread use of oral contraceptives resulting in suppression of ovulation is awaited.

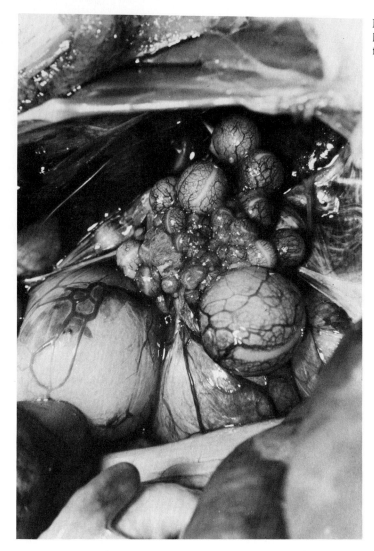

Figure 19–1. A 1-year-old leghorn hen with multiple yolk formation from the left ovary.

PREVENTION

In the United States there are nearly 900,000 hysterectomies performed each year, many with unilateral or bilateral oophorectomies, yet the time trends in ovarian cancer mortality has not changed in the past 20 years. There appears to be no advantage in the removal of one ovary over the opposite as a means of further decreasing the incidence of subsequent ovarian cancer. A normal-appearing ovary preserved at the time of hysterectomy for benign disease does not exhibit a greater tendency for the development of cancer than does any apparently normal ovary.[13] Ovarian cancer following hysterectomy should be judged according to the total number of hysterectomies rather than from retrospective study of cases of ovarian cancer.[14] DeNeef and Hollenbeck pointed out that prophylactic oophorectomy might conceivably save three patients from subsequent ovarian cancer if this were routinely done during 10,000 hysterectomies.[14]

Ovaries that are functioning normally before hysterectomy continue to function completely normally after hysterectomy in women of the 25 to 48 age group according to the report of Beavis et al.[15] The devastating effect of bilateral salpingo-oophorectomy in young women 15 to 30 years has been studied by Johansson and his group. Women with complete oophorectomy were found to have been followed by (1) an increased incidence of cardiac symptoms and nervous diseases as well as an increased use of drugs; (2) a significant increase in the frequency of coronary vascular disease and deaths in ages up to 70 years; (3) an increase in the serum cholesterol and triglycerides; (4) an increase in frequency to fractures, increased osteoporosis, and thinner cortical bone; (4) an increased adrenocortical activity with

significantly increased excretion of 17-ketosteroids and low total estrogens.[16]

At the time of operation for hysterectomy for benign disease in women under the age of 45, the decision to retain the ovaries should be based on their appearance, size, lack of papillary excrescences, and consistency on palpation. Bivalving of the ovary may be carried out to enhance visualization and palpation or wedge biopsy performed for immediate frozen section and later permanent tissue study.

EPIDEMIOLOGY

The woman at risk for developing ovarian cancer has not been defined.[17-21] Also, factors associated with ovarian cancer have not been adequately detailed.[6,22] The main reasons for this are that although there are approximately 17,000 new cases of ovarian cancer each year, ovarian cancer is not a single disease, but a collection of various types, and multidiscipline study of the problem is lacking.

A number of very interesting relationships to cancer of the ovary have been recorded but not explained as yet. Denmark, with an 11.12 rate per 100,000 population, has the highest age-adjusted death rate for ovarian cancer in the world. Sweden with a 9.5 is second and Norway at 8.96 is third with Japan at 1.86 having the lowest age-adjusted death rate in the world. In the United States, white women have a 7.39 age-adjusted death rate for ovarian cancer putting them in the seventh place in the world statistics and nonwhites in the United States with 13th ranking at a 6.05 rate per 100,000 population.[22]

In the United States, a striking geographic differnce in ovarian cancer deaths is present. For a 20-year period (1950-1969), the average annual age-adjusted mortality rates (per 100,000) were calculated from all death certificates in the United States. Impressively high death rates for ovarian cancer are scattered in northern counties, many of which are rural. Rates in the south were generally low.[26-28]

There are many epidemiologic similarities between cancer of the ovary and breast. A twofold excess risk of ovarian cancer occurs among breast cancer patients and vice versa.[23] Females, both black and white, who have an initial cancer of the large intestine or anorectum are at an especially high risk of subsequent cancer of the ovary and cervix.[24] Age-adjusted human breast and ovarian cancer mortalities are significantly and positively correlated with annual per capita consumption of fats and oils.[25]

Women with germ cell malignancies of the ovary are 20 years younger usually when compared to the age (57.7 years) of the patients with the more common cancers. Blacks have a proportionately greater number of gonadal stromal and germ cell cancers and fewer serous cystadenocarcinomas.[2]

A few types of women are known to be at higher risk for developing ovarian cancer in addition to those who have primary cancers of the uterus, breast, and large intestine. There are a few families who have a greater number of ovarian cancers than expected and these are usually of the epithelial type.[29-36] The association of Peutz-Jeghers syndrome and ovarian neoplasms of specialized gonadal stromal origin have been recorded as well as the association of arrhenoblastoma and thyroid adenomas.[36,37]

The defining of the woman at risk for developing ovarian cancer is needed, because if we had the perfect diagnostic aid for detecting ovarian cancer, from a cost effectiveness standpoint it would be difficult to apply to all women.

DIAGNOSIS

The diagnosis of advanced ovarian cancer is common and the preoperative diagnosis of localized ovarian cancer is fortuitous. The percentage of cases classified as localized ovarian cancer under the age of 35 years is 44 percent, 35 to 44 years is 33 percent, 45 to 54 years is 28 percent,

55 to 64 years is 25 percent, 65 to 74 is 25 percent, over 75 years is 24 percent, and for all ages ovarian cancer is localized only in 28 percent of women. For 20 years, the overall percentage trend of cases of ovarian cancer classified as localized has not changed. The earlier diagnosis of ovarian cancer with localized disease is associated with a 72 to 76 percent five-year survival; regional cancer involvement, 32 to 36 percent survival; distant disease spread, 8 to 12 percent survival; for an overall 32 percent five-year relative survival for ovarian cancer.[38]

The symptoms of ovarian cancer are vague and not specific for the disease. The most common symptom is that of abdominal pain that can be of varying intensity, different localities, and with no time pattern. The next most frequent symptom is abdominal swelling that may be described as bloating, fullness, or simply that her clothes are tight fitting (Fig. 19–2). A change in weight, usually weight loss, may be noted and associated with varying degrees of loss of appetite, decrease in ability to consume the usual quantity of food, intermittent nausea, and occasional vomiting with resulting loss of feeling well. With an increasing amount of disease in the pelvis, the symptoms of pelvic pressure, abnormal bleeding, either a change in menstrual pattern or postmenopausal

bleeding, cramps, or obstipation or urinary frequency may be noted. Approximately one-third of women with ovarian cancer are asymptomatic when the diagnosis is made, and 75 percent of them have symptoms of less than six months duration.

The average annual age-adjusted (1970 standard) incidence rates for ovarian cancer per 100,000 population for white women is 14.2 and in black women 10.6. The average annual age-specific incidence rates per 100,000 population, women of all races and areas of the United States combined, 1969–1971 is 35–39, 6.8; 45–49, 23.8; 55–59, 38.5; 65–69, 48.6; and 70–74, 50.8.[39] As there are no specific symptoms of ovarian cancer, as well as the fact that the woman at high risk for ovarian cancer has not been consistently defined, this data stresses the importance of history and physical examination in the perimenopausal and postmenopausal woman. About 60 percent of women with ovarian cancer will be found to have an abdominal or pelvic mass, a third of women with ascites, 25 percent with a diagnosis of either a unilateral or bilateral adnexal mass, and approximately 15 percent being confused with leiomyomata or other pelvic pathology.[40]

The following are indications for surgical ex-

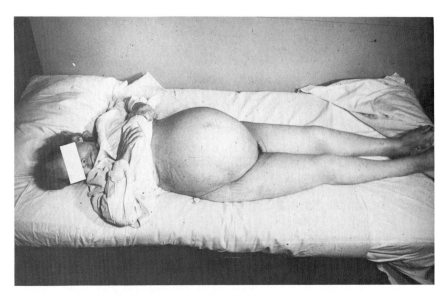

Figure 19–2. A woman with stage III ovarian cancer who complains of diffuse intermittent abdominal cramps, obvious enlargement of the abdomen secondary to ascites, and a loss of appetite. Multiple tumors within the abdomen can be palpated. Lymphatic and vascular obstruction by tumor has resulted in edema of the lower extremities. There has been weight loss in her upper body as seen in her face and hands.

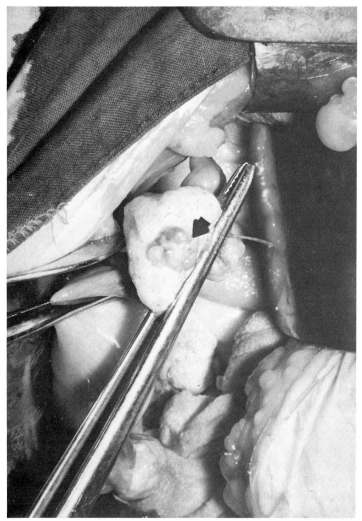

Figure 19–3. The problem with detecting ovarian cancer early by pelvic examination only is seen in this postmenopausal woman with a normal-sized ovary with papillary excrescences on the surface and containing a poorly differentiated endometrioid adenocarcinoma with omental metastases.

ploration and visualization of the ovary: (1) any premenarchal or postmenopausal palpable ovarian tumor. The physiologic changes or cysts of the ovary are not present in women who are not regularly menstruating. Whereas the normal ovary may measure 3 to 4 cm × 2 cm × 1 to 2 cm in size, at the extremes of life, it is about one-half that size and cannot be palpated on examination.[41] The year preceding the menarche and the year following cessation of menstruation are transition periods. In the premenarchal girl the ovary is enlarging and approaching normal size and in the postmenopausal woman the ovary is decreasing in size to its postmenopausal atrophic state. (2) An ovarian tumor around 5 to 6 cm in size that is observed through at least 1 to 2 menstrual cycles. Physiologic cysts of the ovary should regress after one or two menstrual cycles, and the persistence of an ovarian tumor of 5 to 6 cms when examined in the immediate postmenstrual period is suspicious for neoplasia (Fig. 19-3). (3) An ovarian tumor larger than 6 cm should be visualized, as spontaneous regression to normal size is exceedingly uncommon. (4) An ovarian tumor that is consistently solid to hard on palpation has a higher possibility of being associated with neoplasia than a soft or cystic ovary. (5) Symptoms, signs, and pelvic examination which suggest torsion or rupture of an ovarian cyst should be surgically visualized, as acute adnexal events are commonly associated with ovarian neoplasia. (6) Unexplained ascites with the presence of malignant cells in the peritoneal fluid. The ovary is one of the more common sites in women for malignant cells to arise.

Other Diagnostic Procedures

Papanicolaou cytosmears are not reliable to detect early ovarian cancer. Since in advanced disease they are positive in only 10 to 25 percent of women.[40,42]

Although cell samples can be obtained readily by culdocentesis and malignant cells in peritoneal fluid from early ovarian cancer can be seen easily, routine widespread use of peritoneal fluid sampling for the early detection of ovarian cancer is not suggested. Peritoneal fluid cellular analysis for the presence of malignant cells should be performed in women with suspected ascites; adnexal masses, or women in the currently identified high-risk category.

Fine-needle ovarian aspiration biopsy in the diagnosis of ovarian cancer is not advocated because it ruptures the mechanical barrier (the capsule) for spread of cancer cell, and has a high false-negative rate, and even with benign ovarian neoplasm the tumor must be removed.

A final and definitive diagnosis of ovarian malignancy can rarely be made on roentgenographic examination alone. Signs evident on survey films may include abnormal or unusual pelvic or abdominal calcification.[43] Contrast studies are of no help to make the early diagnosis of ovarian cancer, but with advanced disease, excretory uro-

grams may show obstruction or deviation of one or both ureters; impression or deviation of the bowel can be shown on barium enema, or a pelvic soft tissue mass may be shown on either survey or contrast films.

Ultrasound is being utilized in many hospitals and physicians' offices to aid in the detection of ovarian neoplasia and other pelvic pathology. Donald prefers the term sonar for "ultrasonic diagnostic echography." He has repeatedly emphasized that sonar cannot supplant good, clinical examination but may help materially to reinforce or modify the clinician's findings. The information provided indicates macroscopic appearances only and is concerned with tissue density and outlines, their distribution, and fluid content. He further stresses that the pictures must therefore be interpreted in the light of clinical knowledge and common sense. Sonar is no substitute for laparotomy and biopsy in a suspected tumor.[44]

Carcinoembryonic antigen (CEA) is of little value for the early diagnosis of ovarian cancer as is the determination of α-feta proteins (AFP) and serum lactic dehydrogenase (LDH). These tests may be of use in monitoring the response of patients with ovarian cancer to therapy.

Laparoscopy has a place in the investigation and follow-up of cases of ovarian carcinoma. It can be helpful for the differential diagnosis of a pelvic mass after other diagnostic aids have been utilized. Laparoscopy does require general anesthesia, skill in its use, and an appreciation of ovarian neoplasia.

STAGING

Ovarian cancer must be staged properly so that treatment planning and treatment may be carried out, prognosis determined, and therapy evaluated between different regimes and institutions (Table 19-1).[45]

The staging specifies that, with malignant growth limited to one or both ovaries (stage IC) or with pelvic extension (stage IIC), there must be malignant cells present in the peritoneal fluid. Ovarian carcinomas, especially those of epithelial histogenetic background, usually disseminate by multiple implantations on serous surfaces. The disease is known to progress from that confined within an ovary to an increasing number of free-

floating cancer cells in the peritoneal fluid (Figs. 19-9 and 19-10), to a widespread disease process that interferes with gastrointestinal and general metabolic function, to eventual death. Greater amounts of tumor within the peritoneal cavity are usually associated with a poorer prognosis. Malignant cells in the peritoneal fluid must be detected, since they are the earliest evidence of spread beyond the ovary for most ovarian cancers. Thus it is now possible to incorporate cytologic procedures into the clinical care of women with early ovarian cancer, and such procedures can have a direct effect on the treatment and prognosis.

Table 19–1. CLINICAL AND OPERATIVE STAGES OF MALIGNANT OVARIAN TUMORS

Stage I	Growth limited to ovaries.	Stage IIC	Tumor either stage IIA or IIB, but with ascites present or positive peritoneal fluid.
Stage IA	Growth limited to one ovary; no ascites.* (i) No tumor on external surface; capsule intact; (ii) Tumor present on external surface (Fig. 19-5) and/or capsule ruptured.		
		Stage III	Growth involving one or both ovaries (Figs. 19-6 to 19-10) with intraperitoneal metastases outside pelvis and/or positive retroperitoneal nodes. Tumor limited to true pelvis with histologically proved malignant extension to small bowel (Fig. 19-8) or omentum (Figs. 19-16 and 19-24)
Stage IB	Growth limited to both ovaries; no ascites. (i) No tumor on external surface; capsule intact (Fig. 19-4); (ii) Tumor present on external surface and/or capsule(s) ruptured.		
Stage IC	Tumor either stage IA or IB, but with ascites present or positive peritoneal fluid.		
		Stage IV	Growth involving one or both ovaries with distant metastases. If pleural effusion is present, there must be positive cytology to allot a case to stage IV. Parenchymal liver metastasis equals stage IV.
Stage II	Growth involving one or both ovaries, with pelvic extension.		
Stage IIA	Extension and/or metastases to uterus and/or tubes.		
Stage IIB	Extension to other pelvic tissues.		

Approved by the International Federation of Gynaecology and Obstetrics in 1974 and recommended by the American College of Obstetricians and Gynecologists.

*Ascites is peritoneal effusion which in the opinion of the surgeon is pathologic and/or clearly exceeds normal amounts.

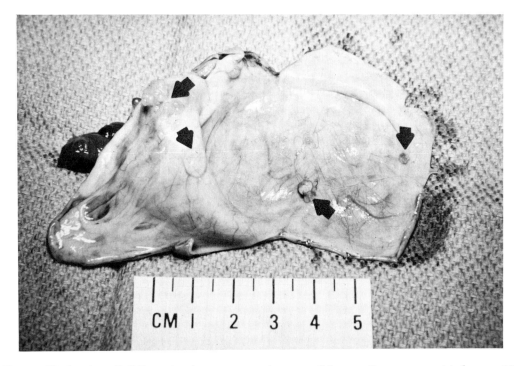

Figure 19–4. A well-differentiated serous cystadenoma of low malignant potential from a 23-year-old woman who had an oophorectomy four years previous for the same tumor.

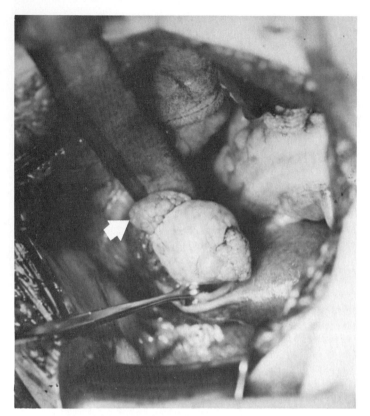

Figure 19–5. A well-differentiated papillary serous cystadenocarcinoma of the right ovary in a 20-year-old woman who is free of disease 18 years following abdominal hysterectomy, bilateral salpingo-oophorectomy, omentectomy, and appendectomy.

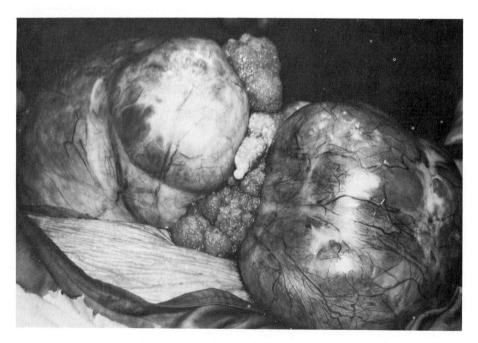

Figure 19–6. Papillary serous cystadenoma (of borderline malignancy) of the right ovary in a 48-year-old woman.

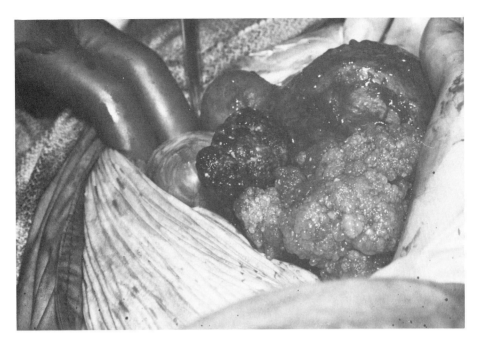

Figure 19–7. The same patient as in Figure 19-6 with a papillary serous cystadenoma of low malignant potential in the left ovary.

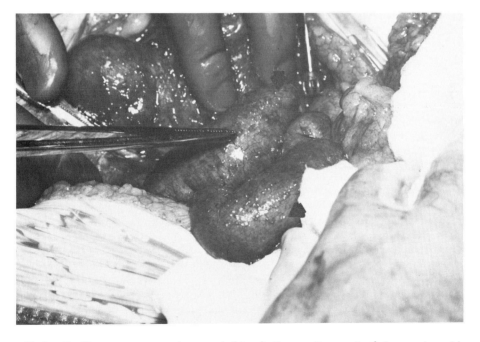

Figure 19–8. Papillary serous cystadenoma (of borderline malignancy) of the ovaries with multiple implants of tumor on small bowel in the woman in Figures 19-6 and 19-7.

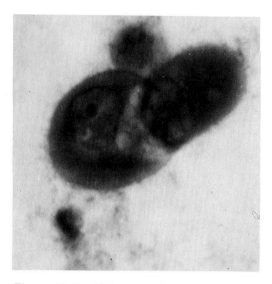

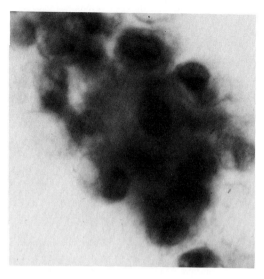

Figure 19–9. Malignant cells seen in peritoneal fluid from patient in Figures 19–6, 19–7, and 19–8. The two cells have enlarged nuclei that are irregular and have thickened rims. Prominent nucleoli are present. There is abundant cytoplasm with a single large vacuole. ×6250.

Figure 19–10. Sheets of atypical cells present in peritoneal fluid of patient in Figures 19–6 to 19–9, with abundant marginal cytoplasm containing large vacuoles. Hyperchromatic and irregular nuclei with overlapping of cells is also observed. ×6250.

CLASSIFICATION

The World Health Organization (WHO) has proposed the histologic classification of ovarian tumors presented in Table 19–2. The classification is based primarily on the microscopic characteristics of the tumors and thus reflects the nature of morphologically identifiable cell types and patterns.[46] WHO justifiably stresses the grade of malignant tumors or a modifying phrase indicating the degree of their differentiation. An appraisal of the appearance of the ovarian stroma both inside the tumor and at its periphery is required. Tumors that show evidence that the stroma is endocrinologically active may be designated by "tumors with functioning stroma." Of great importance to the clinician involved in treatment planning is their statement: "Because ovarian tumors are often composed of combinations of several types that may vary in their biological behavior, it is important that the diagnostic terms chosen include all the varieties encountered and indicate as accurately as possible the proportion and distribution of each; an accompanying description of the microscopic characteristics may be helpful for this purpose."[46]

Ovarian cancer is not one disease but is composed of several cell types that may manifest themselves in different age groups, methods of spread, and racial features, consequently not having the same responses to a therapeutic regimen. In addition to a histologic classification of ovarian tumors, the histogenetic approach to the study of primary ovarian neoplasms clearly demonstrates that all malignant neoplasms of the ovary are not of a single genesis and cannot be treated in a like manner. In a histogenetic classification of ovarian neoplasms as suggested by Abell there are four basic categories (Table 19–3).[47]

The coelomic (germinal) epithelium is represented by the surface cells proper, the small cortical inclusion cysts, and by the rete ovarii and tubular remnants of sex cords in the medulla. The neoplasms that arise from these cells, "epithelial" tumors of the histologic classification, possess the same potential of differentiation toward elements of the paramesonephric (Mullerian) system as do benign hyperplasias and prosoplasias of these cells. Thus we encounter neoplasms in which the epithelium resembles that of the fallopian tube (serous neoplasms), endometrium (endometrial cell or endometrioid neoplasms), and endocervix

Table 19–2. HISTOLOGIC CLASSIFICATION OF OVARIAN TUMORS

I. COMMON "EPITHELIAL" TUMORS
  A. Serous tumors
    1. Benign
      a. Cystadenoma and papillary cystadenoma
      b. Surface papilloma
      c. Adenofibroma and cystadenofibroma
    2. Of borderline malignancy (carcinomas of low malignant potential) (Figs. 19-6 to 19-10)
      a. Cystadenoma and papillary cystadenoma (Fig. 19-4)
      b. Surface papilloma
      c. Adenofibroma and cystadenofibroma
    3. Malignant
      a. Adenocarcinoma, papillary adenocarcinoma, and papillary cystadenocarcinoma (Fig. 19-5)
      b. Surface papillary carcinoma
      c. Malignant adenofibroma and cystadenofibroma
  B. Mucinous tumors
    1. Benign
      a. Cystadenoma
      b. Adenofibroma and cystadenofibroma
    2. Of borderline malignancy (carcinomas of low malignant potential)
      a. Cystadenoma
      b. Adenofibroma and cystadenofibroma
    3. Malignant
      a. Adenocarcinoma and cystadenocarcinoma (Figs. 19-11 to 19-13)
      b. Malignant adenofibroma and cystadenofibroma
  C. Endometrioid tumors
    1. Benign
      a. Adenoma and cystadenoma
      b. Adenofibroma and cystadenofibroma
    2. Of borderline malignancy (carcinomas of low malignant potential)
      a. Adenoma and cystadenoma
      b. Adenofibroma and cystadenofibroma
    3. Malignant
      a. Carcinoma
        (1) Adenocarcinoma (Figs. 19-14 to 19-16)
        (2) Adenoacanthoma
        (3) Malignant adenofibroma and cystadenofibroma
      b. Endometrioid stromal sarcomas

      c. Mesodermal (Mullerian) mixed tumors, homologous, and heterologous
  D. Clear cell (mesonephroid) tumors
    1. Benign: adenofibroma
    2. Of borderline malignancy (carinomas of low malignant potential)
    3. Malignant: carcinoma and adenocarcinoma
  E. Brenner tumors
    1. Benign
    2. Of borderline malignancy (proliferating)
    3. Malignant
  F. Mixed epithelial tumors
    1. Benign
    2. Of borderline malignancy
    3. Malignant
  G. Undifferentiated carcinoma
  H. Unclassified epithelial tumors

II. SEX CORD STROMAL TUMORS
  A. Granulosa-stromal cell tumors
    1. Granulosa cell tumor (carcinoma) (Figs. 19-25 and 19-26)
    2. Tumors in the thecoma-fibroma group
      a. Thecoma
      b. Fibroma
      c. Unclassified
  B. Androblastomas; Sertoli-Leydig cell tumors
    1. Well-differentiated
      a. Tubular androblastoma; Sertoli cell tumor (tubular adenoma of Pick)
      b. Tubular androblastoma with lipid storage; Sertoli cell tumor with lipid storage (folliculome lipidique of Lecene)
      c. Sertoli-Leydig cell tumor (tubular adenoma with Leydig cells, arrhenoblastoma)
      d. Leydig cell tumor; hilus cell tumor
    2. Of intermediate differentiation
    3. Poorly differentiated (sarcomatoid)
    4. With heterologous elements
  C. Gynandroblastoma
  D. Unclassified

III. LIPID (LIPOID) CELL TUMORS

IV. GERM CELL TUMORS
  A. Dysgerminoma (Figs. 19-27 and 19-28)
  B. Endodermal sinus tumor (yolk sac tumor)
  C. Embryonal carcinoma
  D. Polyembryoma

(continued)

Table 19–2.   (cont.)

E.   Choriocarcinoma (chorioepithelioma)
F.   Teratomas
   1.   Immature
   2.   Mature
      a.   Solid
      b.   Cystic
         (1)   Dermoid cyst (mature cystic
             teratoma)
         (2)   Dermoid cyst with malignant
             transformation
   3.   Monodermal and highly specialized
      a.   Struma ovarii
      b.   Carcinoid
      c.   Struma ovarii and carcinoid
      d.   Others
G.   Mixed forms

V.   *GONADOBLASTOMA*
   A.   Pure
   B.   Mixed with dysgerminoma or other form
      of germ cell tumor

VI.   *SOFT TISSUE TUMORS NOT SPECIFIC TO*
    OVARY
   A.   Angiosarcoma
   B.   Rhabdomyosarcoma
   C.   Lymphosarcoma
   D.   Reticulum cell sarcoma
   E.   Leiomyosarcoma

   F.   Fibrosarcoma
   G.   Mesodermal (Mullerian) mixed tumor,
      homologous (carcinosarcoma)
   H.   Mesodermal (Mullerian) mixed tumor,
      heterologous (mixed mesodermal sar-
      coma) (Figs. 19–29 to 19–31)
   I.   Malignant lymphoma
   J.   Mesonephric carcinoma (malignant meso-
      nephroma)

VII.   *UNCLASSIFIED TUMORS*

VIII.   *SECONDARY (METASTATIC) TUMORS*

IX.   *TUMOR-LIKE CONDITIONS*
   A.   Pregnancy luteoma
   B.   Hyperplasia of ovarian stroma and hyper-
      thecosis
   C.   Massive oedema
   D.   Solitary follicle cyst and corpus luteum
      cyst
   E.   Multiple follicle cysts (polycystic ovaries)
   F.   Multiple luteinized follicle cysts and/or
      corpora lutea
   G.   Endometriosis
   H.   Surface-epithelial inclusion cysts (germinal
      inclusion cysts)
   I.   Simple cysts
   J.   Inflammatory lesions
   K.   Parovarian cysts

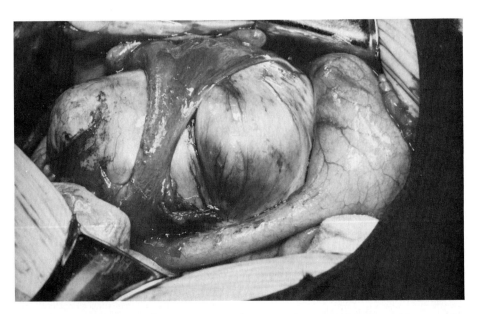

Figure 19–11.   Mucinous cystadenocarcinoma of the ovaries occurring in a 51-year-old woman who had been under medical care for nine months because of intermittent pain in the right lower quadrant of her abdomen. The pain was thought to be due to various intestinal disorders. Note the cecum attached to the right ovary and the appendix encircling the tumor. The right fallopian tube is stretched over the mass.

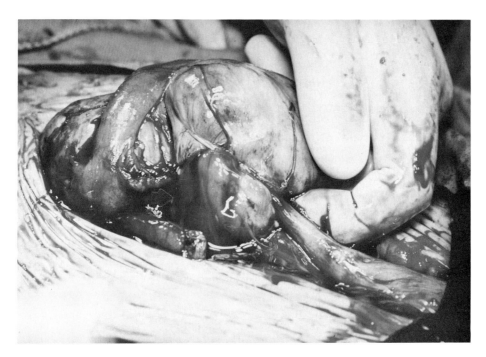

Figure 19–12. After detaching the appendix from the cecum in Figure 19–11, the mass is in the process of being delivered from the pelvis. Another area of bowel attachment, small bowel, is seen next to the index finger. Penetration of the ovarian capsule by disease produced a thinned wall which ruptured during removal and mucin is coming from the tumor.

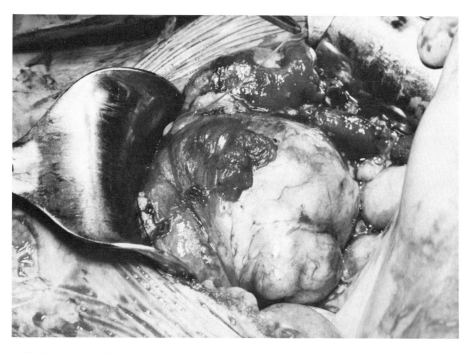

Figure 19–13. The left ovary of the woman in Figures 19–11 and 19–12 is lifted from the cul-de-sac. Multiple areas of bowel adhesions with tumor and parietal peritoneal tumor implants did not prohibit all gross tumor from being removed.

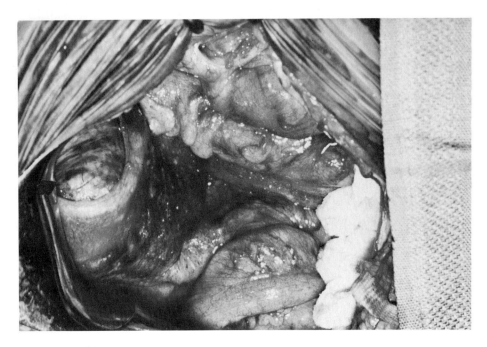

Figure 19–14.   Endometrioid adenocarcinoma of the left ovary in a 73-year-old woman.

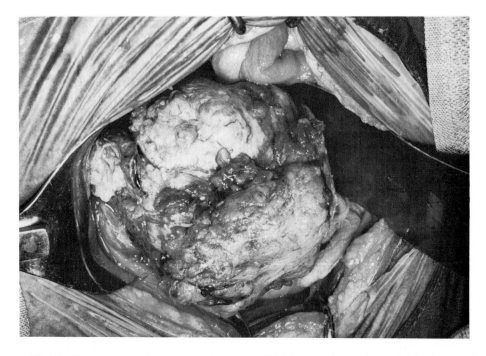

Figure 19–15.   The same patient as seen in Figure 19–14 with the endometrioid adenocarcinoma of the left ovary in the process of being removed from the pelvis.

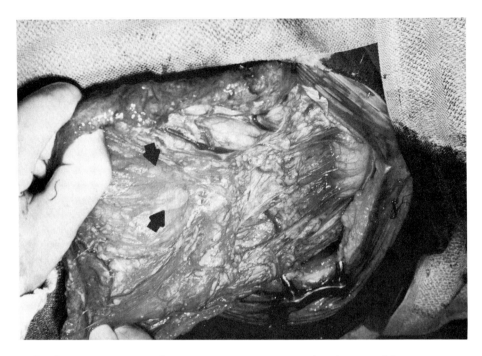

Figure 19–16. The omentum of the patient in Figures 19-14 and 19-15. The omentum contains metastatic nodules and its attachment to the stomach can be seen on the right.

Table 19–3. HISTOGENETIC CATEGORIES OF PRIMARY OVARIAN NEOPLASMS

A   Neoplasms of coelomic (germinal) epithelium and its derivatives

B   Neoplasms of specialized gonadal stroma (sex cords and mesenchyme)

C   Neoplasms of germ cell origin

D   Neoplasms of nonspecialized stroma and heterotrophic elements

---

(mucinous neoplasms). Less frequently, neoplasms in this category consist of a transitional or glandular epithelium which resembles that of the urinary bladder; these are the Brenner tumors. Neoplasms of coelomic epithelium may consist of two or more distinct types of epithelium.

In the category of neoplasms of specialized gonadal stroma Abell includes all lesions that arise from cortical or hilar mesenchyme and from specialized elements in the remants of the sex cords. These are the sex cord stromal tumors of

the histologic classification. These tumors as a group may manifest hormonal activity. If they appear to arise from tissue considered structurally characteristic of the ovary proper, they are classified as granulosa-theca cell neoplasms; whereas, if they arise from hilar structures that are usually associated with testis, they are placed in the Sertoli-Leydig cell group.

In the germ cell category are included all neoplasms that are thought to arise from primitive germ cells and those that may develop in these as secondary cancers.[47]

The neoplasms of nonspecialized stroma include those that arise from tissues common to all organs of the body and thus are not structurally or functionally distinctive.

The distribution of primary ovarian cancer cases based on histogenetic origin are approximately: epithelial type—85 percent of cases and of this percentage approximately 15 to 20 percent will be of borderline malignancy; specialized gonadal stroma (sex cord stromal tumors)—6 percent; germ cell—6 percent, and nonspecialized stroma (soft tissue tumors not specific to ovary)—3 percent.

SPREAD OF OVARIAN CANCER

Ovarian cancer may spread by implantation on peritoneal surfaces (Fig. 19–8), contiguous growth to nearby structures, lymphatic pathways, and least commonly, hematogenously. In his study of autopsies of women with primary ovarian carcinoma of the epithelial type, Bergman[48] noted extraovarian metastases in 88 percent of cases. Direct peritoneal involvement and spread by way of lymphatics were the predominant means of dissemination irrespective of the histologic type and degree of differentiation of the tumor. In advanced disease approximately 50 percent of all women will have pulmonary metastases and 75 percent have lymphatic involvement. Bone and central nervous system metastases each occurs in approximately 2 percent of women with ovarian cancer.[49,50]

Ascites

Ascites is peritoneal effusion which, in the opinion of the physician, is pathologic and/or clearly exceeds normal amounts. The pathophysiology of ascites secondary to ovarian cancer has been subjected to numerous studies. Hirabayashi and Graham discovered that the peritoneal surface, uninvolved by tumor, produces fluid at a rate three to four times that of normal, while the production of fluid from the tumor surface itself is more or less at the rate from the peritoneal surface of a normal patient without tumor. They noted a greater than normal rate of ascitic fluid turnover (inflow-outflow) as compared with the abdominal cavity fluid, which has a considerably less but measurable turnover rate even in the normal individual who has no ascites.[51] Obstruction of diaphragmatic lymphatics with tumor (Figs. 19–9 and 19–10) as well as obstruction of the substernal lymphatic pathways produces a blockage of outflow from the peritoneal cavity and seems to be a cause of ascites in ovarian cancer.[52]

Meyers, with fluoroscopic and roentgenographic observations, demonstrated that intraperitoneal fluid continually follows a circulation through the abdomen. The transverse mesocolon, small bowel

mesentary, sigmoid mesocolon, and the peritoneal attachments of the ascending and descending colon serve as watersheds directing the flow of intraperitoneal fluid. The force of gravity tends to pool peritoneal fluid in dependent peritoneal recesses. Most notable of these is the most caudal and posterior extension of the peritoneal cavity, the pouch or cul-de-sac of Douglas. Four predominant sites of metastases from ovarian cancer correlates with the patterns of flow of ascitic fluid. They are (1) the pouch of Douglas at the rectosigmoid level, (2) the right lower quadrant at the lower end of the small bowel mesentary, (3) the left lower quadrant along the superior border of the sigmoid mesocolon and colon, and (4) the right paracolic gutter lateral to the cecum and ascending colon.[53] The free flow of ascitic fluid containing malignant cells bathes all the visceral and parietal peritoneum, including the diaphragms, of the abdominal cavity.

Lymphatics

The ovary has more and larger lymphatic efferents than any other female pelvic organ. Six to eight principle collecting trunks emerge from the hilus and converge within the mesovarium to form the subovarian plexus. Efferent channels from the fallopian tube and uterine corpus are also incorporated. The drainage trunks ascend along the infundibulopelvic ligament, surrounding the ovarian veins, and cross the ureter for the first time at the level of the external iliac artery. They remain close to the psoas muscle up to the level of the lower pole of the kidney where they abruptly leave the artery and veins to turn medial crossing the ureter and ovarian vessels anteriorly to terminate in aortic nodes. The drainage of lymph from the ovary seems to be almost exclusively in a cephalad direction toward the aortic nodes. Also a collateral lymphatic trunk exists which bypasses the subovarian plexus. It reaches the pelvic wall within the folds of the broad ligament, terminating in the uppermost interiliac nodes.[54]

CAUSE OF DEATH

The major causes of death, particularly of the epithelial type of ovarian cancer relate to intra-abdominal tumor dissemination. Bowel and its mesentary with large peritoneal surfaces is most

commonly involved, producing multiple areas of malfunction, malabsorption, and varying degrees of alteration of peristalsis and obstruction. These women gradually deteriorate over weeks to months and eventually die in electrolyte imbalance, overwhelming septicemia, or cardiovascular collapse all secondary to ovarian cancer. Since the disease has no specific cure in its advanced stage, the various therapies utilized for an extended period of time may contribute to the cause of death in up to 20 percent of women.[55] Also, as many of these women are older, they have various other medical disorders and combined with pulmonary embolism all contribute to the cause of death in another 10 to 15 percent of women dying from ovarian cancer. The hematogenous route is not a common mode of extension but does occur, as demonstrated by isolated parenchymal organ involvement and bone marrow infiltration with tumor.[48,55]

SURGICAL TREATMENT

The primary treatment for ovarian cancer is surgical removal of as much of the tumor as is compatible with the safety of the patient. The preoperative work-up of a patient suspected of having ovarian cancer should always include a careful history, general physical examination, pelvic examination (rectal, vaginal and bimanual), and cervical cytosmear. If there is uterine bleeding, an endometrial tissue aspiration may be carried out. The physical examination should include special attention to the breasts and proctosigmoidoscopy especially in the presence of masses in the left lower quadrant of the abdomen or symptoms that might be confused with a primary bowel lesion. A complete blood count (including platelet count), clean midstream voided urinalysis, and blood chemistries (SMA-12) are necessary.

In a further attempt to document the extent of disease and to determine whether the ovarian tumor is primary or metastatic, roentgenographic study of the chest, upper and lower intestinal contrast studies, should be routinely utilized and usually an intravenous pyelogram performed. Paracentesis or culdocentesis may be performed before operation to obtain a peritoneal fluid cytologic specimen to determine the presence or absence of malignant cells. A lymphangiogram may be useful, particularly when evaluating a prior incidental oophorectomy that was discovered after operation to be a dysgerminoma. Laparoscopy and peritoneoscopy alone are inadequate and improper procedures on which to base treatment planning and treatment for ovarian cancer. If symptoms or roentgenographic studies warrant, some type of preoperative bowel preparation should be utilized.

A vertical skin incision into the abdomen should be utilized which can be extended above the umbilicus to allow adequate examination and biopsy of structures not only in the pelvis but in the upper abdomen.

Physicians opening an abdomen for a suspected or known ovarian tumor should routinely obtain a peritoneal fluid specimen immediately after making the initial incision in the peritoneum and before the peritoneum is completely opened (Fig. 19-17). The amount, color, and character of the peritoneal fluid should be noted. The specimen should be obtained before the peritoneal cavity is contaminated with blood. The peritoneal fluid can be obtained by use of an aspiration syringe and a malleable blunt-tipped cannula (Fig. 19-18). If ascites is not present, a few drops of peritoneal fluid may be aspirated even in a normal abdomen from the cul-de-sac of Douglas, the right lower quadrant in the area of the small bowel mesentary, the left lower quadrant along the superior border of the sigmoid and colon, or lateral to the ascending or descending colon. Only a few drops of peritoneal fluid from these representative areas of the lower abdomen are sufficient to make a predictable cytologic evaluation. Lavage of the peritoneal cavity with so-called "physiologic" solutions is not only usually unnecessary but contraindicated. Excessive fluid placed in the abdomen decreases the number of malignant cells per unit volume from these concentrated sites of tumor cell accumulation. Also, lavage and accompanying complicated and/or time-consuming cell processing may alter the morphology of benign cells and thus make it difficult to differentiate them from malignant cells in various stages of degeneration.

The cytologic specimens should be evenly spread on albumin-coated microscope slides and the slides then promptly put in a glass Coplin jar containing 95 percent ethyl alcohol as a fixative (Fig. 19-19). (A completely frosted slide can be used; cytologic specimens can be quickly placed upon it before immediate fixation. At least one to two direct cytosmears must be obtained on all peritoneal fluid exams.) If sufficient fluid remains in the syringe after the microscope slides have been prepared, the excess fluid can undergo immediate centrifugation (1500 RPM for 5-10 minutes) and the sediment instantly placed on microscopic slides and fixed as mentioned. A good cell concentration will be obtained by this method. The membrane filter method is more

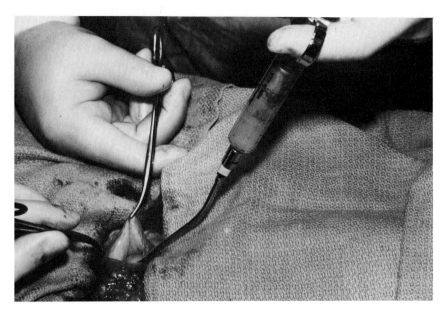

Figure 19–17. Aspiration of a peritoneal fluid cytologic specimen on initial opening of the peritoneal cavity should be performed before it is completely opened.

time consuming and is commonly associated with cell morphologic changes as compared to direct cytosmears, but it should be used in cases where a small volume of peritoneal fluid is obtained or the fluid appears very watery. The slides can remain in the capped Coplin jars with ethyl alcohol until the pathology of the tumor is determined. Should the ovarian tumor be benign, the cytologic specimens may be discarded. If a malignant ovarian tumor is discovered, the cytologic specimens

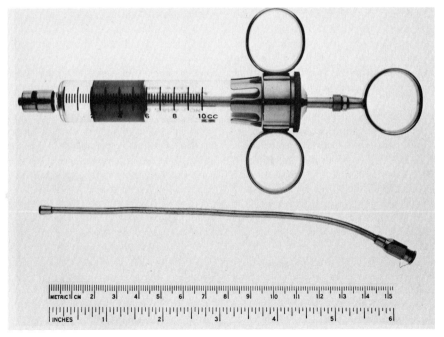

Figure 19–18. The peritoneal fluid specimen is obtained using a 10 cc B-D Sana Lok control syringe with a 6 in. blunt-tipped Abraham-Laryngeal cannula.

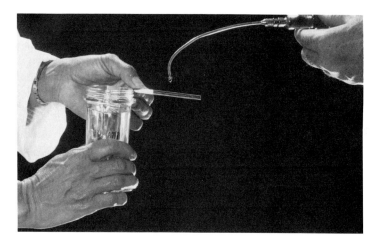

Figure 19–19. One or two drops of peritoneal fluid are placed directly from the syringe and attached cannula to a microscopic slide. The fluid is evenly distributed over the slide with the tip of the cannula and then immediately dropped into the fixative.

should be processed according to Papanicolaou's procedure. All cytologic specimens must eventually be examined under oil immersion.

When operating on women with suspected or known ovarian tumors, physicians should have readily available aspiration syringes, cannulas, microscope slides, and capped Coplin glass jars containing 95 percent ethyl alcohol. The preparation of the slide to receive the peritoneal fluid cytologic specimen should be done a few days before its use, unless a completely frosted slide is used (Figs. 19-20 and 19-21).

A syringe and cannula should be on the operating table and a peritoneal fluid specimen routinely obtained. The quantity of peritoneal fluid has no effect on whether or not malignant cells are present in peritoneal fluid.

Examination of the visceral and parietal peritoneum should include thorough palpation and indicated biopsy. The under surface of the diaphragm should be carefully examined as well as the superior and inferior surfaces of the liver, stomach, pancreas, large and small intestine (Fig. 19-8) and their mesentery, kidneys, pelvic and aortic nodes, and omentum (Fig. 19-16 for metastatic disease.

In the presence of an ovarian tumor and when the diagnosis is not clearly clinically indicated that it is ovarian cancer, frozen-section tissue diagnosis should be performed to determine if it is benign or malignant, or metastatic. Frozen-section diagnosis is especially helpful in the young patient or one desiring pregnancy in the presence of a unilateral tumor. Also frozen section is of great importance in the establishment of the diagnosis of epithelial neoplasms of borderline malignancies (carcinomas of low malignant potential). These women benefit the most in relation to reduction of morbidity and enhanced survival from a primary operation that may include removal of large segments of visceral and parietal peritoneum and perhaps multiple segments of

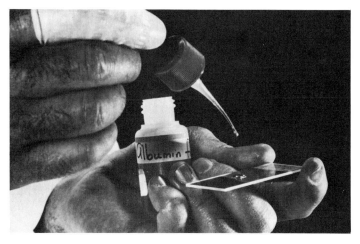

Figure 19–20. An albumin-coated slide should be prepared a few days before it is to be used and is done so by putting one drop of albumin on a properly identified slide.

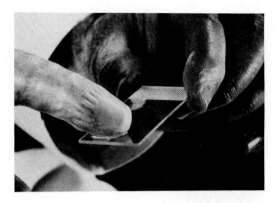

Figure 19–21. The albumin is spread evenly over the slide and any excess briskly wiped off by use of a finger covered with a finger-cot.

small bowel and colon, as well as portions of the bladder and ureters.

Definite palliation may be achieved by the reduction of tumor within the abdomen although survival will not be improved unless all or nearly all of the gross tumor is excised.

The prognosis in ovarian carcinoma is effected by the stage of the tumor at operation, the residual mass after the primary operation, and the histologic type and grade of the tumor.

Omentectomy, partial (removed from the transverse colon) (Fig. 19–45) or total (Fig. 19–16) (removal from the greater curvature of the stomach and transverse colon), is an integral part of proper surgical management for ovarian cancer. In early disease even though the omentum may look to be normal and no nodes are palpable, it should be routinely removed. The omentum freely absorbs malignant cells from the peritoneal fluid and its removal allows for microscopic exam and proper staging of the disease. In more advanced disease an anoxic "omental cake" (Fig. 19–24) should be removed if possible, as this will at least enhance palliative care of the woman. In early disease an appendectomy should also be included as it is in a location and is a site in which microscopic metastases commonly occur.

The para-aortic lymph nodes should be always carefully palpated. In early disease they may be better studied by incision of the parietal peritoneum from the common iliacs toward the bifurcation of the aorta to the renal arteries. Removal of the fat around the anterior and lateral sides of the vena cava as well as the aorta may be performed. In cases where a single enlarged and suspicious lymph node is palpable that node

should be excised and submitted for histopathologic examination. At the same time the use of a proctosigmoidoscope or laparoscope can be utilized for direct examination of the diaphragm.

Treatment of Stage I Ovarian Cancer

Most women with Stage I ovarian cancer should be treated by abdominal hysterectomy, bilateral salpingo-oophorectomy, at least partial omentectomy, and appendectomy (Fig. 19–5).

Malignant cells within an ovarian neoplasm can escape through an intact ovarian capsule into the peritoneal fluid circulation. Tumor excrescences on the external surface of an ovary can exfoliate cancer cells directly into the active peritoneal fluid circulation. All tumor should be removed intact if possible. Accidental rupture of malignant ovarian cysts during surgical removal usually results from already thinned walls due to microscopic penetration by disease or to disease that has perforated the ovarian capsule and attached to nearby structures (Fig. 19–12).

If physicians do not routinely obtain peritoneal fluid cytologic specimens at the time of surgery in women with ovarian tumors, further treatment of stages I and II ovarian cancer will be haphazard, and a meaningful comparison of therapeutic modalities will be impossible. The presence or absence of malignant cells in the peritoneal fluid of a young woman with a unilateral ovarian cancer must be determined before any thought is given to the conservation of ovarian tissue. The presence of malignant cells in the peritoneal fluid of a woman with a grossly involved unilateral ovarian cancer demands removal not only of the other ovary, uterus, and tubes but also of the omentum.

In a woman with a stage IA ovarian cancer limited to one ovary, no ascites, no tumor on the external surface, capsule intact, and the lesion is a well-differentiated or moderately differentiated cancer of the epithelial type, it has not been documented as to what type of further treatment, if any, is required following operation.[56,58] Bisection or wedge biopsy is necessary of the opposite ovary even in a normal-appearing ovary.[59] Only when carcinoma of the ovary is low grade, intracystic, unruptured, nonadherent, and the peritoneal fluid, omentum and appendix are tumor free and occurs in a young woman who is desirous of childbearing can conservative management be considered.

Stage IB and IC ovarian cancer as well as those

poorly differentiated lesions of stage IA, all of the epithelial type, deserve further therapy. Melphalan 7 mg/sq meter/day given by mouth for five days every four weeks is one form of therapy. Another type of therapy is the use of radioactive colloidal chromic phosphorous (^{32}P). It is a beta emitter with an effective radiation ranging from 4 to 6 mm of tissue and its half-life is 14.2 days. It is thought that the colloid is fixed on or near the surface of the peritoneal lining of the abdominal cavity.[60] There is no external radiation hazard unless the material is spilled. At the time of operation, two catheters are placed in the abdomen so that an even distribution of radioactivity throughout the abdomen will take place. Ideally within two to three days postoperatively 10 to 15 millicuries is injected through the catheters into the abdominal cavity.

Treatment of Stage II Ovarian Cancer

Ovarian cancer involving one or both ovaries with pelvic extension, ascites, or malignant cells in peritoneal fluid requires further therapy following operation. Primary surgery should include aspiration of a peritoneal fluid specimen for cytology, abdominal hysterectomy, bilateral salpingo-oophorectomy, omentectomy, appendectomy,

removal of as much as possible of tumor, and a careful abdominal examination to determine extent of disease as previously described. Further therapy after operation can be melphalan 7 mg/sq meter/day given by mouth for five days every four to five weeks alone or combined with pelvic irradiation or pelvic and abdominal irradiation. When pelvic irradiation is utilized, approximately 5000 rads to the midline in five to seven weeks (150 to 200 rads/day) is administered starting no later than four weeks after operation. If abdominal irradiation is added to pelvic irradiation, 3000 rads can be given in four to six weeks with the kidneys and right lobe of the liver protected after a dose of 2000 rads.

Treatment of Stage III and Stage IV Ovarian Cancer

Primary operation should remove as much gross tumor as possible without endangering the life of the patient or producing excessive morbidity. Histologic confirmation of the ovary as the primary site should be established and the clinical extent of the disease within the abdomen determined. At least removal of both ovaries (Figs. 19-22 and 19-23) and the omentum (Fig. 19-24) when most of the gross disease cannot be re-

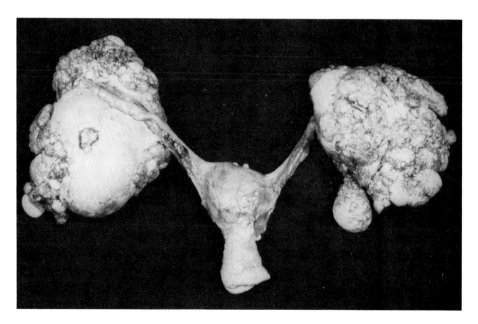

Figure 19–22. Bilateral serous cystadenocarcinoma of the ovaries occurring in a postmenopausal woman.

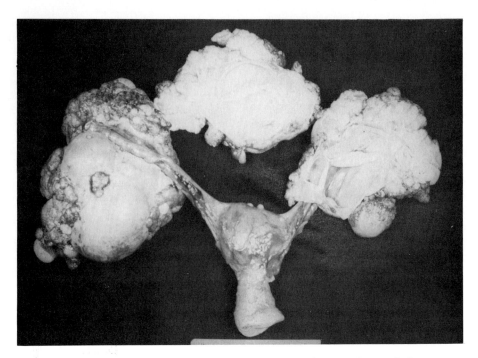

Figure 19–23. Same patient as in Figure 19-22 with the left ovary bisected demonstrating the cystic nature of the tumor with multiple surface papillary excrescences.

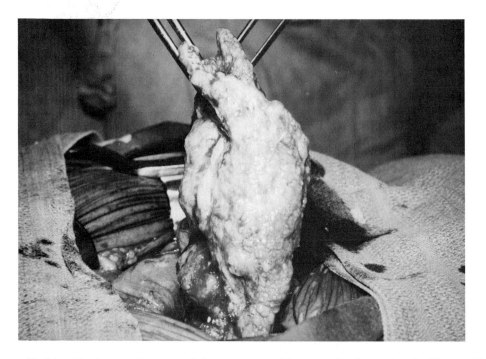

Figure 19–24. Massive involvement of the omentum with cancer in the patient in Figures 19–22 and 19–23.

moved will help in the patient's palliative care. After operative removal of as much tumor as possible, particularly in the tumors of epithelial origin, patients may be divided into optimal or suboptimal categories depending on the greatest diameter of residual tumor or tumors. Optimal is that category such that the size of the largest residual tumor is no greater than 2 cm in diameter. Maintaining the integrity of the gastrointestinal and genitourinary tracts is important in diffuse not completely resectable disease. Patients with advanced ovarian cancer should not undergo extended surgery or pelvic exenteration except in extremely rare instances.

Irradiation therapy has for the most part been abandoned as a treatment for stage III or IV, optimal, suboptimal, or recurrent ovarian cancer of epithelial type. Clinical studies utilizing not only melphalan alone but melphalan with immunotherapeutic agents are currently under clinical investigation and include BCG (bacille Calmette Guerin), irradiated tumor cells, neuramidase-treated tumor cells, corynebacterium parvum (C-parvum), and others. C-parvum is a gram-positive anaerobic bacillus. For optimal disease melphalan may be utilized in a dosage of 7 mg/sq meter/day by mouth for five days every four weeks and in some studies it is being combined with the use of C-parvum 4 mg/sq meter intravenously on day seven following the start of chemotherapy and repeated every four weeks.

Multiple segments of bowel are commonly superficially involved with cancer producing carcinomatosis ileus. The intermittent use of a nasogastric or longer intestinal tube as definitive therapy to decompress the bowel should be considered.

The survival is poor in women with suboptimal stages III and IV and recurrent ovarian cancer, especially of epithelial origin, and for that reason a number of clinical investigations are utilizing different chemotherapy regimens. Some include the combination of hexamethylmelamine 100 mg/sq meter/day by mouth for 14 days and melphalan 5 to 7 mg/sq meter/day for five days, and this combination repeated every four weeks. Also adriamycin 40 to 50 mg/sq meter of body surface can be combined with cyclophosphamide 400 to 500 mg/sq meter of body surface and both given intravenously every three weeks. Melphalan is used in most studies today as the control arm in evaluating any other chemotherapeutic regimen, as a response rate of 30 to 60 percent has been reported.

CHEMOTHERAPY

Chemotherapy is being more commonly utilized today in the management of disseminated ovarian carcinoma because of the continued unsatisfactory results following operation alone and the general failure of irradiation therapy as a sole postoperative modality.[61,62] Alkylating agents used alone give objective regression in approximately 30 to 60 percent of individuals with ovarian cancer. Although chemotherapy has increased the overall survival very little, it has made life more comfortable for a great number of women with ovarian cancer.

Bone marrow suppression is a common adverse effect of chemotherapy for ovarian cancer. Chemotherapy depresses blood cell production and causes abnormalities in neutrophil and platelet function. Immune defenses may also be impaired by the disease itself or as a result of chemotherapy and places the cancer patient with suppressed marrow function in a more susceptible position to serious infection.

A woman with ovarian cancer undergoing chemotherapy may also experience nausea and/or vomiting, diarrhea, stomatitis, alopecia, neurotoxicity, cardiac toxicity, febrile reactions, local tissue necrosis from extravasation of drug, or chemical cystitis. A phenothiazine drug is the preferred antiemetic for vomiting and is most effective when given prophylactically.

During treatment, dietary support to alleviate the effects of chemotherapeutic agents should be considered. Cold bland fluids, ice cream, and milk shakes and mechanically soft foods should be offered. The woman should be adequately hydrated and her food likes and dislikes seriously noted. Highly seasoned, spicy, and acid foods should be avoided. Between treatments a diet that is high in calories and protein should be offered.

Chemotherapy like surgery and radiation therapy must be individualized to the particular patient, stage, and type of ovarian cancer. The height and weight of the woman are utilized in the determination of her body surface area in order to more precisely define drug administration. Treatment modifications that include dose escalation, deescalation, and delays based on adverse

Table 19–4.   ADVERSE EFFECTS CRITERIA

SYSTEM	0	1 =MILD	2 =MODERATE	3 =SEVERE	LIFE 4 =THREAT-ENING
Hematopoietic					
WBC	≥4,000	3,000–3,999	2,000–2,999	1,000–1,999	<1,000
Granulocytes	≥1,500	1,000–1,499	500–999	250–499	<250
Platelets	≥150,000	100,000–149,999	50,000–99,999	25,000–49,999	<25,000
Genitourinary Renal					
BUN mg%	≤20	21–40	41–60	>60	
Creatinine mg%	≤1.2	1.3–2.0	2.1–4.0	>4	
Creatinine clearance	>50 ml/min	35–50 ml/min	20–34 ml/min	<20 ml/min	
Bladder	Normal	Dysuria requiring no treatment (Rx) and/or microscopic hematuria	Dysuria requiring therapy and/or hematuria	Hematuria and drop of Hgb by 2 gm%	
Hepatic (N =Normal) SGOT	N–2N	2N–5N = (2 times normal-5 times normal)	5N–10N	>10N	
SGPT	N–2N	2N–5N	5N–10N	>10N	
Bilirubin	1 mg	1.1–2 mg	2.1–5 mg	>5 mg	
Alkaline phosphatase	N–2N	2N–5N	5N–10N	>10N	
Gastrointestinal					
Stomatitis	Normal	Erythema and enanthema	Ulcers—able to eat	Unable to eat due to ulcerations	
Abdominal pain	None	No treatment needed	Treatment need-ed—helpful	Treatment needed-not helpful	
Constipation	Normal	No treatment needed	Treatment need-ed—helpful	Treatment needed-not helpful	

effects of therapy are an integral part of therapy (Table 19–4).

Currently the most convenient and best first-line chemotherapeutic approach for ovarian cancers of epithelial types is the use of a single alkylating agent such as melphalan. Combination chemotherapy is being investigated in an attempt to obtain a complete remission of disease and for use as a second-line therapy for recurrences. The principles of combination chemotherapy are to use drugs that (1) are active when used alone, (2) have a biochemical basis for suspected synergism, (3) produce toxicity in different organ systems, (4) have different mechanisms of action, (5) produce toxicity at different times following drug administration, and (6) are used in repeated brief courses in order to minimize the immunosuppressive effects.

Table 19-4.   (cont.)

SYSTEM	0	1 =MILD	2 =MODERATE	3 =SEVERE	LIFE 4 =THREAT- ENING
Diarrhea	<3 bowel movements/ day	3-4 liquid stools, no dehydration	>4 liquid stools/ day, needs IV to hydrate	Bloody diarrhea, needs IV and/or blood	
Nausea and vomiting	Normal	Nausea, no vomit- ing	Vomiting, prevent- ed by treatment	Vomiting 6 × day inspite of antiemetics	
Pulmonary	Normal	No symptoms, pul- monary func- tions decreased	Pulmonary symp- toms requiring Rx, no need for assisted ventilation	Assisted ventilation needed	
Cardiac	Normal in all	ECG changes only, or sinus tachy- cardia not to exceed 110 at rest	Arrhythemias, ex- cept ventrical tachycardia and/ or ECG changes	Congestive heart failure, ventri- cular tachycardia, pericarditis, and/or effusion	
Neuromuscular					
Pheripheral nerves	None	Deep tendon reflex- es decreased or absent and/or paraesthesias	Weakness and se- vere paraesthe- sias	Incapacity	
Central nerv- ous system	None	Drowsiness and nervousness	Confusion, anxiety or depression requiring Rx	Convulsions, coma, psychosis	
Skin					
Acute	None	Transient erythema or exanthema	Vesiculation	Ulceration	
Chronic	None	Pigmentation, atrophy, dipilation	Subepidermal fibrosis	Ulceration and necrosis	
Allergy	None	Drug fever <38 C (<100.4 F) Transient rash	Urticaria fever >38 C (>100.4 F), Asthama	Anaphylactic reaction or anaphylactic shock	

In the early stages of ovarian cancer (Stage IC and IIC) and Stage III when all gross disease has been removed, adjuvant chemotherapy should be considered. Micrometastases present at the time of operation are the causes of distant recurrences. The aim of adjuvant chemotherapy is destruction of micrometastases, prevention of clinical metas- tases, and achievement of cure, rather than just delaying the appearance of metastases.

Tobias and Griffiths have succinctly stated that "although the value of chemotherapy in ovarian cancer appears to have been established, little or no progress has been made since the responsive- ness to alkylating agents was first noted more than 20 years ago."[62] The problem is that chemothera- py is limited by the mass of the tumor rather than by its extent.

Physicians who choose to undertake the chemotherapeutic care of a woman with ovarian cancer should do that as a team member with the gynecologic oncologist, for only under those circumstances can there be reasonable assurance of

careful staging, meticulous surgical resection, detailed histologic classification, and exacting follow-up clinical evaluation.

SPECIAL TREATMENT SITUATIONS

In approximately 85 percent of cases, ovarian cancer is of the epithelial type, and when it occurs it is commonly present in perimenopausal or postmenopausal women with an average age of 56. Germ cell neoplasms account for approximately 6 percent of ovarian cancers and occur about 20 years earlier, age 36, than the more common ovarian cancers. Additional problems may arise in some with ovarian cancer as they may be very young children, women desiring a family, and each having a neoplasm of varying degrees of aggressiveness. Children and young adults suspected of having an ovarian neoplasm should have a careful abdominal and rectal examination per-

formed. As the pelvis has limited space available for tumor expansion in young girls, the enlarged ovary is commonly found in the abdomen and can undergo torsion. Ultrasonography at times may be of diagnostic help.

The ideal management of malignant ovarian tumors whether they occur in children, young adults, or in the elderly consists of complete surgical removal. Adequate exploration of the abdomen requires an adequate surgical incision. As previously described, the abdomen must be carefully examined and when combined with comprehensive histologic evaluation of the tumor adequate but not unnecessarily destructive thera-

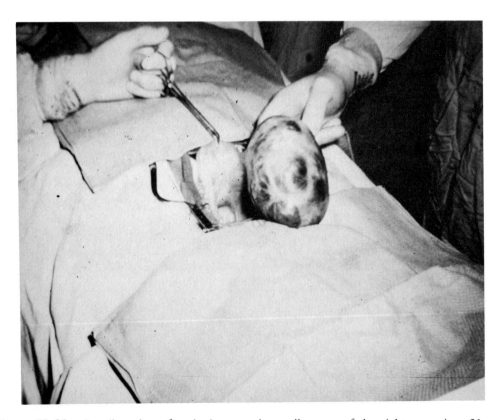

Figure 19–25. A unilateral nonfunctioning granulosa cell tumor of the right ovary in a 21-year-old woman. There was no evidence of extraovarian spread and the mitotic count was low. She was treated by unilateral oophorectomy and has no evidence of disease 15 years later.

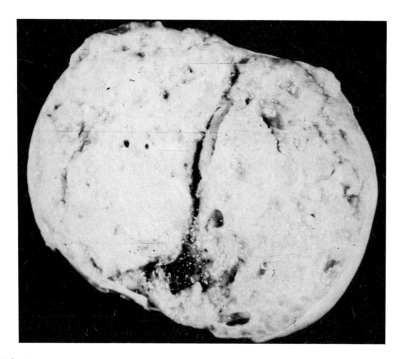

Figure 19–26. The same granulosa cell tumor in Figure 19–25 bisected showing a predominant solid pattern with a few cystic areas.

py can be performed. In children and women desiring additional children, frozen section histologic study can be done at the time of operation and if the diagnosis is still in doubt, the abdomen can be closed awaiting definitive gynecologic pathology consultation.

Sex Cord Stromal Tumors

Granulosa-Stromal Cell Tumors

Granulosa-theca tumors represent approximately 3 percent of ovarian tumors and about 80 percent of sex cord stromal tumors.[63,64] Granulosa-theca tumors occur at all ages with the majority in the age range of 42 to 52 years. Vaginal bleeding is the presenting symptom in over 50 percent of women with granulosa-theca cell tumors.[65] Approximately 80 percent of granulosa cell tumors are stage I disease and 95 percent of all granulosa cell tumors are unilateral (Figs. 19–25 and 19–26). Norris has observed that microscopically, there are as many as 12 histologic patterns in granulosa-theca tumors. He believes the malignancy potential of a thecoma is virtually nil.[66] Dysplasia of the endometrium as well as endometrial cancer can coexist with granulosa cell tumors. Surgical treatment usually includes abdominal hysterectomy and bilateral salpingo-oophorectomy. In children and women desiring children, unilateral oophorectomy with bivalving and wedge resection of the opposite ovary to determine absence of tumor is indicated. If the uterus is left in place, a curettage of the endometrium is mandatory.

The overall prognosis for granulosa cell tumor is approximately 85 to 90 percent five-year survival.[67] Norris cautions that survival data for granulosa tumors must be scrutinized as to the inclusion of adenocarcinomas, if in reality the women died of granulosa tumor, and the proportion of the more benign thecomas included in the series.[66] Fox et al[65] associate the following factors with a relatively poor survival rate: age over 40 and abdominal symptoms at the time of diagnosis, bilateral tumors, extraovarian spread, and numerous mitotic figures in the tumor. Granulosa cell tumor has a propensity for late metastasis, and recurrences often respond well to external irradiation therapy. Those women with widespread disease that does not respond to radiation therapy may be given dactinomycin, 5-fluorouracil, and cyclophosphamide intravenously for five days every four weeks.

Androblastomas: Sertoli-Leydig Cell Tumors and Lipid (Lipoid) Cell Tumors

Sertoli-Leydig tumors are the most common virilizing tumors of the ovary. They are extremely uncommon and probably are one-tenth as frequent as granulosa-theca tumors. They occur most commonly in the ages between 20 and 40 years.[66] They are bilateral in less than 5 percent of cases, and Ireland and Woodruff state the malignancy rate is close to 5 percent.[68] In young patients after appropriate study of the opposite ovary, its preservation as well as that of the uterus certainly seems indicated. At the time of operation should there be clinical evidence of extension or tumor beyond the ovary or if the patient no longer desires children or is beyond the childbearing age, removal of both ovaries and the uterus is indicated. Radiation therapy may be used in diffuse disease and followed by triple chemotherapy (dactinomycin, 5-fluorouracil, and cyclophosphamide) if needed.

Germ Cell Tumors

Germ cell tumors account for approximately 6 percent of all ovarian cancers. Their malignancy potential ranges from an extremely low rate to those of aggressively malignant potential. It cannot be too greatly stressed that multiple tissue sections from each tumor must be meticulously studied in order that the proper cell type is assigned to the tumor, which makes possible knowledgeable treatment planning, treatment, and determination of prognosis for the individual patient.[69]

Dysgerminoma

Dysgerminoma accounts for approximately 2 percent of all primary malignant ovarian neoplasms.[70] Dysgerminomas containing no other germ cell tumor types occur around the age of 20 to 25 years with symptoms referable to an abdominal mass or pain present in over 50 percent of women (Fig. 19-27). Therapy is based on recognition of an ovarian tumor in a young woman followed by surgical exploration. At the time of operation if there appears to be no clinical extension of disease beyond one ovary, para-aortic nodes are not enlarged, as well as no involvement of the opposite ovary as proved by palpation and immediate study of a wedge biopsy, an unilateral oophorectomy may be performed (Fig. 19-28). Asadouiran and Taylor advocate unilateral oophorectomy as a justifiable procedure for treatment of unilateral dysgerminomas when

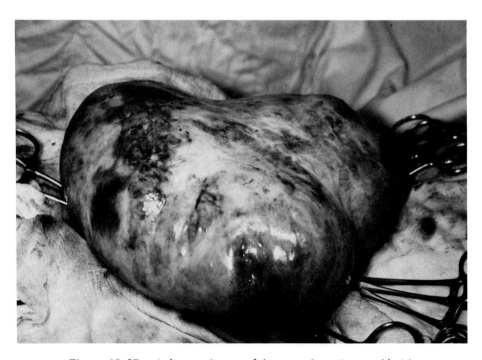

Figure 19-27.   A dysgerminoma of the ovary in a 13-year-old girl.

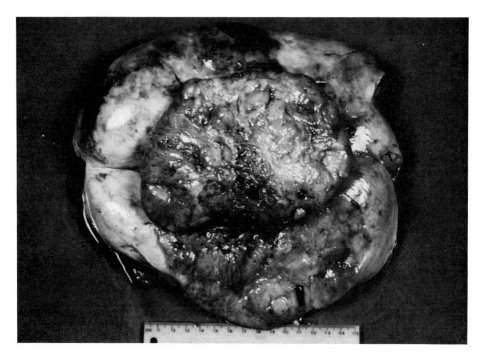

Figure 19–28. A unilateral oophorectomy was performed in the young girl in Figure 19-27. It contained only dysgerminoma with no evidence of spread of disease beyond the ovary. She is free of tumor 11 years later.

preservation of ovarian function is desired. They observed that the 10-year postoperative actuarial survival rate was as good for patients treated by unilateral oophorectomy alone (88 percent) for tumors apparently confined to one ovary as for patients treated more extensively (83 percent).[71]

Dysgerminomas once beyond the ovary may spread by direct extension or by way of the lymphatics to the para-aortic nodes and higher. For disease that has spread beyond one ovary with metastases or recurrent disease moderate doses of external radiation therapy to this most radiosensitive of all ovarian cancers is beneficial.[72]

Lymphangiography is not only effective in evaluating extent of disease but as an aid to follow-up.

Endodermal Sinus Tumors

This uncommon germ cell cancer occurs in young women, average age 18, and in three-quarters of the patients, presents with an abdominal mass and pain. The duration of symptoms may be brief but the tumor size is significant, approximately 15 cm, when found at operation. Although cases clinically thought to be only unilateral disease and

treated with surgery and radiation therapy are associated with the demise of most patients within two years from disseminated disease.[73]

Treatment of endodermal sinus tumors includes abdominal hysterectomy and bilateral salpingo-oophorectomy and prudently removing other tumor bearing areas, followed by chemotherapy. One regimen is the use of vincristine in a dose of 1.5 to 2.0 mg/sq meter body surface area intravenously (IV) either weekly or biweekly for 8 to 12 weeks, dactinomycin 300 to 400 micrograms/sq meter intravenously daily for five days every four weeks, and cyclophosphamide 150 mg/sq meter body surface area intravenously daily for five days every four weeks. The use of triple chemotherapy agents for these rare germ cell tumors appears to significantly enhance survival.[73-76]

Embryonal Carcinoma

Embryonal carcinoma in the past has been not defined microscopically or clinically from endodermal sinus tumor. Kurman and Norris have presented the clinical and pathologic features of embryonal carcinoma of the ovary. They have noted the similarity to that of embryonal carcinoma of the adult testis, and on the basis of histologic and immunohistochemical characteristics, it may be distinguished from endodermal sinus tumor.[77]

The median age was 14 years in Kurman and Norris' study, with an abdominal or pelvic mass plus abdominal pain being present in most young girls with the tumor. Abnormal hormonal manifestations consisting of precocious puberty, irregular vaginal bleeding, amenorrhea, or hirsutism were present in over 50 percent of their patients. Positive pregnancy tests are extremely common even though no pregnancy is present. Clinically, the tumors are large, around 17 cm in size, and may be associated with diffuse disease that includes the retroperitoneal lymph nodes, liver, and lungs. For this reason survival even in early disease is not good, although thought to be better than endodermal sinus tumor. Kurman and Norris carried out an indirect immunoperoxidase method for the localization of human chorionic gonadotropin (HCG) and α-fetoprotein (AFP) on formalin-fixed paraffin-embedded tissue and noted HCG to be positive in all of their study patients and AFP in 70 percent of study patients.[77]

The chemotherapy regimen as detailed for endodermal sinus tumor seems to be promising following ablative tumor surgery.[77,78]

Choriocarcinoma

Primary choriocarcinoma of the ovary is very rare, most examples being metastatic from the uterus. When primary in the ovary, it arises from either an ovarian pregnancy or from neoplastic germ cells. Norris and Chorlton believe the diagnosis is made histologically by placental villi being present or by associated germ cell components.[79] When the patient is premenarchal the diagnosis is obviously easier, as gestational choriocarcinoma is not a consideration. As both primary and metastatic choriocarcinoma are characterized by extensive hemorrhagic necrosis, surgical dissection can be difficult. Surgical removal of as much disease as technically possible is indicated, followed by chemotherapy. One promising regime is the use of dactinomycin 0.5 mg intravenously for five days every three weeks, methotrexate 0.2 mg/kg intravenously daily for five days every three weeks, and chlorambucil 0.2 mg/kg orally daily for five days every three weeks.[79-81]

Teratomas

IMMATURE

Immaure malignant teratoma of the ovary usually occurs around the age of 19 with the complaints of abdominal pain in the presence of a pelvic or abdominal mass. Survival is related to size of tumor and differentiation. Unilateral oophorectomy is indicated in these young patients when the disease is confined to one ovary, is less than 10 cm in size, and is well differentiated. Survival for these women is over 90 percent.[82] Women with ovarian lesions not well differentiated, larger than 10 cm in size, or not confined to one ovary should have an abdominal hysterectomy, bilateral salpingo-oophorectomy, omentectomy, and appendectomy followed by chemotherapy. The drugs dactinomycin, vincristine, and cyclophosphamide may be utilized in the same manner as previously mentioned for endodermal sinus tumor and embryonal carcinoma of the ovary.[83,84]

MATURE (DERMOID CYST WITH MALIGNANT TRANSFORMATION)

Dermoid cysts with malignant transformation occur in less than 1 percent of all dermoids. The dermoid cyst is usually benign, asymptomatic, and not surgically difficult to remove. The diagnosis of malignant degeneration of a dermoid is difficult to make preoperatively as well as at the time of operation. In the presence of dense adhesions or evidence of extraovarian spread, immediate frozen tissue sections of the tumor as well as from areas of adhesions should be performed at the time of a presumed removal of a benign cyst. All gross tumor must be removed if possible. If the diagnosis is established at the time of operation, an en block resection of the cyst with all the adherent viscera seems justified.[85,86] Chemotherapy with the use of the drugs dactinomycin, vincristine, and cyclophosphamide shows promise for diffuse or recurrent disease.

Mixed Forms

The term "mixed germ cell tumor" is applied to neoplasms containing combinations of malignant germ cell elements. They represent no more than 8 percent of malignant germ cell tumors. Kurman and Norris found dysgerminoma to be the most common constitutent followed by endodermal sinus tumor, teratoma, choriocarcinoma, and embryonal carcinoma the least. The most important factors in predicting the prognosis for patients with stage I disease was the size and histologic composition of the neoplasm. They observed that if more than one-third of a stage I neoplasm was composed of endodermal sinus tumor, choriocarcinoma, or grade III teratoma, the prognosis was poor; whereas if the tumor contained less than one-third of these components or contained combinations of dysgerminoma, embryonal carcinoma, or grade I or II teratoma, the prognosis was excellent. All of their patients whose neoplasm was less than 10 cm in maximum diameter survived, regardless of the composition of the tumor.[87]

As a general principal, determination of extent of disease within the abdomen at the time of operation and surgical removal of all disease possible should be performed. In these patients, median age 16 years, unilateral salpingo-oophorectomy should be considered for stage I tumors and frozen-section evaluation of the tumor as well as the opposite ovary will help in arriving at a surgical decision. A woman having metastatic or recurrent disease as well as the mentioned poor prognostic factors should be treated with chemotherapy after operation, one regimen being that utilizing dactinomycin, vincristine, and cyclophosphamide.[87,88]

Gonadoblastoma

Scully reports that the gonadoblastoma may be regarded as an in situ cancer from which dysgerminomas and occasionally other types of invasive germ cell tumor can develop.[89] Dysgerminoma overgrowth is frequent in gonadoblastoma and metastases from this component may occur, as well as from germ cell elements more highly malignant than the dysgerminoma.[90,91] They should be managed in the manner presented for each germ cell type. A patient with a gonadoblastoma and an apparently uninvolved opposite ovary as seen at operation should have chromosome analysis. If the karyogram contains a Y chromosome the remaining gonad represents rudimentary testicular tissue and normal estrogenic function and fertility cannot be expected, so the contralateral ovary plus the uterus should be removed.[90,91] In a normally developed girl with a normal karyogram and the contralateral ovary has been biopsy-proven free of tumor, a unilateral salpingo-oophorectomy may be performed.

Schellhas warns that a patient with gonadal dysgenesis who reveals a Y chromosomal component cytogenetically appears to be at high risk for the development of germ cell tumor and the gonads should be removed.[91]

Soft Tissue Tumors Not Specific to Ovary

This category includes a variety of rare neoplasms that are more commonly found in other parts of the body. The women with these ovarian tumors usually have a palpable pelvic or abdominal mass and experience pain of varying degrees (Fig. 19-29).[63,64,92-98] At the time of surgical operation, the extent of disease should be determined and should include removal of the primary lesion and as much of the metastases as technically possible. Further therapy must be individualized as to the cell type in the ovary and the corresponding usual treatment regimen carried out for the tumor in other parts of the body. Combined modalities of therapy may be carried out as, for example, in mixed mesodermal tumors of the ovary (Figs. 19-30 and 19-31) in which dactinomycin and vincristine are given concomitantly with radiotherapy, followed by a maintenance regimen with cyclophosphamide.[99,100]

Secondary (Metastatic) Tumors

Carcinoma of the breast, genital, and gastrointestinal tract and tumors of the hematopoetic system are most commonly encountered in cancers metastatic to the ovary.[101-103] Determining whether an ovarian enlargement is a primary or metastatic neoplasm begins with the initial history and physical examination of the woman. Symptoms of a gastrointestinal disorder demand appropriate roentgenographic studies of the intestine and also endoscopy. A more regular use of barium enema radiographic examination of the colon and rectum for women with an ovarian tumor would obviate the finding of an unsuspected primary large bowel cancer masking as an adnexal mass or one metastatic to the ovary. Careful breast examination, xeromommography, and breast biopsy are also indicated for a suspicious breast lesion prior to surgical removal of an associated ovarian tumor.

A cancer metastatic to the ovary from advanced endometrial cancer is not unexpected and a curet-

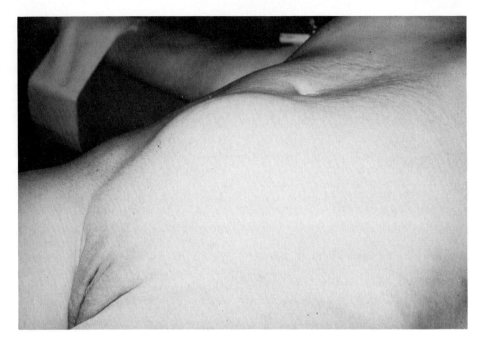

Figure 19–29. A 64-year-old woman with mild lower abdominal pain and a palpable abdominal and pelvic mass.

tage of the uterus before celiotomy in a post-menopausal woman with an ovarian tumor and uterine enlargement would easily determine the primary tumor site.

The operating physician does not want to remove a metastatic unsuspected ovarian tumor and overlook therapy of the primary lesion, therefore a mandatory initial function of the surgeon is to

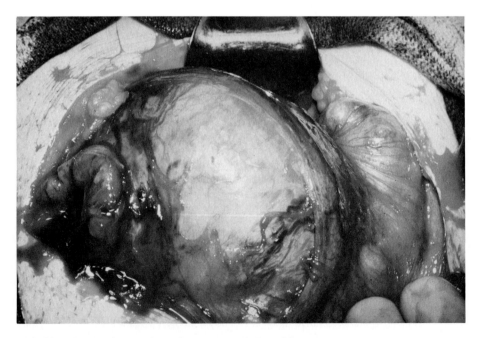

Figure 19–30. A mixed mesodermal sarcoma of the right ovary in the same patient in Figure 19–29.

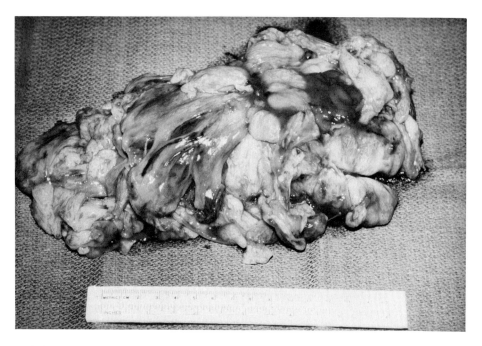

Figure 19–31. The removed ovary containing mixed mesodermal sarcoma from the patient in Figures 19-29 and 19-30.

determine whether the ovarian neoplasm is primary or metastatic. A thorough intra-abdominal examination is indicated with particular emphasis on the pancreas, because with disseminated intra-abdominal pancreatic disease also metastatic to the ovary it may appear as a primary ovarian cancer. The treatment of the metastatic ovarian tumor is obviously secondary to that of the principal tumor site therapy.

FOLLOW-UP OF OVARIAN CANCER PATIENTS

After operation for ovarian cancer the detection of persistent or recurrent disease as well as the monitoring of any further therapy are of prime importance. Efforts to detect persistent or recurrent disease or to monitor therapy must be as equally persistent as those to detect the disease initially. Ultimate survival cannot improve unless surgical efforts are meticulous and the stage of disease determined. Recurrent disease is disease not clinically evident at operation but becomes so six months following operation. Proper assessment as to the presence or absence of malignant cells in peritoneal fluid, the status of the omentum and appendix as to the presence of cancer, and the clinical evaluation of the undersurface of the diaphragm and paraortic lymph nodes is mandatory in early disease.

The early determination of persistent disease following operation and during chemotherapy and/or radiation therapy provides evidence of the futility of continuing that regimen and permits the modification of therapy. Follow-up care of ovarian cancer patients is difficult and many times unreliable if physicians depend solely on palpation and traditional roentgenographic aids, particularly in those women who have had maximum surgical removal.

Methods for Follow-up Care

A history and physical examination that includes a pelvic and rectal exam is the foundation of follow-up care of the ovarian cancer patient. This would include assessment of the patient's weight and its distribution as well as her general well being, appetite, and ability to function at home, work, and socially.

Problems associated with tumor growth would be persistent, progressive ascites and partial intestinal obstruction with mild pain and general debilitation. Repeated paracentesis for symptomatic relief in ovarian cancer presents no risk for the patient and does not significantly lower serum total proteins or albumin.[104] As the tumor may spread over the surface of bowel, the patient may develop inanition and have frequent episodes of nausea and vomiting. The intermittent use of a nasogastric tube is indicated to decompress the bowel. Small frequent feedings are also of benefit, especially when the food is bland, requires little chewing, and is given in small amounts.

Following operation, particularly in those women who were in a severe nutritional deficiency preoperatively, wound healing may present as a problem. After radiation therapy, anemia, lymphopenia, enteritis, colitis, and cystitis may be present and should be identified and treated.

Visualization of Abdomen

Reoperation or reexploration should be considered in three groups of women with ovarian cancer: (1) those who had a biopsy only of the tumor and did not have a complete evaluation of the extent of disease or reasonable tumor reduction surgery was not carried out at the time of initial operation; (2) those who had definitive surgical therapy but with known residual tumor and who were reoperated after chemotherapy or radiation therapy to determine either the resectability of residual tumor or the presence or absence of tumor as a guide to further chemotherapy; and (3) those women who had all known tumor removed at the first operation and who then underwent irradiation therapy or chemotherapy without evidence of recurrence and who require "second-look" procedures to determine the presence or absence of tumor to decide whether to continue or discontinue therapy.[105–108]

Reoperation procedures are not applicable in the presence of clinically advancing tumor.[106] When reoperation is performed the same surgical principles should be carried out as have been detailed at the time of initial operation.

In those patients in whom postoperative adhesions are at a minimum and in whom a more extensive surgical procedure might be associated with significant morbidity or mortality, laparoscopy may be considered.[109] At laparoscopy the abdominal contents can be visualized, peritoneal fluid cellular samples aspirated, and specific biopsies obtained.

Peritoneal Fluid Evaluation

Accurate determination of the stage of the disease process following operation for ovarian cancer can be difficult. The detection of persistent or recurrent disease in an asymptomatic woman without ascites, pleural fluid, or palpable or roentgenographic evidence of tumor is not easy. The efficacy of radiation therapy or chemotherapy in these patients with ovarian cancer is also a hard task.

Culdocentesis has previously been established as a simple, safe, and inexpensive method of obtaining cytologic specimens from the pelvic cavity in ambulatory women.[110,111] After performing a pelvic examination, a speculum is inserted into the vagina and the posterior fornix is visualized. The cervix, if present, is lifted by the anterior blade of the speculum. The posterior fornix of the vagina is then wiped dry with sterile cotton-tipped applicators (Fig. 19-32). Using a number 19 gauge 7.25-in. needle with stylet, the sac of Douglas is deeply entered, usually to the region of the sacrum. The stylet is removed and a 10-ml syringe is used to aspirate the peritoneal fluid specimen as the needle is slowly withdrawn. After placing the specimen on an albumin-coated microscopic slide (Fig. 19-33), it is fixed and stained according to Papanicolaou's procedure. Following removal of the reproductive organs, culdocentesis is performed 1 to 2 cm below the healed vaginal incision, near the midline, in an area free of obvious fibrosis.[112]

Mesothelial (Fig. 19-34) and nonmesothelial cells possessing nuclear characteristics suggestive of, but not conclusive for, malignancy and malignant cells are recorded. A count of 200 cells is made under microscopic oil immersion to describe the various morphologic cellular constituents and for a cytodifferential count. In addition to mesothelial cells (Fig. 19-35), nonmesothelial cells and malignant cells, lymphocytes, polymorphonuclear leukocytes, histiocytes, squamous cells, and erythrocytes are grouped.[113]

McGowan and Bunnag observed that the presence of malignant cells in the peritoneal fluid of women with ovarian cancer in their last week of radiation therapy and during the following month was associated with the death of all women. In women undergoing chemotherapy or being followed after therapy, the finding of malignant cells in three consecutive monthly cytologic specimens was also associated with the death of the patient, usually within 24 months. Malignant cells in the peritoneal fluid, particularly in the earlier stages

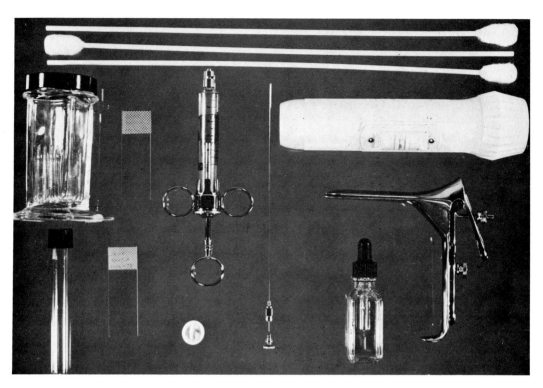

Figure 19–32. Equipment used in culdocentesis. The preparation of the albumin-coated slides is seen in Figures 19–20 and 19–21.

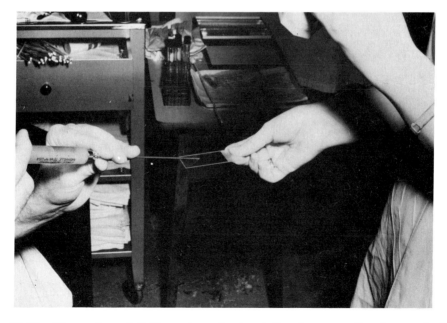

Figure 19–33. The peritoneal fluid specimen is placed directly on an albumin-coated slide. The slides are then promptly placed in a Coplin jar containing 95 percent ethyl alcohol. Any peritoneal fluid remaining in the syringe is put in a capped tube for further studies.

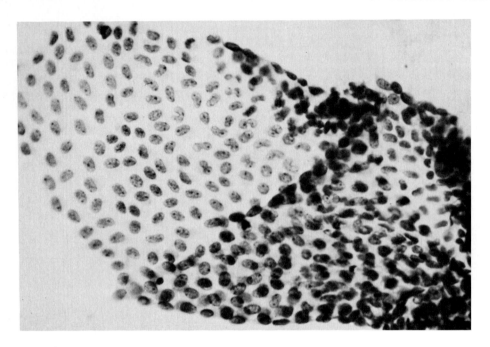

Figure 19–34. A sheet of normal mesothelial cells seen with oil immersion by microscopic examination. These cells were obtained by culdocentesis from a normal woman.

of ovarian cancer, were commonly seen 6 to 23 months before other evidence of recurrent disease appeared (Figs. 19–36 to 19–39). Peritoneal fluid study, especially in those women having the more common types of ovarian cancer, seems to be one of the more practical aids in determining persistent or recurrent disease following the operation, to monitor therapy, and for cytoprognosis (Figs. 19–40 to 19–46).[112]

In women with histologically proven ovarian cancer, McGowan et al have established a diagnostic biochemical pattern for ovarian cancer with a small quantity of peritoneal fluid analyzed by the sequential multiple analyzer 12/60. The peritoneal fluid may be obtained by culdocentesis performed in the physician's office during the patient's regular follow-up care. Calcium, inorganic phosphorous, urea nitrogen, uric acid, cholesterol, total protein, total bilirubin, lactic dehydrogenase (LDH), and glutamic-oxaloacetic acid transaminase (G-OT) levels were elevated above the values contained in control women (Table 19–5). The results suggest that the biochemical pattern of peritoneal fluid may be used to discover early residual or recurrent ovarian cancer, and to monitor therapy.[114]

Radiographic and Related Diagnostic Aids

A chest roentgenogram can aid in the following of a patient with suspected pleural fluid or metastases. A scout film of the abdomen may confirm the clinical impression of intestinal obstruction. An intravenous pyelogram in the postoperative period can reveal an infringement on ureteral drainage that was associated with prolonged mor-

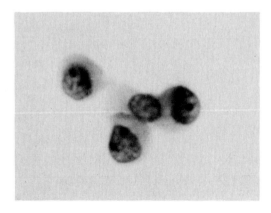

Figure 19–35. Four normal mesothelial cells. ×6250.

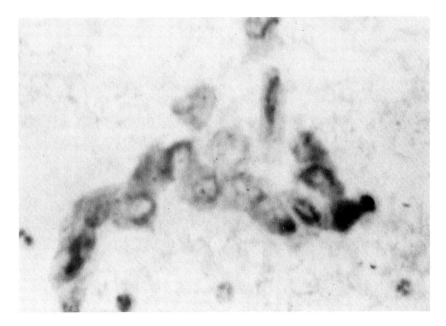

Figure 19-36. A peritoneal fluid cytologic specimen obtained by culdocentesis 3 days after abdominal hysterectomy and bilateral salpingo-oophorectomy for a stage IIA endometrioid carcinoma of the ovary in a 46-year-old woman. Highly atypical cells are noted with some hyperplastic mesothelial cells. ×5000.

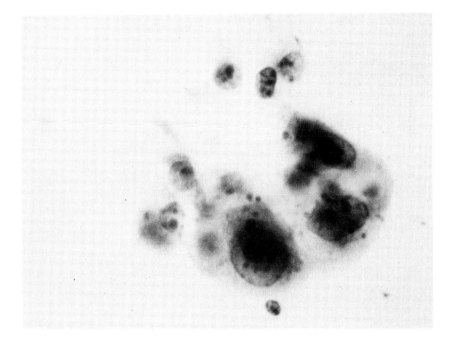

Figure 19-37. A peritoneal fluid cellular specimen from the same patient in Figure 19-36 and obtained 16 months following operation. The patient is asymptomatic without any other evidence of recurrence of disease. This cytologic specimen shows a contrast in the size of cancer cells and mesothelial cells at the top of the group of cells. ×5000.

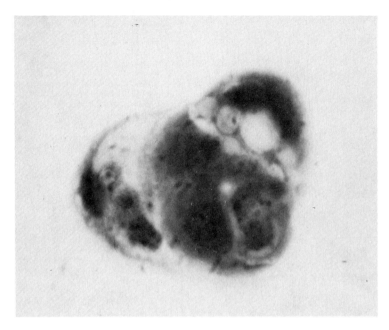

Figure 19–38. A peritoneal fluid cytologic specimen obtained by culdocentesis 22 months after operation (Fig. 19-36) and 6 months after the specimen in Figure 19-37. A very tight group of cancer cells are present. The patient continues to be asymptomatic without any measurable evidence of recurrence of her disease. ×5200.

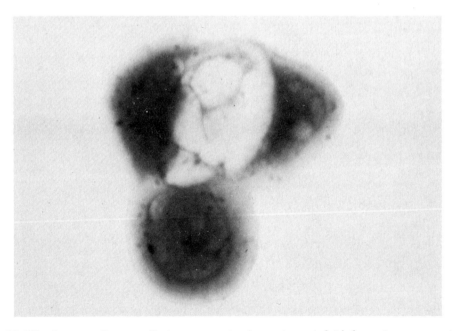

Figure 19–39. Large malignant cells in a group in the peritoneal fluid from the same patient in Figures 19-36 to 19-38. The patient now has symptoms of recurrent disease and this specimen was obtained 25 months after operation (Fig. 19-36). ×5250.

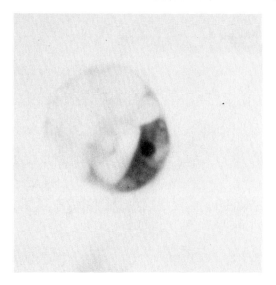

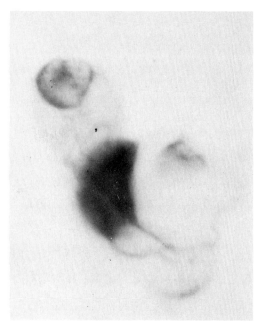

Figure 19–40. A peritoneal fluid cellular specimen obtained from a 55-year-old woman in whom an abdominal hysterectomy, bilateral salpingo-oophorectomy, and partial omentectomy were carried out 12 months previously for a stage III serous cystadecarcinoma. Following operation five day courses of melphalan each month were given to her. This suspicious cell for malignancy contains multivacuolated cytoplasm with a displaced nuclei and prominent nucleoli. ×6250.

Figure 19–41. This cytologic specimen was obtained one month following Figure 19–40 and contains enlarged cells suspicious for adenocarcinoma. Note the multiple cytoplasmic vacuolations and eccentric-placed hyperchromatic nuclei. ×6250.

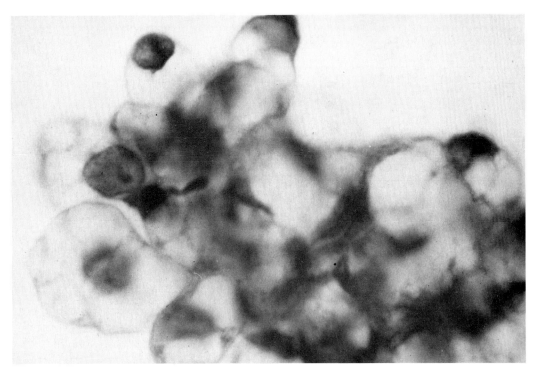

Figure 19–42. A peritoneal fluid cytologic specimen obtained from the same patient in Figures 19–40 and 19–41 22 months after operation. The cells were interpreted as highly suspicious for adenocarcinoma. ×6250.

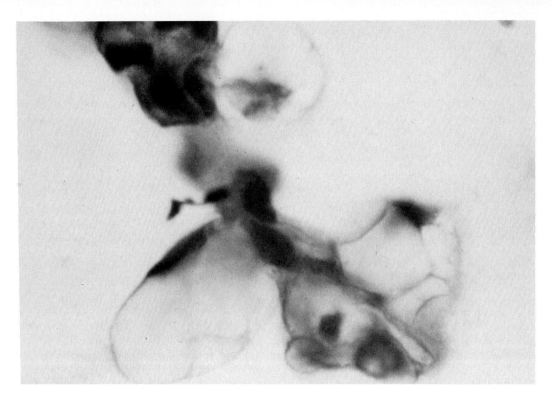

Figure 19-43. Cells consistent with adenocarcinoma of the ovary in the peritoneal fluid of the same patient in Figures 19-40 to 19-42 and obtained 23 months after initial surgery and 21 days before reexploration. She was without symptoms and there was no other evidence of recurrence of her tumor. ×6250.

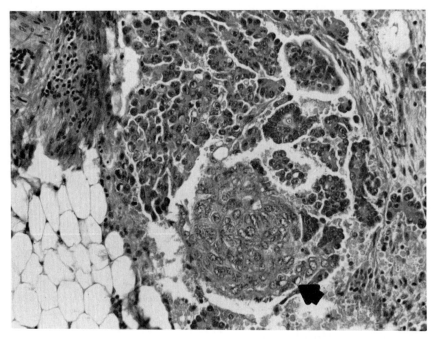

Figure 19-44. Partial omentectomy at initial operation of the patient in Figures 19-40 to 19-43 revealed diffuse metastatic serous cystadenocarcinoma as seen here. ×208.

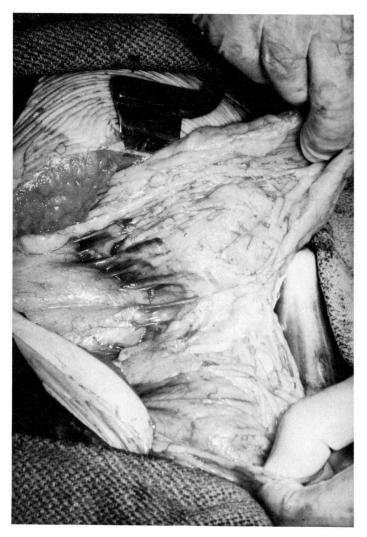

Figure 19–45. The patient in Figures 19–40 to 19–44 had undergone a partial omentectomy at the time of her initial operation. That portion of the omentum remaining at the "second look" operation appeared normal and on microscopic examination contained no cancer.

bidity and temperature elevation secondary to operative removal of the tumor. Atrophy of a kidney following irradiation therapy to the paraaortic nodes in the renal area may be detected on pyelography in a patient complaining of headaches and with an elevated blood pressure. Gastrointestinal radiographic studies are of limited help to the clinician in evaluating the course of the patient.

Ultrasound is of occasional use for the detection of hepatic metastases, abdominal metastases, or ascites.[44]

Liver scans aid in determining parenchymal liver disease as well as in studying the patient who underwent full abdominal irradiation without liver shields and possible radiation hepatitis.

Laboratory Aids

Specific laboratory tests to detect recurrent or persistent ovarian cancer only exist for a few histologic cell types. Since normal carcinoembryonic antigen (CEA) levels may occur in the presence of ovarian malignancy and elevated levels may occur in women who are healthy or have nonmalignant disease, the CEA assay is not a specific test for cancer.[115] CEA levels tend to fall paradoxically during terminal illness.[116] Numerous other tests have been utilized, such as serum lactic dehydrogenase and B protein assay for the detection of ovarian cancer, but are too nonspecific even for cancer in general.

Endodermal sinus tumor (EST) of the ovary

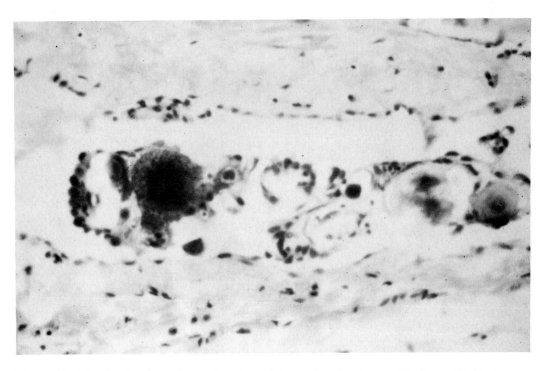

Figure 19–46. At the time of reexploration of the patient in Figures 19–40 to 19–45 the only evidence or recurrence of disease were microscopic deposits in the mesoappendix of a normal-appearing appendix. ×380.

Table 19–5. BIOCHEMICAL PARAMETERS OF PERITONEAL FLUID AND BLOOD FROM CONTROL WOMEN AND WOMEN WITH OVARIAN CANCER[114]

	SMA 12 NORMAL BLOOD RANGE	CONTROL WOMEN: PERITONEAL FLUID	OVARIAN CANCERS: PERITONEAL FLUID
Calcium (mg%)	8.5–10.5	7.0±0.5*	8.2±0.2
Inorganic phosphorus (mg%)	2.5–4.5	2.2±0.7	3.8±0.2
Urea nitrogen (mg%)	10–20	10.9±1.4	18.3±1.5
Uric Acid (mg%)	2.5–8.0	3.8±0.6	5.3±0.3
Cholesterol (mg%)	150–300	64.0±22.5	158.4±9.3
Total protein (gm%)	6.0–8.0	3.2±1.0	5.2±0.1
Total bilirubin (mg%)	0.2–1.0	0.3±0.1	1.0±0.3
LDH (mU/ml)	90–200	128.0±42.3	>630.7±145.0
G-OT (mU/ml)	10–50	12.9±4.8	46.4±8.3

*Mean ± standard error.

produces α-fetoprotein (AFP), and serum AFP quantitations can be used as a marker for these tumors. Serum AFP is unquestionably a valuable parameter in postoperative evaluation and therapy.[117,118] AFP seems to be a reliable tumor marker in both regression and progression of the EST and may therefore be be a prognostic indicator.[73,75] Sell and his group have observed that it is not a perfect text, as there can be only a slight increase in serum AFP concentration with widespread terminal EST tumor growth.[117]

Kurman and Norris have observed α-fetoprotein to be present in embryonal carcinoma of the ovary, so it is not a specific marker for just the endodermal sinus tumor.[77] Also in embryonal carcinoma they observed elevated human chorionic gonadotropin (HCG) levels to be present as evidenced by positive pregnancy tests in most of their women with embryonal carcinoma. Elevated levels of HCG are present in germ cell tumors that are pure choriocarcinomas, thus providing an aid to following these women after therapy. Endodermal sinus tumor, choriocarcinoma, or embryonal carcinoma, when they exist solely in a tumor or when these cell types are mixed, can be followed by these tests and provide the clinician with an aid to monitor the response to therapy in these rare malignant germ cell tumors.[87]

PATIENT SURVIVAL

The overall five-year survival for ovarian cancer is approximately 30 to 35 percent, resulting in almost 200,000 person years lost each year due to the disease. The prognosis in ovarian cancer is effected by the stage of the disease at diagnosis, the success of maximum surgical removal of tumor, and the histologic type and grade of the tumor. The disease is usually diagnosed late, consequently survival is not favorably influenced. With improved surgical staging, delineation of the various histologic tumor types, and coordinated treatment planning, treatment, and follow-up accomplished, the path toward meaningful reduction in the morbidity and mortality of ovarian cancer will be established.

In the process of attempting to improve relative survival rates for ovarian cancer by stressing complete tumor response to therapy, we must also evaluate the individual patient's response to therapy in relation to her pain, general comfort, and ability to resume a near-normal pattern of living at home. In addition, other meaningful responses to therapy for ovarian cancer are that the ascites or pleural effusion are markedly diminished and that the patient's therapy does not produce complications worse than the disease.

In a long-term follow-up of 990 cases of ovarian cancer, Aure et al observed that unilateral tumors had a significantly better prognosis than bilateral tumors, and the occurrence of ascites and malignant cells in the peritoneal fluid in stage I was a bad prognostic sign (Table 19–6).[119] In stages II and III, complete removal of all macroscopic tumor was of great importance (Table 19–7). In women with potentially malignant tumors, they noted that the survival curves showed a small, but steady decline during the entire observation period up to 20 years after primary treatment, and no less than 15 to 25 percent of

Table 19–6. COMPARISON OF SURVIVAL RATES FOR STAGES 1a, 1b, and 1c—ALL HISTOLOGIC TYPES[119]

YR AFTER TREATMENT	5	10	20
1a, low potential malignancy	95*	91	78
1a, carcinomas	69	62	59
1b, low potential malignancy	92	86	86
1b, carcinomas	43	43	43
1c, carcinomas	40	32	32

*Survival rate in %.

Table 19–7. SURVIVAL IN RELATION TO STAGE AND OPERABILITY[119]

Yr After Treatment	TUMOR NOT COMPLETELY REMOVED			TUMOR COMPLETELY REMOVED		
	5	10	20	5	10	20
Stage 1	—	—	—	62*	59	52
Stage 2	15	12	11	50	45	32
Stage 3	8	5	5	30	30	30
Stage 4	5	4	4	—	—	—

*Survival rate in %.

Table 19–8. SURVIVAL RATE FOR
THE DIFFERENT HISTOLOGIC
TYPES—ALL STAGES[119]

YR AFTER TREATMENT	5	10	20
Serous tumors— low potential malignancy	98*	91	75
Mucinous tumors— low potential malignancy	90	88	85
Mesonephroid carcinomas— clear cell	55	55	55
Endometrioid carcinomas	43	39	39
Mucinous carcinomas	40	40	35
Mesonephroid carcinomas— tubular pattern	37	37	37
Serous carcinomas	29	23	19
Undifferentiated carcinomas	17	12	12

*Survival rate in %.

Table 19–9. SURVIVAL RATE IN
STAGE 1 IN RELATION TO
HISTOLOGIC TYPE[119]

YR AFTER TREATMENT	5	10	20
Serous tumors— low potential malignancy	98*	95	78
Mucinous tumors— low potential malignancy	95	92	86
Mesonephroid carcinomas— clear cell	82	82	82
Endometrioid carcinomas	70	67	67
Serous carcinomas	67	53	36
Mucinous carcinomas	64	64	55
Mesonephroid carcinomas— tubular pattern	53	53	53
Undifferentiated Carcinomas	30	24	23

*Survival rate in %.

the women died from cancer (Table 19–8).[119] Among the truly invasive carcinomas, mesonephroid tumors of clear cell type had the best prognosis, and then endometrioid, mucinous, mesonephroid with tubular pattern, serous, and undifferentiated tumors, in that order (Table 19–8). Serous carcinomas had a great tendency to a protracted clinical course with late recurrences up to 20 years after primary treatment (Table 19–9).

Obel, in his study comparing those women with ovarian cancer who survived 10 years to those who did not survive 10 years, observed the expected greater proportion of those with advanced disease in the women not surviving 10 years and this advanced disease occurred more commonly in elderly women. He also noted that women in whom the uterus was not removed at the primary operation had an unusually high rate of metastases to the uterus or the development of a second primary in the uterus. Thus in women with earlier stages of ovarian cancer, hysterectomy should be an integral part of the primary operation.[120] Hart and Norris also found a marked difference in survival between borderline (low malignant potential) and malignant mucinous tumors of the ovary.[121] They strongly recommend preserving the contralateral ovary in a young woman with a borderline mucinous ovarian tumor.[121]

Ovarian adenocarcinoma of mesonephric type is a well-differentiated carcinoma composed of clear or hobnail-type cells resembling renal carcinomas and associated with a very favorable prognosis.[122] In fact, when confined to the ovaries, stage I, it has been observed to have almost as good survival as the tumors of low malignant potential.[123]

Fox and associates, after analyzing their series of 92 cases of granulosa cell tumors of the ovary, state that if no woman dies from any other disease, it would be expected that about 50 percent of women with granulosa cell tumors would be dead within 20 years as a result of the neoplasm.[65] Factors that indicate a relatively poor survival rate are age over 40 at the time of diagnosis, a presentation with abdominal symptoms, a palpable mass that is a solid large tumor or bilateral tumors, extraovarian spread, and numerous mitotic figures in the tumor. It would seem that all granulosa cell tumors should be considered as malignant and that the factors pointing to a poor prognosis are those indicating that a particular tumor has been diagnosed at a late stage in its natural history, either because it has been present for a long time or because it is highly malignant. There are no definite criteria for defining the prognosis in a case in which the tumor has been removed at an early stage in its natural life history (Figs. 19–25 and 19–26).[65]

Pseudomyxoma Peritonei

Pseudomyxoma peritonei is a term used to describe a clinical syndrome of massive accumulation of gelatinous ascites with long survival. This rare condition may be associated with a benign or malignant ovarian tumor and appears years after the primary surgery. The mucinous ascites consists mostly of acid mucopolysaccharides and the epithelium is commonly benign.[124] The patients with the disorder commonly complain of abdominal distention and the disease can produce intestinal obstruction. Long-term survival can be obtained by use of repeated celiotomy and evacuation of as much of the ascites as possible along with the use of an oral alkylating chemotherapeutic agent.

Leukemia Following Treatment for Ovarian Cancer

With greater emphasis on earlier detection of ovarian cancer, proper surgical staging, and maximum surgical removal of tumor combined with the long-term use of chemotherapy, an increasing number of patients developing leukemia following therapy can be expected.[125,126] The total number of reported cases to date is few, but it does emphasize the importance of the occurrence following complete response to ovarian cancer therapy and the need to monitor therapy to permit its cessation when there is no further evidence of disease.

References

1. Cancer Facts and Figures. New York, American Cancer Society, 1978
2. Cramer DW, Cutler SJ: Incidence and histopathology of malignancies of the female genital organs in the United States. Am J Obstet Gynec 118:443, 1974
3. Cutler SJ, Scotto J, Deves SS, Connelly RR: Third national cancer survey—an overview of available information. J Nat Ca Instit 53:1565, 1974
4. Doll R, Muir C, Waterhouse J: Cancer Incidence in Five Continents; vol II. International Union Against Cancer, New York, Springer, 1970
5. Doll R, Payne P, Waterhouse J: Cancer Incidence in Five Continents. International Union Against Cancer, New York, Springer, 1956
6. Lingeman CH: Etiology of cancer of the human ovary: A review. J Nat Cancer Instit 53:1603, 1974
7. The extent of cancer illness in the United States. U.S.P.H.S. Dept HEW No. 547 Washington, D.C.
8. Fraumeni JF, Lloyd JW, Smith EM, Wagoner JK: Cancer mortality among nuns: Role of marital status in etiology of neoplastic disease in women. J Nat Can Instit 42:455, 1969
9. Joly DJ, Lilienfeld AJ, Diamond EL, Bross ID: An epidemiologic study of the relationship of reproductive experience to cancer of the ovary. Am J Epid 99:190, 1974
10. Helmboldt CF, Fredrickson TN: Tumors of unknown etiology. In Hofstad MS, Calneck BW, Helmboldt CF, Ried WM, Yoder HW (eds): Diseases of Poultry, 6th ed. Ames, Iowa, Iowa State University Press, 1972, p 577
11. Gilbert AB: The ovary. In Bell DJ, Freeman BM (eds): Physiology and Biochemistry of the Domestic Fowl. New York, Academic, 1971, p 1163
12. Fathalla MF: Incessant ovulation—a factor in ovarian neoplasia? Lancet 2:163, 1971
13. Fathalla MF: Factors in the causation and incidence of ovarian cancer. Obstet Gynec Surv 27:751, 1972
14. DeNeef JC, Hollenbeck ZJ: The fate of ovaries preserved at the time of hysterectomy. Am J Obstet Gynec 96:1088, 1966
15. Beavis EL, Brown JB, Smith MA: Ovarian function after hysterectomy with conservation of the ovaries in pre-menopausal women. J Obstet Gynaec Brit Commonw 76:969, 1969
16. Johansson BW, Kaij L, Kullander S, et al: On some late effects of bilateral oophorectomy in the age range 15–30 years. Acta Obstet Gynec Scand 54:449, 1975
17. Berg JW, Baylor SM: The epidemiologic

pathology of ovarian cancer. Human Path 4:537, 1973

18. Epidemiology of Ovarian Cancer. Lancet 1:125, 1974

19. James PD: Epidemiology of ovarian cancer. Lancet 1:412, 1974

20. Krain LS: Some epidemiologic variables in ovarian carcinoma. HSMHA Health Report 87:56, 1972

21. Lilienfeld AM, Pedersen E, Dowd JE: Cancer Epidemiology: Methods of Study. The Johns Hopkins Press, Baltimore, Maryland, 1967

22. Segi M, Kurihara M: Cancer Mortality for Selected Sites in 24 Countries. No. 6 (1966-1967). Japan Cancer Society Nov., 1972

23. Henderson BE, Gerkins VR, Pike MC: Sexual factors and pregnancy. In Fraumeni JF (ed): Persons at High Risk of Cancer. New York, Academic, 1975, p 267

24. Newell GR, Krementz ET, Roberts JD: Multiple primary neoplasms in blacks compared to whites. J Nat Can Instit 54:331, 1975

25. Lee AJ: Dietary factors associated with death rates from certain neoplasms in man. Lancet 2:332, 1966

26. Mason TJ, McKay FW: U.S. Cancer Mortality by County: 1950-1969. DHEW Publication No. (NIH) 74-615 Washington, D.C. U.S. Government Printing Office, 1974

27. Mason TJ, McKay FW, Hoover R, Blot WJ, Fraumeni JF: Atlas of Cancer Mortality for U.S. Counties: 1950-1969. DHEW Publication No. (NIH) 75-780. Bethesda, Md., U.S. Dept of HEW, PHS/NIH, 1975

28. Mason TJ, McKay FW, Hoover R, Blot WJ, Fraumeni JF: Atlas of Cancer Mortality Among U.S. Nonwhites: 1950-1969. DHEW Publication No. (NIH)76-1204, U.S. Government Printing Office, Washington, D.C. 1976

29. Fraumeni JF, Grundy GW, Creagen ET, Everson RB: Six families prone to ovarian cancer. Cancer 36:364, 1975

30. Lewis ACW, Davison BCC: Familial ovarian cancer. Lancet 2:235, 1969

31. Li FP, Fraumeni JF, Dalager N: Ovarian cancers in the young. Cancer 32:969, 1973

32. Li FP, Rapoport AH, Fraumeni JF, Jensen RD: Familial ovarian carcinoma. JAMA 214:1559, 1970

33. Liber AF: Ovarian cancer in mothers and five daughters. J Arch Path 49:280, 1950

34. Lynch HT, Guirgis HA, Albert S, et al: Familial association of carcinoma of the breast and ovary. Surg Gynec Obstet 138: 717, 1974

35. Trentni GP, Palmieri B: An unusual case of gonadic germinal tumor in a brother and sister. Cancer 33:250, 1974

36. McCrann DJ, Marchant DJ, Bardawil WA: Ovarian carcinoma in three teen-age siblings. Obstet Gynec 43:132, 1974

37. Jensen RD, Norris HJ, Fraumeni JF: Familial arrhenoblastoma amd thyroid adenoma. Cancer 33:218, 1974

38. Cutler SJ, Myers MH, White PL: Who are we missing and why? Cancer 37:421, 1976

39. The Third National Cancer Survey: Incidence Data. Monograph 41. DHEW Publication No. (NIH) 75-787. Bethesda, Maryland, Biometry Branch, Division of Cancer Cause and Prevention, National Cancer Institute

40. Parker RT, Parker CH, Wilbanks GD: Cancer of the ovary. Am J Obstet Gynec 108:878, 1970

41. Barber HR, Graber EA: The PMPO syndrome. Obstet Gynec 38:921, 1971

42. Jenkins DM, Goulden R: Psammoma bodies in cervical cytologic smears. Acta Cytol 21:112, 1977

43. Teplick JG, Haskin ME, Alvi A: Calcified intraperitoneal metastases from ovarian carcinoma. Am J Roentgenol 127:1003, 1976

44. Donald I: Ultrasound in the diagnosis of ovarian neoplasia. In DeWatteville H (ed): Diagnosis and Treatment of Ovarian Neoplastic Alterations. New York, Elsevier, 1975, p 92

45. Clinical Staging of Gynecologic Cancer. Technical Bulletin. American College of Obstetricians and Gynecologists. Chicago, Aug. 23, 1973

46. Serov SF, Scully RE: Histological Typing of Ovarian Tumours. International Histological Classification of Tumors, No. 9. Geneva, Switzerland, World Health Organization, 1973

47. Abell MR: The Nature and Classification of Ovarian Neoplasms. Proceedings of the

Annual Clinical Conference on Cancer of the Ovary. The Ontario Cancer Treatment and Research Foundation, Windsor, Ontario, University of Windsor, Nov. 1965

48. Bergman F: Carcinoma of the ovary. Acta Obstet Gynec Scandinav 45:211, 1966

49. Fornasier VL, Horne JG: Metastases to the vertebral column. Cancer 36:590, 1975

50. Waddington MM, Martin HL: Convulsive disorder as initial manifestation of ovarian carcinoma. JAMA 192:135, 1965

51. Hirabayashi K, Graham J: Genesis of ascites in ovarian cancer. Am J Obstet Gynec 106:492, 1970

52. Nelson JH, Urcuyo R: Pretreatment staging. Cancer 38:458, 1976

53. Meyers MA: Distribution of intra-abdominal malignant seeding: dependency on dynamics of flow of ascitic fluid. Am J Roent Rad Therapy 119:198, 1973

54. Plentl AA, Friedman EA: Lymphatic System of the Female Genitalia. Philadelphia, Saunders, 1971

55. Julian CG, Goss J, Blanchard K, Woodruff JD: Biologic behavior of primary ovarian malignancy. Obstet Gynec 44:873, 1974

56. Decker DT, Webb MJ, Holbrook MA: Radiogold treatment of epithelial cancer of ovary: late results. Am J Obstet Gynec 115:751, 1973

57. Decker DG, Webb MJ: Prophylactic therapy for stage I ovarian cancer. Gynec Oncol 1:203, 1973

58. Keettel WC, Pixley EE, Buchsbaum HJ: Experience with peritoneal cytology in the management of gynecologic malignancies. Am J Obstet Gynec 120:174, 1974

59. Williams TJ, Dockerty MB: Status of the contralateral ovary in encapsulated low grade malignant tumors of the ovary. Surg Gynec Obstet 143:763, 1976

60. Hilarias BS, Clark DG: The value of postoperative intraperitoneal injection of radiocolloids in early cancer of the ovary. Am J Roentgen Rad Therapy 112:749, 1971

61. Tobias JS, Griffiths CT: Management of ovarian carcinoma. N Engl J Med 294: 818, 1976

62. Tobias JS, Griffiths CT: Managment of ovarian carcinoma. N Engl J Med 294: 877, 1976

63. Fox H, Langley FA: Tumours of the Ovary. Chicago, Year Book, 1976

64. Janovski NA, Paramanandhan TL: Ovarian Tumors. Philadelphia, Saunders, 1973

65. Fox H, Agrawal K, Langley FA: A clinicopathologic study of 92 cases of granulosa cell tumor of the ovary with special reference to the factors influencing prognosis. Cancer 35:231, 1975

66. Norris HJ: Functioning tumors of the ovary. In DeWatteville H (ed): Diagnosis and Treatment of Ovarian Neoplastic Alterations. New York, Elsevier, 1975, p 219

67. Lamont CA, Ashton PW: Observations on granulosa cell tumors. In DeWatteville H (ed): Diagnosis and Treatment of Ovarian Neoplastic Alterations. New York, Elsevier, 1975, p 241

68. Ireland K, Woodruff JD: Masculinizing ovarian tumors. Obstet Gynec Surv 31:83, 1976

69. Norris HJ, Jensen RD: Relative frequency of ovarian neoplasms in children and adolescents. Cancer 30:713, 1972

70. Talerman A, Huyzinga WT, Kuipers T: Dysgerminoma. Obstet Gynec 41:137, 1973

71. Asadouiran LA, Taylor HB: Dysgerminoma. Obstet Gynec 33:370, 1969

72. Afridi MA, Vongtama V, Tsukada Y, Piver MS: Dysgerminoma of the ovary: Radiation therapy for recurrence and metastases. Am J Obstet Gynec 126:190, 1976

73. Kurman RJ, Norris HJ: Endodermal sinus tumor of the ovary. Cancer 38:2404, 1976

74. Ettinger DS, Parmley TH, Owellen RJ, Davis TE: Endodermal sinus tumor. Obstet Gynec 49:53s, 1977

75. Jimerson GK, Woodruff JD: Ovarian extraembryonal teratoma. Am J Obstet Gynec 127:73, 1977

76. Forney JP, Disaia PJ, Morrow CP: Endodermal sinus tumor. Obstet Gynec 45: 186, 1975

77. Kurman RJ, Norris HJ: Embryonal carcinoma of the ovary. Cancer 38:2420, 1976

78. Smith JP: The treatment of embryonal carcinoma of the ovary. In DeWatteville H (ed): Diagnosis and Treatment of Ovarian Neoplastic Alterations. New York, Elsevier, 1975, p 214

79. Norris HJ, Chorlton I: Functioning tumors of the ovary. Clin Obstet Gynec 17:189, 1974

80. Wider JA, Marshall J, Bardin C, Lipsett MB, Ross GT: Sustained remissions after chemotherapy for primary ovarian cancers containing choriocarcinoma. N Eng J Med 280:1439, 1969

81. Gerbie MV, Brewer JI, Tamimi H: Primary choriocarcinoma of the ovary. Obstet Gynec 46:720, 1975

82. Norris HJ, Zirkin HJ, Benson WL: Immature (malignant) teratoma of the ovary. Cancer 37:2359, 1976

83. Malkasian GD, Webb MJ, Jorgensen EO: Observation on chemotherapy of granulosa cell carcinomas and malignant ovarian teratomas. Obstet Gynec 44:885, 1974

84. Disaia PJ, Saltz A, Kagan AR, Morrow CP: Chemotherapeutic retroconversion of immature teratoma of the ovary. Obstet Gynec 49:346, 1977

85. Pantoja E, Ibanez IR, Axtmayer RW, Noy MA, Pelegrina I: Complications of dermoid tumors of the ovary. Obstet Gynec 45:89, 1975

86. Pantoja E, Noy MA, Axtmayer RW, Colon FE, Pelegrina I: Ovarian dermoids and their complications. Obstet Gynec Surv 30:1, 1975

87. Kurman RJ, Norris HJ: Malignant mixed germ cell tumors of the ovary. Obstet Gynec 48:579, 1976

88. Jimerson GK, Woodruff JD: Ovarian extraembryonal teratoma. Am J Obstet Gynec 127:302, 1977

89. Scully RE: Gonadoblastoma. Cancer 25: 1340, 1970

90. Schellhas HF: Malignant potential of the dysgenetic gonad. Obstet Gynec 44:298, 1974

91. Schellhas HF: Malignant potential of the dysgenetic gonad. Obstet Gynec 44:455, 1974

92. Ghosh A: Bilateral fibrosarcoma of the ovary following hysterectomy. Am J Obstet Gynec 112:1136, 1972

93. Cooper JA, Broad AF, Salm R: Primary ovarian lymphoma. J Obstet Gynaec British Commonw 81:571, 1974

94. Long JP, Patchefsky AS: Primary Hodgkin's disease of the ovary. Obstet Gynec 38:680, 1971

95. Azoury RS, Woodruff JD: Primary ovarian sarcomas. Obstet Gynec 37:920, 1971

96. Nieminen U, Numers CV, Porola E: Primary sarcoma of the ovary. Acta Obstet Gynec Scandinav 48:423, 1969

97. Giere JW, Binder RA: Burkitt's lymphoma involving the ovary and jaw. Obstet Gynec 48:63s, 1976

98. Fox HD, Cartinick AN, Shohov P, Zaino EC: Lymphoma of the ovary: a case report and a review of the literature. Gynec Oncol 3:347, 1975

99. Dehner LP, Norris HJ, Taylor HB: Carcinosarcomas and mixed mesodermal tumors of the ovary. Cancer 27:207, 1971

100. Hernandez W, Disaia PJ, Morrow CP, Townsend DE: Mixed mesodermal sarcoma of the ovary. Obstet Gynec 49:59s, 1977

101. Webb MJ, Decker DG, Mussey E: Cancer metastatic to the ovary. Obstet Gynec 45:391, 1975

102. Woodruff JD, Murthy YS, Bhaskar TN, Bordbar F, Tseng S: Metastatic ovarian tumors. Am J Obstet Gynec 107:202, 1970

103. Robboy SJ, Scully RE, Norris HJ: Carcinoid metastatic to the ovary. Cancer 33: 798, 1974

104. Lifshitz S, Buchsbaum HJ: The effect of paracentesis on serum proteins. Gynec Oncol 4:347, 1976

105. Mangioni C, Mattioli G, Natale N: The 'second look' operation in long-term therapy of ovarian malignancies. In DeWatteville H (ed): Diagnosis and Treatment of Ovarian Neoplastic Alterations. New York, Elsevier, 1975, p 153

106. Smith JP, Delgado G, Rutledge F: Second-look operation in ovarian carcinoma. Cancer 38:1438, 1976

107. Symmonds RE: Some surgical aspects of gynecologic cancer. Cancer 36:649s, 1975

108. Tepper E, Sanfilippo LJ, Gray J, Romney SL: Second-look surgery after radiation therapy for advanced stages of cancer of the ovary. Am J Roetgen Radiotherapy 112:755, 1971

109. DeWatteville H: The use of laparoscopy in cases of ovarian cancer. In DeWatteville H (ed): Diagnosis and Treatment of Ovarian Neoplastic Alterations. New York, Elsevier, 1975, p 87

110. McGowan L, Davis RH: Peritoneal fluid cellular patterns in obstetrics and gynecology. Am J Obstet Gynec 106:979, 1970

111. Letko Y: Interet de la culdocentese pour le depistage et la surveillance post-operatoire des cancers de l'ovaire. These presentee a l'universite Claude-Bernard, Lyon, France, Dec. 16, 1975

112. McGowan L, Bunnag B: The evaluation of therapy for ovarian cancer. Gynec Oncol 4:375, 1976

113. McGowan L: A morphologic classification of peritoneal fluid cytology in women. Int J Gynaec Obstet 11:173, 1973

114. McGowan L, Davis RH, Bunnag B: The biochemical diagnosis of ovarian cancer. Am J Obstet Gynec 116:760, 1973

115. Barrelet V, Mach JP: The use and limitation of carcinoembryonic antigen (CEA). In DeWatteville H (ed): Diagnosis and Treatment of Ovarian Neoplastic Alterations. New York, Elsevier, 1975, p 122

116. Khoo SK, Mackay EV: Carcinoembryonic antigen (CEA) in ovarian cancer: factors influencing its incidence and changes which occur in response to cytotoxic drugs. Br J Obstet Gynaec 83:753, 1976

117. Sell A, Sogaard H, Pederson BN: Serum alpha-fetoprotein as a marker for the effect of post-operative radiation therapy and/or chemotherapy in eight cases of ovarian endodermal sinus tumour. Int J Cancer 18: 574, 1976

118. Talerman A, Haije WG: Alpha-feto-protein and germ cell tumors: a possible role of yolk sac tumor in production of alpha-fetopro- tein. Cancer 34:1722, 1974

119. Aure JC, Hoeg K, Kolstad P: Clinical and histologic studies of ovarian carcinoma. Obstet Gynec 37:1, 1971

120. Obel EB: A comparative study of patients with cancer of the ovary who have survived more or less than 10 years. Acta Obstet Gynec Scandavin 55:429, 1976

121. Hart WR, Norris JH: Borderline and malignant mucinous tumors of the ovary. Cancer 31:1031, 1973

122. Norris HJ, Robinowitz M: Ovarian adenocarcinoma of mesonephric type. Cancer. 28:1074, 1971

123. Aure J, Hoeg K, Kolstad P: Mesonephroid tumors of the ovary. Obstet Gynec 37: 860, 1971

124. Sandenbergh HA, Woodruff JD: Histogenesis of pseudomyxoma peritonei. Obstet Gynec 49:339, 1977

125. Sotrel G, Jafari K, Lash AF, Stepto RC: Acute leukemia in advanced ovarian carcinoma after treatment with alkylating agents. Am J Obstet Gynec 47:67s, 1975

126. Reimer RR, Hoover R, Fraumeni JF, Young RC: Acute leukemic after alkylating-agent of ovarian cancer. New Engl J Med 297:177, 1977

Chapter 20

Radiotherapy Treatment of Ovarian Cancer

JOHN G. MAIER, M.D., Ph.D.

Except for patients with clinical stage II ovarian cancer, there is very little solid evidence that radiotherapy is of much value in the treatment of patients with other clinical stages (Table 19–1). This appears to be due in part to the relative radioresistance of most epithelial tumors of the ovary as well as the radiosensitivity of the normal organs that must be included in rather large treatment volumes. In stage I disease where tumors are truly confined to one or both ovaries, surgery should be curative in itself by bilateral oophorectomy. When the tumor has spread to the peritoneal or retroperitoneal areas, the need for shielding the kidneys and liver as well as the tol-

erance of the small intestine precludes adequate tumoricidal doses. Only the pelvic organs are capable of withstanding curative doses or irradiation for the definitive treatment of epithelial ovarian cancers. The dysgerminomas and perhaps the granulosa and thecal cell tumors are more radiosensitive and must be discussed separately. Unfortunately, these more radiocurable tumors are not the major problem and are quite rare.

How often are ovarian cancers confined to the ovary? Let us turn first to the natural history and routes of spread of such tumors in order to define the target volume for radiotherapy.

NATURAL HISTORY AND ROUTES OF SPREAD

At least two-thirds of all patients will have metastatic spread on initial presentation of ovarian cancers. In the M. D. Anderson series,[2,14] 74 percent had metastases beyond the pelvis, 50 percent had ascites, and 21 percent had distant metastases to nodes, lung, bone, or skin on initial presentation. Routes of spread include lymphatic and bloodstream metastases as well as local extension and peritoneal seeding. The former two routes have received much less emphasis than the latter. Most patients present with advanced disease and it is the local extension and seedings that appear to predominate in the findings. Nevertheless, me-

tastases by lymphatic channels should not be ignored.

Figure 20–1 shows a schematic diagram of the lymphatic drainage of the ovaries and Figure 20–2 shows a schematic diagram of lymphatic drainage of the diaphragm. The parenchyma of the ovary has a dense lymphatic network that converges to the hilum of the ovary to form the subovarian lymphatic plexus. This plexus feeds into large collateral trunks that ascend bilaterally along the ovarian vessels and terminate in the para-aortic lymph nodes between the bifurcation of the aorta and the renal pedicles. In addition, accessory ves-

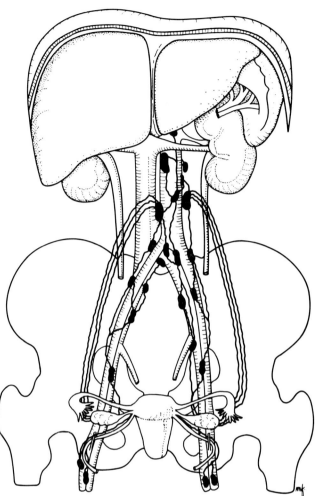

Figure 20–1. Lymphatic drainage of ovaries.

sels drain into the broad ligament toward the lateral and posterior pelvic walls ending in the external iliac and hypogastric lymph nodes. Another group of lymphatics also run along the round ligament and drain into the external iliac and inguinal nodes. Perhaps an even more important lymphatic drainage route is the peritoneal fluid and associated tumor cells draining via lymphatic channels located in the diaphragm. Rosenoff et al[13] have recently reported diaphragmatic metastases in 42 percent of supposed localized ovarian tumors (stage I and II) and in 71 percent of advanced tumors (stage III and IV). Fluid and particles reaching the diaphragm are collected into a network of lymphatic capillaries underneath the mesothelial cell lining of the undersurface of the diaphragm. From here, drainage is either to the upper lumbar para-aortic lymph nodes or through the diaphragm to its subpleural surface. Subse-

quent drainage takes place to the diaphragmatic lymph nodes, which are located adjacent to the pericardium and phrenic nerves. These are mainly on the right and anterior subpleural surface of the diaphragm. From here, drainage is to the retrosternal efferent trunks into the internal mammary group of lymph nodes. Thus, metastases may take place to the peritoneal surface of the diaphragm, the subpleural diaphragmatic lymph nodes, and the retrosternal internal mammary lymph nodes. The explanation for tumor cells in the peritoneal fluid reaching the diaphragm may be a gravity phenomenon when the patient is in the supine position or by changes in the intraperitoneal hydrostatic pressures. In any event, all of these sites must be considered if curative radiotherapy is the aim. Certainly, more commonly we think of local extension of ovarian carcinoma through the capsule to contiguous structures, such as the

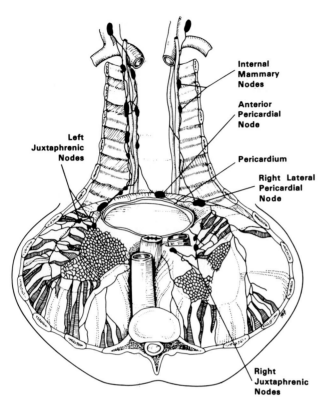

Figure 20–2. Lymphatic drainage of diaphragm.

Internal Mammary Nodes

Anterior Pericardial Node

Pericardium

Right Lateral Pericardial Node

Left Juxtaphrenic Nodes

Right Juxtaphrenic Nodes

tubes, uterus, bladder, and rectosigmoid. The importance of papillary excrescences or penetration of the ovarian capsule has been stressed since the probability of peritoneal seeding increases under these circumstances. Webb et al[17] have shown a progressive decrease in survival within stage I epi-

thelial tumors with surface excrescences on the ovary, occult capsular involvement as suggested by adhesions of the ovarian tumor with contiguous structures, and rupture of the mass at surgical resection.

TREATMENT

Curative radiotherapy implies a cancericidal dose to a specific tumor type as well as accurate localization of the tumor. Determination of such dosage levels to obtain permanent tumor control requires a knowledge of the time-dose relationship for tumor sterilization and the limits of normal tissue tolerance. Unfortunately, the time-dose relationship for ovarian tumor sterilization is poorly understood. In general, the germ cell tumors such as the dysgerminomas are more radiosensitive. In considering the more common epithelial cancers, the endometrioid carcinoma is most radioresponsive and the mucinous carcinoma is least responsive to irradiation. The serous, mesonephric, and undifferentiated carcinomas are somewhat intermediate in their response to irradiation. However, data on exact amounts of dosage required for sterilization are quite lacking. Thus, the doses

employed for such tumors have been somewhat dictated by the limits of tolerance of the normal tissues encompassed by the required treatment volume. To further complicate matters, the necessary treatment volume is not always clear cut because of our inability to correctly identify the location of the tumor target. With this in mind, let us turn to a consideration of the role of radiotherapy in each of the various clinical stages. Comments will be addressed primarily toward treatment of the epithelial tumors.

Stage IA and IB

It is very difficult to make a case for radiotherapy in the treatment of Stage Ia and Ib ovarian cancer. All patients must undergo an abdominal hysterectomy and bilateral salpingo-oophorectomy, peritoneal fluid cytologic study, and should also have an omentectomy. If the staging is correct and the surgery adequate, no tumor should remain. Therefore, there seems little justification for routine postoperative pelvic irradiation. While it is true that the best results reported in the literature for stage I disease range only from 70 to 80 percent cure, the failure is seldom due to local recurrence in the pelvis. Furthermore, early results from the Gynecology Oncology Group[9] randomized prospective study for stage I ovarian cancer show no advantage for postoperative irradiation or postoperative chemotherapy over surgery alone. If postoperative irradiation is given for stage IA and IB disease that has been correctly staged, then doses in the order of 5000 to 5500 rad are recommended in five to six weeks. Pelvic irradiation alone as shown in Figure 20–3 is rec-

ommended. A daily fraction of 180 rad to 200 rad to the midplane of the pelvis is recommended. With ^{60}Co teletherapy, a four-field box technique is employed, with all fields treated daily. In the average patient, 15 × 15 cm anterior and posterior fields are employed with 10 × 15 cm lateral fields. With higher energy accelerators or betatrons, anterior and posterior portals can be utilized with both fields being treated daily five times each week.

Stage II

It is in stage II patients where the tumor also involves the uterus and/or tubes and/or other ovary (IIA) or has extended to other pelvic structures (IIB) that postoperative irradiation appears to have its most significant role. If the staging is correct and tumor is confined to the pelvis, doses of 5000 to 5500 rad in five to six weeks can be safely administered to the pelvis in volumes as shown in Figure 20–3 and as described previously. The fact that cure is possible with local pelvic tumor residual following surgery has been shown in a recent report by Fuks and Bagshaw.[8] A 50 percent cure rate was obtained by pelvic irradiation in a series of 50 patients with initial stage IIB disease where complete surgical removal was not possible. No adjunctive chemotherapy was employed in this study.

Because of the likelihood of intraperitoneal or para-aortic lymph metastases, many authors have advocated abdominal irradiation in addition to pelvic irradiation. This position is somewhat supported by the relatively poor cure rates of 32 percent for patients with ovarian cancer with only regional disease in a large series reported by De-Vita et al.[6] Several techniques are available for administering both pelvic and abdominal irradiation. Large anterior and posterior fields can be administered, as shown in Figure 20–4, with the so-called "abdominal bath" technique. The entire pelvis and abdomen are included from the midobturator foramen of the pelvis to the dome of the diaphragm. A daily fraction of 150 to 160 rad administered five times each week is about the maximum that can be tolerated because of systemic side effects of nausea, vomiting, diarrhea, and bone marrow depression. The dose to the upper abdomen is carried to 3000 to 4000 rad with shielding of the kidneys and liver at 2000 rad to protect these organs from radiation injury. The total dose to the pelvis is usually 5000 to 5500 rad. The total time to administer such irradiation

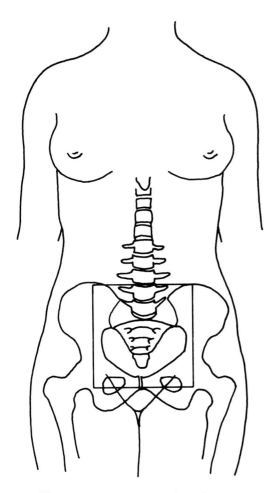

Figure 20–3. Pelvic field irradiation.

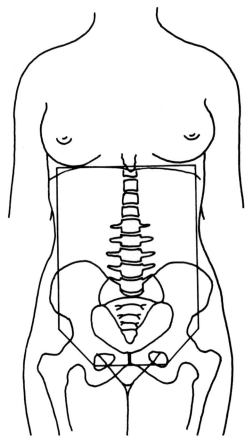

Figure 20–4. Whole abdomen and pelvic field irradiation.

is usually six to eight weeks, which is not entirely satisfactory from a time-dose viewpoint.

The ⁶⁰Co moving strip technique was initially developed in Europe to improve the time-dose relationship for large abdominal fields. This technique was refined by Delclos[4] for ovarian cancers. The moving strip technique allows the delivery of a tumor dose of 2600 to 2800 rad in 12 doses. This technique can be used with any megavoltage unit by proper correction of the depth dose and penumbra effect. The abdomen and pelvis is divided into contiguous segments or strips of 2.5 cm, as shown in Figure 20–5. Both anterior and posterior strips are treated daily. The treatment field is increased by one strip every two days until four strips (10 cm) have been treated. Then the 10 cm segment is moved up every two days (2.5 cm) until the last strip is reached. The field is then reduced progressively by one strip (2.5 cm). On the last two days of treatment, a single 2.5 cm strip is irradiated. A total time period of 30 to 40 days is required to treat the entire abdomen from the pelvic floor to the diaphragm. In this time interval, a tumor dose of 2600 to 2800 rad measured at the midline along a sagital plane is delivered. This dose in this time seems to have a greater biologic effect than the "abdominal bath" technique, where doses in the order of 3000 to 4000 rad are administered in 45 to 60 days. However, one randomized prospective study by Fazekas and Maier[7] showed no significant difference in tumor effects between the two methods,

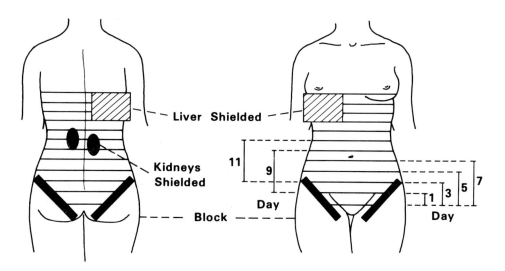

Figure 20–5. ⁶⁰Co Moving strip technique.

with slightly less toxic effects from the moving strip technique.

The technique of the moving strip was developed primarily for ^{60}Co teletherapy. The technique must be modified to avoid cold spots when using a 4 MeV photon beam of a linear accelerator. Smoron[15] has evaluated the dose distribution and developed a method of strip staggering so that the posterior surface line projects to the center of the anterior opposed strip. Marks et al[12] have developed an inexpensive technical aid with a plexiglas strip gradient to more accurately reproduce the treatment field. This system makes it unnecessary for the patient to keep the strip marking on for seven to eight weeks.

Arcangeli et al[1] have recently developed a chessboard-like technique of abdominal and pelvic irradiation that takes advantage of the reproductive patterns of the intestinal cells and the slowly or nonproliferative cancer or connective tissue cells. Bone marrow depletion still remains a problem with this system.

Stage III

In stage III disease, the abdomen is commonly treated in addition to the pelvis because of the high incidence of subsequent recurrent tumor in this area, even though the initial clinical and surgical findings do not demonstrate disease outside the pelvis. Even though the need for shielding the kidneys and the liver severely limits the dose to the upper abdomen, it is hoped that suboptimal doses of irradiation may have an effect on microscopic or occult tumor cells, if present, in the upper abdomen. There is little question for the need of abdominal irradiation. However, when the metastatic tumor enlarges, the capacity for sterilization with irradiation becomes more difficult. As might be expected, the best results have been found when all or most of the tumor has been removed. Many institutions do not utilize postoperative irradiation when residual masses larger than 2 cm are present, due to the poor results with irradiation.

Delclos[5] has reported a 57 percent five-year no-evidence-of-disease (NED) rate for epithelial cancer of the ovary when no residual tumor remained after surgery. When residual tumor masses remained but were under 2.0 cm, a 27.5 percent five-year NED rate was obtained. This fell to 17 percent for masses 2 to 4 cm, and 10 percent for masses 4 to 6 cm. There appeared to be some

improvement in survival by giving an additional boost dose of 2000 rad to the pelvis in two weeks with standard fields, following moving strip technique to the entire abdomen and pelvis. There was no significant increase in morbidity by the additional treatment.

The value of lymphangiography for ovarian cancer has received relatively little attention until recently. Fuks and Bagshaw[8] reported findings in a series of 83 patients with malignant ovarian tumors who underwent lymphangiograms. It is not too surprising that 40 percent of stage III patients and 50 percent of stage IV patients demonstrated metastatic lumbar para-aortic nodal metastases. However, 21 percent of stage I and II patients demonstrated positive metastatic disease in retroperitoneal lymph nodes. Because of this finding along with the diaphragmatic metastatic potential, they have proposed a new type of treatment field for elective irradiation for stage I and II patients as shown in Figure 20-6. Such a field includes the pelvic and para-aortic lymph nodes, the medial portions of the diaphragm, and the subpleural diaphragmatic lymph nodes for patients with stage I and II carcinoma of the ovary.

Stage IV

Obviously, the primary treatment for advanced disease is chemotherapy and/or immunotherapy with supplementary irradiation for symptomatic areas. Limited fields of irradiation can be quite helpful in relieving ureteral or colon obstruction as well as painful pelvic masses or metastatic bone lesions.

Combination Radiotherapy and Chemotherapy

Very few planned studies have been conducted to determine whether irradiation employed with chemotherapy is better than either modality alone following appropriate surgery. Most reports are a bewildering retrospective analysis of patients treated by irradiation, in which adjunctive chemotherapy was utilized in some manner. In some instances, the drugs were utilized for radiotherapy failures and in most reports, a wide variety of different stages and histologic types are reported with small numbers of patients in the different categories. Thus, when the pattern of drug employment is considered and the small numbers of

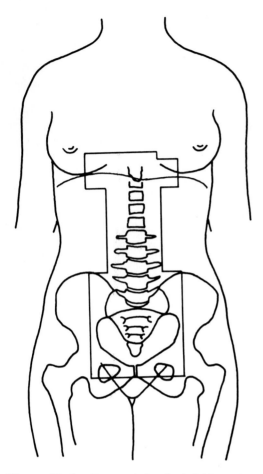

Figure 20–6. Proposed Stanford field irradiation for ovarian cancer.

histologic types for each of the various stages, the reports become meaningless. Often the special histologic category of low malignant potential is not even mentioned. Obviously, a few patients with this histologic category in an appropriate treatment category could markedly enhance results. The Gynecology Oncology Group initiated a prospective randomized study in 1971 for stage III epithelial ovarian cancers comparing radiotherapy alone, radiotherapy followed by melphalan, melphalan followed by radiotherapy, and melphalan alone. The study is incomplete but preliminary data shows no significant difference in survival thus far in the four treatment groups. The group treated by radiotherapy alone does show a lower survival rate, but many of these patients did not receive doses beyond 3500 rad to the pelvis. Randomized prospective studies in stage III disease by Johnson et al[10] comparing

total abdominal irradiation and cyclophosphamide vs cyclophosphamid alone have shown no significant difference. Similar studies with thiotepa[11] as an adjuvant to radiotherapy following surgery have shown no difference.

Germ Cell Tumors

The most interesting of the germ cell tumors of the ovary is the dysgerminoma, as it is identical to the seminoma in histologic appearance and response to irradiation. Less than 12 percent show bilateral involvement at presentation, but 20 to 30 percent are found to have spread beyond the ovary. The spread is primarily by lymphatic pathways similar to seminomas and may show progressive involvement of the retroperitoneal lymph nodes, the mediastinum, and supraclavicular nodes. Lymphangiography is most helpful in ascertaining such spread. In young women desiring subsequent pregnancy and unilateral involvement alone, the question of ipsilateral pelvic irradiation on the involved side along with lumbar para-aortic irradiation arises. Under such circumstances, significant scattered irradiation may occur to the contralateral ovary. This may be as much as 10 percent of the ipsilateral pelvic dose depending on the radiation equipment. Because of the potential of mutations to the contralateral ovary, such irradiation is not recommended. Thus, under the circumstances of unilateral involvement, a careful examination at the time of surgery is indicated, including bivalving and biopsy of the contralateral ovary for close gross inspection. Lymphangiography and sampling of para-aortic lymph nodes is indicated. If these procedures are not done at the time of initial unilateral oophorectomy, a second operative procedure is necessary. When elective irradiation is given to the pelvic and para-aortic lymph nodes in the absence of gross disease, doses in the range of 2000 to 2500 rad in two to three weeks are sufficient for tumor sterilization. However, grossly involved nodes may require 3000 to 4000 rad. When peritoneal implants have taken place, whole abdominal and pelvic irradiation is required either with the abdominal bath technique or moving strip technique as described previously. When retroperitoneal lymph nodes are involved, it is recommended that the mediastinum and supraclavicular nodes also be electively irradiated. An elective dose of 2000 to 2500 rad is recommended in such cases. Results of treatment appear to be quite satisfactory, but are related to the stage of the disease. Thoeny et al[16] have reported a 70 percent survival at five years. Brody[3] reported a 95 percent five-year survival for unilateral tumors, encapsulated and mobile. When the tumor is ruptured, adherent, or associated with ascites, the five-year survival dropped to 78 percent and 33 percent with metastases.

The rarity of other germ cell tumors, such as embryonal carcinoma and teratocarcinoma, make evaluation of the role of radiotherapy most difficult. In general, the moderate radiosensitivity of the kidneys and liver preclude adequate whole abdominal irradiation with these more radioresistant tumors.

Other Ovarian Cancers

Granulosa cell cancer and thecal cell tumors are thought to be more radiosensitive than epithelial tumors. Although granulosa cell cancers occur late, Delclos[5] reports 36 percent five-year survival in 15 patients given postoperative irradiation. Three of the survivors had advanced disease.

References

1. Arcangeli G, Benassi M, DePera V, Paoluzi R, Nervi C: A new fractionation technique of total abdominal irradiation in ovarian cancer. Int J Rad Oncol Bio Phys 1:155–60, 1975

2. Boronow RC: Ovarian cancer. In Rutledge F, Boronow RC, Wharton JT (eds): Gynecologic Oncology. New York, Wiley, 1976, pp 159–176

3. Brody S: Clinical aspects of dysgerminoma of the ovary. Acta Radiol 56:209–230, 1961

4. Delclos L, Braun EJ, Herrera JR, Jr, Sampiere VA, Roosenbeck EV: Whole abdominal irradiation by cobalt-60 moving strip technique. Radiol 81:632–641, 1963

5. Delclos L, Smith JP: Tumors of the ovary. In Fletcher GH (ed): Textbook of Radiotherapy, 2nd ed. Philadelphia, Lea & Febiger, 1973, pp 690–702

6. DeVita VT, Wasserman TH, Young RC, Carter SK: Perspectives on research in gynecologic oncology. Cancer 38:509–525 (suppl no 1), 1976

7. Fazekas J, Maier JG: Irradiation of ovarian carcinomas: A prospective comparison of the open field and moving strip techniques. Am J Roentgenol 120:118–123, 1974

8. Fuks Z, Bagshaw M: The rationale for curative radiotherapy for ovarian cancer. Intl J Rad Oncol Bio Phys 1:21–32, 1975

9. Gynecology Oncology Group. Statistical Report, Philadelphia, June 1976, pp 1–3

10. Johnson CE, Decker DG, Van Herik M: Advanced ovarian cancer—Therapy with radiation and cyclophosphamide in a random series. Am J Roentgenol 114:136–141, 1972

11. Kottmeier HL: Treatment of ovarian carcinomas with thio-tepa. Clin Obstet Gynecol 11:428–438, 1968

12. Marks RD, Scruggs HJ, Wallace K, Hotterstein DF: Technical aid in moving strip abdominal irradiation. Int J Rad Oncol Bio Phys 1:161–164, 1975

13. Rosenoff SH, Young RC, Anderson T: Peritoneoscopy—a valuable tool in ovarian carcinoma. Ann Intern Med 83:37–41, 1975

14. Rutledge F: Treatment of epithelial cancer of the ovary (Mullerian origin). In Rutledge F, Boronow RC, Wharton JT (eds): Gynecologic Oncology. New York, Wiley, 1976, pp 183–199

15. Smoron GL: Strip-staggering: Elimination of inhomogeneity in the moving strip technique of whole abdominal irradiation. Radiol 104:657–660, 1972

16. Thoeny RH, Dockerty MB, Hunt AB, Childs DS, Jr: A study of ovarian dysgerminoma with emphasis on the role of radiation therapy. Surg Gynec Obstet 113:691–698, 1961

17. Webb MJ, Decker DG, Mussey E, Williams TJ: Factors influencing survival in Stage I ovarian cancer. Am J Obstet Gynecol 116:222–230, 1973

Chapter 21

Practical Aspects of Immunology in Gynecologic Cancer

HUGH R. K. BARBER, M.D.

Immunology is making rapid advances and is cutting across all disciplines of medicine. Whether discussed in Jenner's time or at present, the study of immunity is properly the study of resistance to infection. This was the classic definition. It now encompasses a much wider range of phenomenon, and is basically the science of antigens, antibodies and their interactions in vivo and vitro, and the cellular phenomena of recognition of and responsiveness to foreign substances. The term "immunity" recently has taken on a more sophisticated and expanded role and is the property whereby the lymphoreticular system makes a memorized response to an antigenic stimulus. This may result in a state of positive reaction known as sensitization, or in a negative reaction known variously as immunologic tolerance or immunosuppression. Resistance is a complex state arising from properties of the individual, of the community, of race, and of species, but the most striking thing about it is the specific nature of its enhancement in individuals after recovery from specific infection.

As a scientific discipline, *immunology* encompasses immunity dealing with adaptive response to infective agents; *immunochemistry* is concerned with the chemical nature of antigens and antibodies; *immunogenetics* is the area of genetics that deals with antigens, antibodies, and their reactions; and *immunobiology* deals with the activity of the cells of the immune system and their

relationship to each other and their environment. As a biologic science, immunology includes developmental biology, genetics, biochemistry, microbiology, anatomy, and medicine. These basic concepts are fundamental for an understanding of the principles and practice of modern medicine. Table 21-1 compares the recent with the older nomenclature of transplantation immunology (Fig. 21-1).

Modern immunology was started when Jenner discovered that inoculation with cowpox protected man against smallpox. A series of experiments followed, such as the vaccine developed by Pasteur against cholera and the identification of an exotoxin elaborated by diphtheria vaccine by Roux and Yersin. In 1895, Héricourt and Richet[1] attempted to develop an antisera in animals by injecting human tumor cells into them. The results were highly unpredictable with rapid growth of tumors at times, while regression occurred in others. At the turn of the century, Paul Ehrlich[2] proposed the humoral theory of antibody formation. He also hypothesized that malignant neoplasms were antigenic and as such could be recognized by the host as being foreign to it. Unfortunately, he died before he could pursue this work.

The modern era of immunology was born quietly and escaped the notice and attention of the scientific world. The world was locked in a cataclysmic death struggle and the scientific world

Table 21–1. TRANSPLANTATION IMMUNOLOGY

RECENT NOMENCLATURE	OLDER NOMENCLATURE	ADJECTIVE	DEFINITION
Autograft	Autograft	Autochthonous	Tissue transplants within a single individual
Allograft (homologous) allogeneic	Homograft	Allogeneic	Same species but *not* genetically identical
Isograft (isogeneic)	Syngraft	Isogeneic Syngeneic	Transplants between donor and recipient of an inbred strain, or between identical twins (i.e., genetically identical individuals)
Xenograft (xenogeneic)	Heterologous	Xenogeneic	Tissue grafts between a donor and a recipient of different species
Orthotopic graft	Same		Tissue transplanted into its normal anatomical position
Heterotopic graft	Same		Tissue transplanted into an unnatural anatomical position
Histocompatible	Same		A state whereby donor and recipient individuals have an identical complement of tissue antigens, and are mutually able to accept tissue grafts from each other without resultant stimulation of the immune system; refers to the human leukocyte antigens (HL–A)

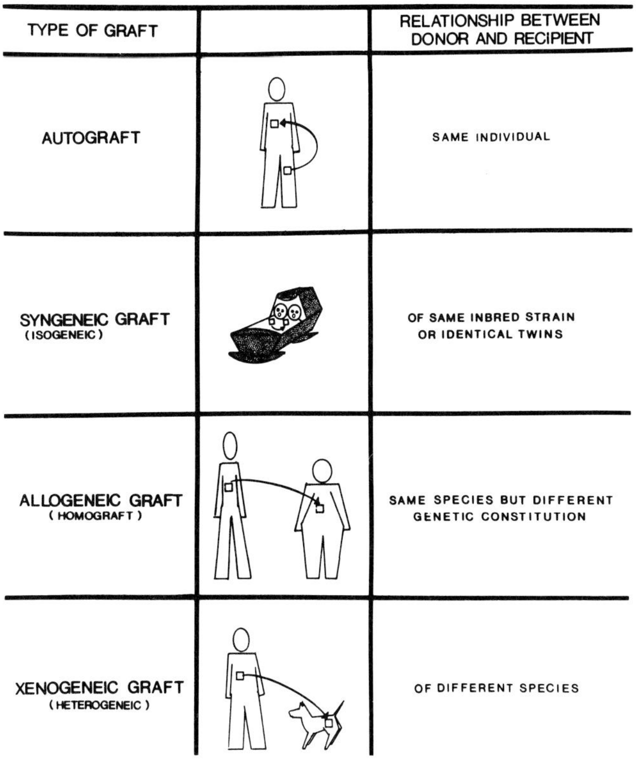

TYPE OF GRAFT		RELATIONSHIP BETWEEN DONOR AND RECIPIENT
AUTOGRAFT		SAME INDIVIDUAL
SYNGENEIC GRAFT (ISOGENEIC)		OF SAME INBRED STRAIN OR IDENTICAL TWINS
ALLOGENEIC GRAFT (HOMOGRAFT)		SAME SPECIES BUT DIFFERENT GENETIC CONSTITUTION
XENOGENEIC GRAFT (HETEROGENEIC)		OF DIFFERENT SPECIES

Figure 21–1. Transplantation of skin.

was engaged in methods for destruction, so that the great war could be brought to an end. It was not prepared to appreciate that Ludwig Gross[3] had identified cancer antigens. His findings were published in a little-quoted, but immensely important, study in 1943. He described the failure of his pedigree (inbred) mice to accept transplants of a specific cancer after they had been immunized with material from the same cancer grown upon other pedigree mice. In 1957, Prehn and Main[4] reported that mice immunized against syngeneic methylcholanthrene-induced (MCA) fibrosarcomas by inoculation of living sarcoma tissue, followed by surgical removal of the growing tumor, were resistant to subsequent grafts of the same tumor. In addition, immunization with normal tissue did not confer resistance to the tumor grafts. The mice that had become resistant to tumors still accepted skin grafts from the primary hosts of these tumors. It was evident that the cancer cell had identical histocompatibility or HL-A antigen as the normal cell of the same host, since this is a characteristic of the host. But the tumor cell had a new antigen in addition and was called the tumor-associated antigen (TAA). The

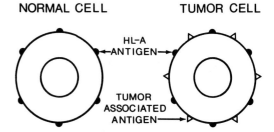

Figure 21–2.   A normal cell and a tumor cell from the same host. The cancer cell has histocompatibility identical to HL-A antigen of the normal cell of the same host, since this is characteristic of the organism. In addition, the cancer cell has a new antigen called tumor-associated antigen (TAA). Modern tumor immunology began with this finding.

observation that the tumor cell possessed the same HL-A antigen (the fingerprint) as the host as well as a new antigen characteristic of the tumor ushered in the modern era of tumor immunology (Fig. 21–2).

IMMUNOLOGY OF CANCER

All vertebrates have a defense mechanism, the immune defense system, that protects them from disease-causing microorganisms. The deliberation and exploration of this defense mechanism has conquered many infectious diseases and has been a major achievement of medical science in terms of preventing suffering and saving lives.

The progressive nature of cancer led the public and physicians alike to believe that human beings were incapable of defending themselves against cancer. A common view was that tumor-associated antigens could not possibly exist, since they would confer a selective disadvantage on the cells that carried them and lead to their immediate elimination by immunologic mechanisms. The observation that neoplasms often metastasize to the lymph nodes was viewed as additional indication that an immunologic defense against cancer could hardly play a role. The same feeling of despair existed about the control of infectious diseases about three decades ago.

In the early 1950s, planned scientific studies of the relationship of immunity to cancer were started. The following contributions were made at that time and advanced the concept of tumor immunology.

1. An abundant supply of highly inbred (syngeneic) animals became available.
2. It became evident that normal tissues as well as tumors could be transplanted to syngeneic recipients (identical twins or members of the same inbred animal strain) and that they were rejected by allogeneic (genetically foreign) recipients.
3. It has been documented that cancers do arouse a specific immune response in the organism in which they appear.
4. Antigenic differences represent the first qualitative distinction between cancer cells and their normal counterparts.

It is well documented now that each animal has antigens on the surface of their cells (human leukocyte antigens, HL-A) that make them genetically different from other members of that species. In the humans these were formerly called alloantigens, but now have been designated as human leukocyte antigens (HL-A). When tissue from one animal is transplanted into another genetically different animal of that species, rejection of the graft is the rule. The HL-A antigens are strong stimulators of an immune response.

This has been observed in humans where skin has been grafted from one human to another, resulting in rejection of the graft. Highly inbred animals (syngeneic) share the same genetic pattern with each other and readily accept grafts from one another. This observation has been confirmed among identical twins. If a tumor is grown in one of these animals and then transplanted to the other syngeneic mate, it is usually rejected, whereas normal skin or other tissue is not. This indicated that the tumor possessed its own antigens that were foreign to the normal tissue of that animal. The result was the development of antibodies against the tumor with rejection of the tumor. Repeated studies showed that cancers do arouse a specific immune response in the organism within which they appear. It confirmed the observation that these antigenic differences represent the first known qualitative distinction between cancer cells and their normal counterparts. The presence of antigens associated with tumor cells were formerly called tumor-specific transplantation antigens (TSTA), because they were demonstrated by transplanting the tumor into another inbred animal. Additional work has shown that the antigens (HL-A) present on normal cells are more potent stimulators of antibodies than are the tumor antigens (TSTA).[5,6]

ANTIGENS

An antigen is a substance that elicits a specific human response when introduced into the tissues of an animal or a human.[7] The term "antigen" is sometimes used loosely to refer to materials such as whole bacteria when these are used to stimulate an immune response. Such organisms contain many hundreds of different antigens, and moreover, it should be noted that even a single antigenic protein molecule may bear on its surface more than one different antigenic determinant. Some workers use the term to refer to any substance that can combine with an antibody, whether or not it is capable of stimulating a specific immune response. High molecular weight molecules of 500,000 or greater with complex polypeptide-carbohydrate or protein structures are among the best antigens. Molecules having a molecular weight of less than 5000 rarely stimulate antibody production. Antigens are defined in terms of what they do rather than what they are. Antigens are divided into the following categories:

Extrinsic: An antigen that is not a constituent of the cell
Intrinsic: An antigen that is a constituent of a cell
Occult: Self-antigen that does not reach antibody forming tissues

Antigens are classified as toxins, A and B isoantigens, heterophil antigens, accessible antigens, haptenes, and adjuvants.

TUMOR ANTIGENS

Tumors have been found to have antigens present on the surface of the tumor cell.[8] They have been designated as tumor-specific transplantation antigens (TSTA) because they were demonstrated by transplanting the tumor into another inbred animal. More recently they have been called tumor-associated antigens (TAA). Tumor antigens have been divided into two groups, i.e., unique antigens or common antigens. Until recently, it was reported that a tumor would have one or the other, but not both, depending on the agent that initiated the response. It is now generally accepted that a tumor may have one or both types of antigens.

UNIQUE ANTIGENS

Animal tumors induced by chemical carcinogens have individual specificity with unique antigens (Fig. 21-3). The same chemical carcinogen painted on different places in the same animal will produce different tumors. Each new tumor has its own specific antigenicity that is not shared with other tumors. The action of the chemical carcinogen appears to be mainly a random interaction with the native cell DNA, resulting in a tumor with unique antigens.

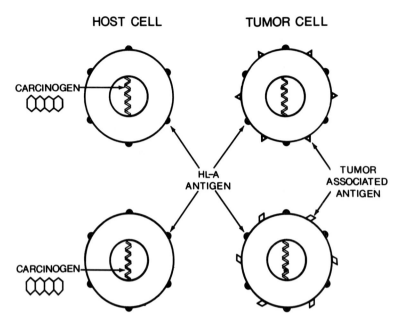

HOST CELL   **TUMOR CELL**

Figure 21–3. Unique antigens—same host. Animal tumors induced by chemical carcinogens have individual antigenic specificity. Recent evidence indicates that chemically induced tumors may possess common antigens as well.

COMMON ANTIGENS

Virally induced tumors appear to carry antigens common to all tumors induced by a given virus, even in animals of different species (Fig. 21–4). Although this is generally true, recent studies indicate that there may be some cross-reacting, some virus tumors having unique antigens as well as common ones, and some chemically induced tumors having common antigens. In some instances, depending on the techniques used, either the common or the individually unique antigens were detected.

The association between viruses and animal tumors has long been appreciated. Nevertheless, despite a great amount of work, there is no documented instance of a virus origin for a tumor. The isolation of the enzyme, reverse transcriptase, may solve this problem. Using this enzyme system, progress has been made in studying myelogenous leukemia.

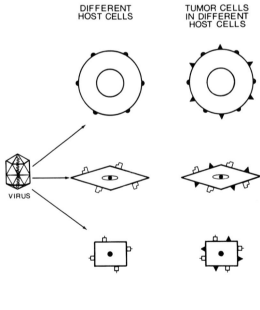

DIFFERENT HOST CELLS   TUMOR CELLS IN DIFFERENT HOST CELLS

VIRUS

⬡ HL–A ANTIGENS OF DIFFERENT HOSTS

▲ TUMOR ASSOCIATED ANTIGENS
(the same in tumor cells of different host cells)

Figure 21–4. Common antigens. All tumors induced by a given virus, even in animals of different species, possess a common antigen. Recently, it has been shown that they may also have unique antigens.

ANTIBODY

An antibody is a substance produced in response to an antigen. An antibody is commonly, if not always, a γ-globulin. All antibody molecules are globulins but not all serum globulins are antibodies. By electrophoretic separation of serum proteins, antibody globulins are localized in the γ-globulin and occasionally β-globulin regions. The antibody portions of the serum globulins are referred to as immunoglobulins.[9] The most important immunoglobulins are immunoglobulin G (IgG), immunoglobulin M (IgM), immunoglobulin A (IgA), immunoglobulin D (IgD), and immunoglobulin E (IgE). The immunoglobulins are produced by the B cells. The thymus-independent cells (B cells) produce the immunoglobulins from the plasma cells and are designated the humoral immunity mechanism. The humoral response is cell free and is mediated by antibody circulating freely in the bloodstream and other body fluids. In order to have a cytotoxic effect, it is necessary to have complement present, as well as an antigen and an antibody. Without complement, free antibody can bind to the antigens on the cell surface but is unable to kill the cell.

BLOCKING OR ENHANCING ANTIBODIES

A blocking antibody is a term used to describe the antibody that reacts (coats) with the antigens on the surface of the cell and prevents an attack by a cytotoxic antibody and/or a reactive killer T cell. The existence of F (ab')$_2$ fragments of IgG, which have blocking activity, have been described in the sera of cancer patients. These fragments were able to inhibit cell-mediated immune reactions in vitro.

UNBLOCKING ANTIBODIES

Certain sera taken from either animals or human patients during the period of tumor remission has been found to increase the cytotoxic effect of immune lymphocytes.[10] The mechanism of the potentiation effect (unblocking or deblocking) is unknown as are the molecules mediating it. If it is correct to assume that the blocking factor is an antigen-antibody complex, the "unblocking" effect of certain sera could be due to antibodies that are bound to the blocking complexes. They could be different from the antibodies of the blocking complexes, or they could be the same antibodies in excess. An antibody may also act as an antigen and if the antibody acting as an antigen is a blocking antibody, it is conceivable that it may produce an unblocking antibody. The blocking factors are considered antigen-antibody complexes (and occasionally free antigen), and therefore, it is anticipated that antibodies to the antigen in such a complex would be unblocking antibodies. The unblocking antibodies may interfere with the attachment of blocking factors to the target cells or to the lymphocytes, may alter the blocking factors, or depress their formation by feedback inhibition. Lymphoid cells may produce unblocking antibodies. The unblocking or deblocking factor may provide a method for monitoring the patients and would be superior to monitoring the blocking factor. This is predicated on the assumption that the disappearance of unblocking serum would occur before the blocking factors are detected. Recently, it has been shown that certain sera can "arm" lymphoid cells from nonimmune donors, so that they become specifically cytotoxic for syngeneic tumor cells. A similar "arming" has been reported in systems involving normal alloantigens rather than tumor-specific antigen.

CELLULAR EVENTS IN AN IMMUNE RESPONSE

The antigen may interact with a macrophage and following this is a processed antigen with the capability of sensitizing a lymphocyte. The sensitized lymphocyte may undergo transformation to a transformed lymphoblast, which may lead to a plasma cell or a sensitized lymphocyte. The plasma cell has the ability to secrete immunoglobulins and is called the humoral response. The

1) INDUCTION

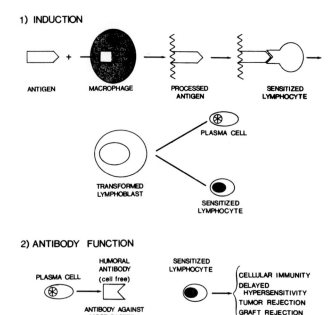

Figure 21–5. Cellular events in an immune response.

sensitized lymphocyte is identified with the cell-mediated response where the antibody remains an integral part of the cell. The sensitized lymphocytes are associated with delayed hypersensitivity reactions and tumor rejection. If the anti-gen is not processed by a macrophage but makes contact with a lymphocyte directly, that lymphocyte is then a tolerant cell and can no longer respond to an antigenic challenge (Fig. 21-5).

COMPLEMENT

Complement is an enzymatic system of proteins that is activated by many antigen-antibody reactions and that is essential for antibody-mediated immune hemolysis and bacteriolysis.[11,12] It also plays a part in several other biologic reactions, i.e., phagocytosis, opsonization, chemotaxis, and immune cytolysis. It consists of a system of at least 11 proteins (9 components) found in different concentrations in normal serum and serves primarily to amplify the effect of the interaction between specific antibody and antigen.

The antibodies react with antigens on the surface of the invading cell and the classical cascade complement chain commences.[13] It ends with the destruction of the cell. An alternate pathway[14,15] has been proposed and supported by recent work. This method is called by either the alternative pathway or properdin pathway. The reaction resulting from this method appeared to set into motion the cytolytic action of complement without relying on cell-bound antibodies to initiate the action. The cascade could be set off by a substance or substances other than an antibody, which is called properdin. This led to the theory of nonspecific resistance mechanism against infection (Fig. 21-6).

DEVELOPMENT OF THE IMMUNE SYSTEM

Pluripotent stem cells originally arise in the yolk sac, and as fetal development progresses, the cells move from the yolk sac to the fetal liver to the adult bone marrow. These pluripotent cells differentiate into the precursor stem cells of all the hematopoietic elements. Certain lymphoid cells are processed in the thymus under stimulation by a thymopoietin hormone. Subpopulations of T

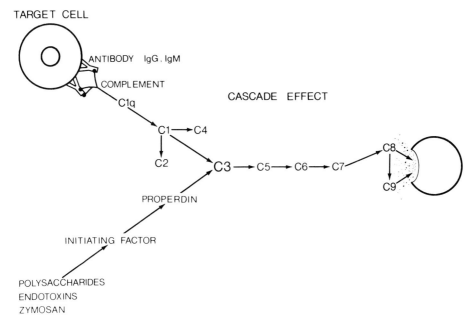

Figure 21-6. Classical complement pathway and its alternate pathway (properdin). In the classic complement pathway, an inciting agent stimulates an antigen-antibody response, which stimulates production of C1, C4, and C2 in the presence of Ca^{2+} and Mg^{2+} which in turn stimulates C3, leading to production of C4 to C9 (chemotaxis). This is a cascade effect. The alternate pathway starts with a polysaccharide or endotoxin, which in the presence of Mg^{2+} leads to the production of properdin C3 proactivator. Enhanced phagocytosis follows production of C3. From C4 to C9, the steps are the same as in the classic pathway.

lymphocytes are produced that liberate a helper T cell factor that stimulates a competent B cell to produce a killer cell (K cell), which can act without complement being present. The subpopulation of T lymphocytes may produce suppressor T cells that inhibit competent B cells from producing immunoglobulins. Lymphoid precursor cells are processed by an alternate pathway in a poorly defined organ in man, but identified as the bursa of Fabricius in the bird by a hormone-like substance, bursin, and differentiate into B lymphocytes. In response to antigenic stimulation processed by macrophages, lymphoblasts are produced and give rise to plasma cells that secrete immunoglobulins. There is another population of circulating lymphocytes that has characteristics of both T and B lymphocytes. These double cells (D cells) represent 2 to 3 percent of circulating lymphoid population. The origin and function of these cells remains to be determined (Fig. 21-7).[16,17]

Since resting T and B cells are morphologically indistinguishable, it has been essential to find certain membrane markers to classify these lymphocyte populations. Spontaneous rosette formation with SRBC (sheep red blood cells) is a characteristic marker for T cells, whereas lymphocytes that have easily detectable membrane-bound Ig (immunoglobulin) determinants are regarded as B cells.

HUMORAL AND CELL-MEDIATED IMMUNE RESPONSES

The immune response takes two forms: (1) a humoral response that is mediated by cell-free fluid containing antibodies that are circulating freely in the bloodstream as well as other body fluids, and (2) a cell-mediated immunity that is carried out by sensitized lymphocytes.

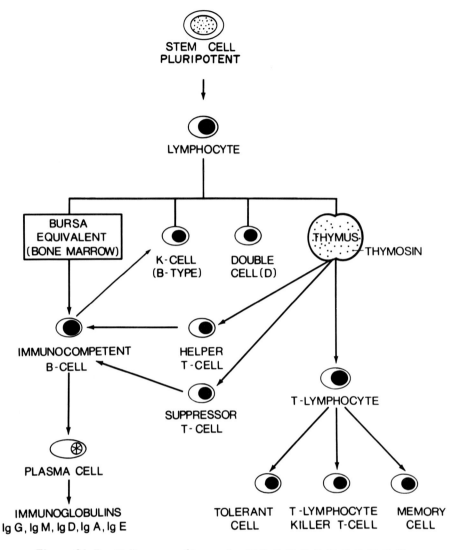

Figure 21-7.   Cell system of immunity (T-Cell, B-Cell, K-Cell, D-Cell).

The humoral response (B cell) is mediated by immunoglobulins. It is cell free and made up of the immunoglobulins IgG, IgM, IgA, IgD, and IgE. In order for this cell-free antibody to have a killing or cytotoxic effect, a third substance in addition to the antigen and antibody is required. This substance, called complement, is made up from several factors present in the normal serum. Without complement, antibody can bind to the antigen on a cell surface but cannot damage or kill the cell. The nature and precise function of complement have only recently been explained. The humoral response offers a defense against most bacteria and some foreign proteins.

The cell-mediated response (T cell) is mediated by sensitized lymphocytes. In the cell-mediated immune (CMI) response, the antibody remains an integral part of the cells that produced it and is a cell-associated antibody. Sensitized lymphocytes carrying such antibody are carried in the lymph to tumor cells where their antibody combines with the antigen determinant on the surface of the tumor cell. The cell-bound antibody then becomes capable of rupturing and killing tumor cells. The mechanisms for this action have not been completely elucidated. The cell-mediated response is particularly important in graft rejection, eliminating viruses as well as intracellular bacterial and cancer cells.

NATURE'S EXPERIMENT TO DEMONSTRATE THE DIFFERENCE BETWEEN HUMORAL AND CELL-MEDIATED IMMUNITY

Any deviation in nature often supplies valuable material for studying normal mechanisms (Fig. 21–8).[18] Nature has supplied such an experiment to study the role of the humoral and cell-mediated response.

A Deficiency of Cell-Mediated Immunity (T Cell)

In DiGeorge's syndrome, there is dysplasia of the thymus and absence of parathyroid glands. The patient has no resistance to viruses or to other agents that are controlled by the cell-mediated immunity system, such as tuberculosis, brucella, leprosy, and certain parasitic diseases. They do not have the immunologic response to develop a delayed hypersensitivity reaction or to reject grafts of foreign tissue. They can produce circulating antibodies and have the ability to respond to bacterial vaccines by developing normal circulating antibodies.

A Deficiency of Humoral Immunity (B Cell)

In the human patient with Bruton type of agammaglobulinemia, there is a deficiency of immunoglobulin synthesis in which IgG is decreased 10-fold and IgA and IgM about 100-fold. They do not give a normal circulating antibody response to bacteria and thus are susceptible to pyogenic infections. These patients do not respond with normal circulating antibody to bactcrial vaccines. The lymphoid tissue in the appendix and Peyer's patches is somewhat reduced and patients do not develop plasma cells and germinal centers in lymph nodes. Nevertheless, the cell-mediated immune mechanisms function normally in these patients, and they can reject grafts and exhibit delayed hypersensitivity to the tuberculin skin test.

Combined Deficiency of T and B Cells

In "Swiss type of agammaglobulinemia," which is an X-linked disease of male children, both cell-mediated and humoral mechanisms are deficient. There is almost complete absence of lymphoid tissue in the body, the thymus is very small, and the lymphoid tissues of the appendix and Peyer's patches are absent. These children cannot make humoral antibodies (immunoglobulins) or develop cell-mediated immune reactions. They suffer from progressive bacterial or viral infection and die within the first two years of life.

In summary, if the thymus is removed from a newborn animal, but the gut-associated lymphoid tissue is not disturbed, the animal cannot reject foreign tissue grafts or fight a virus but has normal resistance to bacterial infection. On the other hand, if the gut-associated lymphoid tissue is destroyed and the thymus kept intact, the animal cannot resist bacterial infection but can reject foreign tissue grafts as well as virus infections.

In addition to the primary immunodeficiency disorders discussed, there are more than 30 phenotypic patterns of immunodeficiency. Among these are selective IgA deficiency disorders, Wiskott-Aldrich syndrome, ataxia telangiectasis, Chédiak-Higashi syndrome, and chronic mucocutaneous candidiasis.

Lymphocyte surface markers have been instrumental in dissecting out the nature of basic defects in primary immunodeficiencies. The significance and understanding of suppressor T cells in the pathogenesis of certain immunodeficiency disorders may help to develop some modalities for the treatment of these patients.

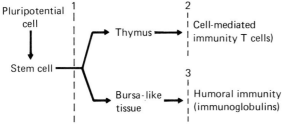

Figure 21–8. Experiment of nature to study the immune deficiency diseases.

1. Swiss agammaglobulinemia
   Good's syndrome
2. DiGeorge's syndrome
3. Bruton's agammaglobulinemia

THE IMMUNE DEFENSE SYSTEM

If tumor cells possess antigens on their surfaces capable of stimulating a specific immune response, why does cancer continue to grow in the presence of a mechanism designated to control its growth?[19] The explanation may be that the rate of growth exceeds the capacity of the immune response. However, from studies in animals, more specific reasons are known for the failure of the immune response to prevent the start and growth of cancer. These are discussed in the next section.

FAILURE OF THE IMMUNE RESPONSE

Immunosuppression

There are many factors that contribute to immunosuppression. Among these are aging, the neoplastic process itself, anticancer drug therapy, radiation therapy, genetic defects, neonatal thymectomy and, to a lesser extent, antibiotics, anesthetics, analgesics, and hypnotics. In reality, it is often difficult to separate the contributions of drugs and disease in bringing about this state of immunosuppression.

Immunologic Tolerance

In a broad sense, immunologic tolerance may represent a specific form of immunosuppression. It is usually associated with the exposure to an antigen during embryonic or early neonatal life before the immune system has matured. The latter then fails to recognize the antigen as nonself and is incapable of mounting an immune response to it. Since cancer is considered to arise from a single cell clone, the tolerance theory for the progress of cancer is offered as an explanation. Work on choriocarcinoma bears out this theory. When this occurs, the host is not immunologically tolerant in general but only for that specific tumor antigen.

Immune Paralysis

The preferred term currently in use is "acquired tolerance." It is induced by injecting very small or very large doses of antigen and persisting so long as that antigen remains in the body. In clinical practice, immune paralysis has been suggested to occur in the host with large tumors. Following the removal of such a large tumor mass, the host exhibits resistance to the reimplantation of their own tumor cells. This suggests that the intrinsic failure of the immune response was not the cause of the original lack of immune reaction. Rather, the temporary paralysis observed was due to the fact that the system was unable to cope with too big a challenge.

Immunologic Enhancement

This results in an increased growth of the tumor in animals. The observation was made in animals transplanted with grafts of foreign cancer cells and then given injections of antiserum against the cancerous cells. It was anticipated that the grafts of foreign cancer cells would be promptly rejected. However, it was found that not only were the cancer cells tolerated but often were found to grow more rapidly. How can this be explained? It is conceivable that what the antibody produced and then injected was an enhancing or blocking antibody as opposed to a cytotoxic antibody. These antibodies may have coated the tumor in the same manner as could be done by covering the tumor with a layer of cream. This would prevent the killer lymphocytes from attacking the tumor. The protective coating (by blocking or enhancing antibodies) would serve to protect the tumor. The process of immunologic enhancement is more complicated than described but was presented in this manner for a simplistic explanation. Immunologic enhancement has indirectly been shown to play a role in humans with choriocarcinoma.

Immunoselection

Cancer develops from a clone of cells. The cell has tumor antigens on the surface and as the tumor grows the bulk of cancer cells have the same type of antigens. During the course of many generations, mutations may occur and certain cells may have more of the original antigen present and stimulate a greater antibody production. These cells will attract more antibodies and may be eliminated from the cell population, leaving cells with weaker antigens as survivors. The result may be a colony of cells with weak antigens followed by a relatively slow growth of tumor at first. It is conceivable that this may even lead to tolerance as described earlier. After a period of time the tumor cell develops autonomy and progressively greater invasive properties.

Antigen Modulation

This is a temporary change in antigenicity reflecting an adaptational alteration in an entire population of cells. In summary, it can be stated that as soon as antibody is present, cancer cells of certain animal leukemias cease synthesizing antigens. As a result, the immunologic defense becomes ineffective. In humans this response has not been documented.

Unknown Factors

The tumor-bearing host may possess factors that depress the immunologic reactivity in a nonspecific way or possibly they may lack factors that are important for such reactivity. This has been suggested by the poor response that the tumor-bearing host develops when tested for delayed hypersensitivity reactions to a variety of antigens. In vitro studies in this group have also shown a decreased ability to transform lymphocytes after stimulation with phytohemagglutinin.

IMMUNOTHERAPY AND IMMUNOPOTENTIATION

Immunotherapy is the treatment of disease by active or passive immunization.[20] Immunity is the property whereby the lymphoreticular system makes a memorized response to an antigenic stimulus. This may result in a state of positive reaction known as sensitization, or in one of negative reaction (diminished or absent) known variously as immunologic tolerance, immunologic paralysis, or immunosuppression. It is not strictly correct, therefore, to follow common usage of the word immunization as synonymous with sensitization or stimulation.

The most efficient cures of diseases that our philosophy can conceive involve the *potentiation of normal,* biophysical, or biochemical processes or the *countering of abnormal processes* that lead to, or accompany, disease. Cancer presents few examples of this ideal at present, but studies of what has become known as host resistance are clearly an early step in this apparently logical direction. These are multitudinous factors, such as intercellular communication, metabolic peculiarity, biochemical selection, and hormonal requirement possibly involved in host resistance. The immune activities of the lymphoreticular system have received the greatest attention and will be the main topic of this discussion.

It is a tribute to the prepared mind of scientists that they observed that cancer regression occasionally followed when the host had an infection. Bacille Calmette Guérin (BCG), an antituberculosis vaccine introduced in 1921, is under controlled observation at present in the field of im-

munotherapy. For more than 100 years, the disappearance of cancer after severe infection has been reported. Coley in the early 1900s noted the disappearance of cancer following a severe streptococcus infection.[25,26] He therefore began to treat cancer patients with a variety of bacterial toxins, but despite a few promising results, found no consistent therapeutic benefit. Interest in the use of toxins as an immunopotentiator waxed and waned until the present time. Clinically, the observation was made and repeatedly observed that those patients with empyema following pneumonectomy for lung cancer did better than those who had an uncomplicated postoperative course. In addition, it has been reported that the simultaneous injection of certain bacteria with an antigen increased the immune response to the antigen. Tubercle bacilli were found to be among the most effective bacterial adjuvants for immune stimulation. Complete Freund's adjuvant is a water-in-oil emulsion adjuvant in which killed, dried tubercle bacilli are suspended in the oil phase. This adjuvant is especially effective in stimulating cell-mediated immunity and in some animals, i.e., guinea pig, potentiates production of certain immunoglobulin classes.

For orientation purposes an outline for the immunotherapy of cancer is presented as follows:[21]

I. Active immunization against cancer
    A. Active immunization *against oncogenic virus*

B. Active immunization *against cancer cells*
1. Autochthonous or autologous cells
2. Allogeneic cells
3. Attenuated cells
4. Soluble tumor antigens
C. Modification of antigenicity
II. Passive immunization against cancer
A. Passive immunization
B. Adoptive immunization
1. Allogeneic lymphocyte transfer
2. Transfer factor
3. Immune RNA
4. Autologous lymphocytes stimulated in vitro with a mitogen is phytohemagglutinin (PHA)
5. Bone marrow transplant
6. Thymosin

III. Nonspecific and miscellaneous
A. Coley's toxin
B. BCG (bacille Calmette Guérin)
C. Vaccinia, pertussis vaccine, poly-IC
D. MER (methanol extraction residue of BCG)
E. Maruyama vaccine
F. Cornybacterium parvum[22]
G. Levamisole
H. DNCB (dinitrochlorobenzene)
I. Chalones
J. Interferon and interferon inducers
K. Deblocking factor
L. Neuraminidase, vibrocholerae (VCN)
M. Concanavalin A (Con A)
N. Viruses
O. Bone marrow transplants

TUMOR MARKERS

It is obvious that humans arise from a single cell and present in the cell are all the things it needs in its journey through life or at least the machinery to produce it.[23] There are many antigens that appear on the surface of a cell during the lifetime of an individual. Recently it has been reported that chorionic gonadotropins, using the new sensitive radioimmunoassay methods, have demonstrated a positive reaction in 40 percent of all tumors including squamous and adeno type of tissue in both females and males, and that among embryonal tumors this figure climbed over 90 percent.

The carcinoembryonic antigen (CEA) has been demonstrated in the fetal gut in the first and second trimester, but disappears in the third trimester. Later, it is identified in certain endodermal cancers, cirrhotics, and heavy smokers. The question that is raised is what represses the gene controlling this antigen in the third trimester and derepresses the gene later in life?

Stolbach has reported work from his laboratory with the Regan alkaline phosphatase isoenzyme. He found this isoenzyme in the serum of 30 to 40 percent of patients with ovarian cancer and in 50 to 70 percent of malignant fluids from patients with carcinoma of the ovary.

In the laboratory at Lenox Hill Hospital,[24] a common antigenic component has been identified among the common epithelial ovarian cancers, using a double immunodiffusion technique and

by immunofluorescence methods. Heterologous antisera produced by pools of ovarian carcinoma tissues have reacted consistently and specifically with tissues of origin in immunodiffusion and immunofluorescence tests. Fresh ovarian tissue was taken directly from the operating room, ho-

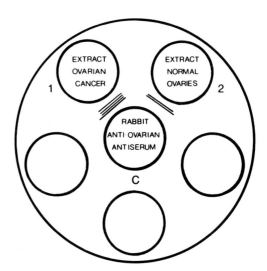

Figure 21–9. Immunodiffusion Test. Schematic representation showing reactivity of rabbit antiovarian tumor serum against soluble antigen extract of ovarian carcinomas and a pool of normal ovaries. Additional precipitin lines are seen with ovarian cancer pools.

mogenized, and tissue homogenates were mixed with complete Freund's adjuvant and emulsified by sonication at 4 C. This emulsion was injected into New Zealand, white, virgin female rabbits. The sera was collected after an appropriate time interval. The highly absorbed sera showed no reaction with normal ovarian tissues, normal human serum components, and various other neoplasms. These investigations have suggested the presence of a specific antigenic component in carcinoma of the ovary. This antigen did not cross-react with the carcinoembryonic antigen (CEA), ferritin, and was not revealed in fetal tissues (Figs. 21–9 and 21–10).

It has been repeatedly reported that a piece of tumor removed from the parent tumor and explanted close to it will probably grow, but the same piece of tumor explanted at a distance from the parent tumor may or may not grow. The tumor explanted close to the parent tumor was protected. Evidence indicated that a cloud of antigen-antibodies surrounded the parent tumor and served as enhancing or blocking antibodies. A study of peritoneal fluid was undertaken to isolate these factors. Peritoneal effusion of patients with ovarian cancer contain sizable amounts of free and complexed immunoglobulins. By means of salt precipitation procedures and Amicon ultrafiltration techniques, it was shown that, by lowering the pH, antibodies could be eluted from the surfaces of tumor cells. Antibodies were recovered that after purification and concentration displayed a high degree of specificity against ovarian carcinoma cells. In indirect immunofluorescence, immunoglobulins recovered from peritoneal effusions showed bright cytoplasmic staining with tissue cultures and fresh suspensions of ovarian cancer cells but not of normal ovaries of nonovarian tumors. Immunoglobulins isolated

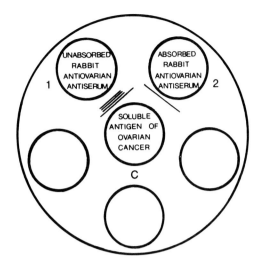

Figure 21–10. Immunodiffusion Test. Schematic representation, using soluble antigen of ovarian cancer against unabsorbed and absorbed antiserum. There is a single line of reactivity against ovarian carcinomas remaining after absorption with extracts of normal ovaries.

from fluids of benign ovarian cysts or from effusions of nonovarian tumors were negative in immunofluorescence tests. Autologous antibodies recovered from peritoneal effusions will be hopefully utilized in sensitive radioimmunoassay tests that are greatly needed for early detection of ovarian cancer, the leading cause of death from gynecologic neoplasia.

The author wishes to thank Mrs. Marcia Miller for her assistance in the preparation of this manuscript; and the medical illustrator, Margaret Ryon Uibel, Department of Medical Photography, Lenox Hill Hospital, New York City.

References

1. Héricourt J, Richet C: De la serotherapies dans le traitement du cancer. CR Acad Sci [D] (Paris) 121:567, 1895

2. Ehrlich P: On immunity with special reference to cell life. Proc R Soc Lond (Biol) 66:424, 1906

3. Gross L: Intradermal immunization of C3H mice against a sarcoma that originated in animals of the same line. Ca Res 3:326, 1943

4. Prehn RT, Main IM: Immunity to methylchlolanthrene-induced sarcomas. J Natl Ca Inst 18:769, 1957

5. Sell S: Immunology, Immunopathology and Immunity. New York, Harper & Row, 1972

6. Roitt I: Essential Immunology. London, Blackwell Scientific Publications, 1972
7. Dumonde DC: Tissue specific antigens. Adv Immunol 5:30, 1965
8. Terethia SS, Katz M, Rapp F: New surface antigen in cells transformed by simian papovavirus SV-40. Proc Soc Exp Biol Med 119:896, 1965
9. Bernier GM: Structure of human immunoglobulins. Prog Allergy 14:1, 1970
10. Hellström KE, Hellström I: Cellular immunity against tumor antigen. Adv Cancer Res 12:167, 1969
11. Alper CA, Rosen FS: Genetic aspects of the complement system. Adv Immunol 14:252, 1971
12. Cochrane CG: Initiating events in immune complex injury. In Amos B (ed): Progress in Immunology. New York, Academic, 1971, p 143
13. Gewurz H: The immunobiologic role of complement. In Good RA, Fisher DW (eds): Stamford, Conn, Sinauer Associates, Inc, 1971
14. Lepow IH, Rosen FS: Pathways to complement systems. N Engl J Med 286:942, 1972
15. Naff GB: Editorial: Properdin—Its biologic importance. N Engl J Med 287:716, 1972
16. Gupta S: Cell surface markers of human T and B lymphocytes. N Y State J Med 76:24, 1976
17. McKhann CF, Yarlott MA: Tumor immunology. Ca 25:187, 1975
18. Weir DM: Immunology For Undergraduates, 3rd ed. Baltimore, Williams and Wilkins, 1976
19. Barber HRK: Immunobiology for the Clinician. New York, Wiley, 1977
20. Currie GA: Eighty years of immunotherapy: A review of immunological methods used for the treatment of human cancer. Br J Ca 26:141, 1972
21. McKhann CF, Gunnarsson A: Approaches to immunotherapy. Cancer 34:1521, 1974
22. Israel L, Halpern B: Le Corynebacterium parvum dans les cancers avances: Premiere evaluation de L'activité therapeutique de cette immuno-stimuline. Nouv Presse Med 1:19–23, 1972
23. Barlow JJ, Bhattacharya M: Tumor markers in ovarian cancer: Tumor-associated antigens. Seminars in Oncology. 2:203, 1975
24. Dorsett BH, Ioachim HL, Stolbach L, Walker J, Barber HRK: Isolation of tumor specific antibodies from effusions of ovarian carcinomas. Int J Cancer 16:777, 1975
25. Coley WB: The treatment of malignant tumors by repeated inoculations of erysipelas, with a report of original cases. Am J Med Sci 105:487, 1893
26. Coley WB: Late results of the treatment of inoperable sarcoma with mixed toxins of erysipelas and Bacillus prodigiosus. Trans Am Surg Ann 19:27, 1901

Glossary of Immunologic Terms

Active immunotherapy. *Active immunotherapy* may be divided into two groups, i.e., specific immunogens and nonspecific adjuvants. Active specific immunotherapy is attempted by the immunization of a tumor-bearing patient with autologous altered (radiation, chemical) tumor cells. Nonspecific immunotherapy attempts to augment antitumor immunologic activity with nonspecific stimulants such as BCG or phytohemagglutinin.

Accessible antigens. *Accessible antigens* are antigens of self that are in contact with antibody-forming tissues and to the host that is normally tolerant.

Adjuvant. An *adjuvant* is a substance which when mixed with an antigen enhances its antigenicity.

Agglutinins. *Agglutinins* are antibodies that produce aggregation or agglutination of a particulate or insoluble antigen.

Allogeneic. *Allogeneic* pertains to genetically dissimilar individuals of the same species or refers to tissues originating in different individuals of the same species or in members of a different inbred strain.

Allogeneic inhibition. In vitro damage to cells caused by contact with genetically dissimilar cells is termed *allogeneic inhibition.* When two antigenetically different lymphocytes are cultured in the presence of phytohemagglutinin (a substance that activates lymphocytes), there is a mutually damaging effect. It is the opposite of syngeneic preference.

Alpha fetoprotein (AFP). *AFP* is synthesized in the fetus by perivascular hepatic parenchymal cells. It is found in a high percentage of patients with hepatomas and malignant teratomas, especially of the endodermal sinus type.

Anamnestic response. An *anamnestic response* is a recall mechanism, an accelerated response of antibody production to an antigen which occurs in an animal that has previously responded to the antigen. It is synonymous with secondary immune response.

Anergy. *Anergy* is a deficiency in the response to agents normally inducing an immune response, especially delayed hypersensitivity.

Antibody. An *antibody* is a specific globulin (immunoglobulin) produced in response to stimulation by an antigen and capable of reacting specifically with that antigen.

Antigen. An *antigen* is a substance that is capable of inducing the production of specific immunity. The antigens may be extrinsic, i.e., an antigen that is not a constituent of the cell, intrinsic, i.e., an antigen that is a constituent of the cell, or occult, i.e., a self-antigen that does not reach antibody-forming tissues.

Antigen-determinant (Epitope). The *antigen-determinant* refers to the small three-dimensional configuration of the everted surface of the antigen molecule that combines with a specific antibody.

Antigenic reversion or conversion. This term refers to the antigenic change in adult cells such that the antigenic profile reverts from the adult form to one existing in immature or fetal cells. Such reversion may follow neoplastic changes.

Ataxia-telangiectasia. This is a familial disease of children characterized by recurrent sinopulmonary infection, telangiectasis in the bulbar conjunctivae, on the ear, and in the antecubital space. A mask-like facies is also characteristic. IgA and IgE are deficient and cellular immunity is often deficient as well, which is demonstrated by phytohemagglutinin stimulation of cultured lymphocytes and by tests for delayed hypersensitivity. There is a high incidence of malignant tumors of lymphoid tissue. These patients are unique in that they have an elevated α-fetoprotein titer.

Autochthonous. Refers to tissues of any sort originating in the same host or tumor borne by the host of origin.

Autologous. *Autologous* means derived from the subject itself.

B cell or B lymphocyte. *B cells* or *B lymphocytes* are bone marrow cells. These cells mediate humoral immunity and are thymus-independent cells. In the avian species these cells are derived from the Bursa of Fabricius; in man, no discrete bursa has been identified.

Binding site. This is a term used for an antibody-combining site and of other sites of specific attachment of macromolecules to one another.

Blast transformation. *Blast transformation* refers to the transformation of small lymphocytes with minimal cytoplasm, condensed nuclei, and few cytoplasmic organelles to a lymphoblast characterized by abundant cytoplasm, numerous organelles, and a large nucleus with multiple nucleoli. It may be induced by a number of mitogens.

Blocking factor (enhancement antibody). A *blocking factor* refers to a humoral antibody or an antigen-antibody complex that acts as a noncytotoxic antibody. Instead of damaging the cell, it coats it with a protective covering so that neither complement or "killer" lymphocytes can attack the cell.

Cancer detection. The smallest tumor that can be detected clinically or detected by x-rays is usually about 1 cu cm (about 1/16 cu inch) in size and weighs about 1 gm (approximately 1/30 oz). A tumor of this size contains at least a billion cells (10^9) and has the capacity for spread.

Cancer epidemiology. *Cancer epidemiology* is the study of the incidence and distribution of human cancers in relation to a variety of environmental and intrinsic factors.

Cancer etiology. *Cancer etiology* is the study of the causes of cancer.

Carcinoembryonic Antigen (CEA). *CEA* is an antigen found originally in fetal tissues of entodermal origin as well as in malignant tumors of adult tissues of entodermal origin. It probably results when a gene is derepressed by some stimulus. Since other tissues have been found to have CEA present, it is possible that the CEA molecule has more than one antigenic surface determinant.

Cell-Mediated Immunity (CMI). *CMI* is a specific immunity that is mediated by small lymphocytes, which are thymus dependent and are referred to as T cells as opposed to the thymus-independent cells which are called B cells. The T cells are probably the most important cells in cancer immunity and organ rejection.

Chalones.   *Chalones* are a group of naturally occurring substances that are sensitized by cells and that appear to be important in the regulation of cell division as well as in differentiation of such normal cell types as epidermal cells, liver and kidney cells, granulocytes, and certain other cell types. Since the antimitotic effect of these substances is tissue specific and since they are essentially nontoxic, they would appear to represent an almost ideal group of substances for use in the suppression of growth of those tumors that have lost an ability to synthesize their own chalones but remain sensitive to their inhibitory effects.

Chediak-Higashi syndrome.   This syndrome is a disease of children inherited as an autosomal recessive. The disease is characterized by pale skin probably due to the decreased pigmentation that approaches albinism. The skin, hair, and eyes lack pigment. There is progressive cranial and peripheral neuropathy. Hepatomegaly may be predominant. There is an increased susceptibility to infection. Lymphoma may occur. There is a defect of granulopoiesis and the neutrophil leukocytes contain abnormally large lyosomal granules which may be 8 to 10 times their normal size. A specific immunologic abnormality has not yet been demonstrated.

Chimerism.   A state in which two or more genetically different populations of cells coexist is called a *chimerism*.

Clonal selection theory of acquired immunity of Burnet.   This theory suggests that immunity and antibody production are functions of clones of mesenchymal cells. Each clone is able to react immunologically with a small number of antigens and each cell is immunologically competent because it carries on its surface a receptor that is able to react with a given antigen.

Clone.   A *clone* is a population of cells derived from a single cell by asexual division.

Complement.   A *complement* is a system of serologically nonspecific proteins present in fresh normal serum that are necessary for the lysis or death of cellular antigens in the presence of antibody.

Congeneic (Co-isogenic, Congenic) strains.   Strains of animals bred to approach genetic identity with each other except for different alleles as one locus, especially a histocompatibility locus, are *congeneic strains*.

Cytophilic antibody.   A globulin component of immune serum which becomes attached in vitro to certain normal cells in such a way that these cells are subsequently capable of specifically absorbing antigens.

Deblocking antibody.   A *deblocking antibody* is capable of overcoming the inhibitory effect of blocking factor, thereby permitting immunologic destruction of malignant cells.

Delayed hypersensitivity.   See **Cell-Mediated Immunity**.

DiGeorge's syndrome.   This syndrome defines a deficiency state only of the cell-mediated immune mechanism, with a deficiency of lymphoid cells from those areas of the spleen and lymph nodes that are under thymic control.

Dinitrochlorobenzene (DNCB).   DNCB is a drug used to test for cell-mediated immunity. When applied to the skin it acts as a haptene attaching to a protein in the skin producing an antigen that has the potential to sensitize lymphocytes. The challenge in two weeks produces a marked local response in a patient with good cell-mediated immunity.

Enhancement antibody.   See **Blocking Factor**.

Freund's adjuvant.   *Freund's adjuvant* may be either complete, i.e., Freund's water-in-oil emulsion of mineral oil, plant waxes, and killed tubercle bacilli used to incorporate with antigen to stimulate antibody production; or incomplete, i.e., Freund's mixture without tubercle bacilli.

Graft-vs-Host reaction.   In the presence of an immune deficient host, the graft may produce lymphocytes that react to the host antigen, producing hepatosplenomegaly, lymphopenia, diarrhea, and skin rash. In the very young, a disease that develops after injection of allogenic lymphocytes into immunologically immature experimental animals producing a similar picture plus the failure to thrive and often death is called "runt disease" (allogeneic disease).

Haptene.   A partial antigen that contains at least one of the determinant groups of an antigen is referred to as a *haptene*. It can react specifically with antibodies, but in itself does not induce the formation of antibodies unless it is complexed with a carrier molecule such as a protein.

HL-A antigens (Human Leukocyte Antigen).   HL-A is a genetic locus containing two, closely linked groups of several alleles, i.e., subloci. It is present on the cell membranes of all nucleated cells and plays a major role in determining graft rejection.

Humoral immunity. This type of immunity pertains to the body fluids, in contrast to cellular immunity. It is initiated by the thymus-independent B cells. These B lymphocytes proliferate and differentiate into plasma cells that secrete immunoglobulins (IgG, IgM, IgA, IgD, and IgE).

Immunogen. An antigen that induces a specific immunologic response is called an immunogen.

Immunologic surveillance. As described by Sir F. MacFarlane Burnet, effective *immunologic surveillance* depends on tumor-specific antigenic determinants being present on the surfaces of neoplastic cells, which enable these altered cells to be recognized as "nonself" and destroyed by immunologic reactions.

Interferon. An *interferon* is a protein that is released by cells in response to virus infection. It represents nonspecific immunity.

Lymphokine. Substances released by sensitized lymphocytes when they come in contact with the antigen to which they are sensitized are called *lymphokines.* There are at least four mediators of cellular immunity, including transfer factor (TF), lymphocyte transforming activity (LTA), migration inhibition factor (MIFO), and lymphotoxins (LT).

Macrophage. A *macrophage* is a large mononuclear phagocyte. In the tissues this cell may be designated a histiocyte and in the blood, a monocyte. An antigen must contact or pass through a macrophage before it can become a processed antigen with the ability to encounter and then sensitize a small lymphocyte.

Migration inhibition factor (MIF). MIF refers to a lymphokine that is produced when a sensitized lymphocyte is cultured in the presence of an antigen to which it is sensitized. MIF inhibits the migration of these lymphocytes.

Mitogen. A *mitogen* is a substance that induces lymphocytes to undergo blast transformation, mitosis, and cell division (causing mitosis or cell division).

Mixed lymphocyte (leukocyte) culture (MLC). The transformation of small lymphocytes to blast cells, with synthesis of DNA, in mixed cultures of blood leukocytes from normal allogeneic individuals is a *MLC.* The magnitude of the reaction reflects the degree of disparity between histocompatibility antigens of the two donors. In identical twins neither set stimulates the other, whereas in unrelated pairs, there is almost always stimulation of each cell by the other. The degree of stimulation is analyzed either morphologically by blast transformation or biochemically by measuring tritiated thymidine incorporation into newly synthesized DNA.

Overgrowth Stimulating Factor (OSF). This factor can cause normal cells in culture to adopt the appearance and growth habit of the transformed cell. Stimulated cells revert to normal when the OSF is removed.

Phytohemagglutinins. *Phytohemagglutinins* are lectins extracted from the red kidney bean, *Phaseolus vulgaris* or *Phaseolus communis.* They can be purified to yield a glycoprotein mitogen that stimulates lymphocyte transformation and causes agglutination of certain red cells. It is a method for estimating the pool of thymus-dependent lymphocytes (T cells).

Pokeweed Mitogen (PWM). PWM is a mitogen extracted from the pokeweed plant and can be purified to yield a glycoprotein. The pokeweed mitogen stimulates blast formation of both B and T cells.

Postcapillary venules. In immunology, *postcapillary venules* are the blood vessels found in the thymus-dependent area of the lymph node, characterized by prominent high endothelial lining cells. Lymphocytes leave the blood via the postcapillary venules in the lymph nodes.

Pyroninophilic cells. *Pyroninophilic cells* show red cytoplasm when stained with methyl-green pyronin stain. The reaction indicates the presence of large amounts of cytoplasmic RNA and therefore of very active protein synthesis. It is characteristic of protein-secreting cells such as plasma cells.

Reverse transcriptase (RNA dependent-DNA polymerase). This recently isolated factor can transcribe the base sequence of a viral RNA onto a DNA strand, in vitro. It is now possible to test human cancers for association with any one of a number of RNA viruses.

Syngeneic. *Syngeneic* pertains to genetically identical or near-identical animals, such as identical twins or highly inbred animals.

Syngeneic preference. Unlike allogeneic inhibition, *syngeneic preference* represents improved growth in syngeneic recipients.

T-Lymphocyte (T Cell). Lymphocytes that have matured and differentiated under thymic influence, have been termed thymic-dependent lymphocytes or *T lymphocytes.* These cells are primarily involved in the mediation of cellular immunity, as well as tissue and organ rejection.

Tolerance. *Tolerance* commonly results from prior exposure to antigens and refers to the failure of antibody response to a potential antigen following exposure to the antigen.

Transfer factor. (See **Lymphokines**). *Transfer factor* is a heat labile, dialyzable extract of human lymphocytes that is capable of conferring specific antigen reactivity to the donor.

Tumor angiogenesis factor (TAF). *TAF* represents the induction of the growth of blood vessels due to a stimulant released by tumor cells. The growth of the tumor parallels the development of new blood vessels.

Waldenström's macroglobulinemia. This disorder is usually seen in elderly males and is characterized by paraproteinemia of IgM type, lym-phoid tissue enlargement, splenomegaly, hemorrhagic tendency, and depression. It is similar to myelomatosis, with a proliferation of lymphocytes rather than plasma cells and is characterized clinically by bleeding from the nose and gums. The disease is monoclonal, but occasionally has antibody activity, e.g., a rheumatoid factor. The course of the disease is more benign than that of myelomatosis.

Wiskott-Aldrich syndrome. This syndrome is a sex-linked recessive disease of infants characterized by hemorrhagic diathesis, eczema, and recurrent infections. It is a combined defect of cell-mediated and humoral immunity. Malignant lymphoma may occur.

Xenogeneic (Heterologous). *Xenogeneic* pertains to individuals of different species.

Chapter 22

Gestational Trophoblastic Disease

CHARLES B. HAMMOND, M.D.
HERBERT J. SCHMIDT, M.D.
ROY T. PARKER, M.D.

Gestational trophoblastic neoplasms (choriocarcinoma and related tumors) are malignant tumors arising from the trophoblast of human pregnancy.[1] These are relatively rare malignancies, but even though unusual diseases, they have received widespread attention in the past 20 years. This attention seems to be due to several factors. For example, these tumors are grafts of malignant fetal chorionic tissue on a maternal host; they invariably produce a protein hormone, human chorionic gonadotrophin; the production of this hormone is directly related to the number of viable tumor cells present; and these malignancies are very sensitive to a variety of chemotherapeutic agents.[2] All of these features, plus the fact that most patients with these tumors, even those with metastases, can be cured, have led to intensive interest and investigation.

Prior to the introduction of chemotherapy, the survival rate for patients with trophoblastic malignancies was universally poor. However, Hertz and co-workers at the National Institutes of Health (1956) began an era of drug treatment that initiated progressive improvement in salvage of these patients. Today, essentially all patients can be cured. The methodology of treatment, the avoidance of irreversible toxicity, and the preservation of intact reproductive structures have dramatically altered the prognosis for a once highly fatal disease.[1,3-7]

This chapter will review the concept of adequate diagnosis and therapy for patients with trophoblastic neoplasms. "Benign" trophoblastic neoplasm (hydatidiform mole), the details of malignant trophoblastic disease, and an address of the controversial issues in diagnosis and therapy will be presented. For further reviews, the reader is referred to the monographs by Bagshawe,[8] Park,[9] and Hertig.[10]

HISTORY OF GESTATIONAL TROPHOBLASTIC NEOPLASIA

Table 22-1 presents some of the important historic landmarks in the understanding of gestational trophoblastic neoplasia (GTN).[11] These diseases have been known since antiquity and often have been poorly understood. GTN is a useful general term, as our current understanding presents these diseases (hydatidiform mole, invasive mole, and choriocarcinoma) as a spectrum of single disease. As will be reviewed in detail, the documentation of one of the forms of this tumor is pertinent for early diagnosis. The patient is best followed by sensitive assays of human chorionic gonadotrophin, which enable the physician to monitor the biologic activity of the process.

Table 22-1 does not attempt to enter the modern era of the study of trophoblastic disease. The

Table 22–1.   EARLY HISTORY OF GESTATIONAL TROPHOBLASTIC
NEOPLASMS

400 BC	Hippocrates: earliest description of hydatidiform mole, "dropsy of the uterus."	1895	Felix Marchand: demonstrated these tumors to be sequelae of pregnancy, abortion, or mole; also described proliferation of synctium and cytotrophoblast.
600 AD	Aetius of Armida: described "bladder-like" objects filling the uterus.		
1700	William Smellie: first related terms "hydatid" and "mole."	1903	Teacher: confirmed Marchand's work and negated Sanger's sarcoma theory.
1827	Velpeau and Boivin: first recognized hydatids as cystic dilatations of chorionic villi.	1929	Fels, Ehrhart, Reossler, and Zondek: demonstrated excess gonadotrophic hormone in the urine of patients with hydatidiform mole.
1889	Max Sanger: coined term "sarcoma uteri deciduocellulae" as malignant tumor derived from decidua of pregnancy.		

contributions of Hertz and co-workers in the evolution of chemotherapy, studies of Hertig, Sheldon, Brewer, and Park investigating pathologic changes, and the significant contributions of Brewer, Bagshawe, Lewis, Goldstein, and others will be discussed in detail in the sections that follow.

PATHOLOGY

Gestational trophoblastic neoplasms include hydatidiform mole, invasive mole (chorioadenoma destruens), and choriocarcinoma (chorionepithelioma). It is a useful general term because it may be applied when the precise histologic nature of the disease may not have been full established or thought to have changed.[2,9,12] Since the development of systemic chemotherapy, one need not have representative tissues from either the uterus or disseminated metastases to start treat-

Table 22–2.   GESTATIONAL TROPHOBLASTIC NEOPLASMS—FLOW OF DISEASE

	INCIDENCE	MORBIDITY	MORTALITY	OUTCOME
HYDATIDIFORM MOLE	1/1200 pregnancies	Moderate, (sepsis, hemorrhage, toxemia)	Low	80+% spontaneous remission after evacuation; 15+% progression to malignancy requiring therapy
CHORIOADENOMA DESTRUENS (INVASIVE MOLE)	1/15,000 pregnancies, anteceded by hydatidiform mole	Major (sepsis, hemorrhage, uterine perforation, loss of reproductive capacity)	15% (prechemotherapy) even with hysterectomy	
CHORIOCARCINOMA	1/40,000 pregnancies, 50% after hydatidiform mole, 50% after (term pregnancy —25%; abortion, ectopic—25%)	Major	Nonmetastatic— 60% (prechemotherapy); Metastatic—98% with surgery and loss of reproductivity (prechemotherapy)	

ment. The main contribution of a pathologic diagnosis is the documentation that the patient has a
tumor fitting under the broad classification of gestational trophoblastic neoplasms. Although a
patient's prognosis may be affected to a certain
degree by the histology of the tumor, the biologic
activity of the tumor is better determined by
monitoring human chorionic gonadotrophin
(HCG) excretion and following the clinical course
of the patient, rather than relying on the prognostic implications of pathologic material.

Table 22-2 outlines the natural history of the
various gestational trophoblastic neoplasms from
data prior to chemotherapy. Each of these tumors
will be considered separately in the section that
follows, and this discussion is limited to preg-
nancy-related tumors of the trophoblast (excluding nongestational trophoblastic tumors of ovary,
testicle, or embryonal rests).

Hydatidiform Mole

Hydatidiform mole is an abnormal pregnancy
characterized grossly by cystic swelling of the placental villi and usually associated with the absence
of an intact fetus (Fig. 22-1). Most hydatidiform
moles are recognizable by their gross appearance,
but some moles are small and may seem grossly to
be ordinary abortions. This is particularly true
when "molar change" is present on the curettings
from early therapeutic abortion. Microscopically,
they may be identified as moles with the three
classic findings of edema of the villus stroma, diminution of the villus vasculature, and proliferation
of the trophoblast (Fig. 22-2). Frequently, differentiation must be made between the "transitional mole" with a few large villi but no undue
trophoblastic proliferation, the blighted ovum
with simple hydropic change of the villus, and, on

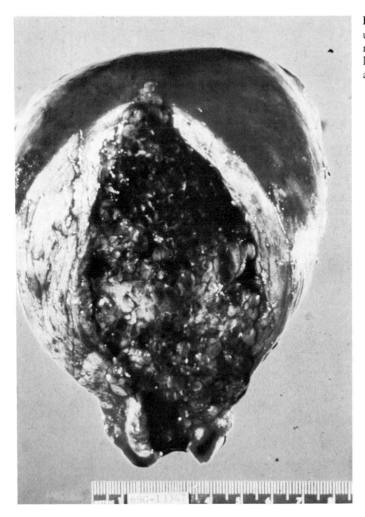

Figure 22-1. An extirpated
uterus containing a hydatidiform
mole. Note the typical "grape-
like" vesicles of varying shapes
and sizes filling the uterine cavity.

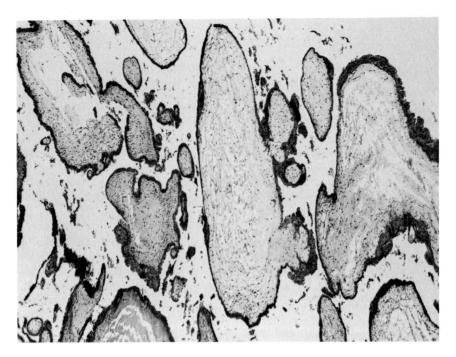

Figure 22–2. A microscopic view of a hydatidiform mole characterized by well-developed villi with stromal edema, minimal trophoblastic proliferation, and scanty vascular support.

occasion, a normal first trimester pregnancy that has relatively large villi.[12,13] It is suggested that if at any time there is doubt as to whether a particular pathologic specimen shows molar change, HCG testing be utilized in the follow-up interval.

Several authors have studied the degree of trophoblastic proliferation associated with the villi of hydatidiform mole in an attempt to predict the likelihood that an individual patient will develop persistent, malignant disease. Hertig and Sheldon in 1947, reviewed 200 patients with molar pregnancy in an attempt to provide such a correlation.[13] From that study, the more abundant, varied, and complex the trophoblast that surrounded the villus, the worse the prognosis for the patient. However, this cannot be decided absolutely for an individual patient, as recently confirmed in a study of 350 patients from Duke University Medical Center.[14] A safe general statement is that among large groups of patients with hydatidiform moles, the likelihood of malignant sequelae developing is increased in patients whose trophoblastic cells showed increased proliferation and anaplasia. Unfortunately, metastatic choriocarcinomas have developed from moles that appeared to be entirely "benign." For this reason, it remains critically important to obtain

accurate, sensitive gonadotrophin assays in all patients who have had hydatidiform moles.

Invasive Mole (Chorioadenoma Destruens)

Invasive mole is a hydatidiform mole that has invaded the myometrium or other structures or, on occasion, metastasized. The pathologic pattern of the hydatidiform mole is maintained (Fig. 22–3). It is difficult to make this diagnosis on the basis of curettage material since adequate myometrium is rarely obtained; the diagnosis is made pathologically less frequently now than formerly, since fewer hysterectomies are performed in patients with trophoblastic disease. Invasive mole is reported in 10 to 15 percent of patients who have had primary molar pregnancy. Invasive mole penetrates the myometrium and may be associated with uterine rupture and hemoperitoneum. Metastases of trophoblastic neoplasia may contain invasive mole, but the vast majority will show choriocarcinoma, regardless of the morphology of the uterine tumor.[15] There is little reason to extirpate peripheral metastases to establish the morphology of that lesion.

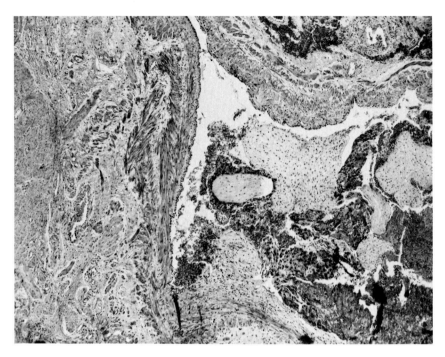

Figure 22–3. A microscopic view of an invasive mole (chorioadenoma destruens). Here the pattern of the hydatidiform mole is maintained, but loses the characteristic of being a surface lesion by penetrating the myometrium.

Invasive mole will be discovered promptly in patients who are being adequately monitored after evacuation of molar pregnancies. Problems of irregular bleeding, failure of uterine involution, and most importantly, failure of steady regression of HCG all signal the likelihood of an invasive mole. Therapy should be promptly instituted in the face of these clinical findings and failure of regression of the HCG titer.

Choriocarcinoma

Choriocarcinoma is a pure epithelial tumor composed of syncytiotrophoblastic and cytotrophoblastic cells.[9,12,13] It may accompany or follow any type of pregnancy. It has been estimated that choriocarcinoma is preceded by hydatidiform mole in approximately 50 percent of patients, the remainder occurring after term pregnancy, abortion, or ectopic pregnancy. An incidence rate of 1 in 40,000 pregnancies is currently accepted for the United States. Histologically, there is no persistence of the villus structure, only sheets or foci of trophoblasts are seen (Fig. 22–4).[9] It may be hazardous to make the diagnosis of choriocarcinoma on curettage specimens, since foci of trophoblast may be dislodged from underlying villi that are present and would be identified if the full uterine specimen were available.[12,15] This is also true in isolated sections of the myometrium that show only trophoblast and in which the villus pattern of invasive mole may have collapsed during fixation and sectioning.

Interpretation of trophoblastic tissue following or accompanying an otherwise normal pregnancy may be extremely difficult. When a curettage is done for postpartum bleeding, it is most important to process histologically all the material obtained, since such specimens may reveal only small, isolated areas of choriocarcinoma.

Hertig has commented upon the histologic similarity of the trophoblastic pattern in very early human pregnancy and in choriocarcinoma. This strong similarity may lead to diagnostic problems. Careful search usually reveals the pattern of the villus in the tissue of early normal pregnancy. One should also be aware that choriocarcinoma can arise from ectopic pregnancy. The appearance of cells at the placental site, whether in the tube or elsewhere, occasionally may raise the suspicion of choriocarcinoma, although it often represents

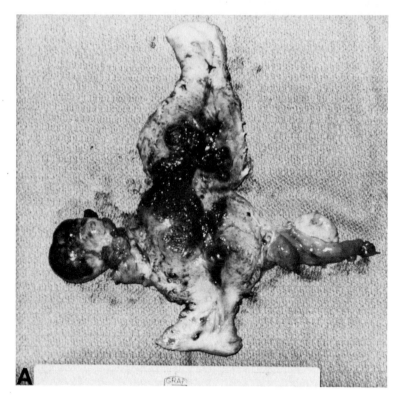

Figure 22–4A. Gross appearance of choriocarcinoma involving the major portion of the uterine fundus. The deep invasion and vascular penetration is obvious. The rubbery consistency is clinically similar to an old organized hematoma.

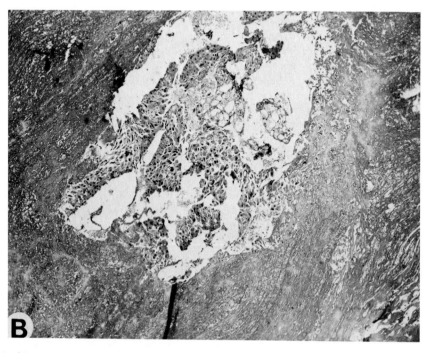

Figure 22–4B. A microscopic view of choriocarcinoma. Here the villus pattern is absent. Anaplastic trophoblastic cells penetrate the myometrium and are surrounded by necrosis and hemorrhage.

only a tangential section through the floor of the placenta.[9,12,13,15] In any of these confusing situations HCG testing may aid greatly the diagnosis and documentation of need for therapy.

Choriocarcinoma, with its exuberant trophoblastic growth and its lack of villus architecture, is usually seen in the metastases of trophoblastic disease.[15] Such areas of trophoblastic growth may be seen in any organ in the body and present the classic pathologic findings seen in the uterus. The pathologic diagnosis of choriocarcinoma in any site should be an immediate signal to institute further treatment, although gonadotrophin excretion is a critical factor for confirmation and further management.[2]

The clinical diagnosis of choriocarcinoma may be very difficult.[2,7] Local uterine disease will present usually as irregular bleeding in a postpartum patient, but the interval may be years from the last known antecedent pregnancy. It may be suspected on curettings obtained in the management of such bleeding. Choriocarcinoma may present only as a finding of distant metastatic disease. Again, this may be immediately after a pregnancy or delayed by a long interval of time. In any woman in the reproductive years, in whom there is unexplained metastatic disease, gestational trophoblastic neoplasia should be suspected. Confirmation may be obtained by measuring HCG and excluding intercurrent pregnancy.

The histopathologic categorization of gestational trophoblastic neoplasms is fraught with problems. If a tissue diagnosis of invasive mole or choriocarcinoma can be made with certainty, therapy should be instituted promptly. If the histopathologic diagnosis is that of primary hydatidiform mole, the patient should be monitored with serial gonadotrophin assays to determine the presence of postmolar malignant disease (20 percent) or whether she is in the larger group (80 percent) for whom uterine evacuation is curative. Any attempt to decide an individual patient's prognosis on the basis of aborted or curetted molar tissue is accompanied by a high risk of error. There are many examples of patients with "benign" hydatidiform mole who progress to metastatic choriocarcinoma. Conversely, there have been many other patients with excessive trophoblastic proliferation in association with molar pregnancy who were cured by simple uterine evacuation. The biologic activity of the tissue and the possible later development of malignancy are much more accurately followed by serial HCG titers in the postmolar interval. Many excellent articles are available summarizing the histopathologic study of the various types of trophoblastic neoplasia.[9,12,13,15]

HUMAN CHORIONIC GONADOTROPHIN ASSAY

Normal and neoplastic human trophoblastic tissues produce a gonadotrophic hormone that seems immunologically and biologically identical. This hormone, human chorionic gonadotrophin (HCG), has been shown to be elaborated in essentially all patients with gestational trophoblastic neoplasms.[1,2] The amount of HCG produced is related to the amount of trophoblastic tissue in the patient.[4] Thus, accurate HCG quantification, coupled with histopathologic determination, permits early diagnosis and affords an efficient method of monitoring the effects of treatment and the diagnosis and follow-up of remission. Precise, sensitive, and accurate assays are required if tragic consequences are to be avoided.

Biologic, immunologic, and radioimmunologic assays for HCG are of major importance in the diagnosis and management of patients with trophoblastic disease. HCG is a glycoprotein composed of alpha and beta subunits. As noted previously, the amount of HCG present is directly related to the number of trophoblastic cells, and the HCG of trophoblastic neoplasia and normal pregnancy are "identical to date." Methods of measurement vary in specificity and sensitivity, and a few are listed in Table 22-3. The earlier assays for detecting HCG in serum or urine utilized small animals and were dependent upon the biologic activity of the material. Such assays include mouse uterine weight, rat uterine weight, ventral prostate, and ovarian hyperemia. The Klinefelter assay of mouse uterine weight, using Kaolin concentrates of 24 hour urines, provides detection of HCG and pituitary LH and FSH. These assays are time consuming and expensive but provide a sensitive and reliable test. Immunoassay (pregnancy testing) has been widely adapted as a commercial enterprise. Immunologic pregnancy tests are quantitative only when positive, and then with considerable variability in dilutional assay. Most pregnancy tests are positive only when HCG is greater than 500 to 1000 international units per liter of urine. They do not extend down to the normal range of pituitary LH

Table 22–3.   ASSAY TECHNIQUES FOR
HCG DETERMINATIONS

TEST	HCG SPECIFIC	HCG SENSITIVITY
Immunologic commercial	no	≥700–5,000 IU/liter
Pregnancy test (latex agglutination and inhibition)	(LH, HCG)	
Biologic assay (mouse uterine weight)	no (LH, HCG)	0.5–10 (5 muu/liter)
Radioimmunologic		
LH-HCG whole molecule	no	<5 mIU/ml
Beta subunit HCG	yes	<5 mIU/ml

*Note that only the Beta subunit radioimmunoassay is HCG specific.

nor to the lower levels of detectability for HCG in patients with trophoblastic disease.[1,2,14] *Thus, pregnancy tests are helpful if positive but worthless if negative.*

Recently, radioimmunoassay has been applied to the measurement of HCG in serum and urine. Initial radioimmunoassays cross-reacted HCG and pituitary LH,[18] but the more specific radioimmunoassays to the beta subunit chain of HCG allow the separation of HCG from LH.[19] The sensitivity of this assay is adequate to detect HCG at very low levels (less than 5 mIU/ml) and has become a superior test for the diagnosis, treat-

ment, and follow-up of patients when trophoblastic disease is suspected.

Beta subunit radioimmunoassays or HCG-LH radioimmunoassays may not be available in a community. In that event the physician should contact a commercial laboratory equipped for this purpose or contact one of the trophoblastic disease centers in his area. It is vital that the physician understand the assay being reported and its level of sensitivity.

It is again stressed that a precise, sensitive, and available HCG assay is mandatory in the diagnosis and therapy of patients with trophoblastic disease.

CLINICAL MANAGEMENT OF HYDATIDIFORM MOLE

Studies of patients with hydatidiform mole indicate that, aside from a lower incidence, molar pregnancy in the United States follows a clinical pattern similar to that found elsewhere in the world.[14] Older pregnant patients must be considered to have a greater likelihood of molar pregnancy, whereas teen-agers do not. Parity does not seem to alter the occurrence rate of molar pregnancy and does not influence the development of malignant trophoblastic disease after molar pregnancy. While it was initially suggested by Bagshawe,[20,21] more recent studies do not tend to support that maternal blood type relates to the development of molar pregnancy.

Symptoms of Hydatidiform Mole

Symptoms of primary molar pregnancy include delayed menses, abnormal uterine bleeding (89

percent), nausea and vomiting (15 percent) and preeclampsia (12 percent) (Table 22–4). Disproportionate uterine size was noted, with 46 percent having uterine size excessive for gestational dates, but 16 percent having a uterus normal in size for dates, and 38 percent having a uterus smaller than expected for the gestational duration. Theca-lutein cyst formation of the ovary, from excessive HCG, has been reported in 15 percent of patients with intact molar pregnancy (Fig. 22–5).[1,22]

Diagnosis of Hydatidiform Mole

Primary hydatidiform mole is most often diagnosed by abortion of vesicular tissue and usually this means a delayed diagnosis. With increased suspicion, however, newer techniques can allow this diagnosis to be achieved at an earlier

Table 22–4. HYDATIDIFORM MOLE—
SIGNS AND SYMPTOMS
(347 PATIENTS)*

	(PERCENT)	
Bleeding	89	
Nausea-vomiting	14	
Toxemia	12	
Pain (abdominal)	10	
Hyperthyroidism	1	
Uterine size	46	large-for-dates
(at evacuation)	38	small-for-dates
	16	normal-for-dates
Ovarian enlargement	14	
(≥8 cm)		Theca-lutein cysts

Prognostic implications initial exam: significant increase of malignant sequelae in patients with both large-for-dates uterus and ovarian enlargement (>50%).
*From Curry et al: Obstet Gynec 45:1 1975.

date.[1,16,22] Techniques for diagnosis, currently recommended, include repetitive HCG determinations, ultrasonography, and amniography.

A single *HCG determination* cannot be considered diagnostic for molar pregnancy, even if very high levels are present. Delfs has shown that unusually high levels of HCG may be seen in normal pregnancy and a single determination thus may be confusing.[23] Repeated assays that fail to show a decline of HCG from very high levels, as would be expected after 80 to 90 days of normal pregnancy, are suggestive of hydatidiform mole. Other endocrine tests (serum leucine aminopeptidase, human placental lactogen, estrogen, progestin) have not been of major assistance in diagnosis for an individual patient.[22]

Ultrasound scanning is a useful diagnostic tool for patients with primary molar pregnancy. Gray scale techniques seem to be most reliable in the hands of a competent ultrasonographer. Greater availability of equipment and further training of personnel will allow this technique to be more widely utilized. (Fig. 22–6).

Amniography is a procedure that can be performed in most hospitals with readily available materials and diagnostic x-ray equipment. Once the uterus has reached 14 weeks in size, a needle is inserted into the uterus by percutaneous abdominal wall puncture under local anesthesia. A small volume of radio-opaque dye (review for iodide allergy) is instilled into the uterus and a plain abdominal x-ray is taken. Molar pregnancy yields a classic "honeycomb" pattern (Fig. 22–7).

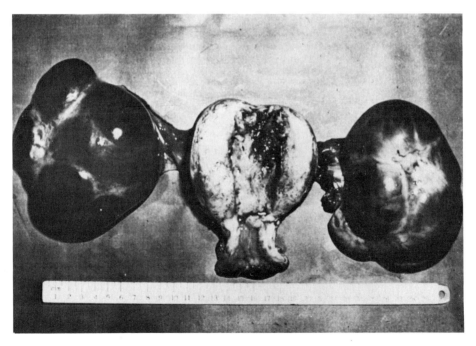

Figure 22–5. Large bilateral theca-lutein cysts of ovaries due to excessive HCG stimulation in primary mole. These spontaneously resolve as the amount of circulating HCG diminishes and disappears.

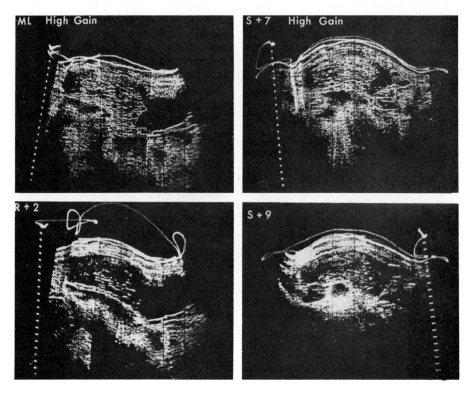

Figure 22–6A. A longitudinal ultrasound scan revealing the usual echo pattern of a hydatidiform mole.

Evacuation of Hydatidiform Mole

The techniques for evacuation of molar pregnancy have included D&C, hysterotomy, and hysterectomy. More current recommendations have deleted hysterotomy unless major hemorrhage occurs.[1,16,22] Suction dilatation and curettage offers a safe, rapid, effective method of termination of the mole for nearly all patients with primary molar pregnancy. The ease and safety of the procedure is noteworthy and problems have been minimal. Blood loss is usually modest. It is recommended that all patients be evacuated of molar pregnancy by suction dilatation and curettage with a laparotomy set available for patients with a large uterus (greater than 12 weeks size). Intravenous Pitocin is begun after a moderate amount of tissue has been removed. After suction curettage, gentle sharp curettement should be done and the tissue from the decidua basialis studied separately. With this technique, we have safely evacuated uteri as large as 28 weeks gestation. Recent studies have suggested that hys-

terotomy is no longer appropriate for the evacuation of the usual patient with hydatidiform mole because of a greater incidence of persistent malignant disease after evacuation of molar pregnancy by this method.[14] It is recognized that many of the patients who had hysterotomy also had significant uterine enlargement, a factor that seems related to a higher rate of persistent disease.[14] Suffice it to say, that most patients may be handled by suction dilatation and curettage.

Primary hysterectomy may be selected as the operative procedure of choice in molar pregnancy if the patient has completed childbearing, since there is a 20 percent chance of subsequent malignant sequelae after a primary mole, and a 1 to 3 percent chance of a subsequent molar pregnancy if the uterus remains in place and the patient again conceives. However, hysterectomy does not negate the need for careful clinical follow-up and HCG testing, as one study has suggested a 3.5 percent chance of malignant sequelae despite removal of the uterus.[14] Other techniques of evacuation such as prostaglandins are being evaluated.

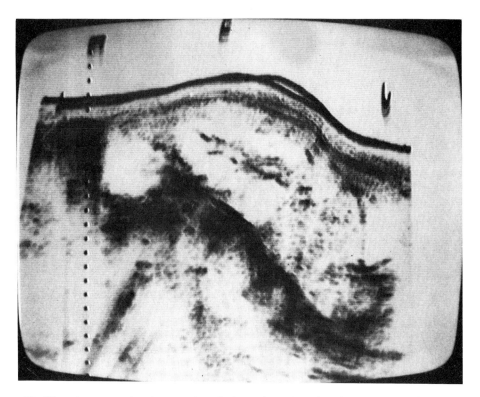

Figure 22–6B. A gray scale ultrasound technique depicting the characteristic echo pattern of a hydatidiform mole. (Courtesy of Dr. A.F. Haney)

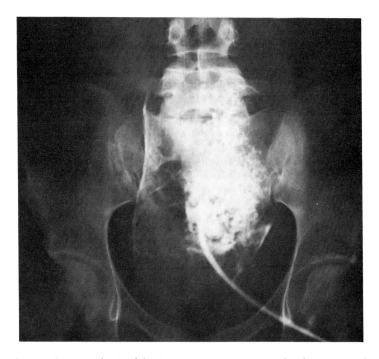

Figure 22–7. An amniogram obtained by intrauterine injection of radio-opaque dye revealing the classic radiologic "honeycomb" appearance of a molar pregnancy.

Prophylactic Chemotherapy

We have elected not to recommend prophylactic chemotherapy except in selected patients, since toxicity may be severe and malignant sequelae may not be prevented.[2,14,16,24] Of the patients with primary mole, 80 percent or more will achieve spontaneous remission following evacuation of the uterus and not need to be exposed to such toxic agents. Several reports have proven that methotrexate does not provide any significant prophylactic benefit. Goldstein and others have reported that actinomycin-D is quite effective when given as prophylaxis against the malignant sequelae of molar pregnancy.[25] If prophylactic chemotherapy is used, we feel it should be restricted to actinomycin-D treatment of patients who are at great risk for malignant sequelae (patients with both large-for-dates uterus and bilateral ovarian enlargement, or patients in whom follow-up is anticipated to be poor). This remains a debatable point. We now know of several patients who have died of toxicity from prophylactic Methotrexate administered in less than ideal settings.

HCG Testing and Follow-up of Molar Pregnancy

Human chorionic gonadotrophin (HCG) can be detected in serum and/or urine in essentially all patients with hydatidiform mole or with malignant trophoblastic disease if a sensitive assay technique is utilized. Despite this knowledge, some physicians continue follow-up of patients who have had molar pregnancy by utilizing only routine pregnancy tests. Pregnancy tests, biologic or immunologic, require urinary HCG concentrations of more than 500 to 1000 IU/liter of urine to give a positive result. Aproximately 25 percent of patients with malignant trophoblastic disease have been found to have urinary HCG concentrations that are elevated, but less than this 500 to 1000 IU/liter level and thus would be missed by pregnancy tests only. Therefore, pregnancy tests are of use only when positive but are of no value in assessing accurately the course of the disease when negative. In this setting a sensitive bioassay or radioimmunoassay for HCG must be utilized.

Recommendations for follow-up after evacuation of molar pregnancy are as follows:

1. Serial radioimmunoassay or bioassay HCG determinations at one-to-two-week intervals after evacuation of mole until negative 2×. This indicates spontaneous remission. Repeat in one month, then bimonthly for one year. Good contraception is necessary for one year. Oral contraceptives are desirable if there are no other contraindications.
2. Regular physical and pelvic exams at two-week intervals until spontaneous remission indicated, then every three months, thereafter.
3. Chest x-ray at two-to-four-week intervals until spontaneous remission, then every six months for one year.
4. If the HCG titer rises or plateaus during follow-up, prompt institution of chemotherapy is indicated.
5. If metastases are detected at any time, chemotherapy is indicated.

This includes patients who have had evacuation of molar pregnancy by hysterectomy. Recommendations are for:

(1) Regular physical and pelvic examinations at one-to-two-week intervals for continuing evaluation of the status of ovarian regression and to allow prompt detection of vaginal metastatic lesions
(2) Serum radioimmunoassay or bioassay for HCG at one-to-two-week intervals
(3) Chest x-rays at two-to-four-weeks intervals for the early detection of disseminated disease.

Such follow-up is continued until the decision is made to institute therapy for malignancy or until spontaneous remission has been documented.

Most studies of patients who have had primary moles show that 80 to 90 percent of patients will spontaneously achieve negative, sensitive HCG assays after evacuation of mole and resume cyclic menses, and will not have subsequent malignant disease.[14] The rate and constancy of decline of HCG is important. If metastases are detected, or if the HCG titer rises or becomes plateaued, these are signals for the institution of chemotherapy (Fig. 22–8). In prior publications we have recommended that therapy be instituted if the HCG titer is elevated beyond 60 days after termination of the molar pregnancy, however, current data suggest that the rate of decline of HCG, as measured by radioimmunoassay, may be prolonged. It is now recommended that if, on se-

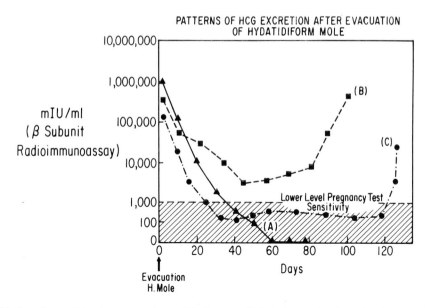

Figure 22–8. A graphic demonstration of follow-up HCG determinations in three patients who underwent evacuation of a hydatidiform mole. Only patient A proceded to spontaneous remission. The HCG level of patient C rapidly fell below the level detectable by the usual pregnancy test sensitivity, plateaued, and then rose rapidly after 120 days. This again demonstrates the importance of the HCG-specific assay (beta subunit), in following the patient who has had a gestational trophoblastic neoplasm.

quential assays, the HCG titer is steadily falling, the patient should be followed and treatment withheld. Therapy would be instituted only in the event of a rising HCG titer or a truly plateaued titer.

If serum HCG declines to nondetectable levels (less than 5 mIU/ml beta subunit radioimmunoassay, in our laboratory) on two successive assays and if the patient is doing well clinically, she is considered to be in "spontaneous remission." The patient who has achieved remission spontaneously should be followed with HCG assays and clinical surveys at 2–3 month intervals for the next year. Good contraception should be utilized for at least one year after molar pregnancy, as the HCG of recurrent trophoblastic malignancy cannot be distinguished from the HCG of intercur-

rent pregnancy. A history of hydatidiform mole places no restriction on the type of birth control used. Oral contraceptive drugs are desirable if there are no contraindications. After one year of negative follow-up, patients may undertake another pregnancy under close supervision. In our experience, successful pregnancy is the usual result, and pregnancy complications are no different than those seen in the general population. It has been estimated that there is a 1 to 3 percent chance of a patient who has had a primary mole having a subsequent pregnancy that is molar.[14] In our series, it would appear that less than one percent of patients who are diagnosed as having achieved spontaneous remission after hydatidiform mole will ever have further problems from trophoblastic malignancy.[14]

EVOLUTION AND STATUS OF CHEMOTHERAPY

In general, both surgery and irradiation for malignant trophoblastic disease have provided less than optimal results. Patients with invasive mole have a significant morbidity from uterine perforation, sepsis, hemorrhage, and occasionally, metastases. Greene reported a mortality of 15

percent in such patients who were treated with surgery alone.[26] The surgical treatment of patients with choriocarcinoma is even less rewarding as a primary therapeutic modality. Brewer and co-workers reported that in patients who already had metastatic choriocarcinoma, surgical therapy was associated with cure in less than 2 percent.[15] The extirpation of metastases was likewise of little assistance. In patients who were thought to have localized uterine disease, hysterectomy yielded only a 41 percent cure rate. Thus, surgical therapy alone is rarely the treatment of choice. Combined surgery with chemotherapy will be discussed in the following paragraph.

Surgical intervention may be indicated in the management of the sequelae of malignant trophoblastic disease. The common indications for supportive surgery are control of hemorrhage, relief of urinary or bowel obstruction, and drainage of abcess.[27] Due to the vascular penetration and hemorrhage often manifested with both local and metastatic trophoblastic disease, it is not surprising that operative therapy for hemostasis may be manditory and life saving. Such surgical procedures rarely cure the patient, but they may keep her alive for the opportunity of curative chemotherapy.

In 1948, Hertz presented data demonstrating that fetal tissues required large amounts of folic acid and that estrogen-induced growth of the genital tract in immature female animals could be inhibited by an antifolate compound. Table 22-5 gives the chronology of the evolution of chemotherapy over the ensuing 25 years. In 1956, Li et al first reported remission in a patient with metastatic choriocarcinoma treated with methotrexate.[3] Many reports have documented successful response of these tumors to a variety of systemically administered chemotherapeutic agents including methotrexate, actinomycin-D, vincaleukoblastin, and 6-Mercaptopurine.[1,2,4,5,16,24,28-30] In addition, there are data that suggest that combination chemotherapy[24] as well as arterial infused chemotherapy[31] may be of significant assistance in the treatment of such patients who are resistant to traditional single-agent chemotherapy.

Acceptable current methods for administering single-agent chemotherapy are listed in Table 22-6[1,4] and for combination chemotherapy[1,2,16,24] in Table 22-7. In general, repetitive courses of the same chemotherapeutic agent (or combination) are administered at intervals, which are frequent enough to continue the oncologic effect of the agent, but infrequent enough to allow resolution of induced toxicity prior to the initiation of the next course of treatment. If therapy is too infrequent, resistent disease will result. If treatment is too frequent, then irreversible toxicity may accrue. Care must be exercised in monitoring

Table 22–5. GESTATIONAL TROPHO-BLASTIC NEOPLASIA—EVOLUTION OF CHEMOTHERAPY

1948	Hertz demonstrated the high folic acid requirements of fetal tissues, and that an antifolic compound, methotrexate (MTX), inhibited estrogen-induced growth of the genital tract in immature animals.
1952	Thiersch: fetal death could be induced by MTX.
1953	Anderson, Bisgard, Greene demonstrated partial beneficial effect of nitrogen mustard on patient with metastatic choriocarcinoma.
1954	Li reported rapid decline of HCG levels in patient treated with MTX for metastatic melanoma.
1956	Li, Hertz, and Spencer treated patient with metastatic choriocarcinoma with MTX, resulting in first reported sustained and complete remission.
1956–66	National Institutes of Health project: multiple reports of effective management and treatment of gestational trophoblastic disease by Hertz, Li, Ross, Lipsett, Odell, Lewis, Goldstein, Hammond, and others.
1966–76	Further refinement in disease identification, categorization, treatment selection and follow-up management, arterial infusion, combination chemotherapy, and the use of surgery and chemotherapy together.

daily the hematologic and hepatic parameters to avoid irreversible toxicity. Therapy is continued with repetitive courses of the same agent, monitoring the progress of the patient by weekly HCG determinations. If the HCG titer fails to decline through two courses of therapy, if it rises significantly with one course of therapy, or if new metastases appear, therapy is altered. Therapy is continued until all HCG has been erradicated. The patient is usually given one full course of chemotherapy after the first normal HCG titer has been returned. Remission is diagnosed when three consecutive weekly HCG titers have been obtained. At that point the patient is moved into the "follow-up" category.

The likelihood of recovery from malignant trophoblastic disease is greatest for the patients treated by physicians who are knowledgeable with the intricacies of the disease process, the

Table 22–6. SINGLE-AGENT CHEMOTHERAPY

1. Actinomycin-D 10-13 mcg/kg IV QD, or Methotrexate 0.2 to 0.4 mg/kg IM QD
   A. Either given in 5-day course
   B. Between course interval 7–10 days, depending on toxicity
   C. Oral contraceptives given for pituitary suppression if not contraindicated

2. Drug is continued with repetitive courses until
   A. Titer is normal (pituitary range) or negative (β-assay)
   B. Switch to alternate drug if
      1. Titer rises (10-fold or more)
      2. Titer plateaus at elevated level after 2 courses of therapy
      3. Evidence of new metastasis appears

3. Safety factors in drug administration—do not begin, continue, or resume a dose of medication (QD during treatment, qid between treatment) if
   WBC < 3,000/cu mm
   Polys < 1,500/cu mm
   Platelets < 100,000/cu mm
   Bun, SGOT, SGPT significantly elevated

4. Remission defined as 3 consecutive normal weekly HCG titers (pituitary range) or negative (β-assay)

5. Follow-up program
   A. HCG titer every 2 weeks 6×; every 4 weeks 4×; then every 2 mo 3×; every 6 mo indefinitely
   B. General P. E., C. x-ray, blood counts every 3 mo for 1 year; then every 6 mo
   C. No pregnancy for 1 year

Table 22–7. COMBINATION CHEMOTHERAPY

1. Methotrexate 10–15 mg IM daily, plus Actinomycin-D 10 mcg/kg IV daily, plus Chlorambucil 8–10 mg PO daily
   A. Given in 5-day courses
   B. Between course interval 12–15 days depending on toxicity
   C. Oral contraception given for pituitary suppression if not contraindicated

2. Drug is continued with repetitive courses as outlined in Table 22-6 (titer rise, plateaus ×2 courses, or increasing metastatic disease evident). Alternate drug choices as follows:
   A. Every 12–15 days: Actinomycin-D 10–12 mcg/kg, IV, daily 5×, plus Velban 2–3 mg IV, BID for 6 doses

   OR

   B. Every 7–10 days: Methotrexate 20 mg (0.2–0.4 mg/kg), IM, daily 5×, plus 6-Mercaptopurine 250 mg PO, daily 5×

   OR

   C. High-dose double agent every 7–10 days: Methotrexate 25 mg (0.2–0.4 mg/kg), IM, QD 5×, plus Actinomycin-D 10–13 mcg/kg, IV, QD, 5×

3. Safety factors in drug administration—do not begin, continue, or resume a dose of medication if
   WBC< 4,000/cmm
   Polys< 1,500/cmm
   Platelets< 150,000/cmm
   BUN, SGOT, SGPT significantly abnormal

4. Remission and follow-up (see Table 22-6)

techniques of chemotherapy, and the management of side effects and toxicity. Adequate HCG testing is mandatory. Excellence in consultative and supportive services are necessary. Several studies have documented the need for precise selection of multiple-agent chemotherapy, surgery, and irradiation therapy. For these reasons, it appears that the opportunity for the patient to recover from malignant trophoblastic disease may be enhanced by treatment in centers that specialize in these forms of therapy.

MALIGNANT TROPHOBLASTIC DISEASE

Diagnosis

Hydatidiform mole precedes malignant trophoblastic disease in approximately 50 percent of patients, and in the remainder there is an antecedent term pregnancy, abortion, or ectopic pregnancy. The usual sign of patients with localized uterine disease is the persistence of irregular bleeding, which follows a lawless pattern, that is not responsive to hormonal therapy, and requires dilatation and curettage. In this manner, histopathologic materials are obtained that may support the suspicion of malignant trophoblastic disease. However, one must remember that a significant percentage of patients with metastatic disease may have no tumor in the uterus. In addition, patients with malignant trophoblastic disease may have that disease deep in myometrium, well beyond the reach of the curette. The index of suspicion is usually greater if such problems occur in proximity to the termination of some type of pregnancy, particularly if it is molar. It is well known, however, that malignant trophoblastic disease may not become manifest by symptoms for a long interval, perhaps years, after the last antecedent pregnancy.[7]

Patients may present with the sequelae of distant metastatic disease. In any woman of reproductive age, unexplained metastases should be considered potentially due to trophoblastic malignancy before the patient is consigned to mere palliative therapy. In patients who have unexplained gastrointestinal or urinary bleeding, pulmonary symptoms, x-ray findings suggesting metastases, and a central nervous system tumor that appears of secondary nature, one should suspect trophoblastic disease and utilize HCG assays for confirmation. If HCG is elevated and there is doubt as to the presence of an intercurrent pregnancy, dilatation and curettage should be performed in this life-threatening situation. Likewise, patients who undergo exploratory surgery with removal of a metastatic lesion should be considered as possibly having this disease, if the pathology does not precisely relate to another known malignant entity. Thus, the unwary pathologist who diagnoses "anaplastic carcinoma" may not be familiar with the histologic patterns of trophoblastic malignancy and make an erroneous diagnosis. HCG testing in suspicious patients can be of significant aid. In this setting, if there is doubt as to the presence of an intercurrent pregnancy, then dilatation and curettage should be considered.[7]

Clinical Staging Studies

Once the diagnosis of malignant trophoblastic disease has been made, it is necessary to categorize the patient's state of illness with clinical studies (Table 22–8). These studies include a thorough general history and physical examination, with pelvic examination and listed tests necessary to detect occult metastatic disease (Fig. 22–9 and 22–10). In addition, arteriographic

Table 22–8.   GESTATIONAL TROPHO-BLASTIC NEOPLASMS

PRIMARY STAGING STUDIES

General history and physical exam with review pathology
Chest x-ray
Isotopic liver and brain scans
EEG
Ultrasound of pelvis
Hepatic and renal function tests, hematology
Thyroid function tests
Initial quantitative gonadotrophin assay (urine)

OTHER STAGING CONSIDERATIONS

Desire for further reproduction
D&C: selected cases
Lumbar puncture for CSF HCG if metastases and no increased CSF pressure
Arteriography: important in selected cases only

studies may be indicated (Fig. 22–11), as may other tests suggested by the patient's symptomatology. It is important to delineate sites of metastases as well as the general status of the patient. Particular reference is made to hepatic and renal function, which are critical in drug toxicity. The patient is categorized as having either nonmetastatic or metastatic trophoblastic disease, sites of metastases or abnormal function are noted and identified, and desires referable to further childbearing are noted. Table 22–9 identifies our present categorization of patients with malignant trophoblastic disease.

Nonmetastatic Trophoblastic Disease

Nonmetastatic trophoblastic disease is defined as disease confined to the uterus without evidence of metastatic lesions. Usually the diagnosis is made during follow-up of a patient after molar pregnancy. In approximately 25 percent of patients, however, the diagnosis is made following other types of pregnancy.[5,6] In either situation, abnormal trophoblastic tissue may be discovered on curettage and when HCG levels are elevated. Initial staging studies, as outlined previously are carried out and the patient's desire for further reproduction ascertained. The possible methods of therapy that can be utilized in patients with nonmetastatic malignant trophoblastic disease are as follows:

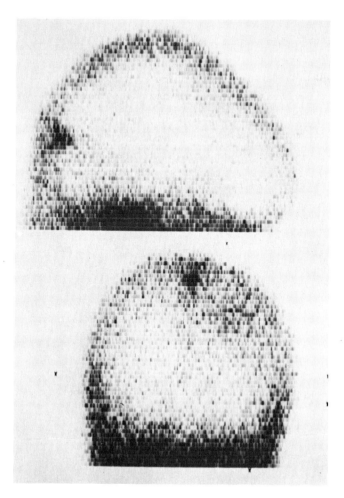

Figure 22–9. A positive brain scan (area of increased uptake) in patient with poor prognosis metastatic gestational trophoblastic disease. (Courtesy of Department of Nuclear Medicine, Duke University Medical Center)

1. Single agent chemotherapy
2. Combination hysterectomy-chemotherapy. Do hysterectomy during first course of chemotherapy (third day), provided patient does not desire further reproduction and that disease is known to exist in the uterus.
3. Arterial infusion chemotherapy: selected cases

If single-agent chemotherapy is elected then it should be administered as outlined in Table 22–6. Therapy must be continued with repetitive courses until HCG excretion is negative. An additional chemotherapy course is given after the first normal titer (weekly determination).

If the patient with nonmetastatic gestational trophoblastic disease does not desire further reproduction, we have suggested that the uterus be removed by abdominal hysterectomy on the third day of the first five-day course of single-drug chemotherapy. It is rarely necessary to remove the ovaries, as metastases to the ovary are rare. The dosages of the drug are identical to those used in patients not being operated upon. Safety parameters noted must be observed. There has been no increase in postsurgical morbidity in patients receiving chemotherapy. Repetitive courses of chemotherapy should be continued in the postoperative period if the HCG titer remains elevated, the same as would have been used had not surgery been performed.

A small percentage of patients with nonmetastatic trophoblastic disease fail to achieve complete remission with systemic chemotherapy. Hysterectomy may well be contraindicated in a young woman of low parity. Pelvic arteriography (Fig. 22–11) can demonstrate trophoblastic disease deep in the myometrium. In such patients, one can consider arterially infused chemotherapy in an attempt to preserve the uterus.[16,27] Intra-

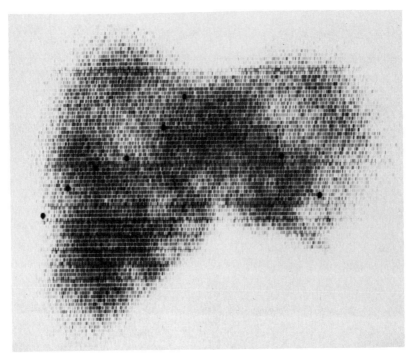

Figure 22–10. Poor prognosis metastatic gestational trophoblastic disease manifest by liver metastases (areas of increased uptake). (Courtesy of Department of Nuclear Medicine, Duke University Medical Center)

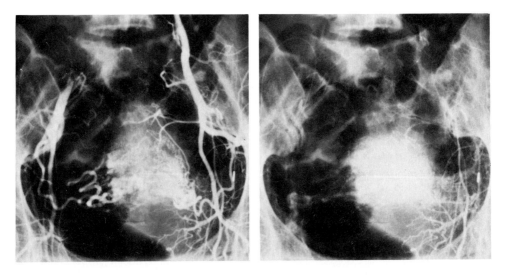

Figure 22–11. Bilateral hypogastric arteriograms. Note enlarged uterine arteries and A-V fistulae in uterus.

Table 22–9. CATEGORIZATION OF GESTATIONAL TROPHOBLASTIC NEOPLASIA

I. *NONMETASTATIC DISEASE: NO EVIDENCE OF SPREAD OUTSIDE OF UTERUS*

II. *METASTATIC DISEASE: ANY SPREAD BEYOND UTERUS*
 A. Good prognosis metastatic disease
  1. Short duration (<4 months)
  2. Low pretreatment HCG titer (<100,000 IU/24 hr)
  3. Metastatis, but *not to brain or liver*
  4. No significant prior chemotherapy
 B. Poor prognosis metastatic disease
  1. Long duration (> 4 months)
  2. High HCG titer (>100,000 IU/24 hr)
  3. Brain or liver metastasis
  4. Significant prior chemotherapy

arterial chemotherapy vs hysterectomy is usually a matter of clinical judgement.

Results of Treatment in Nonmetastatic Disease

Essentially all patients with nonmetastatic malignant trophoblastic disease, of gestational origin, can be cured. Table 22-10 demonstrates our re-sults in a group of 112 patients with nonmetastatic trophoblastic disease. In this and other reports with similar good results, more than 90 percent of the patients were able to preserve reproductive function. There were no toxic deaths, nor were there recurrences after treatment.

The role of combining surgery with chemotherapy in the treatment of these patients is being evaluated. From preliminary studies of these patients, it can be stated that hysterectomy in combination with chemotherapy and followed by further chemotherapy after surgery is curative in patients with trophoblastic disease confined to the uterus. It also appears that combined therapy shortens the duration of treatment in the amount of chemotherapy received and the toxicity that ensues. Further studies will aid in clarification of this approach.

The responsiveness of nonmetastatic trophoblastic disease to the several therapeutic modalities noted would suggest that combination chemotherapy, with its attendant severe morbidity and mortality, is rarely indicated. The hazard of combining surgery with single-agent chemotherapy or even arterially infused chemotherapy is a more acceptable risk in the patients without metastases.

As previously mentioned, the greatest likelihood of cure of nonmetastatic disease is achieved with vigorous therapy under close supervision to

Table 22–10. GESTATIONAL TROPHOBLASTIC NEOPLASIA—NONMETASTATIC DISEASE (DUKE THERAPY 1966–1975)

TYPE OF THERAPY	PRIMARY THERAPY	PRIMARY RX CURE	SECONDARY THERAPY	SECONDARY RX CURE
Single-agent MTX/Act-D	91	84	X	X
Pelvic arterial infusion	1	0	2	2
Elective initial hysterectomy*	15	15	X	X
Indicated initial hysterectomy*	5	5	X	X
Delayed hyster-ectomy* (resistance)	X	X	6	6
Totals	112	104	8	8

*Whenever hysterectomy done, patients continued to receive single-agent chemotherapy (MTX/Act-D) after surgery until no HCG detected; 112/112 (100%) patients were cured; 86/97 (89%) patients who desired to preserve uterus did so.

avoid irreversible toxicity. Chemotherapy should neither be undertaken lightly nor started in a setting in which constant vigilance cannot be maintained.

Metastatic Trophoblastic Disease

In 1956, Li et al reported complete remission in a patient with metastatic trophoblastic disease (choriocarcinoma) treated with methotrexate.[3] This was followed by a 10-year study at the National Cancer Institute by Hertz and his co-workers. This group published a series of reports demonstrating the efficacy of chemotherapy in the treatment of metastatic trophoblastic disease.[1,4-7] They first reported on complete remission of 47 percent of patients treated with methotrexate alone,[1] and later in 74 percent of patients treated with actinomycin-D or methotrexate, sequentially.[4] In addition to proving the efficacy of systemic chemotherapy, these investigators demonstrated that successful results of treatment were influenced significantly by the duration of the disease (prior to institution of therapy), the level of the pretreatment HCG titer, the presence of cerebral or hepatic metastases, and the prior unsuccessful exposure to the chemotherapeutic drugs. When the disease was diagnosed early and treated vigorously, remission rates in excess of 90 percent could be expected. Patients who had extensive disease, treated late in the course of their illness only had a 20 to 30 percent chance of recovery.

Patients with metastatic disease are categorized as follows into good and poor prognostic groups:

I. Metastatic (good prognosis)
    Single-agent MTX or act-D therapy
    Delayed hysterectomy if residual disease
    Combination chemotherapy
    Arterial infusion
II. Metastatic (poor prognosis)
    Combination chemotherapy (MAC) plus
    Whole brain/liver irradiation to 2000 rads
    Delayed hysterectomy if residual disease
    Arterial infusion
    Single-agent chemotherapy

Therapy is based on this initial categorization as well as the previously mentioned factors governing selection of techniques. Table 22-11 outlines our method of therapy in patients with metastatic trophoblastic disease. Patients who have *good*

Table 22-11.   METASTATIC TROPHO-BLASTIC DISEASE— SELECTION OF THERAPY

A. *GOOD PROGNOSIS: SAME AS NONMETA-STATIC*

B. *POOR PROGNOSIS*
    1. High dose combination chemotherapy, MTX, Act-D, Chlorambucil
    2. Irradiation: 2,000–3,000 rads whole brain, liver, or both if metastatic disease present. Given simultaneously with chemotherapy (10–14 days). Also may be used for selected resistant lesions in pelvis and lung when other methods fail (ie, surgery, chemotherapy).
    3. Arterial infusion chemotherapy
    4. Surgery: used as "debulking" procedure in select cases, i.e., resection of isolated accessable resistant metastasis in pelvis, lung, brain.
    5. Other chemotherapeutic agents–Velban, etc.
    6. Alternating single-, multiple-drug regimen.

prognosis metastatic disease are treated initially with single-agent chemotherapy in a manner similar to patients with nonmetastatic disease (see Table 22-6). However, if any one of the poor prognosis findings is present, the patient is initially treated with combination chemotherapy (methotrexate, actinomycin-D, and chlorambucil) (see Table 22-7).

Table 22-12 illustrates the results from our Center utilizing the methodologies of therapy outlined for *good prognosis* metastatic trophoblastic disease. These data demonstrate that of 51 patients with good prognosis metastatic disease, all can be cured; 49 of the patients desired to preserve reproductive ability and 41 of them were able to do so with single-agent, systemic chemotherapy. Two patients had required initial hysterectomy for local uterine problems. Of the 8 patients who were not cured with the primary chemotherapy, 3 were cured by pelvic arterial infusion of drugs, and 5 by delayed hysterectomy for localized uterine disease resistant to systemic treatment. Thus 86 percent of the patients who desired to preserve their uterus for further reproduction were able to do so, and all of the 51 patients were cured with these various therapeutic modalities.

There may be an indication for primary hysterectomy in the treatment of patients with malignant trophoblastic disease in the uterine wall,

Table 22–12. GESTATIONAL TROPHOBLASTIC NEOPLASIA—
GOOD PROGNOSIS, METASTATIC
(DUKE THERAPY 1966–1975)

TYPE OF THERAPY	PRIMARY THERAPY	PRIMARY RX CURE	SECONDARY THERAPY	SECONDARY RX CURE
Single-agent MTX/Act-D	49	41	X	X
Pelvic arterial infusion	X	X	3	3
Indicated 1 degree hysterectomy*	2	2	X	X
Delayed hysterectomy* (resistance)	X	X	5	5
Totals	51	43	8	8

*Whenever hysterectomy done, patients continued to receive single-agent chemotherapy (MTX/Act-D) after surgery until no HCG detected; 51/51 (100%) patients cured; 44/51 (86%) patients who desired to preserve uterus did so.

even when distant metastases are present.[2,16,23,31] A number of investigators are studying the role of hysterectomy in reducing the duration and amount of treatment required. Malignant tissue should be demonstrated in the uterus by curettage, biopsy, or arteriographic visualization. On occasion, arterial infused chemotherapy may be curative for local uterine disease refractory to systemic treatment, even after erradication of peripheral metastases.[31] All of these factors must be considered for the individual patients.

Patients with poor prognosis metastatic disease (Table 22-9) are at major risk for death as well as resistance to standard single-agent chemotherapeutic techniques. Table 22-13 presents data from our Center in treatment of patients with poor prognosis metastatic disease. From 1966 until 1968, patients were treated initially with single-agent chemotherapy and only switched to combination chemotherapy if they failed to achieve remission. With this approach only one of seven patients (14 percent) was cured of her disease. In 1968, we reversed this form of therapy and began to treat initially with combination chemotherapy (methotrexate, actinomycin-D, chlorambucil) (see Table 22-7), and now have a 78 percent complete remission rate.

Patients with demonstrable liver or brain metastases are at risk from hemorrhage from these lesions and the therapy plan is altered to include immediate institution of whole brain or whole liver irradiation in the range of 2000 to 3000 rads simultaneously with combination chemother-

apy.[2,4,16,24] While radiotherapy will not likely cure the patient, bleeding may be avoided and the patient sustained until chemotherapeutic remission can be achieved.[2,4,16,24]

In all patients with malignant trophoblastic disease receiving chemotherapy, treatment must be continued with repetitive courses and the patient's progress monitored by weekly gonadotrophin assays. If a patient fails to show a decline in gonadotrophin secretion through two courses of chemotherapy or fails to achieve a normal HCG titer after four or five courses of one drug, then an alternate method of therapy is used. If toxicity is too severe, then a lesser intensive therapeutic regimen should be considered. Therapy is continued until HCG is erradicated. Usually an additional course of treatment is administered

Table 22–13. GESTATIONAL TROPHO-
BLASTIC NEOPLASIA—
POOR PROGNOSIS, METASTATIC
(DUKE THERAPY 1966–1975)

	NO. OF PTS.	CURE		DIED		
		No.	%	Toxicity	Disease	Total
1966–68*	7	1	14	3	3	6
1968–75†	40	31	78	3	6	9

*Initially treated with single agent MTX/Act-D, and secondarily treated with combination chemotherapy.
†Intially treated with combination chemotherapy.

after the first normal HCG titer, in an attempt to reduce recurrence.

Diagnosis of Remission and Follow-up After Treatment

Treatment of malignant trophoblastic disease must be continued until HCG titers have returned to nondetectable levels on a sensitive assay system (radioimmunoassay or bioassay). All patients treated should be supported with good contraception throughout treatment. The diagnosis of remission is not made until three consecutive, weekly, normal HCG titers have been achieved. We currently have a 3 to 4 percent recurrence rate, while Hertz et al, from the National Cancer Institute, noted an 8 percent recurrence rate after treatment and the diagnosis of remission by these criteria.[1,4] Recurrence, when it occurs, is usually in the first several months after termination of therapy but has been seen as late as three years. Thus, cancer follow-up after treatment is mandatory.

In our Center, we have recommended that HCG titers be performed at two-week intervals during the first three months after termination of therapy, at one-month intervals for the next three months, and at bimonthly intervals for the balance of one year. At that point assays are recommended at six-month intervals, indefinitely. Routine physical examination, chest x-ray, and hematopoietic indices should be surveyed for at least three-month intervals during the first year of observation and semiannually thereafter. An elevation of HCG during this follow-up interval must be investigated closely and managed in a fashion similar to that outlined for the patient with nonmetastatic disease.

After one year of negative follow-up we have allowed patients who have retained reproductive capability to attempt pregnancy if they desire. The best estimates of a second molar pregnancy occurring in the same individual is 1 in 500 pregnancies. In over 100 successful pregnancies in the Duke Center and a similar number accrued by Ross and co-workers from the National Cancer Institute, there does not seem to be other complications in pregnancies occurring after chemotherapeutic treatment for malignant trophoblastic neoplasia. Likewise, there has been no increase in congenital anomaly rates among the infants of these pregnancies. HCG should be measured at three to four weeks after the termination of any type of pregnancy in this setting.

This investigation was supported by Grant Number 1 R18 CA19272-01, awarded by the National Cancer Institute, DHEW.

References

1. Hertz R, Lewis J, Jr, Lipsett MB: Five year's experience with chemotherapy of metastatic choriocarcinoma and related trophoblastic tumors in women. Amer J Obstet Gynec 82:631, 1961
2. Hammond CB, Parker RT: Diagnosis and treatment of trophoblastic disease Obstet Gynec 35:132, 1970
3. Li MC, Hertz R, Spencer DB: Effects of Methotrexate therapy upon choriocarcinoma and chorioadenoma Proc Soc Exp Biol Med 93:361, 1956
4. Ross GT, Goldstein DP, Hertz R, Lipsett MB, Odell WD: Sequential use of Methotrexate and actinomycin-D in treatment of metastatic chorio-carcinoma and related trophoblastic diseases in women. Amer J Obstet Gynec 93:223, 1965
5. Ross GT, Hammond CB, Hertz R, Lipsett MB, Odell WD: Chemotherapy of metastatic and nonmetastatic gestational trophoblastic neoplasms. Texas Rep Biol Med 24:326, 1966
6. Hammond CB, Hertz R, Ross GT, Lipsett MB, Odell WD: Primary chemotherapy for nonmetastatic gestational trophoblastic neoplasms. Amer J Obstet Gynec 98:71, 1967
7. Hammond CB, Hertz R, Ross GT, Lipsett MB, Odell WD: Diagnostic problems of choriocarcinoma and related trophoblastic neoplasms, Obstet Gynec 29:224, 1967
8. Bagshawe LD: Choriocarcinoma: The Clinical Biology of the Trophoblast and its Tumours. Baltimore, Williams and Wilkins, 1969

9. Park WW: Choriocarcinoma: A Study of its Pathology. Philadelphia, Davis, 1971

10. Hertig AT: Human Trophoblast. Springfield, Ill, Charles C Thomas, 1968

11. Ober WB, Fass RO: The Early History of Choriocarcinoma. J Hist Med Allied Sci vol. 16. no. 1, 1961

12. Hertig AT, Mansell H: "Tumors of the Female Sex Organs: I. Hydatidiform Mole and Choriocarcinoma." In: Atlas of Tumor Pathology. Washington, DC, Armed Forces Institute of Pathology, 1956

13. Hertig AT, Sheldon WH: Hydatidiform mole—a pathological-clinical correlation of 200 cases. Amer J Obstet Gynec 53:1, 1947

14. Curry SL, Hammond CB, Tyrey L, Creasman WT, Parker RT: Hydatidiform mole, diagnosis, management, and long-term follow-up of 347 patients. Obstet Gynec 45:1, 1975

15. Brewer JI, Rinehart JJ, Dunbar R: Choriocarcinoma. Amer J Obstet Gynec 81:574, 1961

16. Hammond CB, Lewis JL, Jr: Gestational Trophoblastic Neoplasms. In Davis' Gynecology and Obstetrics, vol 1. Schirra J (ed). Harper and Row, Hagerstown, Md., 1977

17. Hon EH: A Manual of Pregnancy Testing. Boston, Little, Brown, 1961

18. Odell WD, Hertz R, Lipsett MB, Ross BT, Hammond CB: Endocrine aspects of trophoblastic neoplasms. Clin Obstet Gynec 10: 290, 1967

19. Vaitukaitis JL, Braunstein GD, Ross GT: A radioimmunoassay which specifically measures human chorionic gonadotrophin in the presence of human luteinizing hormone. Am J Obstet Gynec 113:751, 1972

20. Bagshawe KD: Choriocarcinoma: The Clinical Biology of the Trophoblast and its Tumours. London, Edward Arnold Ltd, 1969, p 34

21. Bagshawe KD: Choriocarcinoma: The Clinical Biology of the Trophoblast and its Tumours. London, Edward Arnold Ltd, 1969, p 35

22. Goldstein DP, Reid D: Recent developments in management of molar pregnancy. Clin Obstet Gynec 10:313, 1967

23. Delfs E: Quantitative chorionic gonadotropin: Prognostic value in hydatidiform mold and chorioepithelioma. Obstet Gynec 9:1, 1957

24. Hammond CB, Borchert LG, Tyrey L, Creasman WT, Parker RT: Treatment of metastatic trophoblastic disease: Good and poor prognosis. Amer J Obstet Gynec 115: 4, 1973

25. Goldstein DP: Five year's experience with the prevention of trophoblastic tumors by the prophylactic use of chemotherapy in patients with molar pregnancy. Clin Obstet Gynec 13:945, 1970

26. Greene RR: Chorioadenoma destruens. Ann NY Acad Sci 80:143, 1959

27. Lewis J, Jr, Gore H, Hertig AT, Goss DA: Treatment of trophoblastic neoplasms: With rationale for the use of adjunctive chemotherapy at the time of indicated operation. Amer J Obstet Gynec 96:710, 1966

28. Brewer JI, Gerbie AB, Dolkart RE, et al: Chemotherapy in trophoblastic disease. Amer J Obstet Gynec 90:566, 1964

29. Holland JF, Hreshchyshyn MM, Glidewell O: Controlled clinical trials of methotrexate in treatment and prophylaxis of trophoblastic neoplasia. In Abstracts, 10th International Cancer Congress, May 1970, Houston, Medical Arts Publishers, 1970, p 461

30. Lewis J, Jr: Chemotherapy for metastatic gestational trophoblastic neoplasms. Clin Obstet Gynec 10:330, 1967

31. Maroulis GB, Hammond CB, Johnsrude IS, Weed JC, Jr, Parker RT: Arteriography and infusional chemotherapy in localized trophoblastic disease. Obstet Gynec 45: 397, 1975

Chapter 23

Cancer in Pregnancy

LARRY McGOWAN, M.D.

All types of cancer may be associated with pregnancy. Few other medical conditions demand a closer multidiscipline approach in diagnosis and treatment as cancer in a pregnant woman. The obstetrician in his capacity as a primary physician for women is in a unique position to diagnose cancer. The pregnant woman may be making her initial visit to a physician or the first since the birth of her last child for a complete physical examination.

The total number of cancer patients associated with pregnancy seems to be decreasing, probably because the national birth rate is 14/1000 people and is the lowest ever observed in the United States. The small number of many types of cancer associated with the pregnant woman has necessitated reports of few patients extending over many years. As many cancers generally occur in older age groups, their relationship with pregnancy is rare. Diagnostic and treatment methods for the pregnant woman with cancer must take into consideration not only the cancer but the developing intrauterine embryo or fetus.

GENERAL CONSIDERATIONS

The primary purpose of therapy is to cure the patient of cancer. Treatment is directed at destroying the cancer if it is considered curable, preserving the fetus if the cancer patient is terminal, and compromising with both situations when palliation is indicated and the fetus needs to become more mature before its delivery.

A new composite individual is started at the moment of fertilization. However, to survive, this individual needs a very specialized environment for nine months, then extended care for an indefinite period, but from the moment of fertilization a new hereditary composite is formed which, under appropriate conditions will grow into a recognizable personality.[62] Human life is an ongoing process, at least from implantation and most probably from fertilization.

Urine Pregnancy Tests

Within the last few years virtually all laboratories have replaced the old bioassay test for diagnosis of pregnancy with immunologic agglutination tests that detect human chorionic gonadotropin (HCG) in urine; these are more rapid, more reliable, and less expensive than the older methods. The tests offer a high degree of accuracy when the detailed directions are carefully followed and more than two weeks have passed since the missed menstrual period. Slide tests are generally less sensitive than tube tests and are more likely to give false-negative results, especially early in pregnancy. Negative or equivocal tests in suspected early pregnancy, whether done by slide or tube, should be repeated in a week. False-positive tests are rare; they are probably most common due to residues of detergent used to clean the glassware in which the urine was collected.[48]

Cancer Drugs in Pregnancy

The therapeutic value of a drug must be weighed against possible adverse effects on the fetus before or after birth. A lack of obvious adverse effects is not the endpoint as the possibility of unforeseen long-term consequences must be kept in mind. The potential benefit of drug therapy must outweigh the potential hazard, because to assure complete drug safety to all women a physician may have to deny most drug therapy to all women. There is probably no type of drug exposure that cannot be shown to present a potential hazard, however slight. The degree to which an embryo or fetus is adversely affected by drug therapy depends on the type administered, the dosage, and the duration given.

If a drug has a high lipid solubility and/or a molecular weight of less than 1000, it crosses the placenta easily. Most cytotoxic agents used in cancer chemotherapy and immunosuppression have teratogenic potential. Aminopterin given during the first trimester in 52 pregnancies was associated with 34 abortions in Nicholson's study, and malformations were noted in 10 of 12 fetuses that were examined. Methotrexate administered during the first trimester has been reported to have caused malformations of the skull, face, and extremities. Mercaptopurine (Purinethol), azathioprine (Imuran), and large doses of cyclophosphamide (Cytoxan) taken in the first trimester have been associated with a high incidence of abortions.[47]

Almost any drug present in the mother's blood will also be detectable in her milk. The concentration in milk depends on such factors as the concentration in maternal blood, the lipid solubility of the drug, and its degree of ionization. Anticancer drugs can cause bone marrow depression in nursing infants and should be considered a contraindication to breast feeding.

Irradiation During Pregnancy

Irradiation in utero can produce subtle defects that are detrimental to the fetus but are not readily apparent, such as failure to achieve optimal growth and development. Mammography, tumor scanning with gallium 67, and radioactive iodine, particularly iodine 131, should not be used during pregnancy. The latter substance very rapidly crosses the placenta and can destroy the thyroid gland of the fetus, resulting in cretinism. Although in the nonpregnant state, there is thought to be no exposure from mammography to the ovaries and uterus, with an enlarging gestation the usual 0.4 to 1 rads per exposure contradicts routine mammography in the pregnant woman. Sternberg stresses that when a radioisotope procedure is contemplated in a woman of childbearing age, the test should not be performed—as a rule—during the second half of the menstrual cycle, in order to avoid any possibility of an unsuspected early pregnancy. This is particularly important in cases of tests employing radioactive inert gases. For therapeutic applications in nonpregnant women of childbearing age, follow the application of radioactive substances with a course of ovulation-suppressing agents for at least three months. When the husband receives a large dose of radioactive isotope with a proved damage to the chromosomes (phosphorus 32), a six-month course of anticonceptional therapy is indicated.[65]

In Nagasaki, 30 pregnant women exposed to radiation at less than 2000 meters from the hypocenter of the atomic explosion had an average of 43.3 percent perinatal mortality, 68 pregnant women exposed at a distance of 2000 to 4000 meters had only 8.8 percent mortality, and the percentage diminished to 6.3 percent in 113 women exposed at more than 4000 meters from the hypocenter. The incidence of leukemia appears remarkably high after irradiation. In children under 10 years of age in Hiroshima and Nagasaki, the incidence of leukemia was 26 times higher than in a comparative group in a nonexposed area.[32,65] There is a probable teratogenic relationship with acute irradiation with doses higher than 50 rads, and applied to the embryo between the tenth and the fiftieth day of gestation in human subjects. Diagnostic irradiation with less than 25 rads of protracted irradiation seems to have an improbable teratogenic relationship. Individual cases should be separately evaluated and should not be judged on broad generalities.

BREAST

Carcinoma of the breast is the leading cause of death from cancer among women in the United States. The peak incidence is between the ages of 40 and 50, but breast cancer occurs frequently at all ages past 30. The annual incidence of breast carcinoma is about 72 per 100,000 women, and the age-adjusted death rate is about 23 per 100,000 women in this country. In 1978, there will be about 90,000 new cases and 33,800 deaths from breast cancer in American women. It is estimated that 1 out of every 15 American women will develop the disease at some time during her lifetime and that 20 percent of deaths from cancer among women are attributable to breast cancer. There has been no great reduction in the mortality rate of this disease in the past 35 years.[71,72]

One in 35 women with carcinoma of the breast will have pregnancy as a complication, but if the cancer is during the child-bearing years, the figure is 1 in 3; 1 patient in 19 of childbearing age will become pregnant after mastectomy for cancer. The average age of patients with cancer of the breast complicated with pregnancy is 30 to 36 years.[44]

There is evidence that a woman has as much as twice the risk of breast cancer (as compared to the general population) if her family history includes breast cancer in her mother, aunts, or sisters. Marital status and parity also influence the incidence of breast cancer. Single and nulliparous women have a slightly higher death rate from breast cancer than married and parous women. Women with three or more children have a lower risk than women with fewer children.[72]

Diagnosis

The high mortality rate of breast cancer can be most effectively reduced by early detection and adequate surgical treatment. The patient herself is able to discover the early lesions when they are palpable. Regular monthly self-examination of the breast after each menstrual period should be practiced by all women over age 30.

The increased growth of the breast during pregnancy may make the detection of a mass difficult. Failure to examine the breast, misinterpretation, or belittling of the physical findings resulted in delay of tissue diagnosis in approximately two-thirds of women with breast cancer in pregnan-

cy.[44] Routine breast examination should be performed early in pregnancy and postpartum by those providing obstetric care.

Mammography, xeroradiography, is effective in detecting early breast cancer and may be positive before the cancer is palpable. Mammography should not be used as a screening examination in young women except in those women who have a suspicious breast examination. Bone scans utilizing a bone-seeking nuclide, and skeletal x-rays should not be used during pregnancy in order to prevent radiation exposure to the fetus. A posterior and lateral chest roentgenogram with shielding of the abdomen should be obtained in preparation for breast biopsy or radical mastectomy.

The primary complaint in about 80 percent of women with breast cancer is a single nontender firm to hard mass with ill-defined margins, and in approximately 50 percent of cases is found in the upper outer quadrant of the breast. Less frequent and later symptoms are breast pain, erosion, retraction, enlargement, discharge, or itching of the nipples, and redness, generalized hardness, enlargement or shrinkage of the breast. Examination of the breast should be meticulous, methodical, and gentle.

The ultimate diagnosis of breast tumors depends upon examination of tissue removed by surgical biopsy. The safest course is to biopsy all suspicious masses found on physical examination and, in the absence of a mass, suspicious lesions demonstrated by mammography.[71,72]

Clinical Staging

Patients with breast cancer can be grouped into stages according to the characteristics of the primary tumor (T), regional lymph nodes (N), and distant metastases (M). Physical, radiologic, and other clinical examinations, usually including biopsy of the primary lesion, are used in determining the stage, which is based on all information available before therapy.[72]

Stage 1. The tumor is confined to the breast. There may be early signs of skin involvement such as dimpling or nipple retraction, but there are no signs of axillary or distant metastases.

Stage 2. The primary tumor is as in stage 1, but there are movable, suspicious nodes in the ipsilateral axilla.

Stage 3. The primary tumor is infiltrating the skin or chest wall, or the axillary nodes are matted or fixed.

Stage 4. Distant metastases are present.

Treatment and Results

Treatment may be curative or palliative. Curative treatment is advised for clinical stage 1 and stage 2 disease and for selected patients in stage 3. Palliative treatment is recommended for patients in stage 4, for stage 3 patients unsuitable for curative efforts, and for previously treated patients who develop distant metastases or ineradicable local recurrence. Modified radical mastectomy is recommended as the primary treatment of choice in stage 1 and stage 2 lesions.[72] In the overall program of treatment for patients with stage 2 disease (positive axillary nodes), it is essential to keep in mind that most of these patients already have occult metastases elsewhere in the body. Stage 3 lesions are a borderline group and may or may not be suitable for surgical treatment by standard or modified radical mastectomy and must be individualized.

Not only the clinical stage of the disease but the length of gestation should be considered when radiotherapy as an adjunct to radical mastectomy is contemplated. The purposes of preoperative or postoperative radiotherapy in association with modified or standard radical mastectomy are (1) to reduce the incidence of local recurrence from residual cancer in the operative field, and (2) to sterilize metastatic cancer in the internal mammary and supraclavicular lymph nodes. Completely resectable lesions confined to the breast (stage 1) do not call for radiotherapy. On the other hand, stage 2 and stage 3 patients need radiotherapy before or after modified or standard radical mastectomy. Only supervoltage irradiation should be advised as adjunctive therapy. The beneficial results of preoperative radiotherapy are more definite than those of postoperative radiotherapy. Preoperative irradiation reduces the incidence of local recurrence and may improve the 10-year survival rate.[72] In pregnant women with breast cancer and in whom radiation therapy is to be considered, the length of gestation, shielding of the abdomen, and the use of preterm delivery should be included in the decision process for the individual patient.[44]

Chemotherapy as an adjunct to radical mastec-

tomy may be helpful in the therapy of breast cancer in patients with stage 2 and 3 disease who are selected for curative treatment by surgery. Preterm delivery should be performed in those women for whom this course of therapy is needed. The previously mentioned possible teratogenic effects of cytotoxic agents must be considered for the individual patient. Palliative radiotherapy treatment and therapeutic endocrine ablation in women with advanced breast cancer who are pregnant can be delayed a few weeks to permit a preterm viable delivery without altering the survival or morbidity of the mother.

There are sufficient studies in the literature to adequately document that any difference in survival of women with breast cancer associated with pregnancy and those women with breast cancer who are not pregnant is related to the greater difficulties with and later diagnosis of the cancer in women who are pregnant.[41,44] Early diagnosis of breast cancer is the key to improving survival whether the woman is pregnant or not. When cancer is confined to the breast, the five-year clinical cure rate by radical mastectomy is 75 to 90 percent. When axillary nodes are involved, the rate drops to 40 to 60 percent at five years and, by the end of 10 years after radical mastectomy, the clinical cure rate is only about 25 percent in this group of patients. Operative mortality is about 1 percent. The prognosis of carcinoma of the breast occurring during pregnancy or lactation is slightly less because at the time of diagnosis the disease is in a more advanced stage. Following radical mastectomy for stage 1 mammary carcinoma, survival time is unaffected by subsequent pregnancy. If the cancer is completely excised, subsequent pregnancy is not deleterious.[14,58]

Patients with carcinoma of the breast identified during the second half of pregnancy require more individual consideration. Operable lesions should be treated with radical mastectomy. If the lesion is already stage 3 or greater when first seen by a physician, the waiting of a few weeks for fetal maturity to occur to permit a preterm delivery will not decrease the mother's chances of survival or increase her morbidity. After delivery, local and/or systemic treatment may be carried out as indicated. Cancers arising during lactation are treated in a conventional manner after suppression of lactation.

Breast-feeding obviously is contraindicated with concurrent treatment and most likely should be discouraged no matter what the time interval might be from a previous mastectomy. There is concern for transmission of virus-like particles in breast milk to the infant, a possible stimulating effect on preneoplastic cells in the remaining breast as well as the greater difficulties of carrying out self-breast examination by the patient and physician examination during lactation.

Breast cancer patients under age 35 are encouraged to plan pregnancies after a two-to-three-year interval following mastectomy.

Rehabilitation of the woman following surgery for breast cancer should be planned. The Ameri-

can Cancer Society has developed the "Reach to Recovery" program which, at the request of physicians, sends trained volunteers who have had a mastectomy and have adjusted well, to visit mastectomy patients in the hospital. This program along with each hospital's individual rehabilitative programs now brings informative, psychologic, cosmetic, and physical rehabilitation to many women undergoing mastectomy in the United States. Most of the physical and emotional problems related to mastectomy can be offset by planned rehabilitation.

CERVIX

The accessibility, frequent visualization, and increased use of cytology, colposcopy, and biopsy of the cervix during pregnancy establishes this site as one of the more common cancers in pregnancy. Pregnancy can occur at any stage of dysplastic or neoplastic growth. The more advanced the cervical lesion with ulceration and infection, the smaller is the chance of fertilization occurring. An epithet for cervical cancer has been written, yet approximately 7400 American women are currently dying from the disease each year.

Incidence

Cervical carcinoma coexisting with pregnancy occurs once in every 2000 to 6000 women or between .02 and .05 percent. The incidence of pregnancy in carcinoma of the cervix is about 3 percent. The average age of the patient is around 35 years, and the average parity is almost five. Carcinoma in situ and clinically unsuspected invasive cancer of the cervix are found in pregnant and nonpregnant women with about the same frequency. The average age of patients with carcinoma in situ in pregnancy varies between 27 to 35 years.[44]

Early marriage and prompt and numerous pregnancies markedly increase the incidence of invasive cervical cancer and cervical cancer in situ. The disease does not occur unless a certain factor is present and this factor is related to sexual intercourse. The increased incidence among Negroes and those in low social and economic groups appears to result from these same factors. The early and continual anatomical relocation of the squamocolumnar junction appears also to be a factor in the development of the disease.

Symptoms

The majority of patients with invasive cancer of the cervix during pregnancy note persistent vaginal bleeding or staining, but at least 10 to 30 percent have no symptoms.[16] Unfortunately, the bleeding caused by cancer is not different from that caused by complications of pregnancy. The smaller the cervical lesion the fewer the symptoms referrable to the disease.

Diagnosis

All physicians undertaking the care of pregnant women should, in addition to obtaining a history and performing a general physical examination plus pelvic examination, obtain cervical cytosmears. Cytopathology has contributed significantly to the earlier detection of cervical cancer in the pregnant and nonpregnant patient. If an obvious cervical lesion exists, biopsy should be performed. The larger the cervical cancer lesion, the greater the possibility of a false-negative cytosmear. In the absence of an obvious cervical lesion, a single Pap smear taken during pregnancy and reported to be normal is an indication that no further cervical diagnostic procedures need to be carried out during that pregnancy. As to whether the directed biopsy should be obtained in the office or in the hospital, it must be individualized as to the size of the lesion and the duration of the pregnancy. Biopsy of the cervix in a pregnant patient can be associated with hemorrhage, and admission to the hospital for women in the second and third trimesters for cervical biopsy should be seriously considered.

In a woman with no visible cervical lesion and a

cytologic report suggestive of severe dysplasia, carcinoma in situ, or invasive cervical cancer further study is needed.[2] If a skilled colposcopist can be involved in the diagnostic work-up, it is recommended that when colposcopy is performed and an abnormality is visualized, a directed punch biopsy from the most abnormal areas should be performed.[66] In order to rely on the colposcopic biopsy, the following conditions must be satisfied:

1. An abnormality must be seen with an abnormal cytologic smear.
2. The colposcopic biopsy must satisfactorily explain the abnormal smear.
3. The entire lesion must be visible colposcopically.
4. If microinvasion is found on a colposcopic biopsy, conization is necessary to rule out frank invasion.
5. The patient must be reliable to ensure follow-up care.

If any of the five conditions are not satisfied, then the patient should be subjected to conization in order to be certain whether invasive carcinoma is or is not present.[20]

If a skilled colposcopist is not available and if no suspicious lesion is present, the cervix should be stained with Lugol's solution to detect unstained areas on the cervix.[2] If areas are seen that fail to take the stain, punch biopsies or knife biopsies should be taken directly from those areas, and an endocervical curettage performed at the same examination. In patients where no unstained areas are visible on the cervix, conization should be carried out.

When Lugol's solution has been used and the punch biopsy has been taken from abnormal areas, the following conditions must be satisfied.

1. The punch biopsy must explain satisfactorily the abnormal smear.
2. If microinvasion is found on a punch biopsy, conization is necessary to rule out frank invasion.

When the patient has undergone conization, the diagnosis is considered definitive and therapy can be decided accordingly.[2]

In the pregnant woman, it is rare that one needs to resort to performing a classic cone biopsy, because the squamocolumnar junction is usually displaced well out onto the portio vaginalis, which renders the likely cancer-bearing areas more accessible. Because of the maternal and fetal complications associated with conization during pregnancy, conization as a primary diagnostic procedure during pregnancy is to be discouraged. If abnormal cytology is encountered in pregnancy, every alternative to conization must be made in an attempt to reach a satisfactory diagnosis. In an occasional case, however, conization may be required in the pregnant patient. Although conization of the cervix during pregnancy for the diagnosis of preinvasive or invasive cervical cancer has been repeatedly reported as being safe,[34] most series contain patients who abort, have excessive blood loss, experience premature rupture of the membranes with immature birth, have cervical stenosis or an incompetent cervical os due to the procedure.[46,51]

Carcinoma in Situ

Dysplasia and carcinoma in situ of the cervix are unrelated to pregnancy and do not disappear after delivery. The exception to this may occur if the lesions are removed by conization or by trauma associated with labor and delivery.

Pregnancy may occur following conization as the only treatment of carcinoma in situ of the utcrine cervix. The curative rate depends on whether the resected margins are free of pathologic epithelium or not. If cytosmears were repeatedly negative the first year after conization, a new diagnosis of cancer was made in 0.4 percent of women in Bjerre's study.[7] Women with the diagnosis of carcinoma in situ of the cervix established before pregnancy by conization should be placed in a high-risk category and have close obstetric supervision.[46] The size of cervical conization and injury to the internal os will determine the risk of future spontaneous abortion and premature delivery due to cervical incompetence.[51] With a normal cervical cytologic smear during pregnancy, the patient should be allowed to continue to term and deliver by way of the vagina. Definitive management of the patient will depend on the extent of the lesion and the patient's age and desire for more children.[8]

A diagnosis of cervical dysplasia or carcinoma in situ made during pregnancy should not change the management of pregnancy, labor, or delivery.[8] These patients need not be delivered by cesarean section. Serial cytologic exam and colposcopy during pregnancy allow for this conservative approach.[20,44]

Microinvasive Carcinoma

Early stomal invasion, microinvasive carcinoma, or stage IA, is a more frequent diagnosis during pregnancy with the greater use of cervical cytology, colposcopy, and adequate pathologic examination of cervical tissues. Cytology, colposcopy, and punch biopsy of the cervix are not capable of consistently determining microinvasion of the cervix. Knife conization of the cervix and detailed pathologic examination of the specimen are mandatory to make the diagnosis. The factors involved, such as depth of invasion, vascular or lymphatic involvement, or confluence of tongues of disease into the stroma, have not been clearly defined as to what constitutes microinvasion. Most studies use invasion into the underlying stroma from the surface epithelium for a distance of 3 to 5 mm as a consistent criteria for making the diagnosis.[44] The degree of lymphatic involvement by pathologists makes for this determination of less value. Thompson and associates base their management of early invasive cancer of the cervix in pregnancy by using 3 mm of extension of disease into the stroma.[67] They found no positive nodes in 24 women treated by lymphadnectomy and have had no recurrences to date. Also, they were impressed that many patients did not have evidence of residual invasion in the specimen and no patient had evidence of invasion deeper than 3 mm into the stroma. Christopherson et al followed 91 women with microinvasive carcinoma of the cervix for 5 years and 80 patients for 10 years or both until death. Their definition of invasion was no more than 5 mm from the surface epithelium.[18] With one patient lost to follow up after fime years, two patients whose death certificates giving cervical cancer as the cause properly questioned, and one patient with one positive iliac node, they believe simple hysterectomy is the maximal treatment indicated. They state the prognosis of microinvasive carcinoma is similar to that of carcinoma in situ.[18] These studies strongly suggest that women with microinvasion of the cervix should be permitted to carry their pregnancy to term and to deliver vaginally provided there is no obstetric contraindication.[44] Hysterectomy with or without pelvic lymphadnectomy and preserving of the ovaries may be carried out in the postpartum period.[8]

Invasive Cancer of the Cervix

Patients with cancer of the cervix associated with pregnancy should have the same pretreatment evaluation as nonpregnant patients except for those procedures that may produce irradiation damage to the fetus. Understaging during pregnancy is a common error due to the edema, softness, and laxity of the broad ligaments, paracervical, and paravaginal tissues. The clinical stage of invasive cancer during pregnancy is the single most important prognostic criterion. Management of cervical cancer in pregnancy is influenced by stage of the disease, fetal viability in relation to the establishment of diagnosis, the patient and her family's views on her disease, and the influence of therapy on the fetus.[44,68]

There is no significant difference in early stages of invasive cancer of the cervix in pregnancy between the survival rate for primary surgery and radiotherapy in the hands of skilled individuals.[16] The question is not whether irradiation or surgery is the best treatment for cervical cancer, but rather what is best for the patient. An element of selection for surgically treated patients is necessary. Women with stage IB (cancer confined to the cervix and excluding microinvasion) and stage IIA (extension to the vaginal fornix with no obvious parametrial involvement) are probably best treated by radical abdominal hysterectomy and pelvic lymphadnectomy. When a diagnosis is established, definitive therapy is immediately carried out in the first 28 weeks of pregnancy. Usually the uterus does not need to be emptied before proceeding to the radical hysterectomy. Definitive primary surgery permits conservation of the ovaries and negates the possibility of cervical bleeding associated with irradiation-induced abortion.[60] Women with large cervical lesions or for other technical reasons can be managed well with external radiation therapy of approximately 5000 rads to the pelvis and lymph-bearing regions administered in five to six weeks and a single radium application around 4000 rads following spontaneous abortion. The total dosage to the cervical os would be slightly more than 12,000 rads and to the lateral pelvic wall a little over 6000 rads. For the more advanced cervical cancer in pregnancy, stages IIB, III, and IV, the primary treatment is irradiation therapy[22] (Chapter 12 details this therapy). External radiation therapy during the latter part of the second trimester may be associated with a high incidence of microcephalic infants should the radiation therapy not be cancerocidal and produce fetal death. For those very rare patients who do not abort following external irradiation therapy, a modified radical hysterectomy should be performed.

The physician's desire to treat cancer immediately may have to be tempered with the evaluation of fetal maturity. This may require waiting till the thirty-third week of gestation or later for reliable evidence of maturity in those women whose cancer is discovered after the twenty-eighth week of pregnancy. The treatment would be classical cesarean section and radical abdominal hysterectomy with pelvic lymphadnectomy in stages IB and IIA. Classical cesarean section followed by external radiation therapy and radium is indicated for those patients with more advanced stages or who have large cervical lesions or technical or medical problems prohibiting surgery. At the time of operation, it is important to determine the extent of disease, particularly in the para-aortic nodes which would be outside of the standard irradiation field.

Women who deliver vaginally in the first two trimesters of pregnancy do not have a worse prognosis. Numerous studies in which external radiation therapy has produced fetal demise and spontaneous abortion or delivery of a stillbirth demonstrates patient survival is not influenced.[44]

When invasive carcinoma is discovered in the postpartum period, treatment is provided immediately after diagnosis and metastatic evaluation.

HODGKIN'S DISEASE

Hodgkin's disease occurs most commonly in young adults. It is characterized by abnormal proliferation, in one or several lymph nodes, of lymphocytes, histiocytes, eosinophils, and Reed-Sternberg giant cells. It starts most likely as a regional localized process that tends to spread to contiguous lymphatic structures. Accurate measurement of the extent or staging of the disease when first diagnosed is essential for the proper management and prognosis. The "stage" of the disease is important in determining its course, and the histologic pattern also has prognostic value.

Regional unilateral lymphadenopathy (especially swelling of cervical nodes) is usually the presenting sign. The nodes are firm, nontender, and of various sizes. If the mediastinum is involved early, respiratory difficulty may be the initial complaint. Hepatosplenomegaly and constitutional complaints—fever, excessive sweating, fatigue, and pruritus—usually appear late. The blood count may show an absolute lymphocytopenia. Diagnosis is made by lymph node biopsy. The extent of the disease in pregnancy is established prior to therapy by use of chest x-ray, bone marrow biopsy, and liver function tests. In pregnancy the use of lower extremity lymphangiogram or inferior venacavagram, or scintiscan of the liver and spleen should be delayed until the postpartum period. With clinical evidence of disease in the upper abdomen—i.e., a large spleen —exploratory laparotomy and splenectomy may be indicated. The value of staging laparotomy and splenectomy in management of patients with Hodgkin's disease continues to be a controversial topic.[37]

The incidence of Hodgkin's disease is approximately 1 in 6000 deliveries and in women with Hodgkin's disease, the incidence of pregnancy is approximately 18 percent.[44]

Staging of Hodgkin's Disease

Stage 0.   No detectable disease due to prior excisional biopsy

Stage I.   Single abnormal lymph node

Stage II.   Two or more discrete abnormal nodes, limited to one side of diaphragm

Stage III.   Disease on both sides of diaphragm but limited to the lymph nodes, spleen, or Waldeyer's ring

Stage IV.   Involvement of bone, bone marrow, lung parenchyma, pleura, liver, skin, gastrointestinal tract, central nervous system, renal or other sites other than lymph nodes, spleen, or Waldeyer's ring

All stages are subclassified to describe the absence (A) or presence (B) of systemic symptoms.

Previous Therapy, Sterility, and Pregnancy

Young women with Hodgkin's disease treated with radiation therapy to the pelvic area routinely became amenorrheic, frequently developed menopausal symptoms while still in their teens or twenties, and were regularly sterilized. Now that this problem has been recognized, patients with Hodgkin's disease are given the opportunity to have mechanical transposition of the ovaries (away from a potential radiation therapy field), either as part of the initial staging laparotomy or as a separate procedure unrelated to the splenectomy, liver biopsy, or node biopsy. The ovaries may be repositioned in the midline where they can be shielded by means of an external block. Another site of relocation of the ovaries is the anterolateral abdominal wall as near the anterior superior iliac spine as is feasible. Portals can be arranged such that the ovaries receive only scattered radiation from the lateral margin of shaped fields. Under these circumstances the ovary receives about 5 to 8 percent of the normal midplane dose. Successful pregnancies following these procedures have been reported when Hodgkin's disease in the pelvis had been previously treated and repositioning of the ovaries performed.[37] Goodman and associates have reported their results with mantle and para-aortic irradiation in laparotomy-staged patients IA and IIA Hodgkin's disease as being comparable to the results using total nodal irradiation.[24] Thus pelvis irradiation is omitted.

Multiple-drug therapy or single drugs, such as cyclophosphamides and chlorambucil, can induce amenorrhea and sterility when used in the treatment of Hodgkin's disease. In some cases this is reversible.[36,69]

Women who have been in remission of their disease for at least two years before becoming pregnant usually present no special obstetric problems, and this includes those patients who had splenectomy and mechanically transposed ovaries.

Patients with active disease should be advised against pregnancy, not because of any adverse affect of pregnancy on the mother or danger to the fetus but because of the poor prognosis in the mother and associated treatment problems during pregnancy.[44]

Hodgkin's Disease During Pregnancy

Hodgkin's disease per se does not appear to have an adverse affect on fertility, the course of pregnancy, the products of conception, or on labor and the perperium. Conversely, pregnancy seems to have no influence on the course of the disease, neither accelerating it nor providing any protection.[19,37,44]

Hodgkin's disease located above the diaphragm and treated by irradiation has little scattered radiation to the position occupied by the fetus early in pregnancy because of the distance of the uterus from the lower edge of the portal. As pregnancy advances and the uterus becomes an abdominal organ, it comes closer to the lower margins of the field and the dose to the fetus increases.[15,26] With enlargement of the uterus the fetus is maturing and hence more resistant to the effects of radiation. Hodgkin's disease during pregnancy, stages I, II, and III, located in areas of the body which by use of portal size, shielding of the pregnant uterus and ovaries, and distance from the field of irradiation, would seem to be best treated by localized irradiation therapy especially during the first trimester.[19,26]

Lacher has observed that the chemotherapeutic effect of most anticancer agents on human pregnancy in all trimesters has been generally a benign one. In addition he has noted that Hodgkin's disease is chronic and slowly developing, which may allow the physician to delay any therapy until the patient is in the second or third trimester or until the pregnancy is carried to completion. In some instances, the use of chemotherapy cannot be avoided during pregnancy but, if it must be used, it would be better to restrict it to the second or third trimesters.[37]

The treatment of Hodgkin's disease during pregnancy and located in the pelvis must be individualized.[26] Therapy may be delayed until the thirty-third week of gestation when preterm delivery can be carried out. Wells has cautioned that all antineoplastic therapy should be avoided in the first 12 weeks of pregnancy. If drug treatment must be given during this period, mechlorethamine, or vinblastine are preferable. During the second and third trimesters, chemotherapy can be given in full doses, according to these authors, with no more of a toxic effect on the fetus than it has on the mother.[69] When the pelvis must receive the full therapeutic dose of irradiation with approximately 4000 rads in four weeks, spontaneous abortion or premature birth of a stillborn fetus can be anticipated.

LEUKEMIAS

Leukemia is one of the more common fatal malignant diseases in women under the age of 35 years.[45] Therapy for both acute and chronic leukemia has markedly improved over the past few years when measured by one-year survival rates. Acute leukemia of all ages has only approximately a 6 percent five-year survival, which demonstrates that women with leukemia, pregnant or not, have a grim prognosis.

There is no relationship between acute and chronic leukemia and the parity of the patients. The average age of the patient with acute leukemia and pregnancy is 28 years.[44] Fertility is probably reduced in leukemia because of the nature of the debilitating disease and chemotherapeutic agents used in treating the disease may induce sterility. Certainly if leukemia were discovered in the postpartum period or a woman was fortunate to deliver a viable infant, she or her husband should use methods to prevent future pregnancies. This is not recommended because of any deleterious effect of pregnancy on leukemia or leukemia on pregnancy itself, but rather due to the current short survival of women with leukemia.

Many women are treated for "anemia" for several months by various hematinics, while the initial nonspecific constitutional symptoms are ascribed to the pregnancy.[23] The usual fulminate course of acute leukemia, however, soon brings the correct diagnosis to the forefront.[6,44] Most cases of chronic leukemia are diagnosed prior to the onset of pregnancy. Weakness, malaise, anorexia, lassitude, abdominal discomfort are all complaints of pregnant women. Leukocytosis, immature, abnormal white cells in peripheral blood and bone marrow, lymphocytosis, anemia—all establish the diagnosis of leukemia.

The main objective in the medical management is to maintain the disease in remission long enough for the fetus to become viable and to achieve delivery vaginally, unless there is an obstetric indication for abdominal delivery. Pregnant women with acute leukemia may be in need of antibiotics for bacterial infection, platelet concentrates for hemorrhage secondary to thrombocytopenia, and a high fluid intake. Local manifestations of disease, such as severe bone pain,

massive lymph node enlargement interfering with respirations and swallowing, and central nervous system involvement with signs of increased intracranial pressure may be treated successfully with local irradiation and shielding of the abdomen.

In a disease such as acute leukemia with few survivors, the aim of therapy is to maintain the pregnant patient's general condition at least until a healthy baby can be obtained.[44] In the first trimester of pregnancy, the mother should be treated as though she were not pregnant because if treatments are not instituted in the hope of obtaining a remission, the mother is unlikely to survive long enough for the fetus to reach viability. Some mothers have delivered a normal infant following cytotoxic therapy during the first trimester, but the risk of a spontaneous abortion and fetal malformation must be fully explained and acceptable to the patient and her husband.[35] Chemotherapeutic agents are now administered more commonly in dosage related to height and weight of the patient, and treatment modifications are more precisely defined that help to prevent prohibitive toxicity to the patient. This will in turn reduce the risk of spontaneous abortion and fetal malformation.[56] Most authorities now agree that specific antileukemic therapy is beneficial in pregnant women with leukemia and can be safely undertaken after the first trimester.[56]

In chronic leukemia it may be feasable to withhold specific treatment with cytotoxic drugs or irradiation during the first trimester[33] or in certain instances even throughout the pregnancy. In chronic myelocytic leukemia the aim of therapy is palliation of symptoms and correction of anemia. Specific treatment of the anemia is unnecessary, as it is usually corrected by treatment directed at the leukemic process. Local irradiation therapy may be administered at any time with the uterus shielded.[5,57] Busulfan, an alkylating agent, is the drug of choice and has been used throughout pregnancy with usually no effect on the fetus.[52]

MALIGNANT MELANOMA

The uncommon association of malignant melanoma with pregnancy is far overshadowed by the lingering, unsubstantiated impression by many physicians that the malignancy is wildly disseminated by the increased hormones of pregnancy. These malignant neoplastic disorders of the

melanocyte that are nonheritable and spontaneously appear exhibit different shades of color, different sizes and shapes, and different potentials for invasion and metastases. This tumor is the only relatively common human malignant neoplasm that is present on the body surface and can be observed during the early stages of evolution. A pigmented lesion is present before the onset of malignancy in approximately 75 to 85 percent of patients, and at least 50 percent of patients have a lesion present for one year before the development of malignancy.[44]

Malignant melanoma appears in three distinct clinical forms: lentigo maligna melanoma, superficial spreading melanoma, and nodular melanoma. These tumors are defined by their gross and microscopic characteristics correlated with their life history. The specific type of melanoma can only be determined by examination of multiple, carefully selected sites in the primary lesion. A fairly accurate assessment of the patient with malignant melanoma can be made based on classification according to the clinical and pathologic features correlated with the level of histologic invasion of the lesion.

The treatment of malignant melanoma consists of surgical excision. Nearly all lesions except small lentigo maligna melanoma must be excised widely enough so that skin grafting is required. Lymph node dissection is usually not necessary in lentigo maligna melanoma except in rare cases when palpable nodes are present. The same is true of superficial spreading melanoma unless invasion is present. There is considerable controversy regarding the value of prophylactic node dissection for melanoma. Except in more advanced nodular melanoma, the regional nodes are nearly always clinically involved and therapeutic dissection is indicated. As the prognosis is poor with advanced nodular melanoma, regional perfusion with antitumor drugs has been performed both by arterial and endolymphatic routes. Systemic chemotherapy has on occasion produced favorable results. Lentigo maligna and superficial spreading melanomas that do not invade the dermis beyond the papillary level cause death in less than 10 percent of cases. When nodular melanoma is first treated, it usually fills the papillary layer but does not enter the reticular layer and causes death in approximately 45 percent of cases. Regardless of the type of tumor, the mortality rate increases with the depth of invasion at the time of treatment.[50]

Obstetric Implications

The obstetrician should, during the physical exam, observe for nevi on the feet, palms, and genitals, which should be removed because the nevi in these areas have an extremely high incidence of junctional components. In addition, any nevi subject to irritation, as under straps, particularly on the trunk, should be removed. Palpable thickening, rapidly spreading pigmentation, change in pigmentation, peeling, crusting, bleeding, or irritation in a nevus should be excised and examined histologically.

The impression that pregnancy accelerated the growth of malignant melanoma was based on individual case reports in which the histology and clinical stage of the lesion were not defined.[49] Pregnant patients with nondisseminated malignant melanoma are treated by wide surgical excision of the tumor and dissection of the regional lymph nodes as individually determined. This treatment should be individualized for each pregnant patient but should be carried out promptly and at any stage during pregnancy.

The placenta functions as a barrier to maternal cancer cells.[31] Pregnant women with disseminated malignant melanoma may have gross evidence of placental involvement as well as histologic evidence of intervillous and intravillous spread of the disease. Metastatic melanoma may not only spread to the placenta but very rarely to the infant with resulting death of the infant and this is usually associated with villous invasion.[25]

The treatment of the pregnant woman with diffuse malignant melanoma must be individualized as to the general condition of the patient and the stage of pregnancy. Fortunately, with disseminated disease pregnancy rarely takes place and if it occurs during pregnancy, it is commonly associated with fetal demise so the decision as to possibly delaying chemotherapy, regional perfusion with antitumor drugs, or immunologic treatments are extremely infrequent. In general, treatment should be immediate through the first 30 weeks of pregnancy. Should the fetus still be alive at this stage of gestation a preterm delivery can be carried out. Spontaneous vaginal delivery of an immature infant is common with disseminated disease.[44]

The effect of pregnancy on survival in women with melanoma has been subject to five-year survival studies that have minimized the impression of a few dramatic case reports by including them with a larger group. When melanoma is associated with pregnancy, there is no statistical difference between the pregnant and nonpregnant women as far as prognosis is concerned.[44,49,50]

OVARY

Carcinoma of the ovary has been found in all trimesters of pregnancy, postpartum, following spontaneous abortion, and associated with tubal pregnancy. The incidence of all ovarian malignancies coexistant with pregnancy is variously quoted from 2.2 to 5 percent of all ovarian tumors complicating pregnancy. The pregnant patients are much younger than the average ovarian cancer patient. Low parity is common in women with ovarian cancer in pregnancy.[17,44]

The patient with an early ovarian cancer has no signs or symptoms. The most frequent symptoms in women presenting with ovarian cancer are the same whether the pregnancy is present or not. Routine prenatal pelvic examinations account for the discovery of approximately 50 percent of ovarian malignancies with pregnancy.[9] Abdominal pain, painless enlargement of the abdomen out of proportion with the stage of gestation, or the obstruction of labor are common signs and symptoms of the disease.[9]

The most common adnexal mass palpable early in pregnancy is the corpus luteum of pregnancy, which at times may equal but rarely exceeds 6 cm in diameter. Diagnosis of the presence of an adnexal mass by pelvic examination must be made by the obstetrician at the time of the first prenatal visit. Direct inspection of an enlarging ovary 6 cm or more in diameter is indicated in the pregnant woman because a diagnosis of malignancy can never be made without it.

In the reproductive age group, in addition to the more common types of ovarian cancer, serous, mucinous, and endometrioid, there are a greater number of neoplasms of low malignant potential as well as dysgerminomas and granulosa cell tumors. The combination of routine prenatal examination as well as the aforementioned greater frequency of less malignant tumors can account for the discovery of earlier stages of ovarian cancer in pregnancy.[17]

Treatment

The treatment of ovarian cancer associated with pregnancy is the same as in the nonpregnant stage, and that is surgical removal of as much of the cancer as possible.[12] It is important that an adequate surgical incision in the abdomen be performed not only to remove the cancer but to properly explore the abdominal contents, do an omentectomy, and reduce the trauma to the uterus from a small incision and the need for many retractors. The ovarian cancer must be properly staged and sampling of peritoneal fluid for cellular analysis performed. The stage of the disease and histologic type of the lesion are the two most important prognostic criteria (Chapter 19 should be referred to for a more thorough consideration on ovarian cancer). The common epithelial-type tumors and other unusual ovarian malignancies should in the first 28 weeks of pregnancy be managed aggressively. This would usually include bilateral salpingo-oophorectomy, omentectomy, and hysterectomy. Individualization in many cases is necessary. If the pregnancy is in the third trimester, preferably after 32 weeks, a classical cesarean section can be performed during the definitive surgical operation. In the pregnant woman with a low-grade and intracystic or encapsulated ovarian cancer, conservative surgery may be considered, provided there is no evidence of any peritoneal or other spread and the other ovary is normal by wedge resection. Should additional surgery be indicated, it may be combined with classical cesarean section after the thirty-second week of gestation. Chemotherapy or irradiation therapy may be carried out following operation.

Tumors of low malignant potential, as confirmed by frozen section or permanent histologic exam, should have surgical removal of as much disease as possible. During the first 32 weeks of pregnancy, if the uterus itself is not significantly involved or if peritoneal stripping of disease can be carried out the pregnancy may be permitted to continue to term. A second procedure can be performed after the thirty-second week of pregnancy, at which time a classical cesarean section and hysterectomy can be completed.[12]

Dysgerminomas

Over 85 percent of dysgerminomas occur in patients under the age of 30 years.[43] Approximately 15 percent of dysgerminomas occur in women who are either pregnant or in the immediate postpartum period when diagnosed. If the dysgerminoma is confined to one ovary, unilateral oophorectomy is as effective as any other therapeutic modality and associated with a 10-year survival of slightly better than 85 percent.[3] The diagnosis of stage IA dysgerminoma demands exclusion of other histologic elements, normal peritoneal fluid cellular study, no retroperitoneal lymph nodes that are involved with the disease, and the uninvolved ovary has a wedge biopsy that is normal on histologic examination. Evidence of spread of the disease beyond the ovaries in the first two trimesters of pregnancy should be accompanied with surgical removal of the ovaries and hysterectomy, and in the last trimester of pregnancy, usually after 32 weeks, a classical cesarean section prior to operation.[17] Dysgerminoma of the ovary is probably the most radiosensitive ovarian neoplasm and with disease spread beyond the ovaries, external radiation therapy should be used.

Granulosa Cell Tumor

The most important prognostic finding for women with granulosa cell tumors associated with pregnancy is the stage of the tumor at diagnosis. Schwartz and Smith clearly document that in young patients unilateral oophorectomy, if the tumor is limited to one ovary (stage IA), is adequate treatment.[61]

Pregnant women should be permitted, then, to continue to term and deliver vaginally. For patients with ruptured tumors, abdominal radiation should be delayed until a preterm delivery can be accomplished. The relative radiosensitivity of granulosa cell tumors, their low malignant potential when confined to one ovary, and their usual good survival at this stage of disease permit this short delay. Women with tumors in stages IB to IV are treated with abdominal hysterectomy, bilateral salpingo-oophorectomy, and excision of as much of the metastatic disease as possible in the first 28 weeks of pregnancy. A classical cesarean section is to be performed at the time of surgery during the last trimester of pregnancy. Further therapy is carried out as discussed in Chapters 19 and 20.

ADDITIONAL PROBLEMS OF THE PREGNANT WOMAN WITH CANCER

Cancer during pregnancy or in the immediate postpartum period of all types has been reported.[1,4,10,11,21,27–30,36,38–40,42,44,53–55,59,63,70,73] In his monograph on Cancer in Pregnancy, McGowan extensively covers the literature on the subject.[44] No matter what the type of cancer is associated with pregnancy, there are additional common problems in these women. Because of the younger age of pregnant women, malignancy in general is not given the diagnostic consideration that it is in older age groups. Consequently, its diagnosis during pregnancy may be more difficult because the symptoms and physical findings are confused with the superimposed pregnancy. Pregnancy does not accelerate the growth patterns of any cancer in women. Diagnostic procedures utilizing radioisotopes or radiation to the abdomen can usually be delayed to allow fetal maturity and preterm delivery before their use.

Malignancy per se is not likely to jeopardize the normal development of the child and, on the other hand, pregnancy is not likely to alter the prognosis or the course of malignancy. Spontaneous abortions and stillbirths are expected in pregnant women who have a rapidly debilitating disease such as acute leukemia. Adequate treatment of the neoplasm will, at times, terminate a coexisting pregnancy. It is generally conceded that therapeutic abortion does not enhance patient survival for any malignancy associated with pregnancy. Women with active disease or metastatic spread should be urged to wait until at least two years have elapsed without evidence of further spread of the disease before becoming pregnant.

All therapy of a pregnant woman with cancer must take into consideration the stage of the disease, duration of pregnancy and in the case of drug administration, the type of drug, the quantity, and duration utilized. Each woman with malignancy will have to be individually studied following general principles of diagnosis and management and each step thoroughly discussed with the patient, her husband, and close relatives. In the extremely rare instance when a pregnant woman with cancer gives birth to a normal child and succumbs to her disease shortly after, it will be the family's responsibility to raise the child or allow the child to be adopted.

Vaginal delivery of infants is usually anticipated and found to take place without problems even though the infant's mother may have active disease. The infants are rarely involved with the metastatic disease. Spread of cancer to the fetus is usually associated with very widely disseminated disease in the mother. The delivery of a child either by way of the vagina or by cesarean section, before intrauterine development is complete, is common in women with cancer. The preterm delivery of an immature child may be elective to prevent fetal damage during therapy, combined with definitive therapy, as a result of therapy, or secondary to the poor general condition of the mother. Although these children may not develop metastatic disease, they deserve special attention.[13] Breast-feeding in mothers is permitted unless there are pathologic conditions within the breasts, problems with the newborn, the general condition of the mother does not permit, or chemotherapy is being used.

The major medical organizations in the United States involved in the reduction of rates of maternal, perinatal, and infant morbidity and mortality have clearly stated that pregnant women with malignancies contribute significantly to fetal and neonatal morbidity and mortality. They advise the transfer of these obstetric patients prior to the delivery to the most developed (level III) units to assure the immediate availability of comprehensive intensive care for the newborn from the moment of birth.[13]

References

1. Armon PJ: Burkitt's lymphoma of the ovary in association with pregnancy. Brit J Obstet Gynaecol 83:169, 1976
2. ACOG Technical Bulletin: Management of Abnormal Cytology by Colposcopy and/or Conization. No. 38. Am Coll Ob Gyn, Chicago, May, 1976
3. Asadourian LA, Taylor HB: Dysgerminoma. Obstet Gynec 33:370, 1969
4. Barber HRK, Brunschwig A: Carcinoma of the bowel. Am J Obstet Gynec 100:926, 1968
5. Baynes TL, Crickmay GF, Jones RV: Pregnancy in a case of chronic lymphatic leukaemia. J Obstet Gynec Brit Commonw 75:1165, 1968
6. Bhoopathi B, Ostapowicz F, Bazley W: Acute promyelocytic leukemia in pregnancy. Obstet Gynec 41:275, 1973
7. Bjerre B, Eliasson G, Linell F, Soderberg H, Sjoberg N: Conization as only treatment of carcinoma in situ of the uterine cervix. Am J Obstet Gynec 125:143, 1976
8. Boutselis JG: Intraepithelial carcinoma of the cervix associated with pregnancy. Obstet Gynec 40:657, 1972
9. Buttery BW, Beischer NA, Fortune DW, Macafee CAJ: Ovarian tumours in pregnancy. Med J Austr 1:345, 1973
10. Cantin J, McNeer GP: The effect of pregnancy on the clinical course of sarcoma of the soft somatic tissues. Surg Gynec Obstet 125:28, 1967
11. Chamlian DL, Taylor HB: Primary carcinoma of Bartholin's gland. Obstet Gynec 39:489, 1972
12. Chung A, Birnbaum SJ: Ovarian cancer associated with pregnancy. Obstet Gynec 41:211, 1973
13. Committee on Perinatal Health: Toward Improving the Outcome of Pregnancy—Recommendations for the Regional Development of Maternal and Perinatal Health Services. Natl Found - March of Dimes, White Plains, New York, 1976
14. Cooper DR, Butterfield J: Pregnancy subsequent to mastectomy for cancer of the breast. Ann Surg 171:429, 1970
15. Covington EE, Baker AS: Dosimetry of scattered radiation to the fetus. JAMA 209:414, 1969
16. Creasman WT, Rutledge F, Fletcher G: Carcinoma of the cervix associated with pregnancy. Obstet Gynec 36:495, 1970
17. Creasman WT, Rutledge F, Smith JP: Carcinoma of the ovary associated with pregnancy. Obstet Gynec 38:111, 1971
18. Christopherson WM, Gray LA, Parker JE: Microinvasive carcinoma of the uterine cervix. Cancer 38:629, 1976
19. D'Angio GJ, Nisce LZ: Problems with the irradiation of children and pregnant patients. JAMA 223:171, 1973
20. DePetrillo AD, Townsend DE, Morrow CP, et al: Colposcopic evaluation of the abnormal Papanicolaou test in pregnancy. Am J Obstet Gynec 121:441, 1975
21. Duckler L, Cohen HR: Hyperemesis gravi-

darum with gastric carcinoma. Obstet Gynec 45:348, 1975

22. Dudan RC, Yon JL, Ford JH, Averette HE: Carcinoma of the cervix and pregnancy. Gynec Oncol 1:583, 1973

23. Ewing PA, Whittaker JA: Acute leukemia in pregnancy. Obstet Gynec 42:245, 1973

24. Goodman RL, Piro AJ, Hellman S: Can pelvic irradiation be omitted in patients with pathologic stages IA and IIA Hodgkin's disease? Cancer 37:2834, 1976

25. Gillis H, Mortel R, McGavran MH: Maternal malignant melanoma metastatic to the products of conception. Gynec Oncol 4:38, 1976

26. Thomas PR, Peckham MJ: The investigation and management of Hodgkin's disease in the pregnant patient. Cancer 38:1443, 1976

27. Green LK, Harris RE, Massey FM: Cancer of the colon during pregnancy. Obstet Gynec 46:480, 1975

28. Grunberger V: Successful pregnancy after vulvectomy. Wien Klin Woch 85:370, 1973

29. Hardin JA: Cyclophosphamide treatment of lymphoma during third trimester of pregnancy. Obstet Gynec 39:850, 1972

30. Hill CS, Clark RL, Wolf M: The effect of subsequent pregnancy on patients with thyroid carcinoma. Surg Gynec Obstet 122:1219, 1966

31. Holcomb BW, Thigpen JT, Puckett JF, Morrison FS: Generalized melanosis complicating disseminated malignant melanoma in pregnancy: case report. Cancer 35:1459, 1975

32. Hutchison GB: Late neoplastic changes following medical irradiation. Cancer 37:1102, 1976

33. Johnson FD: Pregnancy and concurrent chronic myelogenous leukemia. Am J Obstet Gynec 112:640, 1972

34. Johnstone NR: Pregnancy following conservative management of dysplasia and carcinoma in situ of the uterine cervix. Aust NZ J Obstet Gynaec 14:9, 1974

35. Krueger JA, Davis RB, Field C: Multiple-drug chemotherapy in the management of acute lymphocytic leukemia during pregnancy. Obstet Gynec 48:324, 1976

36. Karlen JR, Sternberg LB, Abbott JN: Carcinoma of the endometrium co-existing with pregnancy. Obstet Gynec 40:344, 1972

37. Lacher MJ (ed): Hodgkin's Disease. New York, Wiley, 1976

38. Lea AW: Pregnancy following radical operation for rectal carcinoma. Am J Obstet Gynec 113:504, 1972

39. Lergier JE, Jimenez E, Maldonado N, Veray F: Normal pregnancy in multiple myeloma treated with cyclophosphamide. Cancer 34:1018, 1974

40. Magee RA, Harley JM, Campbell WA: Clinical report for the years 1970-1972 and a five year review, 1968-1972. Royal Maternity Hospital Belfast, Ireland

41. Mausner JS, Shimkin MB, Moss NH, Rosemond GP: Cancer of the breast in Philadelphia Hospitals, 1951-1964. Cancer 23:260, 1969

42. McCann TO, O'Leary JA, McCaffrey R: Bladder carcinoma in pregnancy. Bull Sloane Hosp Women 13:109, 1967

43. McCarthy TG, Milton PJD: Successful pregnancy after conservative surgery and radiotherapy for disgerminoma of the ovary. Brit J Obstet Gynaec 82:64, 1975

44. McGowan L: Cancer in Pregnancy. Springfield, Ill., Thomas, 1967

45. McLain CR: Leukemia in Pregnancy. Clinic Obstet Gynec 17:185, 1974

46. McLaren HC, Jordan JA, Clover M, Attwood ME: Pregnancy after cone biopsy of the cervix. J Obstet Gynaec Brit Commonw 81&383, 1974

47. Medical Letter: Drugs in Pregnancy. New Rochelle, New York, December 8, 1972

48. Medical Letter: Urine Pregnancy Tests. New Rochelle, New York, January 17, 1975

49. Minawi MF, Hori JM, Donegan WL: Melanoma and pregnancy. Intern J Gynaec Obstet 11:1, 1973

50. Morrow CP, DiSaia PJ: Malignant melanoma of the female genitalia: a clinical analysis. Obstet Gynec Surv 31:233, 1976

51. Nagell JR, Parker JC, Hicks LP, Conrad R, England G: Diagnostic and therapeutic efficacy of cervical conization. Am J Obstet Gynec 124:134, 1976

52. Nolan GH, Marks R, Perez C: Busulfan treatment of leukemia during pregnancy. Obstet Gynec 38:136, 1971

53. Nuss RC, Lee JH: Pregnancy following hemipelvectomy. Obstet Gynec 29:789, 1967

54. Pelosi M, Hung CT, Langer A, Khademi M, Harrigan JT: Renal carcinoma in pregnancy. Obstet Gynec 45:461, 1975

55. Purtilo DT, Clark JV, Williams R: Primary

hepatic malignancy in pregnant women. Am J Obstet Gynec 121:41, 1975

56. Raich PC, Curet LB: Treatment of acute leukemia during pregnancy. Cancer 36:861, 1975

57. Richards HG, Spiers AS: Chronic granulocytic leukaemia in pregnancy. Brit J Rad 48:561, 1975

58. Rissanen PM: Pregnancy following treatment of mammary carcinoma. ACTA Radiol 8:415, 1969

59. Ross MH, Vincent CC: Adenocarcinoma of the jejunum during pregnancy. Obstet Gynec 34:406, 1969

60. Sall N, Rini S, Pineda A: Surgical management of invasive carcinoma of the cervix in pregnancy. Am J Obstet Gynec 118:1, 1974

61. Schwartz PE, Smith JP: Treatment of ovarian stromal tumors. Am J Obstet Gynec 125:402, 1976

62. Shettles LB: When does life begin? JAMA 214:1895, 1970

63. Skinner MS, Sternberg WH, Ichinose H, Collins J: Spontaneous regression of Bowenoid atypia of the vulva. Obstet Gynec 42:40, 1973

64. Stirrat GM: Prescribing problems in the second half of pregnancy and during lactation. Obstet Gynec Surv 31:1, 1976

65. Sternberg J: Irradiation and radiocontamination during pregnancy. Am J Obstet Gynec 108:490, 1970

66. Talebian F, Krumholz BA, Shayan A, Mann LI: Colposcopic evaluation of patients with abnormal cytologic smears during pregnancy. Obstet Gynec 47:693, 1976

67. Thompson JD, Caputo TA, Franklin EW, Dale E: The surgical management of invasive cancer of the cervix in pregnancy. Am J Obstet Gynec 121:853, 1975

68. Wanless JF: Carcinoma of the cervix in pregnancy. Am J Obstet Gynec 110:173, 1971

69. Wells JH, Marshal JR, Carbone PP: Procarbazine therapy for Hodgkin's disease in early pregnancy. JAMA 205:119, 1968

70. Wharton JT, Rutledge FN, Gallager HS, Fletcher G: Treatment of clear cell adenocarcinoma in young females. Obstet Gynec 45:365, 1975

71. Wilson RE: The breast. In Sabiston DC (ed): Textbook of Surgery, 10th ed. Philadelphia, Saunders, 1972

72. Wilson JL: Diseases of the breast. In Krupp MA, Chatton MJ (eds): Current Medical Diagnosis and Treatment. Los Altos, California, Lange, 1976

73. Wolff JR, Lebharz TB: Pregnancy following Wilms' tumor. Am J Obstet Gynec 100:1151, 1968

The Gynecologic Oncology Patient: Restoration of Function and Prevention of Disability

LEO D. LAGASSE, M.D.
MICHAEL L. BERMAN, M.D.
WATSON G. WATRING, M.D.
SAMUEL C. BALLON, M.D.

Statistics compiled by the American Cancer Society suggest that at least 688,000 women will require treatment for invasive gynecologic cancer during the next decade and that two-thirds of these women will survive 5 years.[7] The use of more effective and aggressive approaches to the evaluation and the treatment of these cancers can cure increasing numbers of patients but also can produce disabling complications in some.

The management of patients with serious complications resulting from the treatment of gynecologic cancer is complex and requires care and foresight. Proper prevention and management of disability resulting from intensive radiotherapy or extended surgery require an understanding of both the operative techniques of pelvic reconstruction and the medical problems of bowel dysfunction, starvation, thromboembolism and infection. At the UCLA Medical Center, the City of Hope National Medical Center and other institutions, efforts are increasing the understanding of these complex surgical and medical problems. Techniques now exist to restore vaginal and rectal function. Newer methods of urinary diversion are available. A rational plan of management of the serious complications of intestinal fistula and radiation-induced enteritis has been developed. A coordinated plan for the support of patients with a wide spectrum of severe medical complications who are disabled by the treatment of gynecologic cancer is discussed in this chapter.

PELVIC RECONSTRUCTION

Vaginal Reconstruction

Loss of adequate vaginal function can be seen following treatment for pelvic malignancy because of scarring associated with intensive radiation or after extended operative procedures. A careful, individualized approach can restore vaginal function in many of these patients. A functional and anatomic reconstruction of the vagina ideally results in a moist, smooth surface of normal depth and caliber that covers soft and uninfected surrounding tissues. All of these criteria cannot be met in every patient. If a suitable anatomic space is lined with an adequate cover of grafted skin, the resulting neovagina still may become scarred and rigid. Nevertheless, attempts to restore sexual function should be made, and in many instances such efforts will enable the motivated patient to achieve sexual gratification.

Vaginal reconstruction often is indicated following vaginectomy for localized vaginal neoplasia, when there is radiation damage to the vagina or after pelvic exenteration. The optimal reconstructive procedure and its timing should reflect the needs of the individual patient, the antecedent disease process, and the treatment that necessitated vaginal reconstruction.

Following Vaginectomy with Preservation of Bladder and Rectum

Vaginal reconstruction using a split-thickness skin graft is satisfactory and may be performed at the time of vaginectomy in patients with superficial vaginal cancer. The technique is simple to perform and is similar to that employed in patients with vaginal agenesis.[28,55] In addition to preserving sexual function, vaginal reconstruction permits pelvic examination that can aid in the early diagnosis of recurrence. It facilitates intracavitary radiation if indicated, supports the base of the bladder and thereby prevents bladder dysfunction that can follow vaginectomy.

Management of patients with vaginal stenosis secondary to radiation therapy presents a more difficult problem. Extensive fibrosis and absence of normal tissue planes make elimination of the scar tissue difficult or impossible. At operation, the scar must be excised and the cavity enlarged maximally.[52] In some patients an adequate cavity can be developed by incision of the levator muscles. A split thickness skin graft then is placed and supported for seven days by a soft vaginal pack. It is likely that the grafted skin will survive, but varying degrees of rigidity often remain. No attempt should be made to reconstruct the vagina damaged by radiation until all acute reaction has subsided.

Following Vaginectomy with Removal of Bladder and Rectum

The technique of vaginal reconstruction in patients undergoing pelvic exenteration requires optimal timing of the procedure. Four approaches to this complex problem presently are available:

1. Morley[29] described a vaginal reconstruction procedure that utilizes a split thickness skin graft. About six to eight weeks after exenteration, when the healing pelvic cavity is approximately the size of the vaginal tube, the graft is applied to the bed of granulation tissue and is immobilized for one week by a soft pack. The pack then is replaced by a removable vaginal mold that is worn intermittently until healing is complete. The patient and her husband are counselled and encouraged to resume sexual activity within 2 months following the reconstructive operation. The functional result usually is quite satisfactory, although in some instances the vaginal cavity may decrease progressively in size after placement of the graft. This most commonly occurs with poorly motivated couples who do not resume sexual activity following vaginal reconstruction. Complications associated with this technique include evisceration of free loops of bowel through the perineal defect.

2. The use of an isolated segment of sigmoid colon for vaginal reconstruction was described by Pratt and Smith.[35] By this technique the distal sigmoid colon is mobilized and fixed to the vaginal introitus. The procedure must be performed at the time of the exenteration and usually results in a vagina of satisfactory dimensions. This method is useful in patients who are not candidates for rectal substitution using the sigmoid colon. A major disadvantage of the procedure is the heavy intermittent mucoid drainage experienced by many patients.

3. McCraw et al[27] have developed a technique using gracilis myocutaneous flaps for vaginal reconstruction at the time of pelvic exenteration. The gracilis muscle and overlying skin are brought from the thigh to the perineum through a subcutaneous tunnel. The vascular pedicle to the muscle which also supplies the overlying skin is preserved. Bilateral myocutaneous flaps are dissected and sewn together to form a vaginal tube that is inserted into the open pelvic cavity. The procedure provides a fatty, musculocutaneous tissue mass that serves as a functional vagina. In addition, the neovagina has sufficient bulk to fill a large part of the empty pelvic cavity following pelvic exenteration thereby decreasing the risk of complications related to the raw pelvic floor. The major disadvantage of the procedure is the increase in operative time for the pelvic exenteration. The resulting lower limb scars have not been

debilitating, but may limit early postoperative ambulation. The results of the procedure are promising but further trial is needed.

4. Patients who previously have undergone pelvic exenteration and are free of disease often desire restoration of vaginal function many months or years after operation. Construction of an internal vagina with dissection of the pelvic cavity after extensive fibrosis has occurred neither is feasible nor safe because of the high risk of intestinal or urinary fistulae. Williams[56] described the construction of an external pouch that functions well as a vagina. The steps of the procedure are shown in Figure 24–1. The depth of the pouch is determined by the length of the lateral incisions.[38] While maximal vaginal depth is most desirable, the lateral incision should remain below the level of the clitoris in order to permit intromission. The incisions should be placed as lateral as possible in order to construct a vagina of satisfactory caliber. Obese patients and those with abundant subcutaneous tissue in the region of the vulva are suited best for the procedure, as this tissue permits the formation of a vagina of adequate size. Initially, the vertical angle and the long axis of the neovagina will be more anterior than normal. With use, the vagina will be inclined in a more normal direction.

In our own series of 23 patients undergoing vaginal reconstruction after extensive treatment for pelvic malignancy, a functional vagina was achieved in 18 instances.[52] The remaining 5 patients cannot be evaluated because of recent reconstruction or recurrence of tumor. Split thickness skin grafts have been the procedures of choice in most patients undergoing vaginectomy or pelvic exenteration, while vulvar pouches have proved satisfactory in patients with a contraindication to the formation of an internal vagina. In 5 instances, a combination of two methods was required to obtain a functional result. These involved split thickness skin grafts together with either an external vulvar pouch or a sigmoid colon transplant.

It often is difficult to establish a functional vagina after extensive treatment of a pelvic malignancy. Successful restoration of anatomy is not always possible, and when accomplished is not always associated with complete sexual rehabilitation. Surgical techniques are sufficiently advanced to offer vaginal reconstruction to most of these patients; however, the levels of emotional and sexual adjustment that existed before treatment also are reflected in the final result.

Restoration of Rectal Function

The disability resulting from a permanent colostomy is a major obstacle to the rehabilitation of patients undergoing total or posterior pelvic exenteration. Bacon,[60] Swenson and Bill[45] and others have shown that normal rectal function can be achieved by substituting a segment of sigmoid colon for the resected rectum. The reconstruction can be attempted only if the rectal sphincter can be preserved while providing wide surgical clearance of the tumor. In suitable candidates, rectal substitution, which is performed at the time of pelvic exenteration, can obviate the need for permanent colostomy and decrease the disability that otherwise would result.[24]

The extent of the operative procedure with preservation of the rectal sphincter is outlined in Figure 24–2. Total exenteration involves the en bloc removal of the tumor and adjacent organs, including the rectum, vagina, uterus, adnexae and bladder.[5,6,37,47] The colon is transected superiorly at the recto-sigmoid junction and inferiorly at the rectal sphincter. The descending colon and splenic flexure then are freed from their lateral peritoneal attachments. The most critical portion of the operative procedure is the preservation of adequate blood supply while mobilizing the sigmoid colon. To allow the distal sigmoid to reach the level of the rectal sphincter without tension, the remaining sigmoid colon is mobilized by ligating all but the most superior branches of the inferior mesenteric artery (Fig. 24–3). A wide cuff of mesentery must be mobilized with the sigmoid colon to preserve the blood supply provided by the marginal artery of Drummond. Interruption of this arterial segment usually results in ischemic necrosis of the distal colon.

The transverse colon is transected near the mobilized splenic flexure and the distal segment is brought out through the abdominal wall as a mucous fistula. The functioning transverse colostomy then must be placed immediately adjacent to the mucous fistula (Fig. 24–4). The intervening segment of transverse colon is isolated for use as a urinary conduit as noted in Figure 24–3. The distal portion of the bowel segment to be used as the urinary conduit is closed with a double layer of polyglycolic acid sutures after which the ureters are implanted. The base of the conduit is anchored to the posterior peritoneum and the proximal portion is brought through the anterior abdominal wall as a stoma.

The anastomosis of the sigmoid colon to the

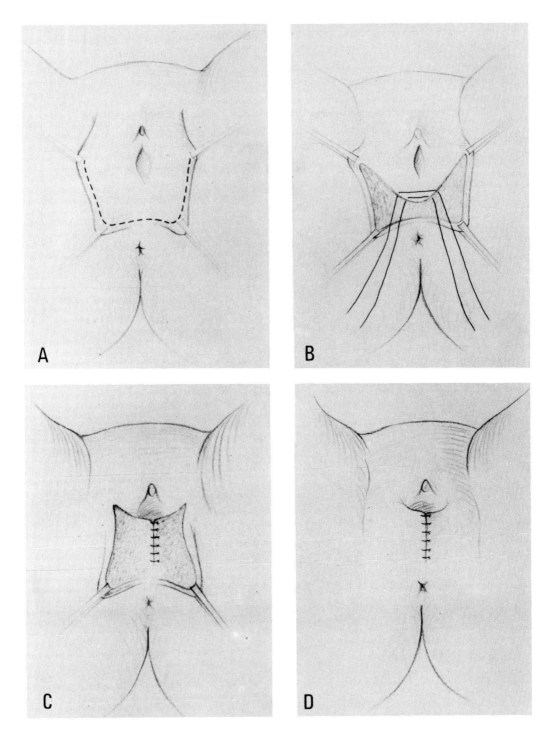

Figure 24–1A. The labia majora are retracted laterally using noncrushing clamps. The U-shaped incision usually is made just medial to the labial-crural fold across the posterior fourchette. The mucosa is undermined posteriorly in the midline to allow mobilization. B. Beginning posteriorly, the medial edges of the incision are approximated using 3-0 interrupted polyglycolic acid sutures. The skin of the labia minora thus is turned inward becoming the posterior vaginal wall as depicted in C. C. The approximation of the medial edges of the incision is now completed and the posterior vaginal wall constructed. D. The lateral edges of the wound are now approximated in the midline. The labia majora thus form an extension and reinforcement of the perineal body. Note that only two layers are used for closure as the placement of a third subcutaneous layer causes the neovagina to be too constricted and rigid for optimum function.

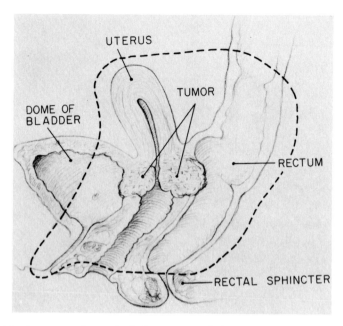

Figure 24–2. Total exenteration to include removal of all structures shown within broken line.

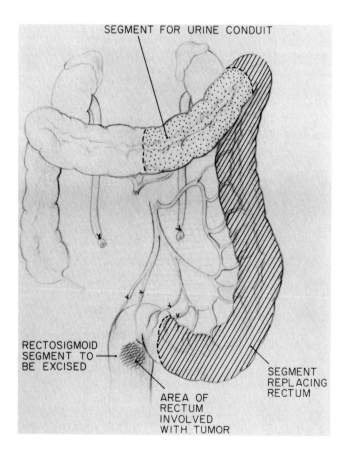

Figure 24–3. Segments of colon to be used for rectal substitution and urine conduit after excision of recto-sigmoid segment.

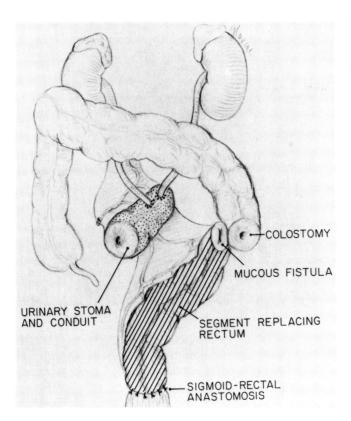

URINARY STOMA
AND CONDUIT

COLOSTOMY

MUCOUS FISTULA

SEGMENT REPLACING
RECTUM

SIGMOID-RECTAL
ANASTOMOSIS

Figure 24–4. Postoperative location of segment replacing rectum. Mucous fistula positioned next to colostomy stoma.

rectal stump is carried out through a perineal approach. The distal sigmoid colon is either drawn through the rectal sphincter, everting the stump of the rectum, or anastomosed through the vaginal introitus. Both methods have been found to be technically satisfactory. A single row of interrupted polyglycolic acid sutures is used to approximate the full thickness of the bowel walls. The vaginal introitus is left partially open to allow drainage and to permit periodic inspection of the colorectal anastomosis.

Closure of the colostomy should be considered four to six months after rectal substitution following evaluation of the colorectal anastomosis and rectal sphincter. A radiopaque contrast medium is instilled in the distal segment to assess the integrity of the anastomosis. Sphincter function is evaluated by instilling saline and then injecting air into the neorectum. The colostomy may be closed after demonstration of a satisfactory sphincteric mechanism and a healed anastomosis. Figure 24–5 shows the segments as they appear after bowel continuity is restored.

Of 25 patients who underwent rectal substitution at the time of pelvic exenteration at UCLA Medical Center and City of Hope, 6 died of tu-

mor, 5 experienced necrosis of the colorectal anastomosis, and 14 have successful anastomosis. Excellent rectal function was established in 12 of the 14 as judged by the presence of the appropriate sensation and good sphincter control without leakage of liquid, solid stool, or gas. Two patients have occasional stool incontinence, which is avoided by the use of enemas. No patient who died of tumor had a recurrence below the colorectal anastomosis. The major problem of rectal substitution is maintaining the viability of the distal transplanted sigmoid colon. When this heals without necrosis, excellent rectal function can be anticipated.

Rectal reconstruction demands increased attention to surgical detail and additional operating time. While not suitable for all patients undergoing exenteration, it can help to restore selected individuals to a more normal life.

Operative Approaches to Urinary Tract Dysfunction

Ureteral Obstruction and Injury

Obstruction or injury of the ureter can result from tumor compression, operative trauma, or

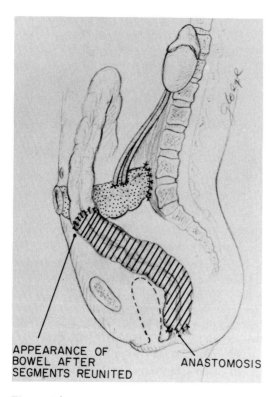

APPEARANCE OF
BOWEL AFTER
SEGMENTS REUNITED   ANASTOMOSIS

Figure 24–5.   Appearance of colon after closure of colostomy and reestablishment of continuity.

the effects of radiation therapy. When bilateral ureteral obstruction results from massive recurrence of a previously radiated and unresectable pelvic tumor, it is appropriate only to provide supportive care and to avoid attempts to relieve the obstruction. Death from progressive uremia with hyperkalemia seems preferable to the agony of prolonged pain and bleeding that will result if urinary diversion is performed in such patients. Operative correction of unilateral ureteral obstruction in patients with known pelvic recurrence also rarely is indicated unless severe infection that is unresponsive to antibiotics develops. Occasional patients with progressive or complete ureteral obstruction in the absence of tumor and those with ureteral fistula will require operation. No single procedure is suitable in all clinical circumstances. Any approach requires knowledge of the location of the injury or obstruction and the overall condition of the patient.

Macaset et al[25] have shown that patients with fistula of the lower third of the ureter are managed best by a neoureterocystostomy, reimplantation of the ureter into the fundus of the bladder.

This technique requires identification of the damaged ureteral segment and transection of the ureter proximal to the site of injury. The spatulated end of the ureter then is anastomosed to the full thickness of the bladder wall. The anastomosis is carried out over a soft ureteral catheter or infant-feeding tube, which usually is left in place for four to five days. Suprapubic drainage is maintained for at least 10 days in patients who have undergone ureteral reimplantation.

If a long segment of the distal ureter is damaged, the bladder can be mobilized and fixed to the psoas muscle, permitting the anastomosis of the shortened ureter directly into the bladder while minimizing tension on the ureterovesical anastomosis. This psoas hitch procedure may be suitable for nonradiated patients, and often can compensate for the loss of several centimeters of ureter. In previously radiated patients with bladder contraction and pelvic fibrosis, the immobility of the bladder can make this procedure impossible.

When the bladder cannot be mobilized sufficiently to compensate for loss of ureteral length, or when injury has occurred to the middle or proximal third of the ureter, an appropriate segment of intestine can be interposed between the ureter and the bladder. This procedure may be associated with postoperative urinary stasis and ureteral reflux that can lead to acute and chronic pyelonephritis.

Transureteroureterostomy is an alternative management of proximal ureteral injury or obstruction.[49] The damaged ureter is transected and brought across the retroperitoneal space to the opposite side. An end to side anastomosis to the uninvolved ureter is carried out. Ureteral catheterization is maintained as with neoureterocystostomy. One disadvantage is seen in the patient with upper urinary infection on the side of ureteral injury. After transureteroureterostomy, the infection can become bilateral and thus jeopardize both kidneys.

Other valuable procedures for the temporary management of ureteral obstruction or fistulae include cutaneous ureterostomy and tube ureterostomy. Unilateral cutaneous ureterostomy can bypass an obstruction up to one year in patients not suited for other procedures because of poor operative condition. Because of the tendency for stenosis at the ureterocutaneous junction, the best candidates for this procedure are those with ureteral dilatation secondary to obstruction. Retrograde infection is a common complication of this procedure. Tube ureterostomy is particularly useful in patients with bilateral ureteral obstruction and advanced uremia who are seen prior to any treatment of their pelvic malignancy. Despite the bilateral nature of the obstruction, this temporizing procedure usually is carried out unilaterally through an extraperitoneal approach. An infant feeding tube is satisfactory and can be left in place for many weeks, during which time radiation therapy can be delivered to the tumor. Should an adequate clinical response result and the obstruction resolve, the urine again can pass into the bladder and the tube can be removed. It may be advantageous to choose the left ureter for tube ureterostomy because of the greater incidence of antecedent right sided pyelonephritis in women and consequent underlying kidney damage. Tube ureterostomy is preferable to nephrostomy, which is associated with a higher incidence of infection and increased discomfort. Nephrostomy may be indicated rarely in the septic patient with complicated ureteral injuries in whom ureteral reimplantation is both dangerous and impractical and in whom adequate contralateral kidney function has been assured.

Urinary Diversion

Urinary diversion is required when the bladder is removed, or when it has been so severely damaged by radiation or tumor infiltration that it cannot be made functional. Early efforts at urinary diversion involved insertion of ureters into the intact colon as a ureterosigmoidostomy or a wet colostomy.[8] This allowed the admixture of the urinary and fecal streams. These methods were not satisfactory because of frequent urinary tract infections, metabolic complications, and incontinence. Studies have revealed higher intraluminal pressures in the intact colon than in the ureter thus leading to ureteral reflux and chronic pyelonephritis.[36,39] Excessive reabsorption of chloride by the bowel mucosa often resulted in hyperchloremic acidosis.[42] In addition, the rectal sphincter often was incapable of preventing urinary loss. Finally, when urine and stool drained through the same bowel segment, the stoma always was difficult to manage.

Bricker[4] first used an isolated loop of ileum as a urinary conduit, thereby avoiding many of the metabolic and infectious complications seen when the intact bowel was used as a urinary reservoir. Until relatively recently, the ileum was used almost exclusively for urinary conduit forma-

tion.[10,43] For many gynecologic cancer patients, another segment of bowel is more appropriate. The majority of patients who require urinary diversion have had extensive radiation therapy and are at high risk to leak at the site of ileal reanastomosis and/or at the ureteroconduit anastomosis.[13] In addition, urine diversion in most gynecologic oncology patients is carried out at the time of a total pelvic exenteration. In these instances, the distal sigmoid usually is transected. This frees a portion of colon for use as a urinary conduit, and avoids the necessity of an additional bowel anastomosis.

Symmonds[46] has demonstrated that the sigmoid colon functions well as a urinary conduit. Although the ability of the colonic mucosa to absorb electrolytes differs from that of the ileum, hyperchloremic acidosis occurs infrequently when either the ileum or colon is utilized as a conduit and not a reservoir.[51] The sigmoid colon usually is redundant and possesses a mobile mesentery that allows optimal placement of the cutaneous stoma. This segment is not always the best choice for a conduit because of prior radiation damage or occasionally inadequate mesenteric length. In addition, adequate resection of the tumor often requires removal of a large portion of the sigmoid colon. Finally, sigmoid colon may be needed for rectal or vaginal reconstruction. Nelson[31] suggested that the transverse colon might be useful as a urinary conduit because the transverse mesocolon is mobile and the large vascular arcades of the middle colic artery are present. In addition, this bowel segment usually is outside the field of prior radiation.

Our own studies suggest that the choice of an appropriate segment depends on many factors and that the ileum, sigmoid colon, or transverse colon may provide a suitable segment of bowel in the appropriate circumstances. In patients undergoing anterior exenteration, ileum is chosen for the urinary conduit. If extensive radiation changes exist, proximal ileum or even jejunum is chosen. A segment of colon is preferred in patients undergoing total exenteration or urinary diversion for relief of radiation-induced obstruction or fistula.

OPERATIVE PROCEDURE

The bowel segment best suited for the conduit is determined. Approximately 20 cm of well-vascularized intestine are isolated to insure at least two large vessels within the mesentery. The intestinal segment is prepared by isolating it from the adjacent bowel and dissecting the surrounding fat from the distal end for a distance of 1 cm. After isolation, the proximal end of the conduit is closed in two layers with polyglycolic acid sutures to avoid leakage at the base of the conduit. The ureters then are mobilized to the level of the pelvic brim with care to preserve the adjacent vasculature of the surrounding peritoneum. The incised end of the ureter then is spatulated by making a 4-mm incision in the long axis. The serosa of the ureter is sutured to the serosa of the intestine with two or three stay sutures in order to stabilize the ureter and allow a more secure anastomosis to the intestine. The intestinal opening is made, and the ureter anastomosed to the full thickness of the intestine with a single row of polyglycolic acid sutures. Before the anterior row of sutures is completed, a ureteral catheter is passed retrograde into the ureteral opening to the pelvis of the kidney, then antegrade into the conduit and out through the stoma where it is fixed. The ureteral anastomosis should be free of tension, and there should be no kinking of the ureter as it approaches the conduit. The base of the conduit then is anchored to the posterior peritoneum. The appropriate stoma site is determined preoperatively by examining the patient in the erect and sitting positions. The area that is chosen should be flat, distant from the abdominal wound or any scar, and so located that the patient can reach the area easily to change the appliance and clean the surrounding skin.

A full thickness core of tissue sufficiently large to admit the conduit without undue constriction is removed from the abdominal wall and the conduit is brought through the opening. The serosa of the bowel then is fixed to the abdominal fascia with interrupted sutures. The stoma is everted and sutured so that the most distal portion protrudes 1 cm above the level of the skin. This allows for the application of a water-tight appliance. The ureteral catheters are transfixed to the abdominal wall and identified as to side of placement. The ureteral catheters usually are removed in four to five days. A temporary appliance is placed before the patient leaves the operating room.

At UCLA Medical Center and City of Hope, 59 patients underwent urinary diversion. The sigmoid colon was used for the conduit in 25 patients, the transverse colon in 24 patient, the ascending colon in 1 patient, and the ileum in 9 patients. Our experience with these 59 patients suggests that the colon functions as well as the ileum for a urinary conduit, and that transverse and sigmoid colon are equally satisfactory. Because most gynecologic patients have been previously radiated, colon conduits may be preferable in many instances.

PREVENTION AND MANAGEMENT OF SERIOUS COMPLICATIONS

Patients treated for advanced gynecologic malignancy are at high risk to develop complications from both the treatment and the recurrence of tumor. New information regarding the prevention and management of these complications has become available. One of these problems concerns the severe catabolic state seen in patients undergoing extensive surgery, radiation, and chemotherapy or when recurrent tumor is present. Parenteral nutrition often is useful in these patients. Another problem is the high incidence of pulmonary thromboembolism in patients with gynecologic malignancies. Preventive measures that promise to reduce the risk of thromboembolism are now available. Other complications can result from small intestinal injuries following radiation therapy. While these injuries still are difficult to manage, the results achieved with carefully planned programs are promising. Finally, an increased incidence of intestinal complications has been noted in patients who have undergone pretreatment operative evaluation for cervical cancer followed by radiation therapy. An operative staging technique devised at UCLA Medical Center promises to reduce the incidence of these complications and to allow the potential benefit of more accurate staging to be assessed.

Total Parenteral Nutrition

The delivery of total nutritional requirements by the intravenous route first was reported by Dudrick et al[11] in 1967. In a study comparing weight and growth of litter-mate puppies, animals given hypertonic glucose and protein hydrolysate as the only source of nutrition showed greater weight gain than control animals maintained on a standard oral diet. Dudrick and others[12] subsequently reported normal development in infants and maintenance of positive nitrogen balance in adults receiving intravenous feedings without oral supplementation. It now is known that nutrients are used as efficiently when given by vein as by mouth.

Normal adults require from 1500 to 3000 calories per day, but have increased caloric needs during illness and following operation.[18,20] When these increased caloric needs are not met, characteristic metabolic events, including the breakdown of fat stores and protein catabolism for gluconeogenesis, occur. Protein depletion can be minimized by providing 3 to 5 percent free amino acids or protein hydrolysate intravenously. Similarly, caloric needs may be met by the intravenous infusion of 10 to 50 percent dextrose solutions containing 340 to 1700 calories per liter. Additional calories may be provided as fat by infusing a 10 percent lipid emulsion derived from soybean oil.[26]

Total parenteral nutrition (TPN) is delivered through a central venous catheter and requires meticulous attention to detail and careful patient monitoring. A large-bore teflon catheter is placed in the subclavian vein and is anchored so that activity does not result in catheter movement. Strict antiseptic technique is maintained during insertion. Radiographic confirmation is required to assure that the catheter tip is in the superior vena cava. Antiseptic measures following catheter insertion include the use of a millipore filter that is changed daily, and avoidance of the venous catheter for withdrawing blood or infusing substances other than nutrients. Nutrient solutions are prepared with meticulous aseptic technique in the hospital pharmacy under laminar flow precautions.

Prior to initiation of TPN, tests of blood-clotting status, liver function, renal function, serum electrolytes, serum proteins, and cardiac status are reviewed. Patients who receive TPN are monitored according to a prescribed protocol that includes temperature and fractional urines taken every six hours, measurements of weight, intake, and output, serum glucose and serum electrolytes daily, complete blood count, prothrombin time, creatinine, calcium, magnesium, and phosphorus twice weekly, total protein, serum albumin, liver function, renal function studies, and serum platelets weekly.

Patients who do not have cardiac, renal, or hepatic disease usually tolerate 3000 to 4000 ml per day of 20 percent glucose and 5 percent ca-

sein hydrolysate. The solutions are delivered by a constant infusion pump, and should be started at a rate of 90 ml per hour. This may be increased to 140 ml per hour over a period of several days. Water soluble and fat soluble vitamins must be given daily, and vitamin K is administered weekly. Calcium, phosphate, and magnesium are replaced daily. The trace elements, zinc and copper, are replaced daily in milligram amounts or weekly as provided by the administration of fresh frozen plasma. Blood transfusions are given as needed to maintain the hematocrit above 30 percent, and sodium and potassium are replaced as needed. Insulin may be required if high serum glucose levels are noted. Patients with severe hepatic, cardiac, or renal disease are given these solutions with great caution because amino acids are poorly tolerated by patients with hepatic impairment and large fluid volumes may be contraindicated in the presence of severe cardiac or renal disease.

Complications of TPN by central venous catheter may be related either to the placement and maintenance of the subclavian catheter or to metabolic disturbances associated with the substances infused.[40] Immediate catheter complications include pneumothorax, air embolism, and trauma to the subclavian vein which may lead to hemothorax, hydrothorax, or subcutaneous hematoma. Later catheter complications include vein thrombosis at the catheter tip and bacterial or fungal sepsis. Metabolic complications of TPN include hyperosmolality, acidosis, electrolyte imbalance, hyperglycemia, hypophosphatemia, and hypoprothrombinemia. Meticulous attention to the metabolic status of patients on total parenteral nutrition should avoid many of these complications.

Indications for parenteral nutrition in oncologic patients include preoperative preparation of the debilitated patient, postoperative support of patients in whom bowel rest is indicated or anorexia persists, dysfunctional gastrointestinal tract associated with radiation therapy, intestinal fistula or obstruction, and nutritional support during intensive chemotherapy or radiation.[9,16] There is a larger group of patients in whom potential benefits of TPN are clear but the risks may outweigh these benefits. Such patients may have sepsis, less severe gastrointestinal dysfunction or may undergo less extensive operative procedures. Some of these patients can be managed by tube feedings; however, others will not tolerate any form of oral alimentation.

Parenteral Nutrition by Peripheral Vein

In an effort to simplify the delivery, to reduce potential hazards, and to broaden the scope of parenteral nutrition, we have used a peripheral rather than a central vein for infusion. The technique is a modification of that used in pediatric patients and utilizes solutions containing 10 percent glucose and 5 percent casein hydrolysate instead of higher concentrations of glucose that invariably lead to peripheral vein thrombosis. Each vein is used for only 48 hours, following which the catheter is moved to another site. Patients receiving parenteral nutrition by peripheral vein require the same monitoring as those on central venous TPN, except that the infusion usually need not be discontinued in the presence of sepsis. The method generally is simpler and therefore more widely applicable. It may be started preoperatively, discontinued during the operation, and then restarted immediately postoperatively The continuous infusion by pump is begun at the rate of 90 ml per hour and gradually increased to maximum volumes tolerated, usually 150 ml per hour.

Over a one year interval, 24 gynecologic oncology patients at UCLA Medical Center requiring nutritional support for indications listed received parenteral nutrition by peripheral vein only, without oral supplementation. Only 2 patients experienced weight loss while under therapy for intervals up to six weeks. There were no complications related to the infusion site or to abnormal metabolic states associated with the substances infused. Anaphylaxis due to an immediate allergic response to infused casein hydrolysate was noted in one patient, and hypoprothrombinemia related to insufficient treatment with vitamin K was noted in another.

Parenteral nutrition by peripheral vein is not intended to replace TPN by central vein. The latter is mandatory in patients with severe hypercatabolic states in whom a maximal rate of weight gain is desired. Nevertheless, peripheral venous supplementation delivers approximately 1800 calories per day in a volume of 3500 ml, and in conjunction with a 10 percent intravenous lipid emulsion may provide an additional 550 to 1100 calories per day in 500 to 1000 ml of fluid.[48] Increasing numbers of oncologic patients being subjected to complex diagnostic and therapeutic measures will benefit from parenteral nutrition.

Prevention of Thromboembolism

Pulmonary embolism is one of the major causes of death and disability in patients undergoing treatment for cancer. Kakkar, at the University of London, has published a noteworthy series of studies dealing with the prevention of deep vein thrombosis and subsequent pulmonary embolism by prophylactic low-dose heparin. These studies and others show that deep vein thrombosis beginning in the popliteal system almost always precedes pulmonary embolism.[21] It has been confirmed that about half the patients with deep vein thrombosis, as diagnosed by I^{125} fibrinogen scans, have no clinical signs or symptoms.[14,30,33] This explains the frequent occurrence of pulmonary emboli in patients with no clinical evidence for deep vein thrombosis. Studies also have shown that about one-half of lower limb deep vein thromboses begin intraoperatively, and the other half postoperatively.[22] The need for the institution of preventive measures prior to operation in patients at risk is clear.

Those patients who develop deep vein thrombosis are at highest risk for pulmonary thromboembolism. In a well-controlled collaborative study, also by Kakkar,[23] of 4196 patients undergoing operation, small doses of heparin begun preoperatively and continued postoperatively reduced the incidence of both deep vein thrombosis and death from pulmonary emboli. The prophylactic use of low-dose subcutaneous heparin did not cause increased intraoperative or postoperative bleeding, but was associated with a significant increase in wound hematoma formation.

Several studies have identified risk factors for deep vein thrombosis in patients undergoing operation. One study has quantified the risk of deep vein thrombosis in patients with known high risk factors (Table 24–1). While precise risk of pulmonary embolism following deep vein thrombosis cannot be determined for the individual patient, the value of low-dose heparin in the prevention of fatal sequelae of this process appears to outweigh the risks associated with its use. As a result, low-dose heparin is given to any gynecologic oncology patient at UCLA Medical Center requiring prolonged immobilization or undergoing major operation, and may be indicated in all high-risk patients undergoing operation.

Patients receiving low-dose heparin therapy do not require extensive monitoring.[2,57] Heparin usually is started the evening prior to operation, and

Table 24–1. INCIDENCE OF DEEP VEIN THROMBOSIS IN 203 POSTOPERATIVE PATIENTS*

CLINICAL DIAGNOSIS	NO. PTS. AT RISK	NO. PTS. WITH DEEP VEIN THROMBOSIS
Prior pulmonary emboli	6	6 (100%)
Prior deep vein thrombosis	19	13 (68%)
Varicose veins	39	22 (56%)
Average age 60 years	59	27 (46%)
Malignancy	59	24 (41%)
Total patients studied	203	62 (31%)

*From Kakkar VV: Am J Surg 120:527, 1970.

is continued every 12 hours for one week or until discharge. The dose of heparin is 5000 international units given subcutaneously in a concentration of 20,000 units per ml. The injection site carefully avoids any planned surgical incision. Routine clotting studies are not performed unless there is a history of bleeding disorder, since changes in these have not been reported when heparin is used as described. If excessive bleeding is noted at any time, heparin is discontinued.

Small Intestinal Injuries

Small intestinal injuries may follow radiation therapy, extensive pelvic operation, or combinations of these therapeutic modalities. Full-course radiation through external pelvic portals can deliver a substantial dose to portions of small intestine resulting in injury from obliterative endarteritis and impaired blood supply. The distal ileum in particular often is heavily irradiated because of its fixed location in or near the pelvis. There is ample evidence that small intestinal loops fixed by adhesions from previous operation also are more susceptible to radiation damage.[19,41] Small intestinal injury with fistula formation can follow pelvic exenteration, especially if preceded by pelvic radiation.

Patients with small intestinal injuries present with a constellation of complaints. The early effects of radiation damage to the small intestine are manifested by diarrhea. The intestine can be so hyperactive as to require hospitalization of the patient, bowel rest, and parenteral restoration of fluid and electrolyte balance. The acute reaction to radiation therapy often responds to strict adherence to a bland, low-residue diet supplemented with narcotic derivatives such as paregoric, which slows intestinal motility. More serious radiation injury is manifest by nausea, vomiting, anorexia, abdominal distention, and often the radiographic findings of dilated loops of small bowel. The clinical picture may be that of bowel obstruction or radiation enteritis. A focus of injured bowel can heal spontaneously; however, obstruction or fistula often results.[17] Patients suffering from radiation damage may develop chronic symptoms including episodic anorexia, nausea, abdominal cramping, and distention, all of which may be associated with normal abdominal roentgenographic findings. There may be progressive weight loss and intermittent bouts suggestive of partial small bowel obstruction. The management of chronic radiation injury often is complex and conservative medical and dietary management almost always are preferable to operative intervention. Prolongation of symptomatic episodes may require parenteral nutrition for maintenance of positive nitrogen balance.

Operative intervention in patients with intestinal injuries is reserved for those patients with clinical evidence of obstruction unrelieved by a trial of conservative therapy, and for certain patients with fistula. Many small intestinal fistulas which drain anteriorly through the abdominal wall and some which drain through the perineum may heal spontaneously following a program of bowel rest and parenteral nutrition. When there is obstruction distal to the fistula, when the individual segment has received previous high doses of irradiation or when the fistula is a perineal one occurring after pelvic exenteration, spontaneous healing is unlikely.[3,44] In these cases operation within 2 weeks of occurrence of the injury may result in improved survival.

Intestinal Fistulae

PREOPERATIVE MANAGEMENT
Initial preoperative management includes contrast studies of the intestinal tract using water-soluble opaque media to localize the site of the fistula and to rule out a colonic fistula (Table

Table 24-2.   10 POINT PROGRAM FOR THE MANAGE-
MENT OF INTESTINAL FISTULAE

Preoperative	I.	Hypaque X rays
	II.	Small bowel tube
	III.	Hyperalimentation
	IV.	Prophylactic antibiotics (gram negative, anaerobic)
	V.	Minimal delay to surgery (usually <14 days)
Intraoperative	VI.	Isolation not excision of damaged segment
	VII.	Mucocutaneous fistulae for defunctionalized segment
	VIII.	Enterocolostomy, side-to-side
	IX.	Cutaneous ileostomy when tumor present
Postoperative	X.	Continue preoperative measures
		A. GI suction (10-14 days)
		B. Hyperalimentation (14-21 days)
		C. Antibiotics (7-14 days)

24-2). While some of the mucosal detail may be lost by using water-soluble media instead of barium, such media precludes the marked peritoneal irritation associated with spillage of barium into the abdominal cavity. After x-rays have been performed, efforts should be made to place a long tube into the small intestine to reduce drainage of small bowel contents through the fistula and to decompress any existing obstruction. At operation, the tube is helpful in identifying afferent and efferent loops of small intestine, and postoperatively it serves to maintain decompression of the small bowel.

Parenteral nutrition should be started as soon as a small bowel fistula is diagnosed. Many of these patients are already poorly nourished because of recent operation, recurrent tumor, malabsorption or obstruction. The usual precautions must be taken to avoid sepsis and to prevent fluid and electrolyte imbalance resulting from the infusion of markedly hyperosmolar solutions. If the patient is febrile, parenteral nutrition by peripheral vein, as previously discussed is preferable to catheterization of a central vein. Prophylactic antibiotics are administered preoperatively in view of the inherent contamination of the surgical field with bowel contents. Because distal small bowel flora are predominantly anaerobic and gram-negative organisms, combination antibiotic therapy is used. Coverage for gram-negative bacteria may consist of an aminoglycoside, a synthetic penicillin, or a cephalosporin compound. Coverage for anaerobic bacteria may consist of either clindamycin, carbenicillin, or chloramphenicol.

The interval between diagnosis of the fistula and operative intervention should be as short as feasible, while allowing for correction of anemia, acid-base problems, electrolyte abnormalities, dehydration and the institution of the steps outlined. Whenever possible, this interval should be less than two weeks.[3]

INTRAOPERATIVE MANAGEMENT

The operative procedure employed in the management of small intestinal fistulae should be designed to reestablish intestinal continuity and minimize the risk of subsequent bowel obstruction or recurrent fistula. Afferent loops of small bowel should be identified early in the procedure by following the course of the indwelling tube. Most fistulae are located in the mid or terminal ileum (Fig. 24-6). The bowel is transected just proximal to the fistula so that maximal length of healthy bowel is preserved. Distally, the transection is made either at the junction of the cecum and ascending colon or across a segment of ileum just proximal to the ileocecal valve, but distal to the damaged segment. It is important that the damaged segment be left in place to prevent other bowel loops from adhering to raw surfaces and becoming damaged.[54]

Both ends of the isolated bowel segment should be brought to the skin as mucous fistulae to prevent closed-loop obstruction. Anastomosis is made between the transected proximal ileum and either ascending or transverse colon (Fig. 24-7). Because the heavily irradiated bowel wall

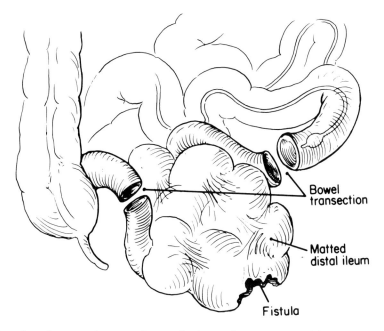

Figure 24–6. Identification of loops of small bowel and transection of bowel proximal and distal to fistula.

frequently may have impaired blood supply, we believe safety of the anastomosis may be improved by employing a side to side technique after closing the ends of the transected ileum and colon. In the patient who is severely debilitated or in whom extensive recurrent tumor is present, cutaneous ileostomy can be used since the procedure is shorter, and is associated with less blood loss and a significantly shorter period of convalescence.

POSTOPERATIVE MANAGEMENT
Patients who have undergone anastomoses should be managed with gastrointestinal suction until active peristalsis and passage of flatus occur. This often requires 14 days or more after operation. Similarly, parenteral nutrition should be continued until oral intake provides sufficient calories to offset negative nitrogen balance. Antibiotics are continued for at least one week postoperatively.

The surgical approach described here appears to offer a better chance of success than resection or primary repair of the fistula, both of which have been associated with high recurrence rates.[44] The importance of complete isolation of the small bowel fistula from the functional intestinal tract is

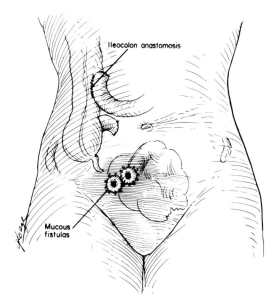

Figure 24–7. Creation of enterocolonic anastomosis and mucous fistulae.

emphasized and failure to do this may result in little improvement in the loss of intestinal contents through the fistula. A side to side anastomosis without isolation from the intestinal stream will not succeed. As significant postoperative morbidity may result from pulmonary problems of atelectasis and pneumonia, and since these conditions can be aggravated by a tube in the nasopharynx for prolonged periods, tube gastrostomy may be included in the operative procedure in an attempt to avoid these complications.

Operative Evaluation of Cervical Cancer

It is axiomatic that therapy will fail if malignancy exists beyond the field of therapy. It follows, therefore, that improved staging efforts that define more accurately the extent of disease are desirable and ultimately could lead to improved survival in patients who currently fail conventional therapy. Numerous reports have shown that patients with cervical cancer treated with operation or radiation aimed at controlling disease in the pelvis alone fail treatment because of the presence of metastases in the aortic lymph nodes or beyond.[1,32,50] Clinical staging is inaccurate in this group of patients. Some patients in whom operative evaluation revealed common iliac or aortic node involvement have received radiation therapy to an extended field, which includes the aortic node chain to the level of the twelfth thoracic vertebra.[15,62] However, it is not yet clear how many of these patients can be salvaged by this treatment.[58]

Transperitoneal operative staging with pelvic and periaortic lymph node sampling when followed by radiation therapy has resulted in a dramatic increase in reported complications as compared with standard radiation therapy in the absence of pretreatment operative evaluation. Piver and Barlow[34] reported 57 percent morbidity and 19 percent mortality from therapy in patients with positive aortic nodes so staged and subsequently treated with pelvic and aortic irradiation therapy using 6000 rads in split doses to the aortic area. Wharton et al[53] also reported increased morbidity in patients so managed, and noted a 17 percent mortality from the combination of surgical staging and radiation therapy. These complications presumably are due to the irradiation of larger volumes of tissue including the periaortic areas, and to the fixation of loops of small intestine by adhesions, especially in the areas of the posterior peritoneal incisions over the aorta and pelvic vessels.

Operative Staging by Extraperitoneal Approach

In an effort to achieve the benefits of operative evaluation while avoiding the high associated morbidity and mortality, we developed an extraperitoneal rather than transperitoneal operative approach that appears to decrease the postoperative formation of adhesions.[59] A lateral vertical incision is made from a point just above the level of the umbilicus and two fingers medial to the left external iliac crest down to the level of the iliac crest and then parallel to the inguinal ligament (Fig. 24-8). The incision is carried through the fascia of the external and internal oblique muscles and the transversalis fascia near the lateral border of the rectus abdominus muscle. The peritoneum is opened anteriorly for a distance of 15 cm to permit abdominal exploration and to rule out intra-abdominal spread. Biopsies are obtained where appropriate and the tumor is palpated to determine correlation with the clinical stage. Peritoneal fluid cytologic specimens are taken at this time. After closing the anterior peritoneum, exposure of the retroperitoneal space is achieved by rolling the peritoneum medially until the left psoas muscle is identified. The round ligament and deep inferior epigastric vessels on the left are ligated to provide better exposure. Retractors are placed in order to expose the aorta and the left-sided vessels. The left ureter is easily identified on the peritoneum and is retracted medially away from the great vessels. Lymph node dissection is then carried out on the left side from the level of

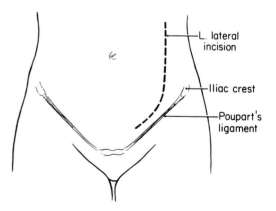

Figure 24–8. Abdominal incision for the extraperitoneal approach to pelvic and periaortic lymphadenectomy.

the second lumbar vertebral body to the inguinal ligament. The specimens are identified separately and submitted for pathological evaluation. The presacral space is visualized easily by this approach, and the lymph nodes in this area are removed. The peritoneum overlying the vena cava and right pelvic vessels is gently lifted in order to expose these vessels and identify the right ureter still attached to the peritoneum. Dissection of the right side is carried out in a fashion similar to that done on the left side. Using the left sided flank incision, it is possible to dissect cleanly the bilateral pelvic, precaval and periaortic nodes. Because of the posterior location of the left periaortic node chain the complete operation is carried out through a left sided incision. The retroperitoneal space is drained with Hemovac suction catheters. The fascia is closed with a single row of non-absorbable sutures.

Of the 80 patients with invasive cervical cancer who underwent operative evaluation, 30 were explored through a transperitoneal approach and 50 through an extraperitoneal approach. While there was no significant difference in estimated blood loss, postoperative stay and interval from operation to onset of therapy in the two groups, there were significantly more pelvic and periaortic nodes sampled in the patients undergoing an extraperitoneal approach (mean 23 versus 11,

$p < .01$). This difference to some extent may reflect the enthusiasm generated by a new surgical technique. Nodes from the periaortic and common iliac areas were positive in 17 percent of patients and from the pelvic area positive nodes were noted in 28.5 percent. Serious intestinal morbidity and mortality was seen only in the group operated through a transperitoneal approach. Ten of the 30 patients in the group operated by the transperitoneal approach developed small intestinal complications 2 to 17 months after radiation which required operative correction. None of the 50 patients explored by the extraperitoneal approach has required subsequent operation for small intestinal injury. Modification of radiation therapy to include the periaortic nodes was made in those patients with common iliac or periaortic node metastases.[60]

The evidence from patients so evaluated suggests that the extraperitoneal approach can provide the needed information without increased morbidity or mortality from the combined surgery and radiation therapy. Whether cancericidal radiation to a field which includes the aortic node chains is in itself an intolerable hazard, and to what extent improved survival can be expected in patients with positive periaortic nodes treated through pelvic and aortic portals are questions which await further study.[62]

References

1. Averette HE, Dudan RC, Ford JH, Jr: Exploratory celiotomy for surgical staging of cervical cancer. Am J Obst Gynec 113: 1090, 1972
2. Ballard RM, Bradley-Watson PJ, Johnstone FD, Kenney A, McCarthy TG: Low doses of subcutaneous heparin in the prevention of deep vein thrombosis after gynecological surgery. J Obst Gynaec Brit Commonw 80:469, 1973
3. Berman ML, Lagasse LD, Watring WG, Moore JG, Smith ML: Enteroperineal fistulae following pelvic exenteration: A 10-point program of management. Gynec Oncol 4:368, 1976
4. Bricker EM: Symposium on clinical surgery: Bladder substitution after pelvic exenteration. Surg Clin No Am 30:1511, 1950
5. Bricker EM, Butcher HR, Jr, Lawler WH, Jr, McAfee CA: Surgical treatment of advanced and recurrent cancer of the pelvic viscera: An evaluation of ten years experience. Ann Surg 152:388, 1960
6. Brunschwig A: Surgical treatment of carcinoma of the cervix recurrent after irradiation or combination of irradiation and surgery. Am J Roent 99:365, 1967
7. Cancer Statistics, 1977. Ca 27:26, 1977
8. Coffey RC: Transplantation of the ureters into the large intestine in the absence of a functioning urinary bladder. Surg Gynec Obst 32:383, 1921
9. Copeland EM, MacFayden BV, Dudrick SJ: Intravenous hyperalimentation in cancer patients. J Surg Res 16:241, 1974
10. Cordonnier JJ, Nicolai CH: Evaluation of

the use of an isolated segment of ileum as a means of urinary diversion. J Urol 83:834, 1960

11. Dudrick SJ, Wilmore DW, Vars HM: Long-term total parenteral nutrition with growth in puppies and positive nitrogen balance in patients. Surg Forum 18:356, 1967

12. Dudrick SJ, Wilmore DW, Vars HM: Long-term total parenteral nutrition with growth, development and positive nitrogen balance. Surgery 64:134, 1968

13. Engel R: Complications of bilateral uretero-ileal cutaneous urinary diversion: 208 cases. J Urol 101:508, 1969

14. Flanc C, Kakkar VV, Clarke MB: The detection of venous thrombosis of the legs using ^{125}I-labelled fibrinogen. Brit J Surg 55:742, 1968

15. Fletcher GH, Rutledge FN: Extended field technique in the management of the cancers of the uterine cervix. Am J Roentgen 114:116, 1972

16. Ford JH: Parenteral hyperalimentation in gynecologic oncology patients. Gynecol Oncol 1:70, 1972

17. Fortner JG: Intestinal fistula after pelvic irradiation and radical surgery. Postgrad Med 50:168, 1971

18. Freeman JB, Lloyd DM: Intravenous hyperalimentation: A review. Can J Surg 14:180, 1971

19. Graham JB, Villalba RJ: Damage to the small intestine by radiotherapy. Surg Gynec Obst 116:665, 1963

20. Greenberg GR, Marliss EB, Anderson GH, et al: Protein-sparing therapy in postoperative patients: Effects of added hypocaloric glucose or lipid. N Engl J Med 294:1411, 1976

21. Kakkar VV, Flanc C, Howe CT, Clarke MB: Natural history of postoperative deep-vein thrombosis. Lancet 2:230, 1969

22. Kakkar VV, Nicolaides AN, Field ES, et al: Low doses of heparin in prevention of deep-vein thrombosis. Lancet 2:669, 1971

23. Kakkar VV, Corrigan TP, Fossard DP: Prevention of fatal postoperative pulmonary embolism by low doses of heparin. Lancet 2:45, 1975

24. Lagasse LD, Johnson GH, Smith ML, et al: Use of sigmoid colon for rectal substitution following pelvic exenteration. Am J Obst Gynec 116:106, 1973

25. Macasaet MA, Lu T, Nelson JH, Jr: Ureterovaginal fistula as a complication of radical pelvic surgery. Am J Obst Gynec 124:757, 1976

26. MacFayden BV, Jr, Dudrick SJ, Maynard AT: Triglycerides and free fatty acid clearances in patients receiving parenteral nutrition using a 10 percent soybean oil emulsion. Surg Gynec Obst 137:813, 1973

27. McCraw JB, Massey FM, Shanklin KD: Vaginal reconstruction with gracilis myocutaneous flaps. Plastic Reconst Surg 58:176, 1976

28. McIndoe AH, Banister JB: An operation for the care of congenital absence of the vagina. J Obst Gynaec Brit Emp 45:490, 1938

29. Morley GW, Lindenauer SM, Youngs D: Vaginal reconstruction following pelvic exenteration: Surgical and psychological considerations. Am J Obst Gynec 116:996, 1973

30. Negus D, Pinto DJ, LeQuesne LP, Brown N, Chapman M: ^{125}I-Labelled fibrinogen in the diagnosis of deep-vein thrombosis and its correction with phlebography. Brit J Surg 55:835, 1968

31. Nelson JA: Atlas of Radical Pelvic Surgery Second Edition, Appleton-Century-Crofts, New York, 1977, 241–257

32. Nelson JH, Jr, Macasaet MA, Lu T, et al: The incidence and significance of para-aortic lymph node metastases in late invasive carcinoma of the cervix. Am J Obst Gynec 118:749, 1974

33. Nicolaides AN, Desai S, Douglas JN, et al: Small doses of subcutaneous sodium heparin in preventing deep venous thrombosis after major surgery. Lancet 2:890, 1972

34. Piver MS, Barlow JJ: High dose irradiation to biopsy confirmed aortic node metastases from carcinoma of the uterine cervix. Cancer 39:1243, 1977

35. Pratt JH, Smith GR: Vaginal reconstruction with a sigmoid loop. Am J Obst Gynec 96:31, 1966

36. Richie JP, Skinner D, Waismann J: The effect of reflux on the development of pyelonephritis in urinary diversion: An experimental study. J Surg Res 16:256, 1974

37. Rutledge FN, Burns BC, Jr: Pelvic exenteration. Am J Obst Gynec 91:692, 1965

38. Schellhas HF, Fidler JP: Vaginal reconstruction after total pelvic exenteration using a

modification of the Williams procedure. Gynecol Oncol 3:21, 1975

39. Scott WW: Methods of urinary diversion in radical pelvic surgery. Clin Obst Gynec 8: 726, 1965

40. Smith BE, Modell JH, Gaub ML: Complications of subclavian vein catheterization. Arch Surg (Chicago) 90:228, 1965

41. Smith JP, Golden PE, Rutledge F: The surgical management of intestinal injuries following irradiation for carcinoma of the cervix. 11th Clinical Conference on Cancer. Cancer of the Uterus and Ovary. Year Book Medical Publishers, Chicago, 1966, p 241

42. Stamey TA: Pathogenesis and implications of the electrolyte imbalance in ureterosigmoidostomy. Surg Gynec Obst 103:736, 1956

43. Swan RW, Rutledge FN: Urinary conduit in pelvic cancer patients: A report of 16 years experience. Am J Obst Gynec 119:6, 1974

44. Swan RW, Fowler WC, Jr, Boronow RC: Surgical management of radiation injury to the small intestine. Surg Gynec Obst 142: 325, 1976

45. Swenson O, Bill AH, Jr: Resection of rectum and rectosigmoid with preservation of the sphincter for benign spastic lesions producing megacolon. Surgery 24:212, 1948

46. Symmonds RE, Gibbs CP: Urinary diversion by way of sigmoid conduit. Surg Gynec Obst 129:687, 1970

47. Symmonds RE, Pratt JH, Webb MJ: Exenterative operations: Experience with 198 patients. Am J Obst Gynec 121:907, 1975

48. Thompson WR: In Meng HC, Wilmore DW (eds): A Symposium on Fat Emulsions in Parenteral Nutrition. Chicago, Ill. American Medical Association, June 1975, p 61

49. Udall DA, Hodges CV, Pearse HM, Burns AB: Transureteroureterostomy: Experience in pediatric patient. Urology 2:401, 1973

50. VanNagell JR, Jr, Roddick JW, Jr, Lowin DM: The staging of cervical cancer: Inevitable discrepancies between clinical staging and pathologic findings. Am J Obst Gynec 110:973, 1971

51. Vitko RJ, Cass AS: Comparison of the absorption of urinary constituents by small and large bowel conduits in dogs. Invest Urol 10:88, 1972

52. Watring WG, Lagasse LD, Smith ML, et al: Vaginal reconstruction following extensive treatment for pelvic cancer. Am J Obst Gynec 125:809, 1976

53. Wharton JT, Jones HW, Day TG, Jr, Rutledge FN, Fletcher GH: Preirradiation celiotomy and extended field irradiation for invasive carcinoma of the cervix. Obst Gynec 49:333, 1977

54. Wheeless CR: Small bowel bypass for complications related to pelvic malignancy. Obst Gynec 42:661, 1974

55. Whitely JM, Parrott MH, Rowland W: Split-thickness skin graft technique in the correction of congenital or acquired vaginal atresia. Am J Obst Gynec 89:377, 1964

56. Williams EA: Congenital absence of the vagina: A single operation for its relief. J Obst Gynecol Brit Commonw 71:511, 1964

57. Williams HT: Prevention of postoperative deep-vein thrombosis with perioperative subcutaneous heparin. Lancet 2:950, 1971

58. Nelson JH Jr, Boyce J, Macasaet M, et al: Incidence, significance, and follow-up of para-aortic lymph node metastases in late invasive carcinoma of the cervix. Am J Obstet Gynecol 128:335, 1977

59. Berman ML, Lagasse LD, Watring WG, Ballon SC, Schlesinger RE, Moore JG, Donaldson RC: The operative evaluation of patients with cervical carcinoma by an extraperitoneal approach. Obst Gynec 50: 658, 1977

60. Bacon HE: Evaluation of sphincter muscle preservation and re-establishment of continuity in the operative treatment of rectal and sigmoidal cancer. Surg Gynec Obst 81:113, 1945

61. Kakkar VV: Deep vein thrombosis of the leg: Is there a "high risk" group? Am J Surg 120:527, 1970

62. Berman ML, Lagasse LD, Ballon SC, Watring WG, Tesler A: Modification of radiation therapy following operative evaluation of patients with cervical carcinoma. Gynec Oncol (In Press)

Chapter 25

The Dying Gynecologic Cancer Patient and Society

LARRY McGOWAN, M.D.

Terminal care utilizing the team approach is the best method of providing continued and integrated medical care for the woman with diffuse metastatic disease and no hope for cure. Terminal care is care given to an individual who is going to die regardless of the use or discontinuance of medical treatment to sustain life processes. Approximately one out of two women with invasive cancers of the female reproductive tract will not survive her disease. The gynecologic oncologist is in an unique position to care for the dying woman because he or she has had the primary responsibility for treatment planning, treatment, and follow-up and, consequently, knows her over months or years as well as possesses the most knowledge of the pathophysiology of her disease. The responsibility for caring for the terminally ill gynecologic cancer patient must also be shared with her obstetrician or gynecologist, general or family practitioner, internist, clergy, medical oncologist, nurses, radiotherapist, and social worker.

It is not the purpose of this section to give an extensive review of the many facets of terminal care and death, as there are many excellent references.[1-7] It is the intent to present some of the more pertinent areas of the terminal care process that especially relate to gynecologic cancers.

DETERMINATION OF DEATH

Gynecologic cancers, because of their chronicity, do not usually arrive at a point at which determination of death is made difficult as a direct result of technologic machines to sustain the signs of life in the severely ill. In women dying of gynecologic cancers, death is a process and not a moment in time. During the process there are a series of physical and chemical changes, starting before the medicolegal definitions of death and continuing afterward.

Although few would disagree that death should rightfully be determined by physicians, as soon as an issue involves the right to life and death, the matter extends beyond just the medical profession.

A reasonable and simple statement to define the death of a woman from gynecologic cancer would be: "She will be considered dead if, in the stated opinion of a physician, based on ordinary standards of medical practice, she has experienced an irreversible cessation of spontaneous respiratory and circulatory functions. If artificial means of support preclude a determination that these functions have ceased, she shall be considered dead if, in the announced opinion of a physician, as based on ordinary standards of medical practice, she has experienced an irreversible cessation of spontaneous brain functions. Death will have occurred at the time when relevant functions ceased."

Some of the criteria a physician may utilize in arriving at determining death are the following.

1. Unreceptivity and unresponsivity. There is a total unawareness to externally applied stimuli and inner need and complete unresponsiveness.
2. No movements or breathing. Observations covering a period of at least one hour by physicians is adequate to satisfy the criteria of no spontaneous muscular movements or spontaneous respiration or response to stimuli such as pain, touch, sound, or light.
3. No reflexes. Irreversible coma with abolition of central nervous system activity is evidenced in part by the absence of elicitable reflexes. The pupil will be fixed and dilated and will not respond to a direct source of bright light.
4. Flat electroencephalogram. Of great confirmatory value is the flat or isoelectric EEG.[8]

ORDINARY AND EXTRAORDINARY CARE

The physicians caring for the woman dying from gynecologic cancer, the gynecologic oncologist and his team, are in the best position to make the determination as to whether ordinary or extraordinary care should be given to their patient. Because of their knowledge of the natural course of the disease and the team approach to continuum of patient care, the distinction between "ordinary" and "extraordinary" means to prolong life when the woman is irremediably ill and death is certain, is very much easier. The identification of therapeutic procedures as ordinary or extraordinary must be made in relation to the patient's condition and prognosis, evaluating the life-potential to be prolonged and the reasonable desires of the patient. We must take all ordinary means to preserve life, even if there is little hope of recovery. We are not obliged to use extraordinary means to prolong life when recovery is no longer possible, although we may do so.[9]

Ordinary means are described as "all medicines, treatments, and operations that offer a reasonable hope of benefit for the patient and can be obtained and used without excessive pain, expense, or other inconveniences."

By extraordinary means are meant "all medicines, treatments, and operations that cannot be obtained or used without excessive expense, pain, or other inconvenience, or which if used would not offer a reasonable hope of benefit." Thus by extraordinary means are all medicines, treatments and operations which will not cure the pathology, but will restrain its progressive destruction; which offer no sure hope of cure, and may involve a significant risk; which, if successful, render the patient incapable of certain functions; which are extremely painful, and which are extremely expensive.

It is important to keep in mind that the criteria for "extraordinary means" are flexible and changing. We must avoid too rigid a categorization of such means. Generally, pain is only temporary, and drugs can be used to minimize its effect. Also, expense is a highly relative factor, and one that receives disproportionate importance. Health care insurance can make medical care available to all, regardless of wealth. Therefore, this is very much a working principal whose terms are subject to continued redefinition. Means of preserving life that are looked upon as extraordinary at a given time or in given circumstances may become quite ordinary and commonplace in a short period of time.[10-15]

In determining when to cease using extraordinary means to prolong life, the woman has the primary right to decide. Physicians, clergy, family, and friends should assist her in making the decision and should help her in the dying process. When a woman is unable to make the decision, for example, due to unconsciousness, the decision devolves usually to the next of kin on the supposition that the next of kin is best able to interpret the wishes of the patient. Vicarious consent is consent given for another by the next of kin. The prerogative to decide may be delegated to her physician. This consent is a presumption (beyond the shadow of a reasonable doubt) that one who cannot give voluntary consent would be willing to do so if she could.

Experimentation on patients without due consent is objectionable. While the notion of totally informed consent may be limited by the ability of the woman, particular care is to be taken in the research (as opposed to the therapeutic) context. All experimental procedures require the consent of the patient or parent or guardian. When the patient is incompetent due to age and/or the gy- necologic cancer disease process, purely experi- mental or research procedures should not be un- dertaken unless the danger is so remote and the discomfort is so minimal that a normal woman would be presupposed to give ready consent.

QUALITY OF SURVIVAL

The kind of life a woman lives with gynecologic cancer is as important as the fact that she is living. Patterson[16] has suggested certain components that go into any consideration of quality should be:

1. Health, the prospect of cure vs failure
2. Function, the ability to work and the quality of performance
3. Comfort, the freedom from pain and the limi- tations to activity
4. Emotional response, self-acceptance, anxiety about the future, and social adjustment
5. Economics, the impact of costs and earning capacity

He further states that subjective responses obviously should not be allowed to replace the objective criteria such as tumor regression and improvement in body metabolism, but we physi- cians should add a measurement of personal value to the criteria by which we judge responses.

Women with advanced pelvic malignancies are usually better able to cope with terminal illness as their disease process evolves slowly. They com- monly not only know that they are dying but they know when they are dying. This gives the patient time to accept the concept of trying to live until she dies, during which time she commonly passes through the stages of denial and isolation, anger, bargaining, depression, and acceptance of her terminal illness. Everyone has the right and the duty to prepare for the solemn moment of death. Unless it is clear, therefore, that a dying woman is already well-prepared for death, it is the physi- cian's duty to inform her of her critical condition or to have some other responsible person impart this information.

Kubler-Ross succinctly states that "it is very important that we as physicians listen carefully to patients when they express their own hope, and that we do not project ours. If a patient has worked at accepting her finiteness and does not want and ask for a prolongation of life, I think we should be able to hear and honor that."[17] She has also observed that any terminally ill patients who can talk in plain English about their own impend- ing death, are usually people who have been able to transcend, to overcome their fear of death. Kubler-Ross further suggests that physicians can best help dying patients by not pushing them through the stages of dying to the stage of accep- tance but rather help them form a concept of death.[17]

Physicians can share in the interdisciplinary pa- tient care team for the gynecologic cancer patient in order:

1. To assist the woman to achieve and maintain maximum independent living and life with dignity until death
2. To aid in reducing the burden of a traumatic life experience by sharing and meeting the expressed needs, physical, emotional, spirit- ual, and social of the cancer patient and her family
3. To minimize the painful and damaging effects of the death of the family member upon the family which remain.

Many women prefer the warm surroundings of their own homes in the last days of their lives. With effective counseling of the patient and the family and with adequate preparations for the needs of the patient, the wishes of the patient can be met.

The Division of Cancer Control and Rehabilita- tion of the National Cancer Institute is currently evaluating on a nation-wide basis the hospice program. The hospice is not a hospital or a nurs- ing home.[18,19] Hospital staffs are oriented toward the treatment, restoration, and recovery of pa- tients. The staff, resources, policies, and proce- dures are, by necessity, concentrated toward and committed to the eradication of disease as the primary objective. A hospice, on the other hand, focuses not on the cure or length of survival of the patient but rather on the quality of that survival. The basic focus of care is the patient and the family, not the disease and its treatment. Nursing and convalescent homes (i.e., extended care facilities) are designed primarily to provide long-term care for the chronically ill and offer nursing care designed for recuperation and/or maintenance. The modern hospice offers services only to the dying cancer patient and her family. The average stay in the hospice inpatient program is from 13 to 18 days. The hospice program represents more the implementation of a philosophy for terminal care rather than simply a program of sophisticated techniques for clinically managing the dying patients. A major emphasis of the philosophy is that many terminally ill cancer patients would prefer to, and thus should be permitted to, die at home. The knowledge that a hospice bed is available in the inpatient facility often makes it possible for the patient to remain at home longer than either the family or the patient considers possible. The inpatient component of a hospice program has the primary goal of involving the patient in the life of other patients, families, staff, and their children, since the most frequently expressed concern of terminal cancer patients is fear of abandonment and isolation. The inpatient hospice strives to create an active, lively community. The environment is structured to provide a home-like atmos-

phere in contrast to a traditional hospital atmosphere.

The goals of a hospice program are to:

1. Ease the physical discomfort of the terminal cancer patient by employing pharmaceutical and advanced clinical techniques for effective symptom control
2. Ease the psychologic discomfort of the terminal cancer patient through programs allowing for active participation in scheduled activities or periods of peaceful withdrawal as determined by the patient
3. Aid in maintaining the emotional equilibrium of the patient and the family as they go through the traumatic life experience of progressive disease and ultimately the final separation of death

Wherever the terminal cancer patient is cared for, either at home, in a hospital, nursing home, or hospice, the philosophy of the purposeful approach to the nursing care plan is the attitude of the nursing personnel. Tennell of Calvary Hospital defines their thoughts, feelings, and actions toward the cancer patient as "be-attitudes." They teach their nursing staff to "be-understanding," "be-supportive," and "be-compassionate."[20]

EUTHANASIA

Eu means "good" or "easy" and *thanatos* means "death" in Greek. Women with incurable gynecologic cancers usually have a chronic disabling course and, on occasion, they or their family will have thoughts or enter into a discussion on euthanasia.

Good physicians for centuries have known the difference between prolonging life and prolonging the act of dying. A kind of euthanasia that can be honorable may be called "death with dignity." We are obliged to procure for any very sick person what is called "ordinary care and ordinary remedy." When this care has reached an evident state of being "extraordinary," the natural course of the disease is simply allowed to run its course. There is nothing dignified about inserting endless needles for multiple transfusions, forced feeding, giving antibiotics to eliminate bronchial pneumonia, or subjecting the dying patient to radiation therapy, operation, or massive toxic and nauseating chemotherapy. It is not euthanasia to give a dying woman sedatives and analgesics for the al-

leviation of pain, when such a measure is judged necessary, even though they may deprive her of the use of reason, or shorten her life.[21] The proper care of the dying woman does not end with the withdrawal of extraordinary forms of treatment. Skilled nursing care and sometimes small amounts of intravenous fluid to keep mucous membranes moist and clean do not prolong life, but they permit death with comfort and dignity. "This is simply proper, tender loving, terminal care."[22] This euthanasia, this kind of care at death, allows such a death to come as a deliverer to those for whom there is no hope, whether of cure, restoration, or continuation of life. It does not allow death to become an inhumane ordeal. The woman dying from cancer is usually not afraid of death but is terribly afraid of being abandoned by her family, physician, or other supporting members of the team. We care for the dying and we humanize death by being present with the dying patient.

A second type of euthanasia is "mercy killing"

and is opposed to the above "death with dignity." It involves the intentional use of medical technology in such a way as to cause death, or at least to speed up death. This type of euthanasia would include giving a terminally ill woman a lethal drug (with the express intention of causing death). It also includes abandonment (or withdrawal) of "ordinary" (reasonable and prudent) medical care. Euthanasia "mercy killing" in all its forms is poor medicine, illegal, and immoral. The failure to supply the ordinary means of preserving life is equivalent to euthanasia. However, neither the physician nor the patient is obliged to use extraordinary means.

There is a third type of euthanasia called "death selection" or "managerial euthanasia." "Managerial euthanasia" is the deliberate termination of lives that are no longer considered "socially useful" (that is, human lives that are considered to be a burden on society). The woman with a relentlessly advancing gynecologic cancer could become the object of physicians' committees or laws of society managing her death. The directly intended termination of any woman's life, even at her own request, is illegal, always morally wrong, and poor medical care.

Physicians who accept responsiblity for the care of cancer patients who have a high death rate, such as invasive gynecologic cancers, must have a broad understanding of the pathophysiology of this variable and sometimes unpredictable disease, plus an awareness of some of the medical ethics surrounding problems such as the death process and terminal care. Leo Alexander's statement[23] (Chief Counsel for the Nuremberg war trials) regarding Nazi medical ethics is pertinent today:

> Whatever proportions these crimes finally assumed, it became evident to all who investigated them that they had started from small beginnings. The beginnings at first were merely a subtle shift in emphasis in the basic attitude of the physicians. It started with the acceptance of the attitude, basic in the euthanasia movement, that there is such a thing as life not worthy to be lived. This attitude in its early stages concerned itself with the severely and chronically sick. Gradually the sphere of those to be included in this category was enlarged to encompass the socially unproductive, the ideologically unwanted, the racially unwanted, and finally all non-Germans. But it is important to realize that

the infinitely small wedged-in lever from which this entire trend of mind received its impetus was the attitude toward the non-rehabilitable sick.[24]

In various states the legislatures are reviewing the need for laws related to "defining death," "death with dignity," "living will," and even active "euthanasia."[9] Physicians by training, experience, and current practice are the only individuals qualified to determine death. Conscientious physicians working in ethical hospitals for many, many decades have cared for the dying woman with extreme dignity. The patient, her family, and her physicians are the most able to make decisions regarding the use of ordinary care or discontinuing the use of extraordinary means for prolonging life. The so-called "living will," which gives written permission for doctors to forego use of extraordinary means should the occasion arise, is certainly superfluous and possibly a teaching mechanism to condition public opinion to accept positive termination of life in cases of incurable illness, such as advanced gynecologic cancer.

Laws relating to definition of death, death with dignity, living will, and euthanasia are unnecessary and should be unalterably opposed. The situations that could eventuate into legislation in these four areas are the following.

1. Inadequate or no efforts by organized medical groups to educate the medical profession and the public as to the former's responsibilities and the latter's abrogation of their rights and their family's to make a reasonable and prudent judgement on the basis of competent medical advice on questions of life and death.

2. Repeated demonstrations to the public of lack of skills or incompetence by the medical profession in medical judgements relating to caring for dying patients with resulting distrust of physicians.

3. If the moral integrity of the medical community is disrupted or abandoned in relation to respect for human life, the state will step in and create laws. Such laws are based on nothing more solid than legal custom or public opinion and are subject to shifts and variations of opinion among judges, lawmakers, and the general public.

J. Englebert Dunphy[22] positively declares that "death is as natural as birth. Regardless of religious belief, when the finality of death arrives, the patient acquires a singular equanimity. Under appropriate circumstances, the anxiety and fear of dying are reduced to a minimum. The role of the physician in accomplishing this goal is unbelievable, but instead of being duped by the illusion of euthanasia, we doctors must hail the spirit that permeates the Home of the Holy Ghost, St. Christopher's Hospice, and many other hospitals and institutions throughout the world. All we need to do is stand up and show the public that we understand."

References

1. Cullen JW, Fox BH, Isom RN (eds): Cancer: The Behavioral Dimensions. New York, Raven Press, 1976
2. Bane JD, Kutscher AH, Neale RE, Reeves RB: Death and Ministry. New York, Seabury Press, 1975
3. McFadden CJ: The Dignity of Life. Huntington, Indiana, Our Sunday Visitor, Inc., 1976
4. Haring B: Ethics of Manipulation. New York, Seabury Press, 1975
5. Wilson JB: Death by Decision: The Medical, Moral and Legal Dilemmas of Euthanasia. Philadelphia, Westminister Press, 1975
6. Shneidman ES: Deaths of Man. Baltimore, Penguin, 1974
7. Kubler-Ross E: On Death and Dying. New York, Macmillan, 1969
8. Institute of Society, Ethics, and the Life Sciences: Refinements in criteria for the determination of death: an appraisal. JAMA 221:48, 1972
9. McHugh JT (ed): Death, Dying and the Law. Huntington, Indiana, Our Sunday Visitor, Inc., 1976
10. Greenhill JP, Schmitz HE: Intraspinal alcohol injections and sympathectomy for pain associated with carcinoma of the cervix: A comparison in 80 cases. Am J Obstet Gynec 31:290, 1936
11. Greenhill JP, Schmitz HE: Intraspinal (sub-arachnoid) injection of alcohol for pain associated with malignant conditions of female genitalia. JAMA 105:406, 1935
12. McGowan L: Ovarian cancer: caring for the terminal patient. Consultant 15:175, 1975
13. McGowan L: Cancer in Pregnancy. Springfield, Ill., Charles C Thomas, 1967
14. Labrum AH: Psychological factors in the etiology and treatment of cancer of the cervix. Clin Obstet Gynec 19:419, 1976
15. Llorens AS: Control of pain in pelvic cancer. Gynec Oncol 4:133, 1976
16. Patterson WB: The quality of survival in response to treatment. JAMA 233:280, 1975
17. Kubler-Ross E: On death and dying. Bull Am Coll Surg 60:12, 1975
18. Liegner LM: St. Christopher's Hospice, 1974. JAMA 234:1047, 1975
19. Holden C: Hospices: For the dying, relief from pain and fear. Science 193:389, 1976
20. Tennell P: The essence of cancer nursing. J Pract Nurs 26:35, 1976
21. O'Donnell TJ: To live—To die. JAMA 228:501, 1974
22. Dunphy JE: On caring for the patient with cancer. Bull Am Coll Surg 61:7, 1976
23. Alexander L: Medical science under dictatorship. N Engl J Med 241:39, 1949
24. Mitscherlich A: Doctors of Infamy: The Story of the Nazi Medical Crimes. New York, Schuman, 1949

Index